Advanced Research in Periodontitis

Advanced Research in Periodontitis

Edited by Norman Waltz

hayle medical

New York

Hayle Medical,
750 Third Avenue, 9th Floor,
New York, NY 10017, USA

Visit us on the World Wide Web at:
www.haylemedical.com

ISBN: 978-1-63241-568-4

Cataloging-in-Publication Data

Advanced research in periodontitis / edited by Norman Waltz.
    p. cm.
Includes bibliographical references and index.
ISBN 978-1-63241-568-4
1. Periodontitis. 2. Inflammation. 3. Dentistry. I. Waltz, Norman.
RK450.P4 A38 2019
617.632--dc23

Table of Contents

Preface

The inflammatory conditions affecting the tissues surrounding the teeth fall under the broad category of periodontal disease. The early stage of periodontal disease is known as gingivitis. In this stage, the gums become red and swollen, and may even bleed. The more severe form of periodontal disease is called periodontitis. In periodontitis, the gums often pull away from the teeth, the bones become weak, and there is a possibility that the teeth may loosen or fall out. Periodontal disease is usually caused by bacteria. Periodontal probe and X-rays are commonly used to diagnose periodontal disease. Root Surface Instrumentation, and scaling and root planing are the common treatment methods. The topics included in this book on periodontitis are of utmost significance and bound to provide incredible insights to readers. It presents researches and studies performed by experts across the globe. This book will prove to be immensely beneficial to students, doctors and researchers in this field.

The researches compiled throughout the book are authentic and of high quality, combining several disciplines and from very diverse regions from around the world. Drawing on the contributions of many researchers from diverse countries, the book's objective is to provide the readers with the latest achievements in the area of research. This book will surely be a source of knowledge to all interested and researching the field.

In the end, I would like to express my deep sense of gratitude to all the authors for meeting the set deadlines in completing and submitting their research chapters. I would also like to thank the publisher for the support offered to us throughout the course of the book. Finally, I extend my sincere thanks to my family for being a constant source of inspiration and encouragement.

Editor

Adiponectin Ameliorates Experimental Periodontitis in Diet-Induced Obesity Mice

Lan Zhang[1,2], Shu Meng[1,2], Qisheng Tu[1]*, Liming Yu[1], Yin Tang[1,2], Michel M. Dard[3], Sung-Hoon Kim[4], Paloma Valverde[5], Xuedong Zhou[2], Jake Chen[1,6]*

1 Division of Oral Biology, Tufts University School of Dental Medicine, Boston, Massachusetts, United States of America, 2 Key Laboratory of Oral Diseases, West China Hospital of Stomatology, Sichuan University, Chengdu, Sichuan, China, 3 Periodontology and Implant Dentistry, New York University College of Dentistry, New York, New York, United States of America, 4 Cancer Preventive Material Development Research Center (CPMDRC) and Institute, College of Oriental Medicine, Kyung Hee University, Dongdaemun-gu, Seoul, Korea, 5 Department of Sciences, Wentworth Institute of Technology, Boston, Massachusetts, United States of America, 6 Department of Anatomy and Cell Biology, Tufts University School of Medicine, Sackler School of Graduate Biomedical Sciences, Boston, Massachusetts, United States of America

Abstract

Adiponectin is an adipokine that sensitizes the body to insulin. Low levels of adiponectin have been reported in obesity, diabetes and periodontitis. In this study we established experimental periodontitis in male adiponectin knockout and diet-induced obesity mice, a model of obesity and type 2 diabetes, and aimed at evaluating the therapeutic potential of adiponectin. We found that systemic adiponectin infusion reduced alveolar bone loss, osteoclast activity and infiltration of inflammatory cells in both periodontitis mouse models. Furthermore, adiponectin treatment decreased the levels of pro-inflammatory cytokines in white adipose tissue of diet-induced obesity mice with experimental periodontitis. Our in vitro studies also revealed that forkhead box O1, a key transcriptional regulator of energy metabolism, played an important role in the direct signaling of adiponectin in osteoclasts. Thus, adiponectin increased forkhead box O1 mRNA expression and its nuclear protein level in osteoclast-precursor cells undergoing differentiation. Inhibition of c-Jun N-terminal kinase signaling decreased nuclear protein levels of forkhead box O1. Furthermore, over-expression of forkhead box O1 inhibited osteoclastogenesis and led to decreased nuclear levels of nuclear factor of activated T cells c1. Taken together, this study suggests that systemic adiponectin application may constitute a potential intervention therapy to ameliorate type 2 diabetes-associated periodontitis. It also proposes that adiponectin inhibition of osteoclastogenesis involves forkhead box O1.

Editor: Michael Glogauer, University of Toronto, Canada

Funding: This project was supported by National Institutes of Health (NIH) grants R01DE16710 and R01DE21464, and the International Association of Dental Research (IADR) and the Academy of Osseointegration (AO) Innovation in Implant Science Award (to J.C.); Ministry of Education, Science and Technology (MEST) grant 2007-0054931 in South Korea (to S.H.K.); NIH grant DK080344 (to L.Q.D.). The funders had no role in study design, data collection and analysis, decision to publish, or preparation of the manuscript.

Competing Interests: The authors have declared that no competing interests exist.

* E-mail: jk.chen@tufts.edu (JC); qisheng.tu@tufts.edu (QT)

Introduction

Periodontitis is an inflammatory disease that involves progressive loss of alveolar bone around the teeth and can result in tooth loss. It is twice as prevalent in diabetics as in non-diabetics, and has been rated as the sixth complication of diabetes [1]. Pathologically and clinically, type 2 diabetes (T2D)-associated periodontitis is more severe than in non-diabetics. Excess white adipose tissue (WAT) in obese is characterized by increased macrophage infiltration and production of proinflammatory cytokines including tumor necrosis factor-α (TNF-α) and interleukine-6 (IL-6) that mediate local and systemic effects on inducing insulin resistance [2]. Indeed, this systemic inflammation and insulin resistance in T2D contributes to the pathogenesis of periodontitis [1,3]. Hence developing an effective therapeutic treatment for T2D-associated periodontitis that can both inhibit bone resorption and decrease inflammation is critically important.

Adipose tissue plays an important role in energy homeostasis by secreting a number of adipokines, among which adiponectin (APN) [4] has been shown to exhibit insulin-sensitizing effects [4–

6], and potent anti-inflammatory properties [7]. Circulating levels of APN are reduced in obesity, T2D or periodontitis [8–11], whereas improvement in hyperglycemia of T2D upon treatment with thiazolidinediones [12,13] or periodontal therapeutic intervention that decreased inflammation, significantly led to increased serum APN levels [14]. Low circulating levels of this adipokine may therefore be related to insulin resistance and poor periodontal status.

Bone metabolism involves the concerted actions of bone resorbing cells called osteoclasts [15] and bone producing cells called osteoblasts [16]. While lack of APN in APN knockout (APN$^{-/-}$) mice did not result in an obvious bone phenotype change [17,18]; when bone was explanted into these mice, noticeable effects of APN on bone metabolism were revealed. Thus, lack of APN led to significant growth retardation of bone explants and increasing osteoclastogenesis [19]. APN has been shown to indirectly stimulate osteoclast differentiation via receptor activator of nuclear factor kB ligand (RANKL) and osteoprotegerin (OPG) expression by osteoblasts [20] and to inhibit osteoclast activity and bone resorption by suppressing RANKL-induced Akt signaling in osteoclasts [19,21]. Furthermore, APN can decrease bone mass by inhibiting osteoblast differentiation and promoting their apoptosis via inducing phosphorylation of Akt which downregulated forkhead box O1 (FoxO1) [22]. In addition APN was shown to increase bone mass by decreasing sympathetic tone [22]. Taken together, the peripheral and central effects of APN on bone metabolism require further investigation.

In this study we established experimental periodontitis in mice to evaluate whether systemic APN infusion could ameliorate periodontal destruction in APN$^{-/-}$ and diet-induced-obesity (DIO) mice, a model of obesity and T2D. Furthermore, we performed *in vitro* studies with osteoclast precursor cells to delineate the molecular mechanisms implicated in APN signaling under osteoclastogenic conditions.

Materials and Methods

Ethics Statement

The animal protocols used in this study were approved by the Institutional Animal Care and Use Committee at Tufts University/Tufts Medical Center (Approved Protocol #B2011-49). All mice were kept in a controlled temperature-and controlled room under a 12 h light, 12 h dark cycle.

Purification of Recombinant APN Protein and Periodontal Pathological Bacteria

pEt15b bacterial expression vector encoding the C-terminal part of human APN (amino acids 106–244) was used to purify globular APN as a His-tagged protein in BL21(D3) bacterial cells as described previously [23]. *Porphyromonas gingivalis* (*P. gingivalis*, ATCC) was cultured and maintained in supplemented tryptic soy broth (ATCC) in an anaerobic chamber with 85% N$_2$, 10% H$_2$, and 5% CO$_2$ at 37°C. 5–0 silk sutures were presoaked in the broth containing (10^8/ml) *P. gingivalis* for 2 days prior to periodontitis induction.

Mice, Experimental Periodontitis Induction, and Systemic APN Infusion

Male APN$^{-/-}$ (Jax #008195), DIO (Stock #380050), and wild-type (WT, Jax #000664) mice were purchased from the Jackson Laboratory (Bar Harbor, ME, USA). DIO mice were fed with 60% high fat diet.

APN$^{-/-}$ mice were randomly divided into 3 groups (n = 5/group): experimental periodontitis (PD), experimental periodontitis with systemic APN treatment (PD+APN), and untreated mice (control). WT mice were divided into 2 groups (n = 5/group): experimental periodontitis (PD), and untreated mice (control). DIO mice were divided into 2 groups (n = 5/group): experimental periodontitis (PD), and experimental periodontitis with systemic APN treatment (PD+APN).

To induce experimental periodontitis [24,25], mice were anesthetized by an IP injection of ketamine (80 mg/kg) and xylazine (10 mg/kg). A 5–0 silk suture presoaked in the bacterial broth for two days was then wrapped around the right and left second maxillary molars and knotted mesio-buccally. Ligatures were changed every other day to maintain sufficient microbial burden.

As the APN half-life is only 2.5 h, APN was administered by systemic infusion in order to guarantee a constant blood concentration. An Alzet micro-osmotic pump (model 1004, Durect Corporation) was subcutaneously inserted in the back of each mouse following periodontitis induction. Sham surgery for osmotic pump insertion was performed in the animal models used in this study (data not shown). The APN concentration in the pump was

1 mg/ml and the pump rate was set at 0.11 µl/h, hence the pump delivered approximately 2.5 µg of recombinant APN per day to each mouse. Mice were euthanized 10 days after periodontitis induction.

Cell Culture and Transfection Experiments

RAW264.7 (ATCC) cells were cultured in RPMI 1640 with 10% fetal bovine serum (FBS, Life Technologies). Cells were serum-starved overnight and treated with receptor activator of NF-κB ligand (RANKL, PeproTech), *E.coli* lipopolysaccharide (LPS, Sigma-Aldrich), or the c-Jun N-terminal kinase (JNK) inhibitor SP600125 (Tocris Bioscience). Transfection of plasmids was performed using Lipofectamine 2000 (Life Technologies) following the manufacturer's recommendations. The pGL3-CtpsK-luciferase reporter vector was constructed in our previous study [19], which contained a 4.0-kb mouse cathepsin K promoter. Plasmid encoding FoxO1 (Flag-FoxO1) was purchased from Addgene (Cambridge, MA). pCMV5 which contained the vector backbone was used as a control plasmid in transfection experiments.

Quantitative Real-Time PCR (qRT-PCR) for mRNA Analyses

Total RNA from RAW264.7 cultures were prepared with an RNeasy Mini Kit (Qiagen) and reverse-transcribed with M-MLV Reverse Transcriptase (Affymetrix) according to the manufacturer's instructions. qRT-PCR assays were performed with USBVeriQuestFastSYBRGreenqPCR Master Mix with Fluorescein (Affymetrix) using a Bio-Rad iQ5 thermal cycler. The mRNA expression levels of target genes were calculated with the comparative cycle threshold method using GAPDH as a control.

WAT was removed from male DIO mice. Total RNA was prepared from tissues with TRIzol reagent (Life Technologies) according to the manufacturer's instructions. Reverse transcription and qRT-PCR assays were performed as mentioned above to detect the expression of TNF-α, interleukin-1 (IL-1), and IL-6 in WAT. Primers used for amplification are listed in Table 1.

Western Blot Analyses

Whole protein lysates were prepared with RIPA lysis buffer (Santa Cruz Biotechnology, Inc.) according to the manufacturer's instructions. Nuclear proteins were purified using a nuclear extraction kit (EMD Millipore). SDS-PAGE electrophoresis and Western blots were performed using Novex 4–20% Tris-Glycine gels (Life Technologies) and 0.45 µm polyvinylidene fluoride membranes (Millipore). Antibodies for nuclear factor of activated T cells c1 (NFATc1, 1:1000) and lamin B1 (1:1000) were purchased from Santa Cruz Biotechnologies. FoxO1 (1:1000), p-JNK (1:1000), and JNK (1:1000) were purchased from Cell Signaling Technology. The secondary antibodies were horseradish peroxidase-linked goat-anti-rabbit IgG (Santa Cruz Biotechnology, Inc.). Blots were visualized using SuperSignal West Dura Extended Duration Substrate (Thermo Fisher Scientific).

Luciferase Assay

Co-transfections of Flag-FoxO1 (or pCMV5 control plasmid) with pGL3-CtpsK-luciferase reporter vector were performed in RAW264.7 cells and 50 ng/ml RANKL was used to induce osteoclastogenesis for 5 days. Then luciferase assay was performed using a Lumat LB9501 luminometer (Berthold Technologies) as described previously [26].

Table 1. Primers used in qRT-PCR analyses.

Gene		Primer Sequence
GAPDH	Forward	5'-AGG TCG GTG TGA ACG GAT TTG-3'
	Reverse	5'-TGT AGA CCA TGT AGT TGA GGT CA-3'
TNF-α	Forward	5'-CAT CTT CTC AAA ATT CGA GTG ACA A-3'
	Reverse	5'-TGG GAG TAG ACA AGG TAC AAC CC-3'
IL-6	Forward	5'-GAG GAT ACC ACT CCC AAC AGA CC-3'
	Reverse	5'-AAG TGC ATC ATC GTT GTT CAT ACA-3'
IL-1	Forward	5'-CCA TGG CAC ATT CTG TTC AAA-3'
	Reverse	5'-GCC CAT CAG AGG CAA GGA-3'
Cathepsin K	Forward	5'-GAA GAA GAC TCA CCA GAA GCA G-3'
	Reverse	5'-TCC AGG TTA TGG GCA GAG ATT-3'
FoxO1	Forward	5'-CTC CCG GTA CTT CTC TGC TG-3'
	Reverse	5'-GTG GTC GAG TTG GAC TGG TT-3'

GADPH, Glyceraldehyde-3-phosphate dehydrogenase; TNF-α, tumor necrosis factor-alpha; IL-6, interleukin-6; FoxO1, forkhead box O1.

In Vitro Osteoclastogenesis and Tartrate-Resistant Acid Phosphatase (TRAP) Staining

Primary cultures of mouse osteoclast precursor cells in the form of bone marrow-derived monocytes/macrophages (BMM) were obtained from 6–8 week-old male WT mouse femurs and tibias as described previously [27]. Briefly, femurs and tibias were flushed with a 25-gauge needle and cultured in α-MEM supplemented with 10 ng/ml monocyte colony-stimulating factor (M-CSF) overnight. The non-adherent cells were collected and layered on Histopaque gradient (Sigma). Cells at the gradient interface were seeded to 96 well plates. Transfection of FoxO1 or pCMV5 control plasmid was performed. Then osteoclastogenesis was induced with 10 ng/ml M-CSF and 50 ng/ml RANKL. The medium was changed every 3 days. After 7 days of induction, cells were fixed and stained for TRAP activity using the K-ASSAY TRACP staining kit (Kamiya Biomedical Company). The osteoclasts were identified as red-stained cells with three or more nuclei. The number of osteoclasts was manually counted in four separate fields at a magnification of 200×. Data were reported as the mean number of osteoclasts in one separate field.

Alveolar Bone Loss Analysis

After euthanasia, the palatal bone samples were dissected and defleshed after 15 minutes in boiling water, immersed overnight in 3% hydrogen peroxide, and stained with 1% methylene blue. The buccal and palatal faces of the molars were photographed at 30× magnification using a dissecting microscope with the occlusal face of the molars positioned perpendicular to the base. The distance from the cementoenamel junction to the alveolar crest was measured at six sites of secondary molar: mesio-buccal, mid-buccal, disto-buccal, disto-palatal, mid-palatal and mesio-palatal using Image-Pro Plus software [24,25].

Histology and TRAP Staining of Bone Specimens

Palatal bone samples were fixed in 4% paraformaldehyde and decalcified in 10% EDTA. Tissue sections were stained with hematoxylin and eosin (H&E), and interdental areas between the first and second molars were examined. The total number of inflammatory cells, mainly polymorphonuclear leukocytes, was manually counted according to its morphology, from 4 separate fields at 400× magnification on H&E-stained sections. Data were

reported as the numbers of inflammatory cells per square millimeter. TRAP staining was performed using Acid Phosphatase, Leukocyte (TRAP) kit (Sigma-Aldrich) according to the manufacturer's instructions. The osteoclasts were identified as red-stained cells with three or more nuclei. The number of osteoclasts was counted from images captured at 200× magnification. Data were presented as the number of osteoclasts per bone surface.

Statistical Analysis

Data are presented as the average ± standard deviations (SD) of 3 or more experiments. Statistical significance was analyzed by one-way ANOVA followed by LSD post hoc test or independent sample t test; and data were considered significant at $P<0.05$.

Results

APN Inhibits Alveolar Bone Resorption and Infiltration of Inflammatory Cells in APN$^{-/-}$ Mice Induced with Experimental Periodontitis

Several lines of evidence have revealed that APN can act directly and indirectly in bone metabolism through complex regulatory mechanisms. To investigate the plausible therapeutic effects of APN on alveolar bone loss, we established experimental periodontitis in APN$^{-/-}$ and WT mice. Our results showed that alveolar bone loss was significantly increased upon induction of experimental periodontitis in male WT and APN$^{-/-}$ mice (Figure 1A, $P<0.05$), indicating that periodontitis was successfully established. Although there was no significant difference in alveolar bone loss between WT and APN$^{-/-}$ mice induced with periodontitis, TRAP-stained palatal bone samples from APN$^{-/-}$ mice with periodontitis exhibited a higher number of osteoclasts than in those derived from WT mice induced with experimental periodontitis (Figure 1B, $P<0.05$). Furthermore, periodontitis induction led to higher infiltration of inflammatory cells in APN$^{-/-}$ mice than in WT mice (Figure 1C, $P<0.05$), suggesting that APN deficiency made mice susceptible to periodontal destruction. Then we administered recombinant APN in APN$^{-/-}$ mice and found that systemic APN infusion significantly decreased alveolar bone loss associated with experimental periodontitis in APN$^{-/-}$ mice (Figure 1A, $P<0.05$). More importantly, systemic APN treatment reduced the number of

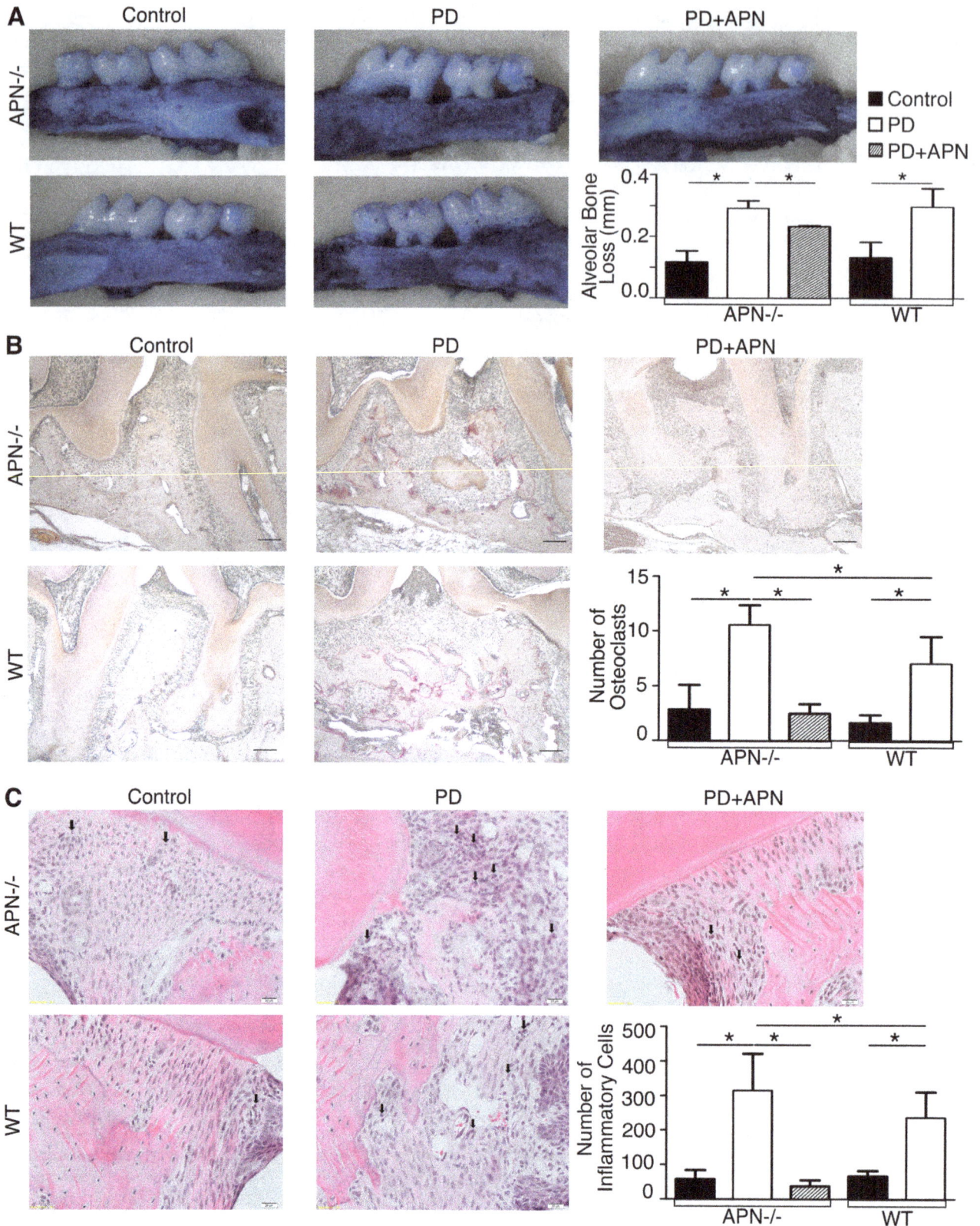

Figure 1. APN Inhibits Bone Resorption and Inflammation in APN$^{-/-}$ Mice Induced With Experimental Periodontitis. (A) Alveolar bone loss was determined in palatal bone samples stained with 1% methylene blue and photographed at 30× magnification using a dissecting microscope with the occlusal face of the molars perpendicular to the base. The distance between the cementoenamel junction and the alveolar crest was measured at 6 sites in APN$^{-/-}$, APN$^{-/-}$+PD, APN$^{-/-}$+PD+APN, as well as WT and WT+PD mice (magnification, ×30). (B) TRAP staining determined the number of osteoclasts (magnification, ×200; scale bars, 500 μm). (C) H&E staining determined the number of inflammatory cells of palatal bone samples in APN$^{-/-}$, APN$^{-/-}$+PD, APN$^{-/-}$+PD+APN, as well as WT and WT+PD mice (magnification, ×400; scale bars, 20 μm; black arrows = inflammatory cells). Data are shown as mean ± SD (n = 5). *$P < 0.05$.

osteoclasts (Figure 1B, $P<0.05$) and infiltration of inflammatory cells (Figure 1C, $P<0.05$) in APN$^{-/-}$ mice induced with periodontitis.

APN Inhibits Alveolar Bone Resorption, Infiltration of Inflammatory Cells and Expression of Proinflammatory Cytokines by WAT in DIO Mice Induced with Experimental Periodontitis

T2D patients are more prone to developing severe periodontitis [1,3]. To mimic the pathological characteristics of periodontitis in T2D patients, we induced experimental periodontitis in DIO mice. DIO mice are a widely studied model of T2D. These mice develop obesity with elevated blood glucose and impaired glucose tolerance when fed a high-fat diet. We then evaluated whether systemic APN infusion could mediate potential therapeutic effects on alveolar bone loss, osteoclast number and infiltration of inflammatory cells in palatal bones of DIO mice induced with periodontitis. Our results revealed that systemic APN infusion significantly downregulated alveolar bone loss (Figure 2A, $P<0.05$), osteoclast number (Figure 2B, $P<0.05$), and the number of inflammatory cells (Figure 2C, $P<0.05$) in DIO palatal bones. We also found that systemic infusion of APN in the DIO-animal model diminished hyperglycemia (data not shown), which was in agreement with the insulin sensitizing properties of APN.

Excess WAT in obesity has been linked to insulin resistance partly through production of proinflammatory cytokines by infiltrated macrophages [2,28]. The insulin resistance and chronic general inflammation in T2D patients could ultimately contribute to periodontitis that is more severe and refractory in T2D patients than in patients without diabetes [1,3]. We then evaluated whether systemic APN infusion affected the mRNA expression of proinflammatory cytokines by WAT isolated from DIO mice with periodontitis. Our results indicated that recombinant APN treatment decreased mRNA expression of the proinflammatory cytokines including TNF-α, IL-1, and IL-6 in WAT isolated from DIO mice induced with periodontitis (Figure 2D, $P<0.05$).

APN Promotes FoxO1 Expression and Nuclear Activation in RANKL-Treated RAW264.7 Cells

FoxO1 is a forkhead transcription factor that acts as the master regulator of energy metabolism [28], and it is highly expressed in insulin-responsive tissues including bone. On one hand, FoxO1 controls glucose metabolism through osteoblasts by regulating the activity of osteocalcin, and on the other it serves as a target of insulin signaling in osteoblasts. Recently APN was also reported to decrease bone mass by decreasing the nuclear levels of FoxO1 in osteoblasts [22]. We then investigated whether APN could also inhibit osteoclastogenesis by directly signaling through FoxO1 in osteoclasts. To that end, we first analyzed the FoxO1 mRNA expression in RAW264.7 cells undergoing RANKL-induced osteoclastogenesis in the presence and absence of APN. We found that the normalized FoxO1 mRNA expression was significantly upregulated in cells treated with APN (Figure 3A, $P<0.05$). As JNK has been implicated in activating FoxO1 by increasing the nuclear fraction of FoxO1 protein [29], we tested whether JNK phosphorylation was induced by APN treatment in RANKL-treated osteoclast-precursor cells. Western blot analysis of whole protein extracts showed that JNK phosphorylation levels were dramatically enhanced by APN treatment in RAW264.7 undergoing RANKL-induced osteoclastogenesis (Figure 3B, $P<0.05$). We then evaluated if these results were consistent with the notion that APN was promoting the activation of FoxO1 upon JNK-phosphorylation. To that end, nuclear extracts from RAW264.7

undergoing RANKL-induced osteoclastogenesis in the presence and absence of APN were subjected to western blot analysis. In these experiments we found that APN treatment significantly increased FoxO1 nuclear protein levels (Figure 3C, $P<0.05$). Cytoplasmic FOXO1 levels were also increased approximately 5-fold in the presence of APN and RANKL (data not shown). However, when cells undergoing osteoclastogenesis were pretreated with the JNK inhibitor SP600125, nuclear FoxO1 levels were significantly decreased (Figure 3C, $P<0.05$). These results supported our hypothesis that APN could activate FoxO1 in a JNK-dependent manner in our in vitro model of osteoclastogenesis.

FoxO1 Over-Expression Inhibits Osteoclastogenesis

To further investigate whether APN-induced FoxO1 activation was partly responsible for the inhibitory effects of APN in osteoclastogenesis, we over-expressed FoxO1 in BMM osteoclast precursor cells undergoing osteoclastogenesis. We then performed TRAP staining to evaluate possible differences in osteoclast formation by comparing untransfected cells, cells transfected with pCMV5 control plasmid or those transfected with Flag-FoxO1 (Figure 4A). Our experiments showed that over-expression of FoxO1 under osteoclastogenic conditions led to the formation of fewer osteoclasts than in untransfected cells or those transfected with the control plasmid (Figure 4A, $P<0.05$).

We then tested whether FoxO1 activation could mediate its inhibitory effects on osteoclastogenesis by altering the activation of NFATc1, the master regulator of osteoclastogenesis. Upon binding of RANKL to RANK, NFATc1 translocates from the cytoplasm to the nucleus and induces osteoclastogenesis by increasing expression of several genes including cathepsin K. Cathepsin K is a cysteine protease expressed predominantly in osteoclasts that is required for their bone resorptive activity. We performed western blot analyses with nuclear extracts isolated from RANKL-treated RAW264.7 cells that were transiently transfected with FoxO1. Our results showed that FoxO1-overexpressing cells undergoing osteoclastogenesis exhibited a dramatic decrease in NFATc1 nuclear expression as compared to those transfected with the control plasmid (Figure 4B, $P<0.05$).

Since cathepsin K expression is normally upregulated by NFATc1 transcription factor during osteoclastogenesis, we investigated whether its expression could be altered by FoxO1 over-expression. Our results indicated cathepsin K mRNA expression was significantly reduced in FoxO1-overexpressing cells undergoing osteoclastic differentiation by RANKL (Figure 4C, $P<0.05$). To investigate whether FoxO1 could mediate those effects by acting on the cathepsin K promoter directly, Flag-FoxO1 and pGL3-CtspK-luciferase reporter vector were co-transfected in RAW264.7 cells undergoing osteoclastogenesis. Results of the luciferase assays showed that cells over-expressing FoxO1 had a lower promoter activity than cells co-transfected with the control plasmid and the pGL3-CtspK-luciferase reporter vector (Figure 4D, $P>0.05$).

Taken together, these results suggest that APN may inhibit RANKL-induced osteoclastogenesis by increasing FoxO1 nuclear protein level and by reducing NFATc1 nuclear localization and activation (Figure 4E).

Discussion

Adiponectin is an adipokine that exhibits insulin-sensitizing effects and potent anti-inflammatory properties [30]. Circulating levels of APN are reduced in obesity and type 2 diabetes [8,9], whereas improvement in insulin sensitivity upon treatment with thiazolidinediones correlated with increased APN levels [12,13].

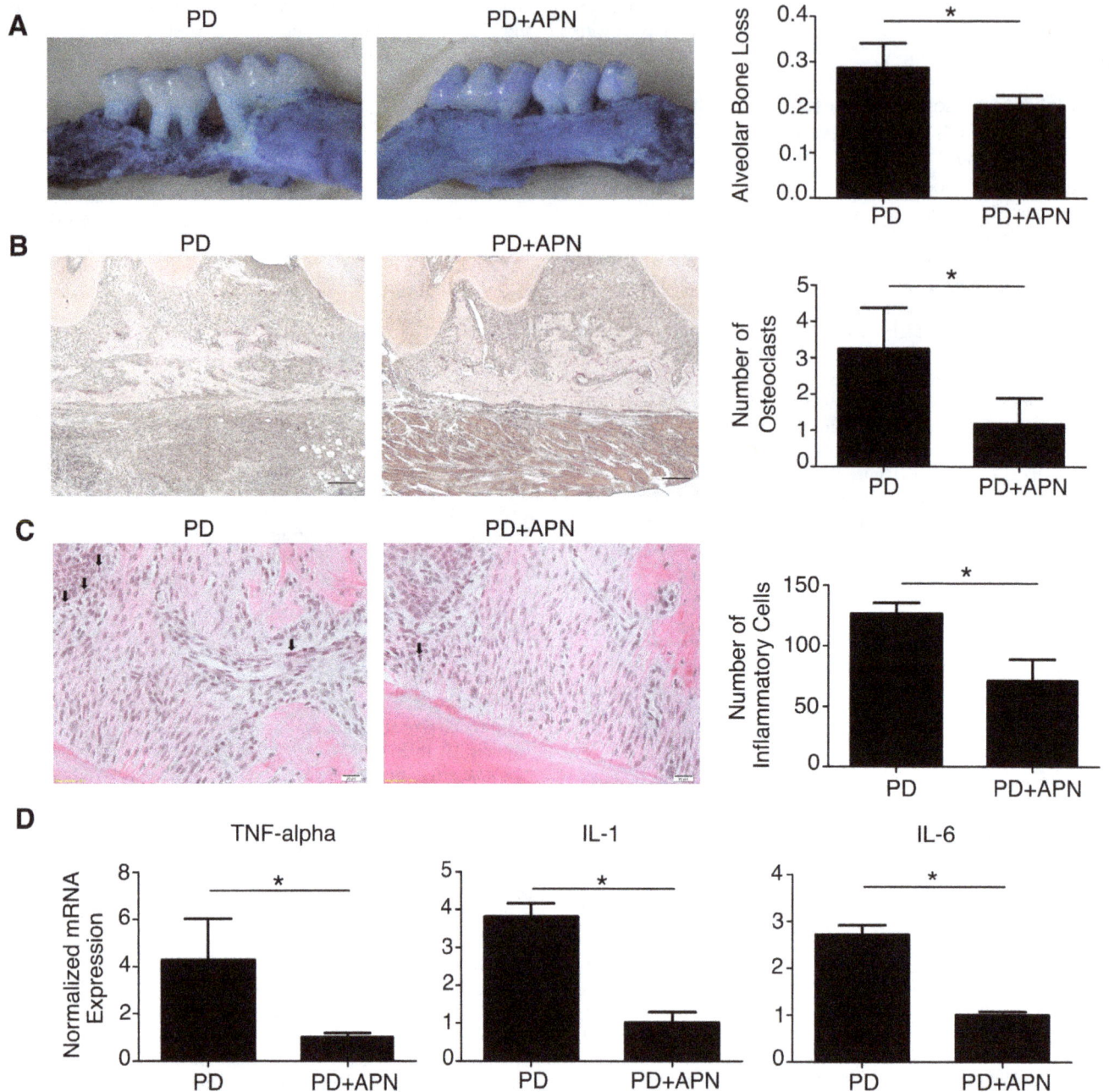

Figure 2. APN Inhibits Bone Resorption and Inflammation in DIO Mice Induced With Experimental Periodontitis. (A) Alveolar bone loss was determined in palatal bone samples stained with 1% methylene blue and photographed at 30× magnification using a dissecting microscope with the occlusal face of the molars perpendicular to the base. The distance between the cementoenamel junction and the alveolar crest was measured at 6 sites in DIO+PD and DIO+PD+APN mice (magnification, ×30). (B) TRAP staining determined the number of osteoclasts (magnification, ×200; scale bars, 500 μm). (C) H&E staining determined the number of inflammatory cells of palatal bone samples in DIO+PD and DIO+PD+APN mice (magnification ×400; scale bars, 20 μm; black arrows = inflammatory cells). (D) qRT-PCR of TNF-α, IL-1, and IL-6 mRNA levels in WAT from DIO+PD and DIO+PD+APN mice, normalized to GAPDH. Data are shown as mean ± SD (n = 5). *$P < 0.05$.

Similarly serum APN levels were lower in patients with periodontitis than in those without the disease [10,11] and periodontal therapeutic intervention significantly led to increased serum APN levels [14]. In this study, we first compared the periodontal destruction between WT and APN$^{-/-}$ mice, and found that periodontitis induction led to more osteoclasts and higher infiltration of inflammatory cells in APN$^{-/-}$ mice. These results suggested that APN deficient mice were more susceptible to

periodontal disease than WT mice, although alveolar bone loss was not significantly different between both groups 10 days after periodontitis induction. Whether this is resulting from the low sensitivity of the method used to measure alveolar bone loss or from compensating effects by other circulating factors needs to be further investigated.

To further determine the therapeutic potential of APN for treating T2D-associated periodontitis, we induced periodontitis in

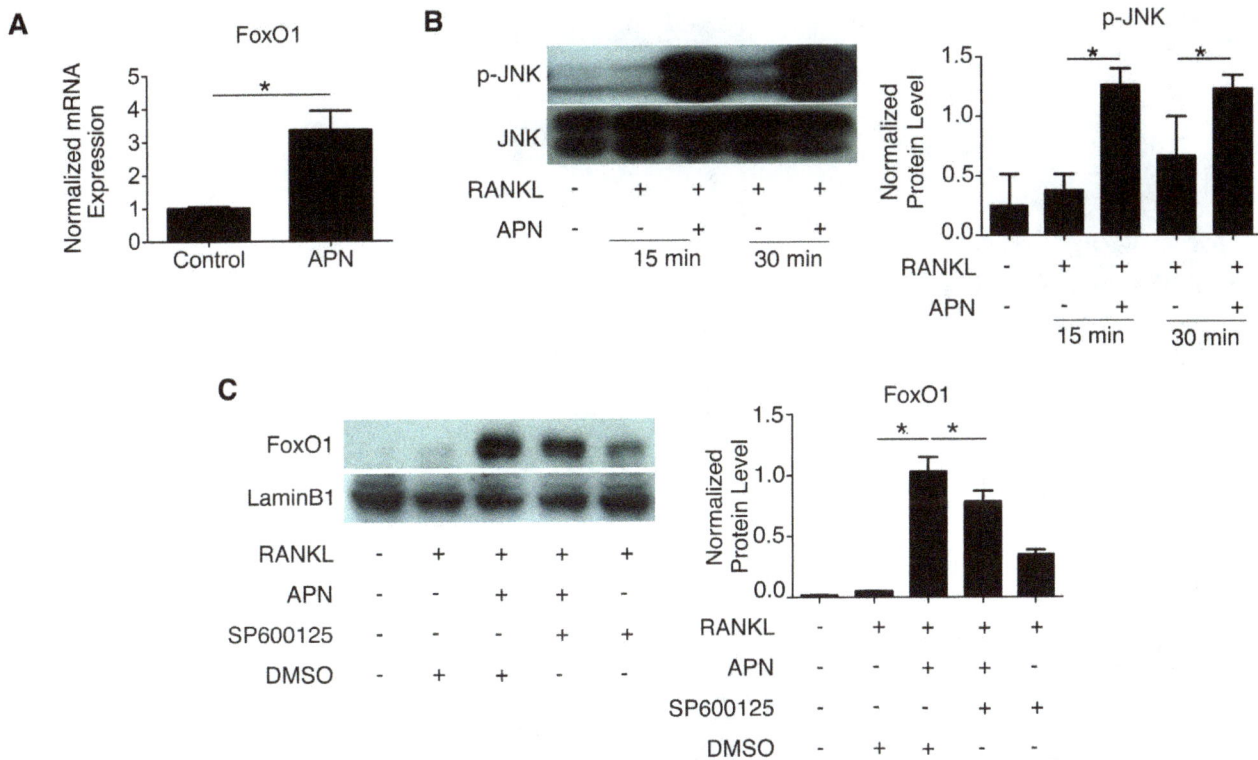

Figure 3. APN Induces FoxO1 and JNK Phosphorylation in RANKL-Treated RAW264.7 Cells. (A) qRT-PCR of FoxO1 mRNA levels in RAW264.7 cells treated with 50 ng/ml RANKL in the absence (control) and presence of 0.5 µg/ml APN treatment for 24 hours. The mRNA level was normalized with those of GAPDH. (B) Western blot for phosphorylated JNK in RAW264.7 cells treated with 50 ng/ml RANKL in the absence or presence of 0.5 µg/ml APN for 15 or 30 minutes. JNK was detected as the loading control. Data are shown as mean ± SD of three independent experiments. *P<0.05. (C) Western blot of FoxO1 nuclear protein extracted from RAW264.7 cells that were treated with 50 ng/ml RANKL in the presence and absence of 0.5 µg/ml APN, with or without prior treatment with the JNK inhibitor SP600125 for 2 hours. DMSO was used to dissolve SP600125. Nuclear Lamin B1 was used as the loading control. Data are shown as mean ± SD of three independent experiments. *P<0.05.

DIO mice, a model of T2D and obesity with elevated blood glucose, impaired glucose tolerance and WAT-associated chronic inflammation. Even in the context of chronic inflammation, systemic APN infusion could decrease alveolar bone loss, osteoclast number and infiltration of inflammatory cells in DIO mice induced with periodontitis. Our *in vivo* results support the notion that APN is potentially beneficial to treat T2D-associated periodontitis based on APN dual roles in inhibiting osteoclastogenic activity and attenuating local inflammation (Figure 5).

In agreement with the ability of APN to inhibit local chronic inflammation in our experimental periodontitis DIO model, we found gene expression levels of proinflammatory cytokines including TNF-α, IL-1, and IL-6 were significantly reduced in WAT tissues. WAT mediated chronic inflammation in diabetics not only contributes to more severe periodontitis [31], but also is implicated in determining insulin resistance through the production of pro-inflammatory cytokines [2,28]. Thus, pro-inflammatory cytokines including TNF-α have been described to decrease circulatory levels of APN and promote chronic inflammation and insulin resistance. Therefore our results point out at beneficial effects of APN not only by inhibiting osteoclastogenesis and alveolar bone loss, but also by reducing chronic inflammation and hyperglycemia in DIO mice induced with periodontitis (Figure 5).

Another important finding of our study is that APN inhibited osteoclastogenesis by directly signaling through FoxO1 in osteoclast-precursor cells undergoing differentiation. FoxO1 is a transcriptional regulator of energy homeostasis [28] that controls glucose metabolism through osteoblasts partly by regulating the

activity of osteocalcin. In addition, insulin signaling targets osteoblasts and inactivates FoxO1 in a PI3K/AKT dependent manner [20,28]. A more recent study found that over-expression of FoxO family factors led to the formation of fewer mature osteoclasts [32]. This latter work was consistent with our results, showing that FoxO1 over-expression in pre-osteoclasts significantly decreased the formation of mature osteoclasts. In addition, APN increased FoxO1 gene expression in RANKL-treated RAW264.7 cells and promoted FoxO1 activation while FoxO1 over-expression decreased NFATc1 nuclear localization. NFATc1 is a master regulator of osteoclastogenesis [33,34], and its nuclear translocation and activation up-regulates gene expression of osteoclastogenic markers hence promoting osteoclast formation. It has been reported that APN not only inhibited NFATc1 induction via AMPK signaling [6], but also by promoting its nuclear exclusion via inhibition of the Akt signaling pathway [19]. Taken together our results indicate that APN activates FoxO1 in osteoclast-precursor cells undergoing differentiation, and that FoxO1 activation inhibit RANKL-induced osteoclastogenesis by restricting NFATc1 transcription functions during osteoclastogenesis.

Whereas APN has been reported to directly inhibit bone formation by decreasing the nuclear levels of FoxO1 in a PI3K/AKT-dependent manner in osteoblasts [22], we have found that APN inhibits RANKL-induced osteoclastogenesis by increasing the nuclear levels of FoxO1 in osteoclast-precursor cells. These results are in agreement with our previous findings that APN inhibits AKT activation in RANKL-induced osteoclasts [19]. In fact, inhibition of AKT by APN has been shown to promote

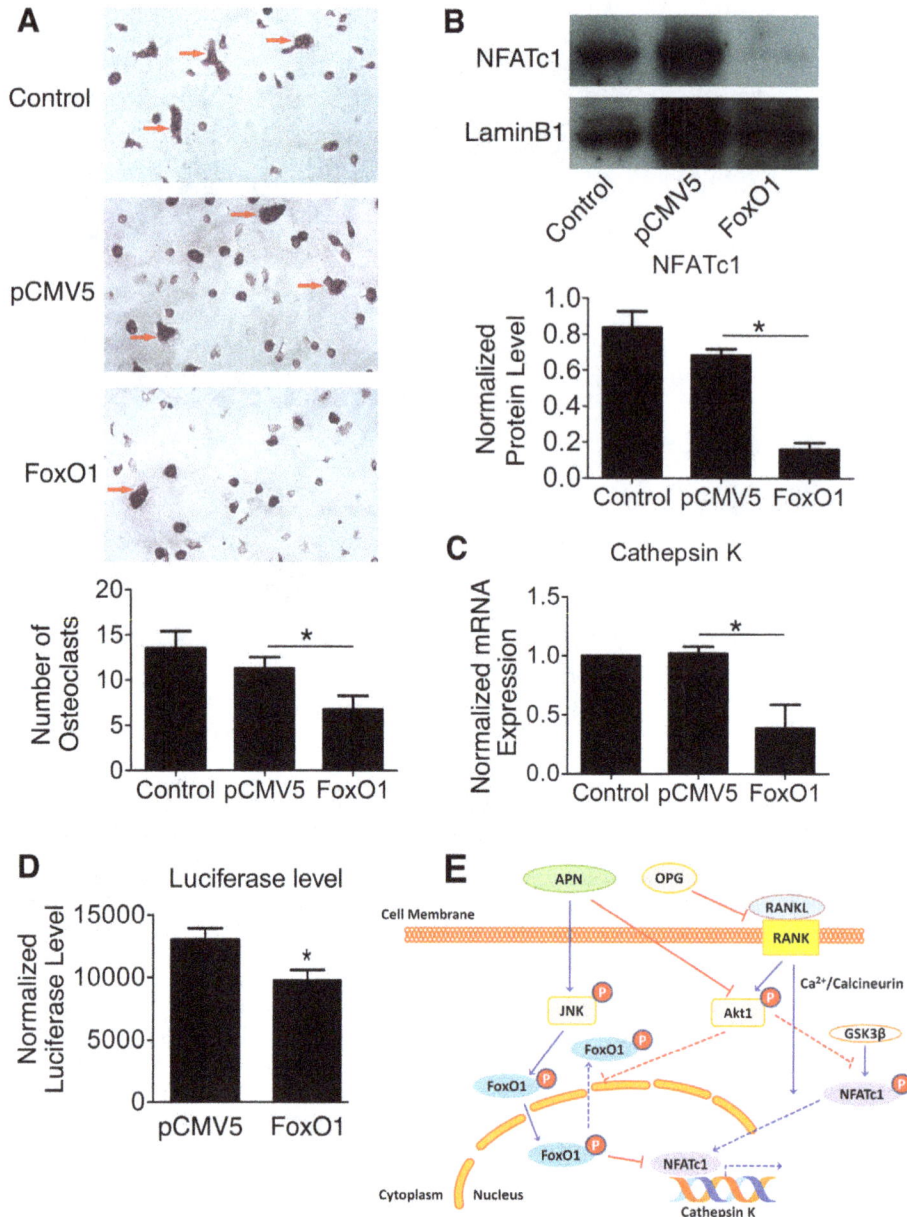

Figure 4. FoxO1 Over-Expression Inhibits RANKL-Induced Osteoclastogenesis by Down Regulating NFATc1. (A) BMMs isolated from WT mice were transfected with or without pCMV5 or Flag-FoxO1, and osteoclastogenesis was induced with 10 ng/ml M-CSF and 50 ng/ml RANKL for 7 days. TRAP staining was performed and the number of osteoclasts was manually counted in four separate fields (magnification, ×200; red arrows = osteoclasts). (B) Western blot for NFATc1 nuclear protein extracted from RAW264.7 cells, which were transfected with or without pCMV5 or Flag-FoxO1. Lamin B1 was detected as the loading control. Data are shown as mean ± SD of three independent experiments. *$P<0.05$. (C) qRT-PCR of cathepsin K mRNA levels in RAW264.7 cells transfected with or without pCMV5 or Flag-FoxO1 during osteoclastogenesis. The mRNA level was normalized to GAPDH. (D) Luciferase assay determined luciferase levels in RAW264.7 cells co-transfected with Flag-FoxO1 or pCMV5 (control) and pGL3-CtspK-luciferase reporter vector. (E) APN inhibition of RANKL-induced osteoclastogenesis through activation of FoxO1 and inactivation of NFATc1. APN promotes FoxO1 activation directly in a JNK-dependent manner and indirectly by inhibiting AKT phosphorylation [19] (data not shown). In the absence of APN, NFATc1, the master regulator of osteoclastogenesis [33,34], is activated by RANKL in a Ca^{2+}/calcineurin-dependent manner. In the presence of APN, NFATc1 nuclear translocation is inhibited indirectly by APN-mediated inhibition of AKT [19] and by a FoxO1-mediated mechanism. Inhibitory signaling by APN is depicted by red lines and stimulatory signaling is represented by blue lines. Dashed lines are used to represent signaling events that are diminished in osteoclast-precursor cells undergoing RANKL-induced differentiation in the presence of APN.

activation of FoxO1 indirectly, via suppressing its AKT-induced nuclear exclusion [29]. As part of our study, we further showed that APN can also activate FoxO1 in a JNK-dependent manner in osteoclast-precursor cells and that JNK-inhibition decreased APN-induced activation of FoxO1 in osteoclast-precursor cells undergoing differentiation. FoxO1 belongs to the O class of the

Forkhead superfamily and is regulated by Akt and JNK signal pathways. The present study and our published work [19] demonstrated that APN activated JNK signaling and suppressed Akt signaling [19], all of which can activate FoxO1. Several reports have previously shown APN can activate JNK in a variety of cell types and tissues to regulate a variety of functions including

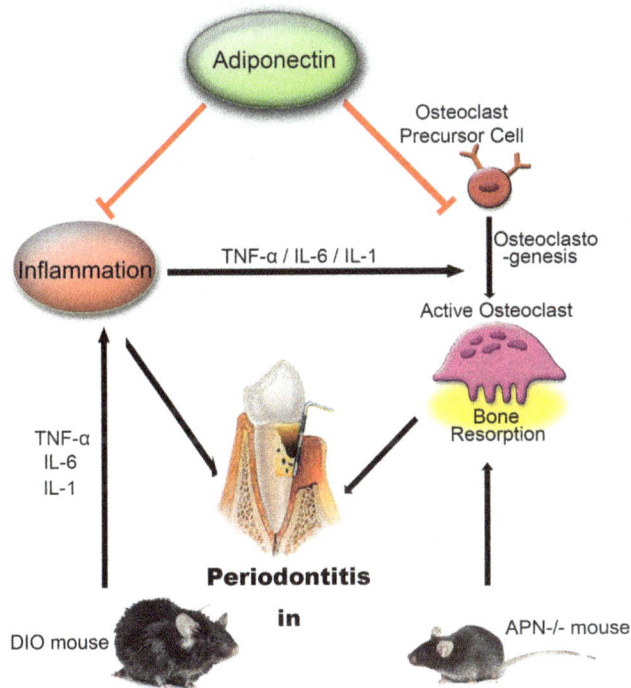

Figure 5. Schematic Diagram of APN Therapeutic Potential in Treating T2DM-Associated Periodontitis. We established experimental periodontitis in APN$^{-/-}$ and DIO mice and treated them with systemic APN infusion. Our results support the notion that systemic administration with APN may constitute a therapeutic strategy to ameliorate T2DM-associated periodontitis due to dual roles of APN at inhibiting osteoclastic activity and hence bone resorption, and at attenuating inflammation.

proliferation and apoptosis. It has been reported that APN regulated the proliferation and apoptosis of C2C12 myocytes, prostate cancer and hepatocellular carcinoma cell lines via activation of JNK [35,36]. In addition osteoblasts [37], chondrocytes [38], endothelial cells [39] and macrophages were also regulated by adiponectin through activation of JNK [40,41] Therefore JNK and Akt signaling pathways may participate in APN-induced FoxO1 activation in osteoclasts. Hence, the different responses to APN in osteoblasts and osteoclasts may be dependent on the signaling pathway that APN activates. Further studies will be needed to characterize the underlying mechanisms involved.

In the present study, we found that APN increases FoxO1 expression in RANKL-treated RAW264.7 cells, but not in the absence of RANKL (data not shown). Although we did not evaluate whether APN by itself activates JNK in the present experiment conditions, other studies reported that APN could regulate the functions of RAW264.7 macrophages via activation of JNK [40,41]. The synergistic effect of APN and RANKL to induce FoxO1 expresssion and JNK activation may be attributed to oxidative stress. Several reports directly suggest that oxidative stress is responsible for RANKL-induced osteoclastogenesis and

bone resorption [42–45] In the presence of oxidative stress, JNK was phosphorylated, and further regulating FoxO1 activity, which is suggested to antagonize oxidative stress [46] Hence APN may inhibit osteoclastogenesis through modulating oxidative stress and further activating JNK and FoxO1 [47].

Although our results point out at APN inhibiting osteoclastogenesis and hence bone resorption *in vitro* and *in vivo*, they do not exclude other mechanisms that can also contribute at preserving alveolar bone integrity. In fact, signaling mechanisms through which APN affects bone metabolism are just beginning to be elucidated. Indeed, the bone phenotype of APN$^{-/-}$ mice was shown to be normal under physiological conditions [17,18]. However, if the effects of long term adaptation and compensation are excluded and the possible effects of mechanical loading on bone metabolism are eliminated through bone explantation assays in APN$^{-/-}$ mice, APN inhibits osteoclastogenesis and promotes osteogenic differentiation [19]. Furthermore, sustained release of APN was also shown to improve peri-implant osteogenesis in ovariectomized rabbits by suppressing osteoclastic activity both *in vivo* and *in vitro* [21]. Importantly, our results do not exclude the possibility that APN not only inhibits osteoclastogenesis, but also promotes alveolar bone formation. In agreement with this view, it has been recently shown that APN signals in neurons of the locus coeruleus, through FoxO1 to decrease the sympathetic tone thereby increasing bone mass by decreasing energy expenditure [22]. This indirect effect on increasing bone mass has been shown to mask the opposing local effects of APN on osteoblasts at decreasing bone mass and circulating osteocalcin levels [22]. Taken together, the direct and indirect role of FoxO1 to inhibit osteoclastogenesis appears to play a dominant role over the opposite effects of APN in osteoclastogenesis through osteoblast regulation of OPG and RANKL levels. In addition, some of the protective effects of APN on alveolar bone loss found in our study may be resulting from APN inhibiting pro-inflammatory cytokines and/or from APN central effects that may increase alveolar bone mass indirectly.

In conclusion, our study supports the notion that APN may constitute a potential intervention therapy to treat T2D-associated periodontitis due to its dual inhibitory effects in bone resorption and inflammation. It also proposes that APN protection from alveolar bone loss associated with periodontitis may occur partly through a JNK-FoxO1 pathway in osteoclasts.

Acknowledgments

We thank Jean Tang for her assistance in tissue sample preparation and histology, and Dana Murray and Jessica Cheng for their help in the preparation of the manuscript. We are grateful to the other members of the Chen lab for discussion and technical help.

Author Contributions

Conceived and designed the experiments: LZ QT JC. Performed the experiments: LZ SM LY YT. Analyzed the data: LZ QT MMD SHK PV XZ JC. Wrote the paper: LZ QT PV JC. Revised/edited the manuscript: LZ SM QT LY YT MMD SHK PV XZ JC.

References

1. Eke PI, Dye BA, Wei L, Thornton-Evans GO, Genco RJ (2012) Prevalence of periodontitis in adults in the United States: 2009 and 2010. J Dent Res 91: 914–920.
2. Bastard JP, Maachi M, Lagathu C, Kim MJ, Caron M, et al. (2006) Recent advances in the relationship between obesity, inflammation, and insulin resistance. Eur Cytokine Netw 17: 4–12.
3. Mealey BL (2006) Periodontal disease and diabetes. A two-way street. J Am Dent Assoc 137 Suppl: 26S–31S.
4. Yamauchi T, Kamon J, Waki H, Terauchi Y, Kubota N, et al. (2001) The fat-derived hormone adiponectin reverses insulin resistance associated with both lipoatrophy and obesity. Nat Med 7: 941–946.

5. Yamauchi T KJ, Ito Y, Tsuchida A, Yokomizo T, Kita S, et al. (2003) Cloning of adiponectin receptors that mediate antidiabetic metabolic effects. Nature 423: 762–769.

6. Yamaguchi N, Kukita T, Li YJ, Kamio N, Fukumoto S, et al. (2008) Adiponectin inhibits induction of TNF-alpha/RANKL-stimulated NFATc1 via the AMPK signaling. FEBS Lett 582: 451–456.

7. Wulster-Radcliffe MC, Ajuwon KM, Wang J, Christian JA, Spurlock ME (2004) Adiponectin differentially regulates cytokines in porcine macrophages. Biochem Biophys Res Commun 316: 924–929.

8. Weyer C, Funahashi T, Tanaka S, Hotta K, Matsuzawa Y, et al. (2001) Hypoadiponectinemia in obesity and type 2 diabetes: close association with insulin resistance and hyperinsulinemia. J Clin Endocrinol Metab 86: 1930–1935.

9. Hotta K, Funahashi T, Arita Y, Takahashi M, Matsuda M, et al. (2000) Plasma concentrations of a novel, adipose-specific protein, adiponectin, in type 2 diabetic patients. Arterioscler Thromb Vasc Biol 20: 1595–1599.

10. Zimmermann GS, Bastos MF, Dias Goncalves TE, Chambrone L, Duarte PM (2013) Local and circulating levels of adipocytokines in obese and normal weight individuals with chronic periodontitis. J Periodontol 84: 624–633.

11. Saito T, Yamaguchi N, Shimazaki Y, Hayashida H, Yonemoto K, et al. (2008) Serum levels of resistin and adiponectin in women with periodontitis: the Hisayama study. J Dent Res 87: 319–322.

12. Maeda N, Takahashi M, Funahashi T, Kihara S, Nishizawa H, et al. (2001) PPARgamma ligands increase expression and plasma concentrations of adiponectin, an adipose-derived protein. Diabetes 50: 2094–2099.

13. Combs TP, Wagner JA, Berger J, Doebber T, Wang WJ, et al. (2002) Induction of adipocyte complement-related protein of 30 kilodaltons by PPARgamma agonists: a potential mechanism of insulin sensitization. Endocrinology 143: 998–1007.

14. Sun WL, Chen LL, Zhang SZ, Wu YM, Ren YZ, et al. (2011) Inflammatory Cytokines, Adiponectin, Insulin Resistance and Metabolic Control after Periodontal Intervention in Patients with Type 2 Diabetes and Chronic Periodontitis. Internal Medicine 50: 1569–1574.

15. Teitelbaum SL (2000) Bone resorption by osteoclasts. Science 289: 1504–1508.

16. Ducy P, Schinke T, Karsenty G (2000) The osteoblast: a sophisticated fibroblast under central surveillance. Science 289: 1501–1504.

17. Shu RZ, Zhang F, Wang F, Feng DC, Li XH, et al. (2009) Adiponectin deficiency impairs liver regeneration through attenuating STAT3 phosphorylation in mice. Lab Invest 89: 1043–1052.

18. Ren W, Li X, Wang F, Qiao JN, Dang SY, et al. (2006) Generation of adiponectin gene knock-out and LacZ gene knock-in mouse model. Prog Biochem Biophys 33: 846–853.

19. Tu Q, Zhang J, Dong LQ, Saunders E, Luo E, et al. (2011) Adiponectin inhibits osteoclastogenesis and bone resorption via APPL1-mediated suppression of AKT1. J Biol Chem 286: 12542–51.

20. Luo XH, Guo LJ, Xie H, Yuan LQ, Wu XP, et al. (2006) Adiponectin stimulates RANKL and inhibits OPG expression in human osteoblasts through the MAPK signaling pathway. J Bone Miner Res 21: 1648–1656.

21. Luo E, Hu J, Bao C, Li Y, Tu Q, et al. (2012) Sustained release of adiponectin improves osteogenesis around hydroxyapatite implants by suppressing osteoclast activity in ovariectomized rabbits. Acta Biomater 8: 734–743.

22. Kajimura D, Lee HW, Riley KJ, Arteaga-Solis E, Ferron M, et al. (2013) Adiponectin regulates bone mass via opposite central and peripheral mechanisms through FoxO1. Cell Metab 17: 901–915.

23. Mao X, Kikani CK, Riojas RA, Langlais P, Wang L, et al. (2006) APPL1 binds to adiponectin receptors and mediates adiponectin signalling and function. Nat Cell Biol 8: 516–523.

24. Amar S, Zhou Q, Shaik-Dasthagirisaheb Y, Leeman S (2007) Diet-induced obesity in mice causes changes in immune responses and bone loss manifested by bacterial challenge. Proc Natl Acad Sci USA 104: 20466–20471.

25. Li CH, Amar S (2007) Morphometric, histomorphometric, and microcomputed tomographic analysis of periodontal inflammatory lesions in a murine model. J Periodontol 78: 1120–1128.

26. Tu Q, Zhang J, Paz J, Wade K, Yang P, et al. (2008) Haploinsufficiency of Runx2 results in bone formation decrease and different BSP expression pattern changes in two transgenic mouse models. J Cell Physiol 217: 40–47.

27. Tu Q, Zhang J, Fix A, Brewer E, Li YP, et al. (2009) Targeted overexpression of BSP in osteoclasts promotes bone metastasis of breast cancer cells. J Cell Physiol 218: 135–145.

28. Kousteni S (2012) FoxO1, the transcriptional chief of staff of energy metabolism. Bone 50: 437–443.

29. Hay N (2011) Interplay between FOXO, TOR, and Akt. Biochim Biophys Acta 1813: 1965–1970.

30. Kadowaki T, Yamauchi T, Kubota N, Hara K, Ueki K, et al. (2006) Adiponectin and adiponectin receptors in insulin resistance, diabetes, and the metabolic syndrome. J Clin Invest 116: 1784–1792.

31. Li H, Xie H, Fu M, Li W, Guo B, et al. (2013) 25-hydroxyvitamin D3 ameliorates periodontitis by modulating the expression of inflammation-associated factors in diabetic mice. Steroids 78: 115–120.

32. Bartell S, Han L, Warren A, Crawford J, Iyer S, et al. (2012) Gain or loss of FoxO function in osteoclasts alter bone mass in mice. ASBMR 2012 Annual Meeting: 284.

33. Takayanagi H, Kim S, Koga T, Nishina H, Isshiki M, et al. (2002) Induction and activation of the transcription factor NFATc1 (NFAT2) integrate RANKL signaling in terminal differentiation of osteoclasts. Dev Cell 3: 889–901.

34. Hirotani H, Tuohy NA, Woo JT, Stern PH, Clipstone NA (2004) The calcineurin/nuclear factor of activated T cells signaling pathway regulates osteoclastogenesis in RAW264.7 cells. J Biol Chem 279: 13984–13992.

35. Miyazaki T, Bub JD, Uzuki M, Iwamoto Y (2005) Adiponectin activates c-Jun NH2-terminal kinase and inhibits signal transducer and activator of transcription 3. Biochemical and Biophysical Research Communications 333: 79–87.

36. Saxena NK, Fu PP, Nagalingam A, Wang J, Handy J, et al. (2010) Adiponectin modulates c-Jun N- terminal kinase and mammalian target of rapamycin and inhibits hepatocellular carcinoma. Gastroenterology 139: 1762–1773.

37. Luo XH, Guo LJ, Yuan LQ, Xie H, Zhou HD, et al. (2005) Adiponectin stimulates human osteoblasts proliferation and differentiation via the MAPK signaling pathway. Exp Cell Res 309: 99–109.

38. Kang EH, Lee YJ, Kim TK, Chang CB, Chung JH, et al. (2010) Adiponectin is a potential catabolic mediator in osteoarthritis cartilage. Arthritis Research & Therapy 12: R231.

39. Bobbert P, Antoniak S, Schultheiss HP, Rauch U (2008) Globular adiponectin but not full-length adiponectin induces increased procoagulability in human endothelia cells. Journal of Molecular and Cellular Cardiology 44: 388–394.

40. Park PH, Huang H, McMullen MR, Bryan K, Nagy LE (2008) Activation of cyclic-AMP response element binding protein contributes to adiponectin-stimulated interleukin-10 expression in RAW 264.7 macrophages. J Leukoc Biol 83: 1258–1266.

41. Subedi A1, Kim MJ, Nepal S, Lee ES, Kim JA, et al. (2013) Globular adiponectin modulates expression of progammed cell death 4 and miR-21 in RAW 264.7 macrophages through the MAPK/NF-KB pathway. FEBS Letters 587: 1556–1561.

42. Bullon P, Morillo JM, Ramirez-Tortosa MC, Quiles JL, Newman HN, et al. (2009) Metabolic syndrome and periodontitis: is oxidative stress a common link? J Dent Res 88: 503–518.

43. Manolagas SC (2010) From estrogen-centric to aging and oxidative stress: a revised perspective of the pathogenesis of osteoporosis. Endocr Rev 31: 266–300.

44. Toker H, Ozdemir H, Eren K, Ozer H, Sahin G (2009) N-acetylcysteine, a thiol antioxidant, decreases alveolar bone loss in experimental periodontitis in rats. J Periodontol 80: 672–678.

45. Manolagas SC, Almeida M (2007) Gone with the Wnts: beta-catenin, T-cell factor, forkhead box O, and oxidative stress in age-dependent diseases of bone, lipid, and glucose metabolism. Mol Endocrinol 21: 2605–2614.

46. Galli C, Passeri G, Macaluso GM (2011) FoxOs, Wnts and oxidative stress-induced bone loss: new players in the periodontitis arena? J Periodontal Res 46: 397–406.

47. Nakanishi S, Yamane K, Kamei N, Nojima H, Okubo M, et al. (2005) A protective effect of adiponectin against oxidative stress in Japanese Americans: the association between adiponectin or leptin and urinary isoprostane. Metabolism 54: 194–199.

2

Mobilization of Endothelial Progenitors by Recurrent Bacteremias with a Periodontal Pathogen

Moritz Kebschull[1,2], Manuela Haupt[2], Søren Jepsen[1], James Deschner[1], Georg Nickenig[2], Nikos Werner[2]*

1 Department of Periodontology, Operative and Preventive Dentistry, University of Bonn, Bonn, Germany, 2 Department of Internal Medicine II, University of Bonn, Bonn, Germany

Abstract

Background: Periodontal infections are independent risk factors for atherosclerosis. However, the exact mechanisms underlying this link are yet unclear. Here, we evaluate the in vivo effects of bacteremia with a periodontal pathogen on endothelial progenitors, bone marrow-derived cells capable of endothelial regeneration, and delineate the critical pathways for these effects.

Methods: 12-week old C57bl6 wildtype or toll-like receptor (TLR)-2 deficient mice were repeatedly intravenously challenged with 10^9 live *P. gingivalis* 381 or vehicle. Numbers of Sca1+/flk1+ progenitors, circulating angiogenic cells, CFU-Hill, and late-outgrowth EPC were measured by FACS/culture. Endothelial function was assessed using isolated organ baths, reendothelization was measured in a carotid injury model. RANKL/osteoprotegerin levels were assessed by ELISA/qPCR.

Results: In wildtype mice challenged with intravenous *P.gingivalis*, numbers of Sca1+/flk1+ progenitors, CAC, CFU-Hill, and late-outgrowth EPC were strongly increased in peripheral circulation and spleen, whereas Sca1+/flk1+ progenitor numbers in bone marrow decreased. Circulating EPCs were functional, as indicated by improved endothelial function and improved reendothelization in infected mice. The osteoprotegerin/RANKL ratio was increased after *P. gingivalis* challenge in the bone marrow niche of wildtype mice and late-outgrowth EPC *in vitro*. Conversely, in mice deficient in TLR2, no increase in progenitor mobilization or osteoprotegerin/RANKL ratio was detected.

Conclusion: Recurrent transient bacteremias, a feature of periodontitis, increase peripheral EPC counts and decrease EPC pools in the bone marrow, thereby possibly reducing overall endothelial regeneration capacity, conceivably explaining pro-atherogenic properties of periodontal infections. These effects are seemingly mediated by toll-like receptor (TLR)-2.

Editor: Gian Paolo Fadini, University of Padova, Medical School, Italy

Funding: The study was funded by the German Research Foundation (DFG KFO208 TP6 & TP9). The funders had no role in study design, data collection and analysis, decision to publish, or preparation of the manuscript.

Competing Interests: The authors have declared that no competing interests exist.

* E-mail: nikos.werner@ukb.uni-bonn.de

Introduction

Cardiovascular diseases are the leading cause of mortality in the western world. Their underlying pathological condition is atherosclerosis [1]. Risk factors for the development or acceleration of atherosclerosis include established predictors identified in the Framingham study [2], but also chronic infections, most notably periodontitis, a highly prevalent chronic inflammatory condition of the tooth-supporting tissues caused by specific periodontal pathogens in a susceptible host [3,4].

There is ample evidence from epidemiological studies suggesting that periodontal infections are an independent risk factor for atherosclerosis [5–7]. Despite the overall modest association, the consistency of data across different study populations, exposures and outcome variables suggests that these findings are not spurious or attributable to confounders.

In the past, several potential mechanisms for a periodontal-cardiovascular link have been proposed (for review, see [6,8]). These are conceptually based on the fact that the sizable ulcerated epithelium of the periodontal pockets [9] mediates persistent, recurrent bacteremia with pathogens (for review, see [10]). The mechanisms include direct effects of periodontal pathogens or their components on vascular cells, auto-immune reactions, and oxidative stress. A causative link of infections with activation of the innate immune system, and increased atherogenesis is strongly suggested by recent studies demonstrating the necessity of pattern-recognizing receptors, e.g. the Toll-like receptors, for atherosclerotic lesion formation [11–16]. Specifically, it was shown that TLR2, the receptor recognizing a principal pathogen in human periodontitis, the gram-negative anaerobe *Porphyromonas gingivalis*, is critical for both the effects of the pathogen in the oral cavity [17,18] and in atherogenesis [19,20]. Interaction of *P. gingivalis* fimbriae with TLR2 is necessary to mediate invasion of the pathogen into endothelial cells, where it was shown to persist and replicate [21], and eventually induce endothelial dysfunction [22].

A critical first step in atherogenesis is the activation of vascular endothelial cells and the development of endothelial dysfunction with subsequent apoptosis of endothelial cells [23]. Cross-sectional studies have demonstrated increased endothelial dysfunction in otherwise healthy patients with periodontitis [24,25]. Periodontal therapy could improve endothelial dysfunction [26]. However, the pathways underlying these effects are not yet fully understood.

Vascular health is maintained by healthy endothelium that can in part be regenerated by circulating endothelial-regenerating cells (e.g. Sca1+/flk1+ progenitors) [27]. Numbers of these regenerating cells are associated with endothelial function [28] and cardiovascular outcomes [29]. Impaired endothelial regeneration after endothelial cell damage – as known to be elicited by periodontal pathogens [30] - is closely connected to the development of atherosclerotic lesions [31].

However, no mechanistic studies evaluating the effect of periodontal infections on endothelial regeneration have been conducted so far. The data available to date are limited to a single, cross-sectional study showing increased endothelial progenitor cell (EPC) counts in otherwise healthy periodontal patients when compared to controls without periodontitis [32], and an intervention study in the same population that showed a decrease of CD34 positive cells by periodontal therapy [33]. Importantly, these studies were neither designed nor suitable to prove causality, or to investigate the underlying mechanisms of a potential association.

Therefore, in this study we evaluated the effects of infection with the periodontal model pathogen *P. gingivalis* on numbers of different endothelial progenitor cell populations in an *in vivo* model. We aimed to evaluate whether progenitor cell numbers were in fact higher in infected groups than controls, and to determine the biological significance of this finding.

Materials and Methods

Ethics Statement

All animal experiments were performed in accordance with institutional guidelines and the German animal protection law. The study protocol was approved by the appropriate authority (North-Rhine Westphalia State Environment Agency (*Landesamt für Natur, Umwelt und Verbraucherschutz*/LANUV), Recklinghausen, Germany, permit no #8.87-50.10.35.08.013).

Mice

Female, 12-week-old C57bl6 mice (Charles River, Sulzfeld, Germany) or age- and gender-matched TLR2−/− mice (a kind gift of Dr. Sabine Specht, Bonn) were used for this study. The animals were maintained in a 22°C room with a 12-hour light/dark cycle and received chow and water *ad libitum*. The mice were killed at day 12, and blood and tissue samples were recovered immediately. To account for potential gender-specific effects in the wildtype mice, we also tested several age-matched male mice, with very similar results than in female mice (data not shown).

Bacteria

Porphyromonas gingivalis strain 381 (a kind gift of Dr. Evie Lalla, New York, NY, USA) was cultured under anaerobic conditions, as described previously [34].

In vivo Infection (Bacteremia Model)

2×10^9 live *P. gingivalis* resuspended in 200 µl saline or saline alone (control) were injected into the tail veins on days 0, 2, 4, 6, 8, and 10.

Flow Cytometry

Peripheral blood was collected from the inferior vena cava at sacrifice. Bone marrow cells were flushed from both femurs using sterile saline.

After red blood cell lysis (BD Pharm Lyse, BD, Heidelberg, Germany) and blocking of the Fcγ II/III receptors (CD16/CD32, BD), the viable lymphocyte population was assessed for the expression of Sca-1-FITC (BD Pharmingen) and vascular endothelial growth factor receptor-2 coupled to PE (VEGFR2/flk-1, BD). Isotype-identical antibodies served as controls (BD). Analyses were run on a BD FACScalibur flow cytometer (BD), data were analyzed using FloJo (Treestar, Ashland, OR, USA).

Data were presented as %gated, relative to levels found in control mice.

Preparation of Spleen-derived Mononuclear Cells

Spleens were minced and gently homogenized. The resulting single cell suspension was fractionated using Ficoll (Percoll, Biochrom, Berlin, Germany) gradient centrifugation.

Preparation of Circulating Angiogenic Cells (CAC)

1×10^6 spleen-derived mononuclear cells were seeded into fibronectin-coated (Sigma-Aldrich, St. Louis, MO, USA) 24-well plates in 500 µl of endothelial basal medium 2 (Lonza) with supplements. After 7 days in culture, cells were assayed for Dil-Ac-LDL uptake and lectin staining (UEA-1, Sigma-Aldrich). Per well, 5 high-power fields were analyzed by a blinded observer (author MH) for Dil-Ac-LDL+/lectin+ staining.

Preparation of CFU–Hill

CFU-Hill were cultured from splenic MNCs, as described [35,36]. In brief, 1×10^7 cells were seeded on 6 cm dishes in complete EBM-2 medium, after 48 hours, 1×10^6 non-adherent cells were collected and replated on fibronectin-coated 24-well plates for 7 days. CFU-Hill were counted by a blinded observer (author MH) using a phase-contrast microscope using a mosaic of 10×10 high power fields.

Preparation of Late-outgrowth EPC

Late-outgrowth EPC were grown from splenic MNCs, as described [37,38]. In brief, 1×10^7 cells were seeded in complete EBM-2 medium on a 6 cm dish, non-adherent cells were removed after 48 hours, and cells were cultured for a total of 21 days. Colonies were identified by visual inspection using phase-contrast microscopy. Results of the dichotomous decision (presence of differentiated colonies) by a blinded observer (author MH) were statistically tested using Fishers exact test.

In vitro Infection

1×10^5 phenotyped [39] late-outgrowth EPC were seeded in 6 cm dishes in EBM-2 medium with growth supplements, but without antibiotics. 5×10^6, 1×10^7, or 5×10^7 live *P. gingivalis* 381 were added, corresponding to a multiplicity-of-infection (MOI) of 50, 100, or 500 bacteria per EPC. The infection was maintained for 24 hours.

ELISA

Bone marrow supernatants were produced by flushing both femurs with chilled saline and subsequent removal of bone marrow cells by centrifugation. Levels of RANKL and osteoprotegerin protein were assessed using commercially available ELISAs (#DY462 and #DY805, R&D Systems, Abingdon, UK) and normalized for total protein content, as assessed by Bradford assay.

Quantitative RT-PCR

Total RNA was isolated using Trizol reagent (Invitrogen, Carlsbad, CA) and subsequent spin-column purification (RNeasy

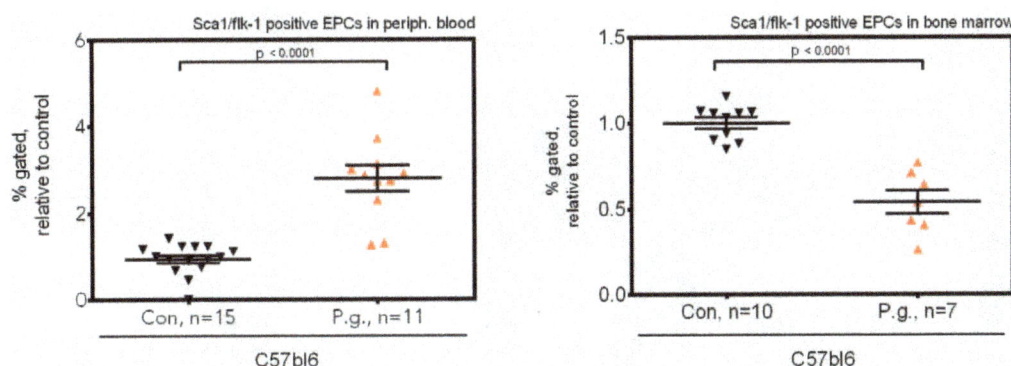

Figure 1. Bacteremia with P. gingivalis leads to mobilization of Sca1/flk1 progenitors from the bone marrow into peripheral blood of wildtype mice. Sca-1/flk1 progenitor cells (EPC) were quantified by flow cytometry in peripheral blood (left panel) or bone marrow (right panel) of C56bl6 wildtype mice after intravenous application of the periodontal pathogen P. gingivalis or saline (control). Data are presented as mean percentages of gated cells ± SEM normalized to control, statistical testing was performed using unpaired t-tests.

Mini Kit, Qiagen, Hilden, Germany), reverse-transcribed using Superscript III (Invitrogen) and analyzed using Taqman chemistry (Applied Biosystems, Foster City, CA, USA) using the probes Mm00441906_m1 for RANKL, Mm01205928_m1 for osteopro-tegerin, and Mm99999915_g1 for GAPDH on a ABi 7500 Fast cycler (Applied Biosystems). Data were analyzed using the ∆∆ct method.

Aortic Ring Preparation and ex vivo Measurement of Endothelial Function

To assess endothelial function ex vivo, vasoconstriction and endothelium-dependent and –independent vasodilation were measured in isolated organ baths, as described previously [40]. In brief, the thoracic aorta was carefully dissected, adventitial tissue was removed, and 3 mm segments were prepared for investigation (3–4 replicates/mouse) in organ baths filled with oxygenated modified Tyrode buffer at 37°C. After administration of a resting tension of 10 mN, drugs were added in increasing concentrations and cumulative concentration response curves were recorded. We used 20 and 40 mM KCl and 1 nM –10 μM phenylephrine to induce aortic ring contraction. 10 nM –100 μM carbachol were then added to assess endothelium-dependent vasodilation after precontraction with phenylephrine. Finally, endothelium-independent vasodilation was assessed by application of 1 nM –10 μM nitroglycerine. At each drug concentration, a plateau phase was observed before addition of a higher dose of the drug. Before addition of the next substance, drugs were washed out.

Reendothelization after Defined Carotid Artery Injury

Reendothelization was assessed in an electric injury model of the common carotid artery, as described previously [41]. In brief, on day 7 of the experimental protocol, a defined area of 4 mm length of the distal common carotid artery was denuded of endothelium using a bipolar microregulator.

The extent of endothelial repair was measured after 5 days by staining of the denuded areas by intravenous injection of 50 μl Evan's blue dye (5% in saline). The yet unrepaired area – stained blue by the dye – was quantified by a blinded observer (author MH) using a calibrated stereomicroscope and expressed as percentage of the total injured area. Data are presented relative to the mean unrepaired are in sham-infected control animals.

Statistical Analysis

All data were analyzed using GraphPad Prism V (GraphPad, San Diego, CA, USA). Normality of data was assessed using d'Agostino K^2 tests, where appropriate. For normally distributed data, in comparisons of two groups, two-tailed, unpaired or paired (analysis of circulating angiogenic cells) t-tests were used, for comparisons of three or more groups, one-way ANOVA and *post-hoc* Tukey tests or two-way ANOVA with *post-hoc* Bonferroni tests were utilized. Late-outgrowth EPC experiments yielding dichotomous decisions were analyzed by Fishers exact test. All data are presented as means ± SEM. A p-value of <0.05 was considered significant.

Results

In C57bl6 wildtype animals, recurrent bacteremia with *P. gingivalis* did not impair clinical status of the animals, but lead to strongly increased peripheral count of Sca1+/flk1+ progenitors (control vs. test: 1.0±0.09 vs. 2.80±0.30, p<0.0001) with concomitantly decreased counts in bone marrow (control vs. test: 1.0±0.03 vs. 0.54±0.06, p<0.0001; figure 1). This increase in progenitor counts was dependent on the numbers of periodontal pathogens injected (data not shown).

Spleen-derived early and late-outgrowth endothelial progenitor population counts were also increased by *P. gingivalis* bacteremia. Specifically, numbers of Dil-Ac-LDL+/lectin+ circulating angiogenic cells (CAC) were increased more than 5-fold in the infected group (control vs. test: 6.2±0.55 vs. 38.66±2.28 double-positive cells/HPF, p<0.0001; figure 2), numbers of CFU-Hill were increased (control vs. test: 1.00±0.18 vs. 2.71±0.19 CFU/HPF (normalized to control), p=0.0002; figure 3a), and almost all infected mice yielded differentiated late-outgrowth EPC, whilst those in the control group showed no late-outgrowth EPC development after 21 days in culture (figure 3b).

To assess the biological functional relevance of the observed strong increases in counts of the different endothelial progenitor populations, we determined the impact of a recurrent bacteremia and subsequent progenitor mobilization on endothelial function and reendothelization.

Endothelium-dependent vasodilation, a measure of endothelial function, was significantly improved in the bacteremia group (figure 4, left panel). Endothelium-independent vasodilation on the other hand was similar in the bacteremia and the control group (figure 4, right panel).

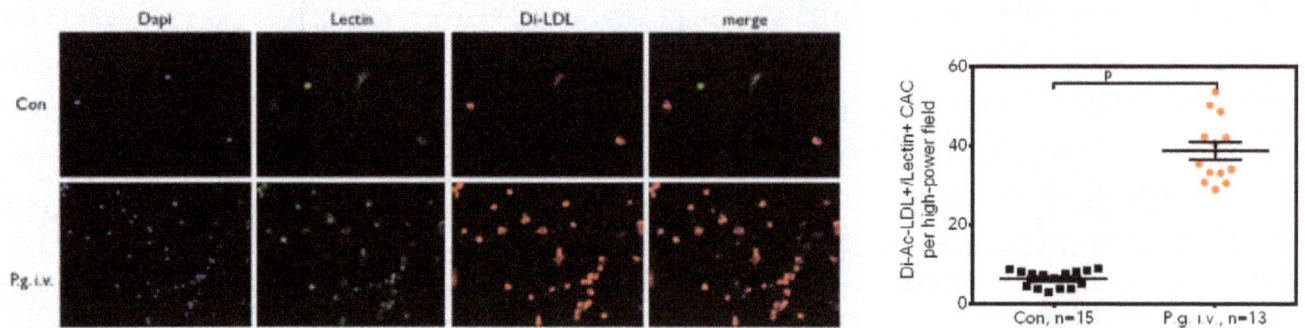

Figure 2. Bacteremia with P. gingivalis leads to increased numbers of circulating angiogenic cells (CACs) in wildtype mice. Strongly increased counts of Dil-Ac-LDL+/Lectin+ spleen-derived CACs in *P. gingivalis* infected mice. Data are presented as means of five high-power fields/mouse $\pm$ SEM, statistical testing was performed using paired t-tests to account for day-to-day staining variability.

Similarly, reendothelization after electric/thermic denudation of the endothelium of the common carotid artery was improved in the bacteremia group characterized by high numbers of peripheral progenitors (figure 5).

Lastly, we assessed how critical mediators of bone marrow cell mobilization were affected by *P. gingivalis* infection and the subsequent strong mobilization of progenitors from bone marrow into peripheral blood.

In the bone marrow niche, we found an increased osteoprotegerin/RANKL protein ratio in *P. gingivalis* infected mice (control vs. test: 0.27 ± 0.03 vs. 0.51 ± 0.05, p = 0.0035; figure 6a). In line with this observation, an increased osteoprotegerin/RANKL mRNA ratio ($+339\pm0.18\%$ at MOI 100, p<0.0001) was observed in *P. gingivalis* infected late-outgrowth EPC *in vitro* (figure 6b).

Finally, we evaluated the molecular pathway underlying the demonstrated mobilization and concomitant depletion of functional endothelial progenitors by recurrent bacteremia with the periodontal pathogen *P. gingivalis*. Unlike most gram-negative species, *P. gingivalis* was described to primarily utilize toll-like receptor (TLR)-2, rather than TLR4, to invade into host cells and exert its primary biological effects. Indeed, in mice deficient in TLR2, we could not observe the pronounced mobilization found in C56bl6 wildtype mice (figures 7&8). In line with these observations, the aforementioned increase in osteoprotegerin/RANKL protein ratios in the bone marrow niche of *P. gingivalis* infected mice was not found in the absence of TLR2 (figure 9). These data indicate that the observed biological effects on

progenitor mobilization are in fact primarily mediated by interactions of *P. gingivalis* with the TLR2 receptor.

Discussion

Here, we show that recurrent bacteremias with the periodontal model pathogen *P. gingivalis* induce Sca1+/flk1+ endothelial progenitor mobilization from the bone marrow into the peripheral circulation *in vivo* and result in higher levels of both early and late EPC, distinct progenitor cell subtypes with dissimilar properties [42]. These data corroborate reports from a cross-sectional study showing higher peripheral EPC counts in otherwise healthy periodontal patients [32]. Increased levels of endothelial progenitors have also been associated with other inflammatory conditions exhibiting similarities in pathobiological mechanisms with periodontal infections, such as rheumatoid arthritis [43], or in situations of acute tissue damage, such as myocardial infarction [44–47], percutaneous coronary intervention [48], or excessive exercise [49].

The infection-induced mobilization was dependent on the presence of toll-like receptor 2 (TLR2), the receptor primarily mediating the invasion of *P. gingivalis* into host cells [11], seemingly a prerequisite for exerting its biological effects. These data are in line with prior observations of reduced periodontal infection-mediated atherosclerosis in a mouse model deficient in TLR2 [19,20] and point to a potential role for TLR2 as a therapeutic target in host modulation [50]. Still, it needs to be noted that since

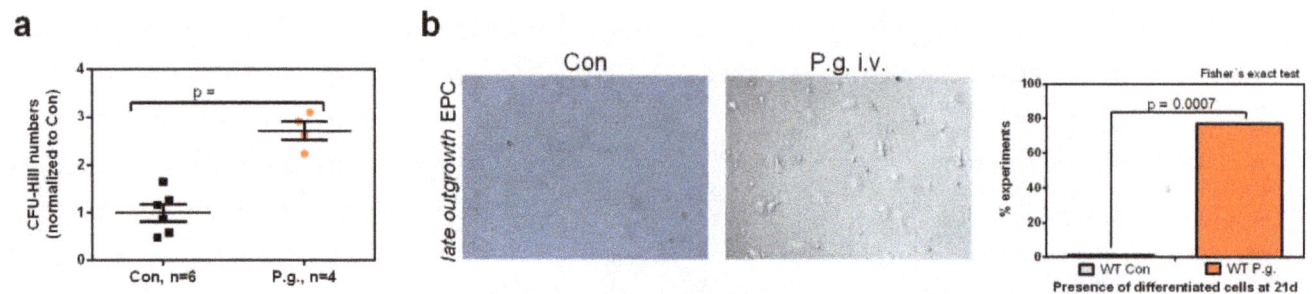

Figure 3. Bacteremia with P. gingivalis leads to increased numbers of CFU-Hill and late-outgrowth EPC in wildtype mice. (a) Increased numbers of CFU-Hill, (b) high proportion of presence of differentiated late-outgrowth EPC in *P. gingivalis* infected mice. Data are presented as mean colony counts $\pm$ SEM relative to controls (CFU-Hill) or as numbers of experiments yielding differentiated colonies (late EPC). Data were analyzed using unpaired t-tests (CFU-Hill) or Fishers exact test (late EPC).

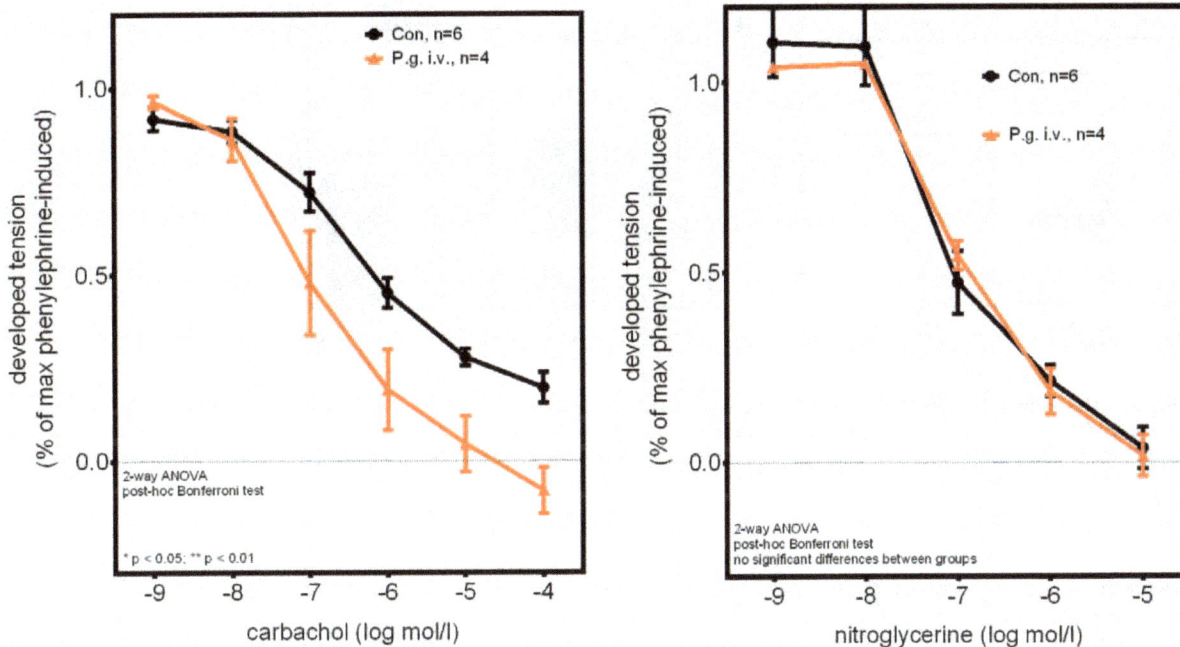

Figure 4. Improved endothelium-dependent vasodilation in P. gingivalis infected mice (left panel). No difference between groups in endothelium-independent vasodilation (right panel). Data are presented as means of 3–4 aortic ring preparations/mouse ± SEM. Statistical testing was performed using 2-way ANOVA and post-hoc Bonferroni tests.

TLRs play a vital role in host defense, there exist several challenges that future TLR-targeting drugs need to overcome [51]. Importantly, our data suggesting a specific reaction towards the periodontal pathogen also corroborate reports showing that unspecific acute systemic inflammation *per se* does not lead to increased mobilization of endothelial progenitors [52].

The beneficial effects of acute bacteremia with the periodontal pathogen on endothelial function and reendothelization point to a functional relevance of mobilized endothelial progenitors. Our group has previously demonstrated that increased levels of endothelial progenitors by systemic transfusion in fact significantly improve endothelial function [40].

In addition to the hitherto demonstrated beneficial effect of regenerating progenitors, the observed significantly improved endothelial-dependent vasodilation in infected mice could also be attributed in part to the excessive vasodilatation in sepsis [53]. However, it must be noted (i) that our treatment regimen did not at all induce a septic shock, a prerequisite for abundant NO production and vasodilatory state, and (ii) that we also demonstrated an improved re-endothelization in the infected group, an outcome independent of endothelial vasodilatory state.

Thus, the observed enhanced mobilization of endothelial progenitors leads to a short-term functional improvement, likely acting as a counter-measure against pathogen-mediated endothelial damage. However, since during the course of periodontal

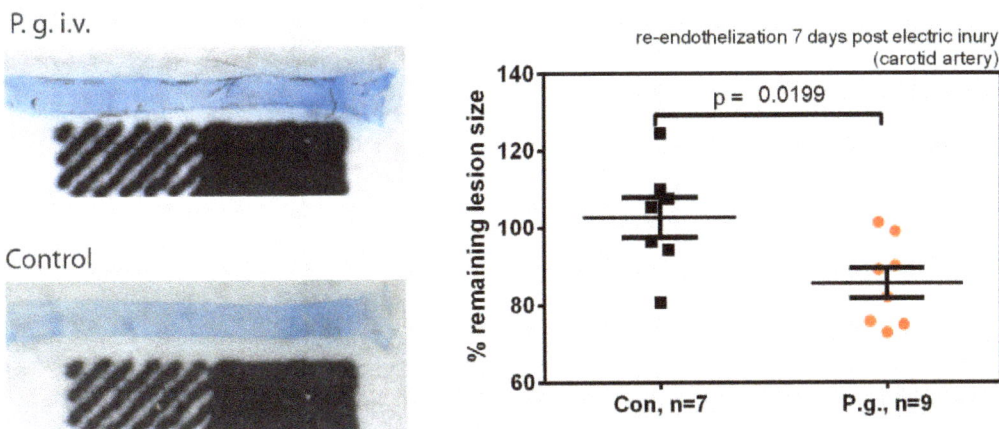

Figure 5. Improved reendothelization in P. gingivalis infected mice 5 days after electric injury of the common carotid artery. Data are expressed as proportions of non-regenerated to regenerated areas relative to saline-treated controls. Micrographs show representative results, dark blue areas mark denuded areas. Data are presented as means ± SEM, statistical testing was performed using an unpaired t-test.

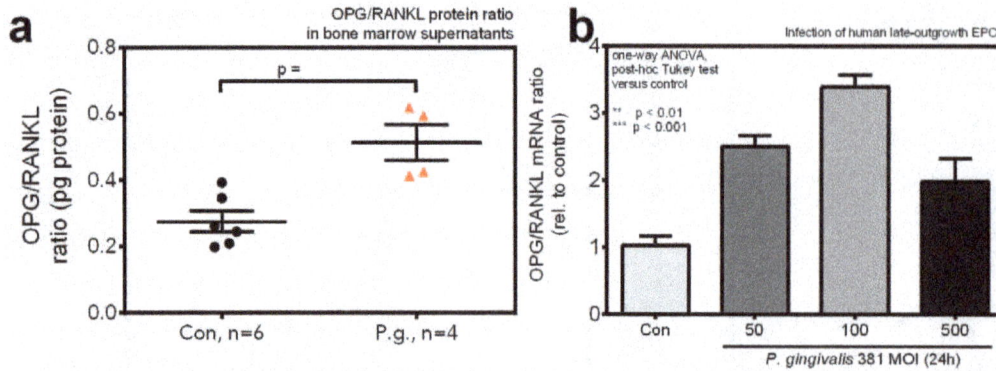

Figure 6. Increased osteoprotegerin/RANKL protein ratio within the bone marrow nice in P. gingivalis infected mice (a), increased osteoprotegerin/RANKL mRNA ratio in P. gingivalis infected late-outgrowth EPC *in vitro* (b). Osteoprotegerin induces bone marrow cell retention and expansion, RANKL triggers mobilization. Increased osteoprotegerin/RANKL ratios may counter act a strong mobilization and depletion of bone marrow EPC. Data are presented as means ± SEM, statistical testing was performed using an unpaired t-test (protein data) and ANOVA and post-hoc Tukey test (mRNA data). MOI, multiplicity-of-infection (ratio of prokaryotic/eukaryotic cells).

infections, bacteremia with periodontal pathogens is a frequent event [10], recurrent mobilization of bone marrow-derived cells may conceivably deplete bone marrow pools over time, thereby reducing the overall regenerative potential and facilitating atherogenesis. Still, to adequately test for the long-term consequences of our observations in the present, acute bacteremia model, appropriate atherosclerosis models need to be employed [54].

To further assess the mobilization of progenitors, we examined in mice infected with *P. gingivalis* the levels of RANKL, a cytokine triggering mobilization [55] and osteoprotegerin, a decoy receptor for RANKL that is known to mediate bone marrow cell expansion and retention that was recently established as a biomarker for cardiovascular prognosis and mortality [56,57]. Importantly, we found increased osteoprotegerin/RANKL ratios in the bone marrow niche of infected wildtype mice. In this work, we have defined this niche as a 'cellular and molecular microenvironment that regulates (...) the engagement of specific programs in response to stress', as proposed by Ehninger and Trumpp [58]. Contrastingly, in TLR2-deficient mice showing no mobilization, the ratio was unchanged. In this context, it needs to be mentioned that the number of control animals in this comparison was rather low (n = 3) due to the sparse availability of the knockout animals. This finding is unexpected, since an increased ratio is indicative for increased retention and decreased mobilization of bone marrow

cells [55]. Here, is could possibly act as a counter measure against the conceivable bone marrow cell depletion by recurrent bacteremias. In fact, our group has previously shown that increased systemic progenitor levels in response to physical training are accompanied by similarly increased, and not diminished, levels in the bone marrow [59].

In line with these observations in vivo, we could demonstrate in vitro that infection of human late-outgrowth EPC with *P. gingivalis* also increases the osteoprotegerin/RANKL ratio. Interestingly, the increase was less pronounced at multiplicities of infection in the range associated with apoptotic changes in endothelial cells [30], an observation in line with reports of decreased osteoprotegerin production in endothelial cells with activated p53 [60]. Increased systemic osteoprotegerin/RANKL ratios after intravascular application of *P. gingivalis* LPS have been reported before [61].

Interestingly, this is in contrast to the well-established osteoclastic phenotype dominated by increased RANKL over osteoprotegerin levels [62] that is found in periodontal lesions that are primarily characterized by bone resorption [63]. We attribute this discrepancy of effects triggered by *P. gingivalis* to the apparent strong differences in cellular composition of the different tissue compartments. The pathogen in the systemic circulation is most likely to encounter endothelial cells and progenitors or vascular smooth muscle cells, potent producers of osteoprotegerin when

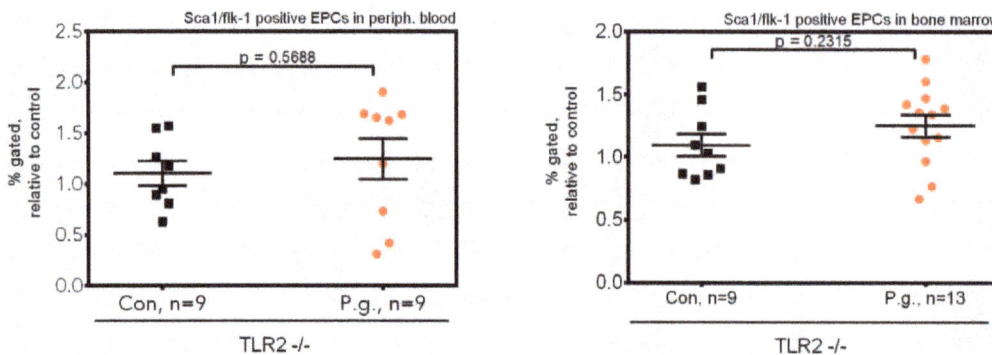

Figure 7. Sca1+/flk1+ progenitor mobilization is TLR2-dependent. In mice deficient in toll-like receptor (TLR)-2, the receptor primarily mediating the invasion of *P. gingivalis* into host cells, no increased mobilization of Sca1+/flk1+ progenitors was observed. Data are presented as mean percentages of gated cells ± SEM normalized to control, statistical testing was performed using unpaired t-tests.

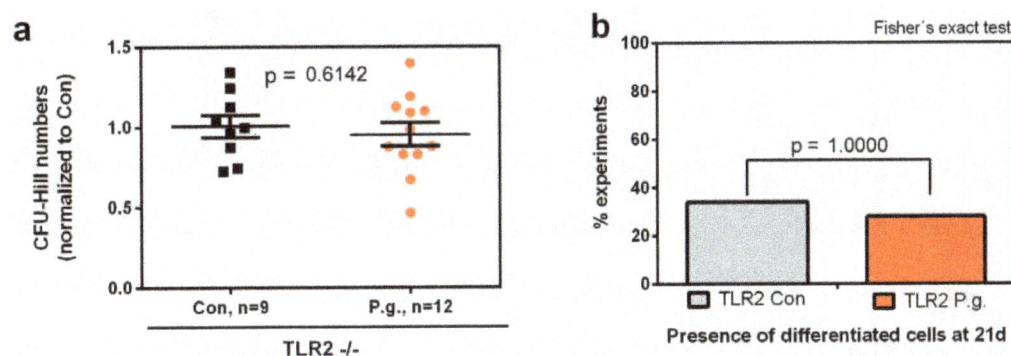

Figure 8. CFU-Hill and late-outgrowth mobilization is TLR2-dependent. No significant differences in CFU-Hill numbers (a) and the proportion of presence of differentiated late-outgrowth EPC (b) in *P. gingivalis* infected TLR2-deficient mice. Data are presented as mean colony counts ± SEM relative to controls (CFU-Hill) or as numbers of experiments yielding differentiated colonies (late EPC). Data were analyzed using unpaired t-tests (CFU-Hill) or Fishers exact test (late EPC).

activated [64], whilst in the periodontal tissues, the pathogens are in intimate contact with bone stromal cells and infiltrating mononuclear cells, such as T-cells, all of those are known to predominantly produce RANKL [65,66].

On the other hand, osteoprotegerin, but not RANKL, was recently shown to induce endothelial cell and ECFC activation and to improve microvessel formation in vitro [67,68] – therefore, it must also be considered that the observed increase of the systemic osteoprotegerin/RANKL ratio might as well constitute another counter-measure against vascular damage inflicted by the pathogen.

When judging the inferences drawn from our data, it must be, however, noted that the utilized acute model of bacteremia with a periodontal model pathogen is neither a model of atherosclerosis nor of periodontitis. It merely mimics the bacteremia known to be a feature of active periodontal disease [6,10,69,70], and allows for exact determination of the effects exerted by these bacteria on bone marrow-derived progenitor mobilization.

An oral model of periodontal infection in atherosclerosis-prone mice [54] is more likely to adequately mimic human periodontal disease and its effects on atherosclerosis progression. However, these models all rely on genetically modified mice prone to develop atherosclerosis in due course, potentially not ideal models to shed light onto the underlying pathobiology of associations found in otherwise healthy subjects suffering from periodontitis.

Subsequent studies in adequate models of chronic challenge with periodontal pathogens are necessary to evaluate whether the observed strong mobilization of endothelial progenitors from the bone marrow into the peripheral circulation induced by bacteremia with *P. gingivalis* will in fact lead to depletion of progenitor pools and subsequently reduced overall regeneration capacity. Alternatively, it is possible that the acute shortage of progenitors in the bone marrow is effectively countered by increasing osteoprotegerin/RANKL levels leading to stem cell expansion and retention, eventually resulting in increased EPC levels in peripheral blood and bone marrow nice, as found after repeated physical exercise [59].

These studies will unequivocally show whether, to what extent, and by what mechanisms endothelium-regenerating cells are involved in increased atherogenesis mediated by periodontal infections.

Taken together, we show that in an acute model of periodontal infection recurrent bacteremias lead to strong, TLR2-dependent mobilization of endothelial progenitors from the bone marrow to the circulation. In the short term, these cells improve endothelial function and reendothelization. Long-term studies in atherosclerosis models are needed to determine whether this recurrent mobilization is relevant for the reported increased atherosclerosis in periodontitis.

Acknowledgments

The authors thank Dr. Sabine Specht, Institute for Medical Microbiology, Immunology and Parasitology, University of Bonn, for the TLR2 deficient mice, and Dr. Evie Lalla, Columbia University College of Dental Medicine, New York, NY, USA for the *Porphyromonas gingivalis* strain 381. The authors acknowledge the excellent technical assistance of Kathrin Paul, Annika Bohner, Catharina Peseke, and Isabel Paez-Maletz.

Author Contributions

Conceived and designed the experiments: MK JD SJ GN NW. Performed the experiments: MK MH. Analyzed the data: MK MH NW. Wrote the paper: MK NW.

References

1. Libby P, Ridker PM, Maseri A (2002) Inflammation and atherosclerosis. Circulation 105: 1135–1143.
2. Borden WB, Davidson MH (2009) Updating the assessment of cardiac risk: beyond Framingham. Rev Cardiovasc Med 10: 63–71.
3. Darveau R (2010) Periodontitis: a polymicrobial disruption of host homeostasis. Nat Rev Microbiol 8: 481–490.

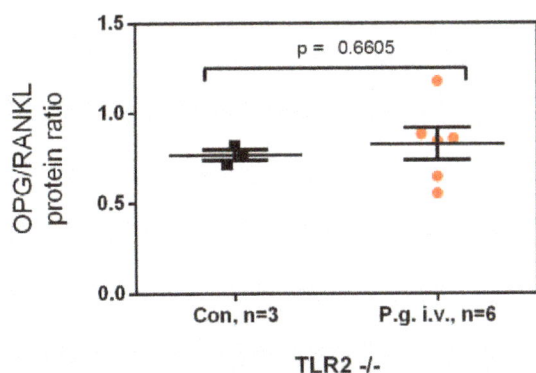

Figure 9. No differences in osteoprotegerin/RANKL ratio in the bone marrow niche of P. gingivalis infected vs. control mice deficient in TLR2. Data are given as means ± SEM, data were analyzed using an unpaired t-test.

4. Pihlstrom BL, Michalowicz BS, Johnson NW (2005) Periodontal diseases. Lancet 366: 1809–1820.

5. Dietrich T, Jimenez M, Krall Kaye EA, Vokonas PS, Garcia RI (2008) Age-dependent associations between chronic periodontitis/edentulism and risk of coronary heart disease. Circulation 117: 1668–1674.

6. Kebschull M, Demmer RT, Papapanou PN (2010) "Gum bug, leave my heart alone!"–epidemiologic and mechanistic evidence linking periodontal infections and atherosclerosis. J Dent Res 89: 879–902.

7. Lockhart PB, Bolger AF, Papapanou PN, Osinbowale O, Trevisan M, et al. (2012) Periodontal Disease and Atherosclerotic Vascular Disease: Does the Evidence Support an Independent Association?: A Scientific Statement From the American Heart Association. Circulation.

8. Hayashi C, Gudino CV, Gibson FC 3rd, Genco CA (2010) Review: Pathogen-induced inflammation at sites distant from oral infection: bacterial persistence and induction of cell-specific innate immune inflammatory pathways. Mol Oral Microbiol 25: 305–316.

9. Hujoel PP, White BA, Garcia RI, Listgarten MA (2001) The dentogingival epithelial surface area revisited. J Periodontal Res 36: 48–55.

10. Iwai T (2009) Periodontal bacteremia and various vascular diseases. J Periodontal Res 44: 689–694.

11. Hajishengallis G, Wang M, Bagby GJ, Nelson S (2008) Importance of TLR2 in early innate immune response to acute pulmonary infection with Porphyromonas gingivalis in mice. J Immunol 181: 4141–4149.

12. Liu X, Ukai T, Yumoto H, Davey M, Goswami S, et al. (2008) Toll-like receptor 2 plays a critical role in the progression of atherosclerosis that is independent of dietary lipids. Atherosclerosis 196: 146–154.

13. Madan M, Amar S (2008) Toll-like receptor-2 mediates diet and/or pathogen associated atherosclerosis: proteomic findings. PLoS One 3: e3204.

14. den Dekker WK, Cheng C, Pasterkamp G, Duckers HJ (2010) Toll like receptor 4 in atherosclerosis and plaque destabilization. Atherosclerosis 209: 314–320.

15. Michelsen KS, Wong MH, Shah PK, Zhang W, Yano J, et al. (2004) Lack of Toll-like receptor 4 or myeloid differentiation factor 88 reduces atherosclerosis and alters plaque phenotype in mice deficient in apolipoprotein E. Proc Natl Acad Sci U S A 101: 10679–10684.

16. Zimmer S, Steinmetz M, Asdonk T, Motz I, Coch C, et al. (2011) Activation of endothelial toll-like receptor 3 impairs endothelial function. Circ Res 108: 1358–1366.

17. Zhang P, Liu J, Xu Q, Harber G, Feng X, et al. (2011) TLR2-dependent modulation of osteoclastogenesis by Porphyromonas gingivalis through differential induction of NFATc1 and NF-kappaB. J Biol Chem 286: 24159–24169.

18. Burns E, Eliyahu T, Uematsu S, Akira S, Nussbaum G (2010) TLR2-dependent inflammatory response to Porphyromonas gingivalis is MyD88 independent, whereas MyD88 is required to clear infection. J Immunol 184: 1455–1462.

19. Gibson FC 3rd, Genco CA (2007) Porphyromonas gingivalis mediated periodontal disease and atherosclerosis: disparate diseases with commonalities in pathogenesis through TLRs. Curr Pharm Des 13: 3665–3675.

20. Hayashi C, Madrigal AG, Liu X, Ukai T, Goswami S, et al. (2010) Pathogen-mediated inflammatory atherosclerosis is mediated in part via Toll-like receptor 2-induced inflammatory responses. J Innate Immun 2: 334–343.

21. Rodrigues PH, Belanger M, Dunn W Jr, Progulske-Fox A (2008) Porphyromonas gingivalis and the autophagic pathway: an innate immune interaction? Front Biosci 13: 178–187.

22. Honda T, Oda T, Yoshie H, Yamazaki K (2005) Effects of Porphyromonas gingivalis antigens and proinflammatory cytokines on human coronary artery endothelial cells. Oral Microbiol Immunol 20: 82–88.

23. Sima AV, Stancu CS, Simionescu M (2009) Vascular endothelium in atherosclerosis. Cell Tissue Res 335: 191–203.

24. Amar S, Gokce N, Morgan S, Loukideli M, Van Dyke TE, et al. (2003) Periodontal disease is associated with brachial artery endothelial dysfunction and systemic inflammation. Arterioscler Thromb Vasc Biol 23: 1245–1249.

25. Mercanoglu F, Oflaz H, Oz O, Gokbuget AY, Genchellac H, et al. (2004) Endothelial dysfunction in patients with chronic periodontitis and its improvement after initial periodontal therapy. J Periodontol 75: 1694–1700.

26. Tonetti MS, D'Aiuto F, Nibali L, Donald A, Storry C, et al. (2007) Treatment of periodontitis and endothelial function. N Engl J Med 356: 911–920.

27. Kirton JP, Xu Q (2010) Endothelial precursors in vascular repair. Microvasc Res 79: 193–199.

28. Werner N, Wassmann S, Ahlers P, Schiegl T, Kosiol S, et al. (2007) Endothelial progenitor cells correlate with endothelial function in patients with coronary artery disease. Basic Res Cardiol 102: 565–571.

29. Werner N, Kosiol S, Schiegl T, Ahlers P, Walenta K, et al. (2005) Circulating endothelial progenitor cells and cardiovascular outcomes. N Engl J Med 353: 999–1007.

30. Roth GA, Ankersmit HJ, Brown VB, Papapanou PN, Schmidt AM, et al. (2007) Porphyromonas gingivalis infection and cell death in human aortic endothelial cells. FEMS Microbiol Lett 272: 106–113.

31. Werner N, Nickenig G (2006) Clinical and therapeutical implications of EPC biology in atherosclerosis. J Cell Mol Med 10: 318–332.

32. Li X, Tse HF, Yiu KH, Jia N, Chen H, et al. (2009) Increased levels of circulating endothelial progenitor cells in subjects with moderate to severe chronic periodontitis. J Clin Periodontol 36: 933–939.

33. Li X, Tse HF, Yiu KH, Li LS, Jin L (2011) Effect of periodontal treatment on circulating CD34(+) cells and peripheral vascular endothelial function: a randomized controlled trial. J Clin Periodontol 38: 148–156.

34. Pollreisz A, Huang Y, Roth GA, Cheng B, Kebschull M, et al. (2010) Enhanced monocyte migration and pro-inflammatory cytokine production by Porphyromonas gingivalis infection. J Periodontal Res 45: 239–245.

35. Ito H, Rovira, II, Bloom ML, Takeda K, Ferrans VJ, et al. (1999) Endothelial progenitor cells as putative targets for angiostatin. Cancer Res 59: 5875–5877.

36. Hill JM, Zalos G, Halcox JP, Schenke WH, Waclawiw MA, et al. (2003) Circulating endothelial progenitor cells, vascular function, and cardiovascular risk. N Engl J Med 348: 593–600.

37. Ingram DA, Mead LE, Tanaka H, Meade V, Fenoglio A, et al. (2004) Identification of a novel hierarchy of endothelial progenitor cells using human peripheral and umbilical cord blood. Blood 104: 2752–2760.

38. Yoder MC, Mead LE, Prater D, Krier TR, Mroueh KN, et al. (2007) Redefining endothelial progenitor cells via clonal analysis and hematopoietic stem/progenitor cell principals. Blood 109: 1801–1809.

39. Steinmetz M, Nickenig G, Werner N (2010) Endothelial-regenerating cells: an expanding universe. Hypertension 55: 593–599.

40. Wassmann S, Werner N, Czech T, Nickenig G (2006) Improvement of endothelial function by systemic transfusion of vascular progenitor cells. Circ Res 99: e74–83.

41. Brouchet L, Krust A, Dupont S, Chambon P, Bayard F, et al. (2001) Estradiol accelerates reendothelialization in mouse carotid artery through estrogen receptor-alpha but not estrogen receptor-beta. Circulation 103: 423–428.

42. Medina RJ, O'Neill CL, Sweeney M, Guduric-Fuchs J, Gardiner TA, et al. (2010) Molecular analysis of endothelial progenitor cell (EPC) subtypes reveals two distinct cell populations with different identities. BMC Med Genomics 3: 18.

43. Jodon de Villeroche V, Avouac J, Ponceau A, Ruiz B, Kahan A, et al. (2010) Enhanced late-outgrowth circulating endothelial progenitor cell levels in rheumatoid arthritis and correlation with disease activity. Arthritis Res Ther 12: R27.

44. Massa M, Rosti V, Ferrario M, Campanelli R, Ramajoli I, et al. (2005) Increased circulating hematopoietic and endothelial progenitor cells in the early phase of acute myocardial infarction. Blood 105: 199–206.

45. Leone AM, Rutella S, Bonanno G, Abbate A, Rebuzzi AG, et al. (2005) Mobilization of bone marrow-derived stem cells after myocardial infarction and left ventricular function. Eur Heart J 26: 1196–1204.

46. Wojakowski W, Tendera M, Michalowska A, Majka M, Kucia M, et al. (2004) Mobilization of CD34/CXCR4+, CD34/CD117+, c-met+ stem cells, and mononuclear cells expressing early cardiac, muscle, and endothelial markers into peripheral blood in patients with acute myocardial infarction. Circulation 110: 3213–3220.

47. Brehm M, Ebner P, Picard F, Urbien R, Turan G, et al. (2009) Enhanced mobilization of CD34(+) progenitor cells expressing cell adhesion molecules in patients with STEMI. Clin Res Cardiol 98: 477–486.

48. Banerjee S, Brilakis E, Zhang S, Roesle M, Lindsey J, et al. (2006) Endothelial progenitor cell mobilization after percutaneous coronary intervention. Atherosclerosis 189: 70–75.

49. Goussetis E, Spiropoulos A, Tsironi M, Skenderi K, Margeli A, et al. (2009) Spartathlon, a 246 kilometer foot race: effects of acute inflammation induced by prolonged exercise on circulating progenitor reparative cells. Blood Cells Mol Dis 42: 294–299.

50. Hajishengallis G (2009) Toll gates to periodontal host modulation and vaccine therapy. Periodontol 2000 51: 181–207.

51. Cole JE, Mitra AT, Monaco C (2010) Treating atherosclerosis: the potential of Toll-like receptors as therapeutic targets. Expert Rev Cardiovasc Ther 8: 1619–1635.

52. Padfield GJ, Tura O, Haeck ML, Short A, Freyer E, et al. (2010) Circulating endothelial progenitor cells are not affected by acute systemic inflammation. Am J Physiol Heart Circ Physiol 298: H2054–2061.

53. Sommers MS (2003) The cellular basis of septic shock. Crit Care Nurs Clin North Am 15: 13–25.

54. Lalla E, Lamster IB, Hofmann MA, Bucciarelli L, Jerud AP, et al. (2003) Oral infection with a periodontal pathogen accelerates early atherosclerosis in apolipoprotein E-null mice. Arterioscler Thromb Vasc Biol 23: 1405–1411.

55. Calvi LM, Adams GB, Weibrecht KW, Weber JM, Olson DP, et al. (2003) Osteoblastic cells regulate the haematopoietic stem cell niche. Nature 425: 841–846.

56. Venuraju SM, Yerramasu A, Corder R, Lahiri A (2010) Osteoprotegerin as a predictor of coronary artery disease and cardiovascular mortality and morbidity. J Am Coll Cardiol 55: 2049–2061.

57. D'Amelio P, Isaia G, Isaia GC (2009) The osteoprotegerin/RANK/RANKL system: a bone key to vascular disease. J Endocrinol Invest 32: 6–9.

58. Ehninger A, Trumpp A (2011) The bone marrow stem cell niche grows up: mesenchymal stem cells and macrophages move in. The Journal of Experimental Medicine 208: 421–428.

59. Laufs U, Werner N, Link A, Endres M, Wassmann S, et al. (2004) Physical training increases endothelial progenitor cells, inhibits neointima formation, and enhances angiogenesis. Circulation 109: 220–226.

60. Secchiero P, Corallini F, Rimondi E, Chiaruttini C, di Iasio MG, et al. (2008) Activation of the p53 pathway down-regulates the osteoprotegerin expression and release by vascular endothelial cells. Blood 111: 1287–1294.

61. Lu HK, Yeh KC, Wu MF, Li CL, Tseng CC (2008) An acute injection of Porphyromonas gingivalis lipopolysaccharide modulates the OPG/RANKL system and interleukin-6 in an ovariectomized mouse model. Oral Microbiol Immunol 23: 220–225.

62. Graves D (2008) Cytokines that promote periodontal tissue destruction. J Periodontol 79: 1585–1591.
63. Taubman MA, Valverde P, Han X, Kawai T (2005) Immune response: the key to bone resorption in periodontal disease. J Periodontol 76: 2033–2041.
64. Zhang J, Fu M, Myles D, Zhu X, Du J, et al. (2002) PDGF induces osteoprotegerin expression in vascular smooth muscle cells by multiple signal pathways. FEBS Lett 521: 180–184.
65. Belibasakis GN, Reddi D, Bostanci N (2010) Porphyromonas gingivalis Induces RANKL in T-cells. Inflammation.
66. Reddi D, Bostanci N, Hashim A, Aduse-Opoku J, Curtis MA, et al. (2008) Porphyromonas gingivalis regulates the RANKL-OPG system in bone marrow stromal cells. Microbes Infect 10: 1459–1468.
67. Benslimane-Ahmim Z, Heymann D, Dizier B, Lokajczyk A, Brion R, et al. (2011) Osteoprotegerin, a new actor in vasculogenesis, stimulates endothelial colony-forming cells properties. J Thromb Haemost.
68. McGonigle JS, Giachelli CM, Scatena M (2009) Osteoprotegerin and RANKL differentially regulate angiogenesis and endothelial cell function. Angiogenesis 12: 35–46.
69. Kinane DF, Riggio MP, Walker KF, MacKenzie D, Shearer B (2005) Bacteraemia following periodontal procedures. J Clin Periodontol 32: 708–713.
70. Lockhart PB, Brennan MT, Sasser HC, Fox PC, Paster BJ, et al. (2008) Bacteremia associated with toothbrushing and dental extraction. Circulation 117: 3118–3125.

3

Comparing the Bacterial Diversity of Acute and Chronic Dental Root Canal Infections

Adriana L. Santos[1], **José F. Siqueira Jr.**[2]*, **Isabela N. Rôças**[2], **Ederson C. Jesus**[4], **Alexandre S. Rosado**[1], **James M. Tiedje**[3]

1 Institute of Microbiology Prof. Paulo de Góes, Federal University of Rio de Janeiro, Rio de Janeiro, Brazil, 2 Department of Endodontics and Molecular Microbiology Laboratory, Estácio de Sá University, Rio de Janeiro, Brazil, 3 Center for Microbial Ecology, Michigan State University, East Lansing, Michigan, United States of America, 4 Laboratory of Soil Microbiology, EMBRAPA, Seropédica, Brazil

Abstract

This study performed barcoded multiplex pyrosequencing with a 454 FLX instrument to compare the microbiota of dental root canal infections associated with acute (symptomatic) or chronic (asymptomatic) apical periodontitis. Analysis of samples from 9 acute abscesses and 8 chronic infections yielded partial 16S rRNA gene sequences that were taxonomically classified into 916 bacterial species-level operational taxonomic units (OTUs) (at 3% divergence) belonging to 67 genera and 13 phyla. The most abundant phyla in acute infections were *Firmicutes* (52%), *Fusobacteria* (17%) and *Bacteroidetes* (13%), while in chronic infections the dominant were *Firmicutes* (59%), *Bacteroidetes* (14%) and *Actinobacteria* (10%). Members of *Fusobacteria* were much more prevalent in acute (89%) than in chronic cases (50%). The most abundant/prevalent genera in acute infections were *Fusobacterium* and *Parvimonas*. Twenty genera were exclusively detected in acute infections and 18 in chronic infections. Only 18% (n = 165) of the OTUs at 3% divergence were shared by acute and chronic infections. Diversity and richness estimators revealed that acute infections were significantly more diverse than chronic infections. Although a high interindividual variation in bacterial communities was observed, many samples tended to group together according to the type of infection (acute or chronic). This study is one of the most comprehensive in-deep comparisons of the microbiota associated with acute and chronic dental root canal infections and highlights the role of diverse polymicrobial communities as the unit of pathogenicity in acute infections. The overall diversity of endodontic infections as revealed by the pyrosequencing technique was much higher than previously reported for endodontic infections.

Editor: Jack Anthony Gilbert, Argonne National Laboratory, United States of America

Funding: This study was supported by grants from Conselho Nacional de Desenvolvimento Científico e Tecnológico (CNPq), and Fundação Carlos Chagas Filho de Amparo à Pesquisa do Estado do Rio de Janeiro (FAPERJ), Brazilian Governmental Institutions. The funders had no role in study design, data collection and analysis, decision to publish, or preparation of the manuscript.

Competing Interests: The authors have declared that no competing interests exist.

* E-mail: jf_siqueira@yahoo.com

Introduction

Apical periodontitis is a common bacterial biofilm-induced disease that develops around the apex of the dental root and is caused primarily by root canal (endodontic) infection [1]. The disease can manifest itself as different clinical presentations. The asymptomatic (chronic) form is more common and seldom poses a medical problem of significant magnitude, even though evidence is mounting that it contributes to the total oral infectious burden and thus may influence systemic health [2]. Moreover, the typical symptomatic form - the acute apical abscess - can spread from the original site of infection to sinuses and other facial spaces of head and neck and cause serious life-threatening complications [3].

Apical periodontitis has a heterogeneous etiology, where no single species can be considered as the main endodontic pathogen and multiple bacterial combinations play a role in disease causation [4]. Thus far, no strong evidence of the specific involvement of a single species with any particular sign or symptom of apical periodontitis has been found. While some Gram-negative anaerobic bacteria have been suggested to be involved in symptomatic disease [5,6,7], the same species are also present in somewhat similar frequencies in asymptomatic cases [8,9,10]. Nevertheless, community profiling molecular studies have suggested that the structure of bacterial communities follows specific patterns according to the clinical condition [11,12]. This suggests that some bacterial community structures may predispose to acute infections instead of the presence of a specific group of species. However, these studies were based on cloning and Sanger sequencing [12], denaturing gradient gel electrophoresis [11] and terminal restriction fragment length polymorphism [12] approaches, all of which are recognized to have the limitation of revealing only the most dominant community members.

Massively parallel DNA pyrosequencing techniques have become widely available over the last years and is now regarded as one of the leading sequencing technologies for 16S rRNA-based bacterial diversity analyses [13]. The technology provides a large number of reads in a single run, resulting in unprecedented greater sampling depth. This allows for detection not only of the dominant community members, but also of the low-abundant microbial populations, the so called "rare biosphere" [13,14].

Numerous recent studies have used pyrosequencing of 16S rRNA gene to profile the diversity of bacterial communities from diverse environments, including hydrothermal vents of a deep marine biosphere [14,15] and soil [16,17]. This technology has also been applied to the analysis of the human microbiota associated with healthy or diseased sites [18,19,20,21,22], including the oral cavity [23,24,25,26]. These studies disclosed a much larger breadth of bacterial diversity than previously anticipated. So far, only a couple of studies have used this technology to investigate dental root canal infections [27,28]. However, one was an early study reporting on the ability of the method to unravel the microbiota of 7 infected cases exhibiting different clinical presentations [27], while the other investigated the apical root canal microbiota of teeth with chronic apical periodontitis [28].

Deciphering the composition of the microbiota associated with any infectious disease is of utmost important for a better understanding of the disease pathogenesis and for the establishment of more effective therapeutic protocols. Therefore, the present study was undertaken to evaluate and compare the bacterial diversity of the microbiota associated with acute (abscesses) and chronic dental root canal infections by using a high-throughput multiplexed 16S rRNA gene barcoded pyrosequencing approach.

Results

Of the pyrosequencing reads that passed the quality control, 13,905 were from acute root canal infections and 13,552 from chronic infections. The average length of the sequences was about 210 bp after trimming the primers.

Overall, 13 phyla were represented in endodontic infections (Figure 1). Of the major phyla, *Firmicutes* (52%), *Fusobacteria* (17%) and *Bacteroidetes* (13%) were the most abundant in acute infections, while *Firmicutes* (59%), *Bacteroidetes* (14%) and *Actinobacteria* (10%) were the most abundant in chronic infections (Figure 1). Five of the detected phyla, namely *Firmicutes*, *Bacteroidetes*, *Fusobacteria*, *Actinobacteria* and *Proteobacteria*, collectively constituted more than 90% of the microbiome. Except for *Spirochaetes* (2.6%), each of the other phyla corresponded to less than 1% of the sequences. About 2% of the sequences could not be assigned to any bacterial phylum. In terms of prevalence, members of *Firmicutes* were found in all cases. *Fusobacteria* were much more prevalent in acute (8/9, 89%) than in chronic cases (4/8, 50%). *Bacteroidetes* occurred in 7/9 (78%) acute and 7/8 (87.5%) chronic cases, while representatives of *Actinobacteria* were present in 7/9 (78%) acute and 5/8 (62.5%) chronic cases.

Overall, sequences were assigned to 67 different genera. Of these, acute and chronic infections were represented by 49 and 47 genera, respectively. The most abundant genera in acute cases were *Fusobacterium* (19%), *Parvimonas* (11%) and *Peptostreptococcus* (10%). *Fusobacterium* was also the most prevalent (8/9, 89%), followed by *Parvimonas*, *Dialister* and *Atopium* (all detected in 7/9 cases, 78%). Twenty genera were exclusively detected in acute infections, all of them in both low abundance and prevalence. Eleven genera were found in more than 50% of the acute cases (Figure 2).

The most abundant genera in chronic cases were *Phocaeicola* (12.5%), *Eubacterium* (12%) and *Pseudoramibacter* (10%). *Eubacterium* and *Mogibacterium* were the most prevalent (both in 6/8, 75%), followed by *Pseudoramibacter* (5/8, 62.5%) and *Phocaeicola* (4/8, 50%). Eighteen genera were found exclusively in chronic infections, all of them in both low abundance and prevalence. Only 5 genera were found in more than 50% of the chronic cases (Figure 2). About 3% of the sequences could not be classified at the genus level and were placed at the next highest possible resolution level.

For OTUs at 3% distance (species level), 916 different phylotypes were detected. Of these, 651 phylotypes were found in acute cases and 430 in chronic cases. The percentage of species-level taxa shared in acute and chronic groups was 18% (165 species) (Figure 3). The mean number of OTUs at the 3% dissimilarity level present per acute case was 114 (range, 56 to 225) compared to 71 OTUs (range, 42 to 104) in chronic cases. Data regarding shared genera are available as supporting information (Figure S1). Table 1 depicts data from diversity and richness estimate calculations. Calculation of Shannon estimator of diversity at 3% difference revealed that acute infections were significantly more diverse than chronic infections, with no overlap of the 95% CIs. Using the ACE nonparametric estimator of richness, it was possible to observe that there are a predicted 1,466 species-level OTUs in the acute cases and 1,031 in the chronic cases. Based upon Chao1, there is an average of 1,090 and 857 species-level OTUs in acute and chronic infections, respectively. The shapes of the rarefaction curves confirmed that acute infections are more diverse than chronic infections (Figure S2). Rarefaction curves also indicated that bacterial richness in acute and chronic infections is not yet completely revealed by the number of sequences analyzed. Although a high interindividual variation in bacterial communities was revealed by PcoA and cluster analyses, there was a trend for many samples to group together according to the type of infection (acute or chronic) (Figure 4).

Discussion

The present findings indicate that there is a significantly higher diversity of bacteria in acute dental infections (abscesses) when compared to asymptomatic chronic infections. This significantly increased diversity may be an important aspect of acute infections and the possibility exists that the microbiota present in these cases may contain harmful bacterial species contributing to the severity of symptoms. Also, as a highly diverse polymicrobial infection, incalculable synergistic interactions between multiple bacterial species are expected and can result in increased pathogenicity. Therefore, the ability of the community to cause disease is very likely to be related to collective pathogenicity and is coherent with the current trend to categorize the bacterial community as the unit of pathogenicity for many endogenous diseases [29,30,31].

A recurrent theme in endodontic microbiology research is the desire to find the major pathogen responsible for acute disease. This study failed to disclose a single specific taxon associated with acute infections. Actually, many bacterial taxa were either exclusive or much more prevalent/abundant in acute infections than in chronic cases. Most of these taxa were rather in low abundance and may have passed unnoticed in previous culture and molecular studies. The present results suggest that the composition of the bacterial community can be much more important to the development of acute symptoms than the mere presence of a potentially pathogenic species. It is also possible to speculate that those species found in higher prevalences or exclusively in acute cases play a decisive ecological role in determining the virulence of the consortium. Because none of these taxa were found in all cases, the possibility of functional redundancy in the pathogenic community is suspected.

Previous studies comparing acute and chronic infections have suggested that some species are more related to acute symptoms [5,6,7,32], more species are found per individual acute case than per chronic case [11,12], and some community profiles are more related to disease severity [11,12]. Most of these findings were also evident and expanded in the present study using deep-coverage

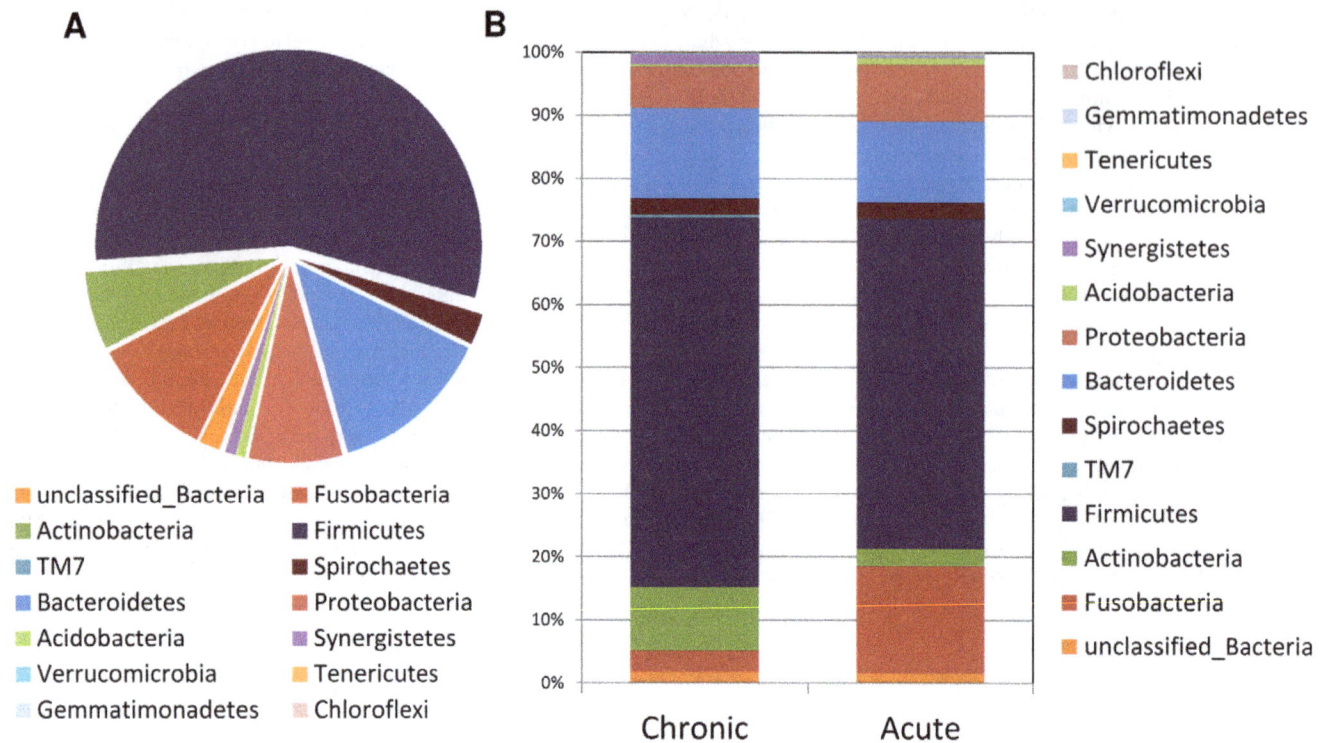

Figure 1. Relative abundance of the different bacterial phyla in acute and chronic dental root canal infections. *A,* overall data. *B,* data according to the clinical condition. Phylogenetic classification was based on Ribosomal Database Project Classifier analyses.

pyrosequencing. Taken together, these data reveal that acute infections have a more complex microbiota and interactions between the numerous community members may be critical for the development of symptoms.

A marked interindividual variability in the composition of the bacterial communities was observed. Each individual harbored a unique endodontic microbiota in terms of species richness and abundance. This is in agreement with previous molecular studies using community profiling techniques [11,33,34]. The fact that the composition of the microbiota differs consistently between individuals suffering from the same disease denotes a heterogeneous etiology for apical periodontitis, where multiple communities can lead to similar disease outcomes. Despite this interindividual variability, most samples showed a tendency to group together according to the presence of symptoms. This suggests that there may exist some patterns of community structures related to distinct clinical conditions.

Our overall findings revealed 67 genera belonging to 13 phyla in primary endodontic infections. A recent comprehensive compilation of findings from previous culture and molecular studies demonstrated that more than 460 bacterial species/phylotypes belonging to 100 genera and 9 phyla have been detected in the different types of endodontic infections [35]. The present findings strongly indicate that these numbers may have been grossly underestimated. Application of barcoded parallel pyrosequencing to the study of endodontic infections provided a view of the bacterial diversity associated with apical periodontitis at a much deeper level. This is in consonance with an early study of root canal infections using pyrosequencing [27]. Nonetheless, irrespective of the depth of analysis, true diversity was still greater than that identified in this study, as revealed by diversity and richness estimators and rarefaction curves.

Of the 13 phyla represented in this study, *Verrucomicrobia* and *Gemmatimonadetes* had not been previously reported in endodontic infections. Of the major phyla, *Firmicutes* and *Bacteroidetes* were the most abundant and prevalent, which is in agreement with previous studies using culture methods or cloning and Sanger sequencing [12,36,37]. Noteworthy was the fact that members of the *Fusobacteria* phylum were much more adundant and prevalent in acute than in chronic infections. A species of this phylum – *Fusobacterium nucleatum* – has been frequently identified in acute endodontic infections [7,38,39,40].

The vast majority of the species-level phylotypes occurred at very low levels. This confirms the great potential of pyrosequencing analysis to reveal the rare biosphere. At this stage, it is not possible to infer a role for these bacteria in the community. However, it is widely recognized in microbial ecology that even low-abundant members might serve as keystone species within complex communities [41,42]. Low-abundant members may hold the potential to become dominant in response to shifts in environmental conditions [41]. Finally, a consistent understanding of the ecology and pathogenicity of a microbial community requires the thorough knowledge of every component involved, including identification of species present at low levels in the environment [29].

It has been shown that factors such as the number of sequences analyzed and the sample size can influence the species richness and the overall diversity [43,44]. Therefore, one must assume that microbial community analyses based on the traditional cloning and Sanger sequencing are limited to identification of the most abundant taxa in a sample. The greatest advantage of the pyrosequencing approach over the traditional cloning and sequencing method is that a much larger number of 16S rRNA sequence reads can be obtained in a single run, providing a huge

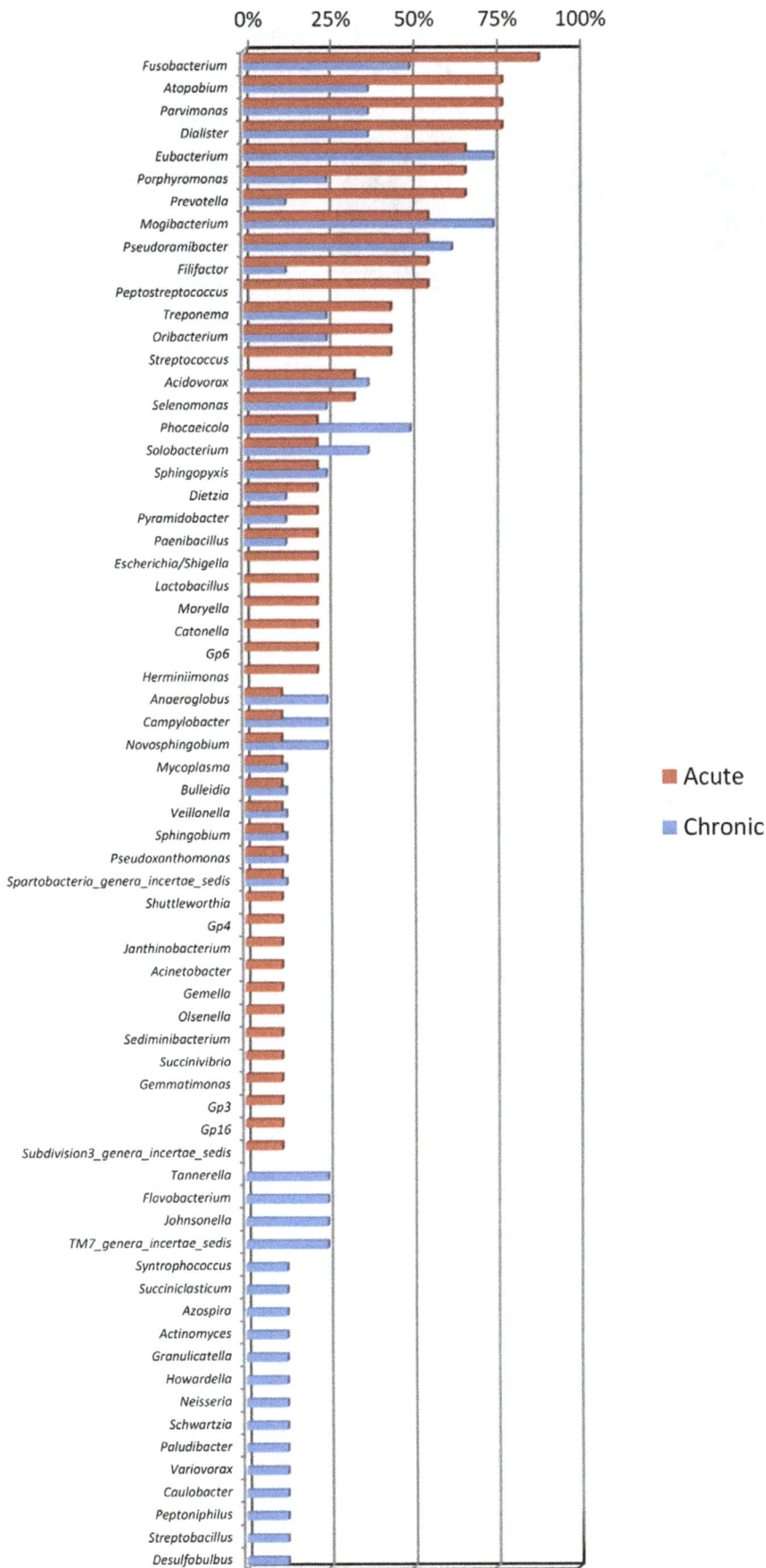

Figure 2. Prevalence of the different genera detected in samples from acute and chronic dental infections.

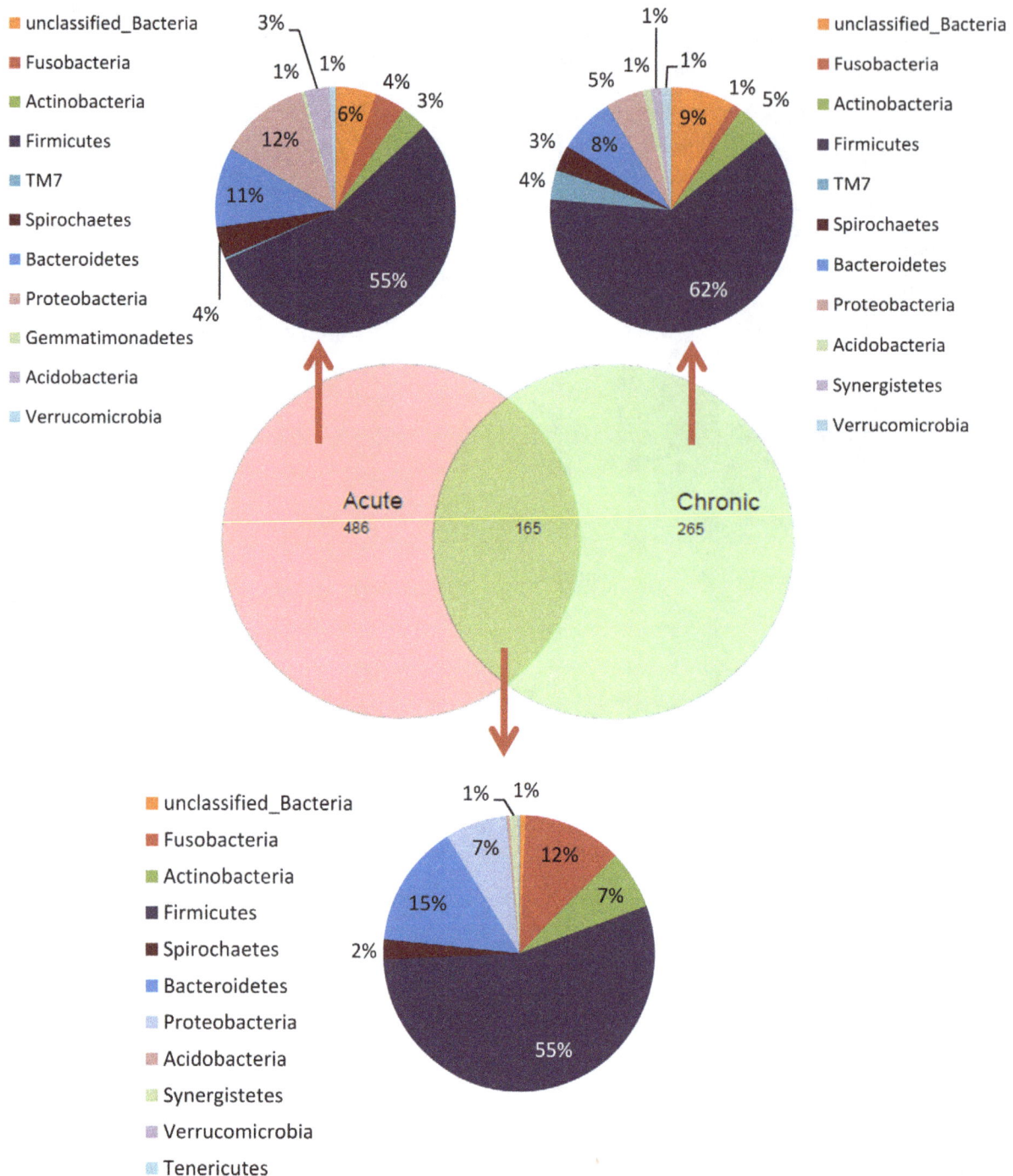

Figure 3. Venn diagram for overlap between observed OTUs at 3% divergence in acute and chronic dental root canal infections. The number of OTUs exclusively found in acute samples was 486 and in chronic samples was 265. The number of OTUs shared between acute and chronic infections was 165. Percentage of shared OTUs was 18%. Data are also represented by the phyla which the detected OTUs belong to. Data regarding genera are shown as supplementary material.

coverage depth. Moreover, the pyrosequencing approach also avoids the biases inherent to the cloning procedure. Nevertheless, the short length of reads generated by this high-throughput technology may represent a limitation in terms of bacterial taxonomy characterization. Even so, it has been shown that reads spanning particular variable regions of the 16S rRNA gene can still be highly informative and that despite the shorter read lengths, the pyrosequencing approach provides a description of the

microbiome that is in good agreement with that provided by the cloning and Sanger sequencing approach [25,45]. In order to avoid overestimates when analyzing short sequence reads, we abided by the recommendations of Kunin et al. [13], who recommended a stringent quality-based trimming of the reads and a cut-off value for identification no greater than 97%. However, about 2% of bacterial taxa were unclassified, which can be considered as high at the phylum level. The possibility exists that

Table 1. Sequencing data and diversity estimate calculations for bacterial taxa in acute and chronic dental root canal infections.

	Acute	Chronic
Total number of sequences	13,905	13,552
Total OTUs at 3% difference (phylotypes)	676	443
Total OTUs at 5% difference (phylotypes)	555	352
Shannon estimator at 3% difference (95% CI)	4.12 (4.09; 4.15)	3.95 (3.92; 3.97)
Shannon estimator at 5% difference (95% CI)	3.86 (3.83; 3.89)	3.85 (3.83; 3.88)
Chao1 estimator of richness at 3% (95% CI)	1,090 (972; 1,250)	857 (712; 1,072)
Chao1 estimator of richness at 5% (95% CI)	922 (819; 1,065)	668 (554; 844)
ACE estimator of richness at 3% (95% CI)	1,466 (1,342; 1,612)	1,031 (921; 1,165)
ACE estimator of richness at 5% (95% CI)	1,184 (1,081; 1,308)	800 (710; 913)
ESC [Cx =1 - (Nx/n); Nx =unique sequences/n = total sequences]	0,62	0,65

this may be probably not due to unknown bacterial phyla, but to sequencing errors, short sequencing reads or PCR artifacts.

In conclusion, our findings using the massive parallel pyrosequencing analysis of dental root canal samples revealed that the bacterial diversity associated with acute infections is higher than chronic infections. It is also reasonable to conclude that the severity of disease (intensity of signs and symptoms) may be related to the bacterial community composition. This means that the disease outcome is a result of a summation of attributes of a pathogenic community. Further studies evaluating the activity and pathogenic potential of the endodontic bacterial communities should be encouraged using methods such as proteomics, transcriptomics and metabolomics. The overall diversity of endodontic infections as revealed by the pyrosequencing technique was much higher than previously anticipated.

Materials and Methods

Case description, sample taking and DNA extraction

The study protocol was approved by the Ethics Committee of the Estácio de Sá University, Rio de Janeiro, and written informed consent was obtained from the patients. Samples were taken from 17 patients who had been referred for root canal treatment or emergency treatment to the Department of Endodontics, Estácio de Sá University. Only single-rooted teeth from adult patients (ages ranging from 18 to 62 years), all of them having carious lesions, necrotic pulps and radiographic evidence of apical periodontitis (bone destruction around the dental root apex), were included in the study. Selected teeth showed an absence of periodontal pockets deeper than 4 mm. Eight asymptomatic cases were diagnosed as chronic apical periodontitis and nine cases were diagnosed as acute apical abscesses. Diagnosis of acute apical abscess was based on the presence of spontaneous pain, exacerbated by mastication, and localized or diffuse swelling, along with fever, lymphadenopathy, or malaise.

In cases of chronic apical periodontitis, samples were obtained from the root canals under strict aseptic conditions, which included rubber dam isolation and a two-step disinfection protocol of the operative field with 2.5% NaOCl as previously described [11]. Endodontic files with the handle cut off and paper points used for sampling the root canals were transferred to cryotubes containing TE buffer (10 mM Tris-HCl, 1 mM EDTA, pH 7.6) and immediately frozen at −20°C. Abscesses were sampled by aspiration of the purulent exudate from the swollen mucosa over

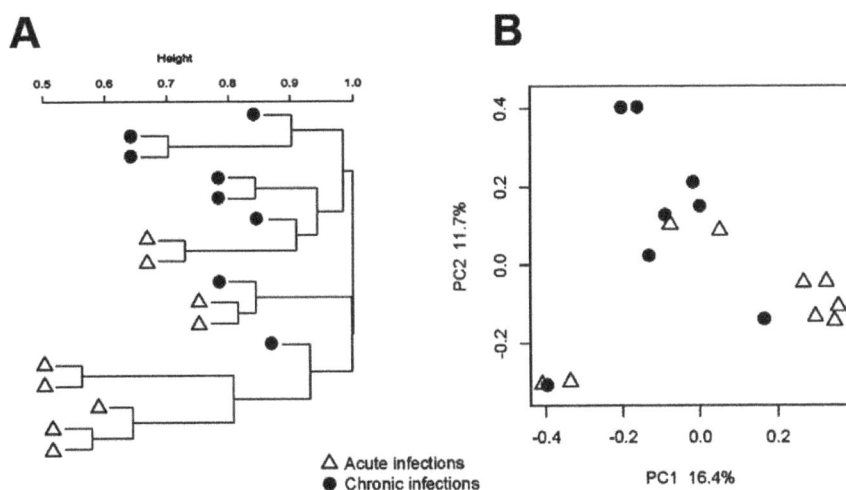

Figure 4. Cluster (A) and PCoA (B) analyses of acute (symptomatic) and chronic (asymptomatic) dental root canal infections.
Although a high interindividual variability can be observed, some samples tended to group together according to the type of infection.

each abscess. The overlying mucosa was disinfected with 2% chlorhexidine solution, and a sterile disposable syringe was used to aspirate pus, which was immediately injected into cryotubes containing TE buffer and frozen at $-20°C$. DNA was extracted from clinical samples using the QIAamp DNA Mini Kit (Qiagen, Valencia, CA) according to the manufacturer's instructions. To maximize DNA extraction from Gram-positive bacteria, a step of pre-incubation with lysozyme for 30 min was added.

Pyrosequencing

Partial 16S rRNA gene sequences were amplified from clinical samples using the barcoded-primer approach to multiplex pyrosequencing. Polymerase chain reaction (PCR) amplification of the V4 region of the 16S rRNA gene was performed using 8-bp barcoded degenerate eubacterial primers 563F and 802R (http:// pyro.cme.msu.edu/pyro/help.jsp). PCR mixtures were as described elsewhere [17]. Equimolar amplicon suspensions were combined and subjected to pyrosequencing using a Genome Sequencer FLX system (454 Life Sciences, Branford, CT) at the Michigan State University Genomics Technology Support Facility.

Sequence processing and statistical analysis

Raw sequences were processed through the Ribosomal Database Project (RDP) pyrosequencing pipeline (http://wild-pigeon.cme.msu.edu/pyro/index.jsp). Sequences were excluded from the analysis if the read length was less than 150 bp, if the minimum average exponential quality score was lower than 20 (Average Qscore of 20 for 16S sequences) or if the primer sequences contained errors (about 13%). Qualified sequences were clustered into operational taxonomic units (OTUs) defined by a 3% distance level using complete-linkage clustering and these were assigned to phyla using the RDP-II classifier at a 50% confidence threshold [46]. The sequences obtained in this study were uploaded and are availableat the Sequence Read Archive (SRA) at URLhttp://www.ebi.ac.uk/ena/data/view/ERP000669. Sequences that could not be classified into a phylum at this level of confidence were excluded from subsequent phylum composition analyses.

A total of 27,457 partial 16S rRNA sequences were obtained from the clinical samples. Phylum composition was determined by taxonomic assignment performed by Classifier [46] with default parameters via the RDP II web site. Multiple sequence alignments for each sample were performed with Infernal Aligner (with the default parameters) via RDP II web site [47]. Based on the alignment, a distance matrix was constructed by the Mothur v 1.17.3 package [48] with the default parameters using the Jukes-Cantor model option [49]. These pairwise distances served as inputs for clustering the sequences into OTUs. The clusters were made at a 3% dissimilarity cut off and served as OTUs for generating predictive rarefaction models and for making calculations of the richness indices Ace and Chao1 [50] and Shannon's diversity index [51]. These analyses were made using Mothur v 1.17.3 package [48]. A 3% distance-level OTU matrix was used to calculate a distance matrix with the Bray-Curtis distance. This matrix was submitted to clustering and principal coordinates analysis (PCoA) according to Kindt and Coe [52]. The algorithm used for clustering was the complete linkage algorithm. These analyses were performed with the package vegan [53] for program R (http://www.R-project.org/).

Supporting Information

Figure S1 Venn diagram for overlap between observed OTUs at the genus level in acute and chronic dental root canal infections.

Figure S2 Rarefaction curves used to estimate richness of acute and chronic dental root canal infections. The vertical axis shows the number of OTUs at 3% and 5% divergence expected to be disclosed after sampling the number of sequences shown on the horizontal axis.

Author Contributions

Conceived and designed the experiments: ALS JFSJ INR. Performed the experiments: ALS INR. Analyzed the data: ALS JFSJ ECJ. Contributed reagents/materials/analysis tools: JFSJ INR ASR JMT. Wrote the paper: ALS JFSJ. Obtained biospecimens: INR.

References

1. Siqueira JF, Jr. (2011) Treatment of endodontic infections. London: Quintessence Publishing.
2. Caplan DJ, Chasen JB, Krall EA, Cai J, Kang S, et al. (2006) Lesions of endodontic origin and risk of coronary heart disease. J Dent Res 85: 996–1000.
3. Robertson D, Smith AJ (2009) The microbiology of the acute dental abscess. J Med Microbiol 58: 155–162.
4. Siqueira JF, Jr. (2002) Endodontic infections: concepts, paradigms, and perspectives. Oral Surg Oral Med Oral Pathol Oral Radiol Endod 94: 281–293.
5. Sundqvist G (1976) Bacteriological studies of necrotic dental pulps [Odontological Dissertation no.7]. Umea, Sweden: University of Umea.
6. Gomes BP, Lilley JD, Drucker DB (1996) Clinical significance of dental root canal microflora. J Dent 24: 47–55.
7. Siqueira JF, Jr., Rôças IN (2009) The microbiota of acute apical abscesses. J Dent Res 88: 61–65.
8. Baumgartner JC, Watkins BJ, Bae KS, Xia T (1999) Association of black-pigmented bacteria with endodontic infections. J Endod 25: 413–415.
9. Siqueira JF, Jr., Rôças IN, Souto R, de Uzeda M, Colombo AP (2000) Checkerboard DNA-DNA hybridization analysis of endodontic infections. Oral Surg Oral Med Oral Pathol Oral Radiol Endod 89: 744–748.
10. Rôças IN, Siqueira JF, Jr. (2008) Root canal microbiota of teeth with chronic apical periodontitis. J Clin Microbiol 46: 3599–3606.
11. Siqueira JF, Jr., Rôças IN, Rosado AS (2004) Investigation of bacterial communities associated with asymptomatic and symptomatic endodontic infections by denaturing gradient gel electrophoresis fingerprinting approach. Oral Microbiol Immunol 19: 363–370.
12. Sakamoto M, Rôças IN, Siqueira JF, Jr., Benno Y (2006) Molecular analysis of bacteria in asymptomatic and symptomatic endodontic infections. Oral Microbiol Immunol 21: 112–122.
13. Kunin V, Engelbrektson A, Ochman H, Hugenholtz P (2010) Wrinkles in the rare biosphere: pyrosequencing errors can lead to artificial inflation of diversity estimates. Environ Microbiol 12: 118–123.
14. Sogin ML, Morrison HG, Huber JA, Mark Welch D, Huse SM, et al. (2006) Microbial diversity in the deep sea and the underexplored "rare biosphere". Proc Natl Acad Sci U S A 103: 12115–12120.
15. Huber JA, Mark Welch DB, Morrison HG, Huse SM, Neal PR, et al. (2007) Microbial population structures in the deep marine biosphere. Science 318: 97–100.
16. Roesch LF, Fulthorpe RR, Riva A, Casella G, Hadwin AK, et al. (2007) Pyrosequencing enumerates and contrasts soil microbial diversity. ISME J 1: 283–290.
17. Teixeira LC, Peixoto RS, Cury JC, Sul WJ, Pellizari VH, et al. (2010) Bacterial diversity in rhizosphere soil from Antarctic vascular plants of Admiralty Bay, maritime Antarctica. ISME J 4: 989–1001.
18. Koren O, Spor A, Felin J, Fak F, Stombaugh J, et al. (2011) Human oral, gut, and plaque microbiota in patients with atherosclerosis. Proc Natl Acad Sci U S A 108(Suppl 1): 4592–4598.
19. Sundquist A, Bigdeli S, Jalili R, Druzin ML, Waller S, et al. (2007) Bacterial flora-typing with targeted, chip-based Pyrosequencing. BMC Microbiol 7: 108.
20. Wu GD, Lewis JD, Hoffmann C, Chen YY, Knight R, et al. (2010) Sampling and pyrosequencing methods for characterizing bacterial communities in the human gut using 16S sequence tags. BMC Microbiol 10: 206.
21. Dethlefsen L, Huse S, Sogin ML, Relman DA (2008) The pervasive effects of an antibiotic on the human gut microbiota, as revealed by deep 16S rRNA sequencing. PLoS Biol 6: e280.
22. Dowd SE, Sun Y, Secor PR, Rhoads DD, Wolcott BM, et al. (2008) Survey of bacterial diversity in chronic wounds using pyrosequencing, DGGE, and full ribosome shotgun sequencing. BMC Microbiol 8: 43.

23. Lazarevic V, Whiteson K, Hernandez D, Francois P, Schrenzel J (2010) Study of inter- and intra-individual variations in the salivary microbiota. BMC Genomics 11: 523.

24. Zaura E, Keijser BJ, Huse SM, Crielaard W (2009) Defining the healthy "core microbiome" of oral microbial communities. BMC Microbiol 9: 259.

25. Nasidze I, Quinque D, Li J, Li M, Tang K, et al. (2009) Comparative analysis of human saliva microbiome diversity by barcoded pyrosequencing and cloning approaches. Anal Biochem 391: 64–68.

26. Keijser BJ, Zaura E, Huse SM, van der Vossen JM, Schuren FH, et al. (2008) Pyrosequencing analysis of the oral microflora of healthy adults. J Dent Res 87: 1016–1020.

27. Li L, Hsiao WW, Nandakumar R, Barbuto SM, Mongodin EF, et al. (2010) Analyzing endodontic infections by deep coverage pyrosequencing. J Dent Res 89: 980–984.

28. Siqueira JF, Jr., Alves FR, Rôças IN (2011) Pyrosequencing analysis of the apical root canal microbiota. J Endod 37: 1499–1503.

29. Siqueira JF, Jr., Rôças IN (2009) Community as the unit of pathogenicity: an emerging concept as to the microbial pathogenesis of apical periodontitis. Oral Surg Oral Med Oral Pathol Oral Radiol Endod 107: 870–878.

30. Kuramitsu HK, He X, Lux R, Anderson MH, Shi W (2007) Interspecies interactions within oral microbial communities. Microbiol Mol Biol Rev 71: 653–670.

31. Costerton JW (2007) The biofilm primer. BerlinHeidelberg: Springer-Verlag.

32. Haapasalo M, Ranta H, Ranta K, Shah H (1986) Black-pigmented *Bacteroides* spp. in human apical periodontitis. Infect Immun 53: 149–153.

33. Siqueira JF, Jr., Rôças IN, Debelian GJ, Carmo FL, Paiva SS, et al. (2008) Profiling of root canal bacterial communities associated with chronic apical periodontitis from Brazilian and Norwegian subjects. J Endod 34: 1457–1461.

34. Machado de Oliveira JC, Siqueira JF, Jr., Rôças IN, Baumgartner JC, Xia T, et al. (2007) Bacterial community profiles of endodontic abscesses from Brazilian and USA subjects as compared by denaturing gradient gel electrophoresis analysis. Oral Microbiol Immunol 22: 14–18.

35. Siqueira JF, Jr., Rôças IN (2009) Diversity of endodontic microbiota revisited. J Dent Res 88: 969–981.

36. Sundqvist G (1992) Associations between microbial species in dental root canal infections. Oral Microbiol Immunol 7: 257–262.

37. Munson MA, Pitt-Ford T, Chong B, Weightman A, Wade WG (2002) Molecular and cultural analysis of the microflora associated with endodontic infections. J Dent Res 81: 761–766.

38. Chavez de Paz LE (2002) *Fusobacterium nucleatum* in endodontic flare-ups. Oral Surg Oral Med Oral Pathol Oral Radiol Endod 93: 179–183.

39. Williams BL, McCann GF, Schoenknecht FD (1983) Bacteriology of dental abscesses of endodontic origin. J Clin Microbiol 18: 770–774.

40. Sundqvist G, Johansson E, Sjogren U (1989) Prevalence of black-pigmented bacteroides species in root canal infections. J Endod 15: 13–19.

41. Sogin ML, Morrison HG, Huber JA, Welch DM, Huse SM, et al. (2006) Microbial diversity in the deep sea and the underexplored "rare biosphere". Proc Natl Acad Sci U S A 103: 12115–12120.

42. Huse SM, Dethlefsen L, Huber JA, Welch DM, Relman DA, et al. (2008) Exploring microbial diversity and taxonomy using SSU rRNA hypervariable tag sequencing. PLoS Genet 4: e1000255.

43. Schloss PD, Handelsman J (2005) Introducing DOTUR, a computer program for defining operational taxonomic units and estimating species richness. Appl Environ Microbiol 71: 1501–1506.

44. Rajilic-Stojanovic M, Smidt H, de Vos WM (2007) Diversity of the human gastrointestinal tract microbiota revisited. Environ Microbiol 9: 2125–2136.

45. Huse SM, Dethlefsen L, Huber JA, Mark Welch D, Relman DA, et al. (2008) Exploring microbial diversity and taxonomy using SSU rRNA hypervariable tag sequencing. PLoS Genet 4: e1000255.

46. Wang Q, Garrity GM, Tiedje JM, Cole JR (2007) Naive Bayesian classifier for rapid assignment of rRNA sequences into the new bacterial taxonomy. Appl Environ Microbiol 73: 5261–5267.

47. Cole JR, Wang Q, Cardenas E, Fish J, Chai B, et al. (2009) The Ribosomal Database Project: improved alignments and new tools for rRNA analysis. Nucleic Acids Res 37: D141–145.

48. Schloss PD, Westcott SL, Ryabin T, Hall JR, Hartmann M, et al. (2009) Introducing mothur: open-source, platform-independent, community-supported software for describing and comparing microbial communities. Appl Environ Microbiol 75: 7537–7541.

49. Jukes TH, Cantor CR (1969) Evolution of protein molecules. In: Unro HNM, ed. Mammalian protein metabolism. New York: Academic Press. pp 21–132.

50. Chao A, Bunge J (2002) Estimating the number of species in a stochastic abundance model. Biometrics 58: 531–539.

51. Shannon CE, Weaver W (1949) The mathematical theory of communications. Urbana: University of Illinois Press.

52. Kindt R, Coe R (2005) Tree diversity analysis. A manual and software for common statistical methods and biodiversity studies. Nairobi: World Agroforestry Centre (ICRAF).

53. Oksanen J, Blanchet FG, Kindt R, Legendre P, O'Hara RB, et al. (2011) Vegan: Community Ecology Package. R package version 1.17-6. The Comprehensive R Archive Network website. http://CRAN.R-project.org/package=vegan. Accessed 2011 Apr 21.

Gene Expression Profiles in Paired Gingival Biopsies from Periodontitis-Affected and Healthy Tissues Revealed by Massively Parallel Sequencing

Haleh Davanian[1]*[◑], Henrik Stranneheim[2◑], Tove Båge[1], Maria Lagervall[3], Leif Jansson[3], Joakim Lundeberg[2], Tülay Yucel-Lindberg[1]

1 Division of Periodontology, Department of Dental Medicine, Karolinska Institutet, Huddinge, Sweden, 2 Science for Life Laboratory, Division of Gene Technology, School of Biotechnology, Royal Institute of Technology (KTH), Solna, Sweden, 3 Department of Periodontology at Skanstull, Stockholm County Council Sweden, Stockholm, Sweden

Abstract

Periodontitis is a chronic inflammatory disease affecting the soft tissue and bone that surrounds the teeth. Despite extensive research, distinctive genes responsible for the disease have not been identified. The objective of this study was to elucidate transcriptome changes in periodontitis, by investigating gene expression profiles in gingival tissue obtained from periodontitis-affected and healthy gingiva from the same patient, using RNA-sequencing. Gingival biopsies were obtained from a disease-affected and a healthy site from each of 10 individuals diagnosed with periodontitis. Enrichment analysis performed among uniquely expressed genes for the periodontitis-affected and healthy tissues revealed several regulated pathways indicative of inflammation for the periodontitis-affected condition. Hierarchical clustering of the sequenced biopsies demonstrated clustering according to the degree of inflammation, as observed histologically in the biopsies, rather than clustering at the individual level. Among the top 50 upregulated genes in periodontitis-affected tissues, we investigated two genes which have not previously been demonstrated to be involved in periodontitis. These included interferon regulatory factor 4 and chemokine (C-C motif) ligand 18, which were also expressed at the protein level in gingival biopsies from patients with periodontitis. In conclusion, this study provides a first step towards a quantitative comprehensive insight into the transcriptome changes in periodontitis. We demonstrate for the first time site-specific local variation in gene expression profiles of periodontitis-affected and healthy tissues obtained from patients with periodontitis, using RNA-seq. Further, we have identified novel genes expressed in periodontitis tissues, which may constitute potential therapeutic targets for future treatment strategies of periodontitis.

Editor: Michael Glogauer, University of Toronto, Canada

Funding: This study was supported by funds from the Swedish National Graduate School in Odontological Science, Swedish Research Council, project number 73XD-15005, the Swedish Patent Revenue Fund, Stockholm County Council and Karolinska Institutet. The funders had no role in study design, data collection and analysis, decision to publish, or preparation of the manuscript.

Competing Interests: The authors have declared that no competing interests exist.

* E-mail: haleh.davanian@ki.se

◑ These authors contributed equally to this work.

Introduction

Periodontitis is a chronic inflammatory disease characterized by the destruction of periodontal tissue. This common disease, primarily initiated by periodontal pathogens, is an outcome of a complex interaction between periodontal microorganisms and the host inflammatory response [1]. The host response involves proinflammatory cytokines, chemokines, prostaglandins, Toll-like receptors and proteolytic enzymes, which have all been demonstrated to play an important role in the pathogenesis of periodontitis [2,3].

Studies have been performed combining *in vivo* and *in vitro* approaches to identify genes responsible for periodontitis. To date, there are a few published microarray studies investigating the gene expression profile in periodontits. One microarray study reported no significant differences in gene expression at different pathological sites in patients with chronic and aggressive periodontitis [4], whereas Kim et al. [5] and Demmer et al. [6] showed a number of genes that were upregulated in periodontitis compared to healthy controls. In addition, Beikler et al. [7] demonstrated that in periodontitis sites, the expression of immune and inflammatory genes was down-regulated following non-surgical therapy. With regard to *in vitro* studies, gene expression profiling has been performed on gingival fibroblasts from inflamed and healthy gingival tissues, for a limited number of inflammatory markers, such as interleukin (IL)-1, IL-6, IL-8, tumor necrosis factor- α (TNF-α) and CD14 [8]. Furthermore, microarray analysis has also been performed on periodontal ligament cells and gingival keratinocytes [9,10]. With regard to disease susceptibility at a genomic level, one genome-wide association study (GWAS) has been conducted in patients with aggressive periodontitis showing an association between aggressive periodontitis and intronic single nucleotide polymorphism rs1537415, which is located in the glycosyltransferase gene GLT6D1 [11].

Despite research investigating periodontitis gene expression profiles through microarray analysis, specific genes responsible for the disease have not yet been found. However, the recent development of massively parallel sequencing has provided a more comprehensive and accurate tool for gene expression analysis through sequenced based assays of transcriptomes, RNA-Sequencing (RNA-Seq). This method enables analysis of the complexity of whole eukaryotic transcriptomes [12] and studies comparing RNA-Seq and microarrays have shown that RNA-Seq has less bias, a greater dynamic range, a lower frequency of false positive signals and higher reproducibility [13,14]. The aim of the present study was to investigate the general pattern of the gene expression profile in periodontitis using RNA-Seq. We also aimed to investigate the local variation in gene expression at site level, comparing periodontitis-affected and healthy gingival tissues obtained from the same patient.

Materials and Methods

Ethics Statement

The study was performed in accordance with the Declaration of Helsinki and the current legislation in Sweden and after approval from the Karolinska Institutet Ethical Research Board. The Regional Ethics Board in Stockholm approved the collection of the biopsies and informed consent was obtained from all patients.

Collection of gingival tissue samples

A total of 10 nonsmoking individuals (20 biopsies), were included in the study. Four patients in the study group had other types of diseases: patient 2 was undergoing investigations for the disease sarcoidosis, patient 3 had diabetes type-2, patient 7 had a history of osteoarthritis and patient 10 was diagnosed with asthma. All participants were examined for periodontal disease and those with a tooth site demonstrating a probing depth ≥ 6 mm, clinical attachment level ≥ 5 mm and bleeding on probing were included in the periodontitis-affected group, according to the clinical parameters previously used as indicators of periodontitis [15,16,17]. During flap surgery, two adjacent gingival biopsies with identical clinical status were harvested from a periodontal pocket affected by periodontitis. The sizes of the specimens were approximately 2×2 mm, and included the connective tissue and the epithelium. In the same subjects, two adjacent gingival biopsies with identical clinical status and of about the same size were also obtained from a clinically healthy gingival pocket. Clinically healthy pockets were defined as sites with no gingival/periodontal inflammation, no bleeding on probing, a probing depth ≤ 3.5 mm and a clinical attachment level ≤ 3.5 mm. One of the biopsies from each site was stored in RNA Later (Applied Biosystems, USA) overnight at 4°C and thereafter stored at -80°C for subsequent RNA isolation. The second biopsy from each site was used for histological and immunohistochemical analysis.

Hematoxylin-Eosin staining

Deparaffinized serial sections of gingival tissues were formalin fixed (4% neutral buffered formalin) and paraffin embedded. For assessment of orientation of the epithelium and connective tissue as well as the degree of inflammation, deparaffinized serial sections (4 µm) were prepared and sections of each biopsy were stained with Hematoxylin-Eosin (H&E). The degree of inflammatory cell infiltration was evaluated by three blinded observers, using a relative scale from 0 to 3, and statistical differences between periodontitis-affected and healthy sites were tested using the Wilcoxon signed-rank test.

Table 1. Patient characteristics and periodontal status.

Patient characteristics			Periodontitis-affected sites			Healthy sites		
Patient	Gender	Age	Probing depth (mm)	Inflammation H&E (0-3) [a, c]	Inflammation CD3 (0-3) [b, d]	Probing depth (mm)	Inflammation H&E (0-3) [a, c]	Inflammation CD3 (0-3) [b, d]
1	M	52	7	3	2	3	2	0
2	M	45	8	1	1	3	1	1
3	M	52	7	3	3	3	1	1
4	F	47	7	3	3	3	1	2
5	F	37	7	2	2	3	1	1
6	M	59	7	2	3	3	2	1
7	F	66	7	2	-	3	0	-
8	M	48	6	2	2	3	0	0
9	M	42	8	3	1	2	1	1
10	F	54	6	2	1	3	1	1

[a] 0 = no evidence of inflammatory infiltration, 1 = slight inflammatory infiltration, 2 = moderate inflammatory infiltration and 3 = severe inflammatory infiltration.
[b] 0 = no CD3 positive cells, 1 = low amount of CD3 positive cells, 2 = moderate amount of CD3 positive cells, 3 = high amount of CD3 positive cells and - = not enough material to perform staining.
[c] Significant difference between periodontitis-affected and healthy sites ($p<0.01$).
[d] Significant difference between periodontitis-affected and healthy sites ($p<0.05$).

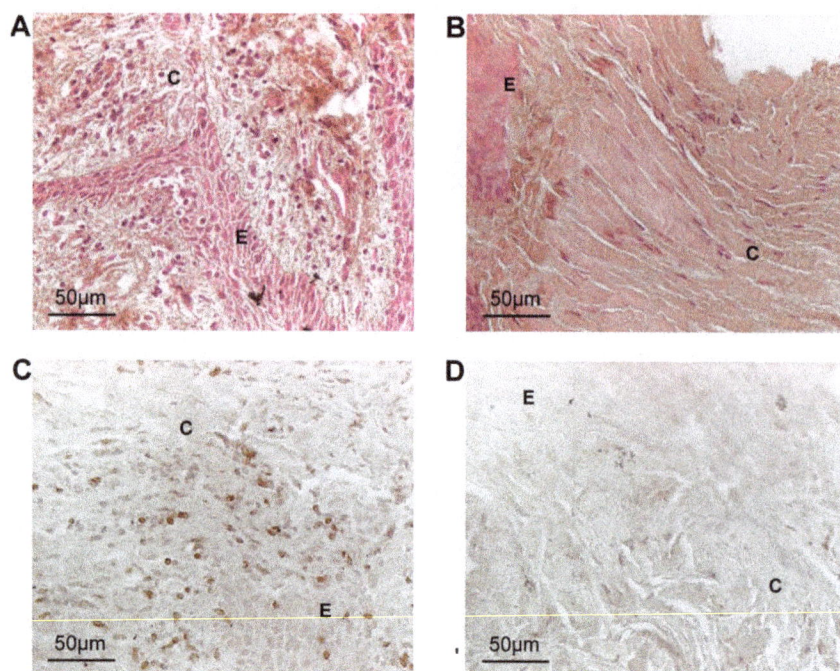

Figure 1. H&E and CD3-stained paraffin-embedded gingival biopsies obtained from one representative patient with periodontitis.
A. H&E staining of inflammatory cells in periodontitis-affected sections. B. H&E staining of inflammatory cells in healthy gingival sections. C. Staining of the T-cell marker CD3 in periodontitis-affected sections. D. Staining of the T-cell marker CD3 in healthy sections. E, epithelium, C, connective tissue.

Immunohistochemical stainings in gingival tissue

For staining of the T cell marker CD3, interferon regulatory factor 4 (IRF4) and chemokine (C-C motif) ligand 18 (CCL18), gingival tissues were rinsed in phosphate buffered saline (PBS) with 0.1% Saponin (PBS-Saponin buffer) for 10 min. After an antigen retrieval procedure, 10 mM Tris, 1 mM EDTA (pH 9.0) for CD3 and 0.01 M Citrate acid (pH 6.0) for IRF4 and CCL18, sections were blocked in 1% H_2O_2 in PBS-Saponin for 60 min at room temperature (RT) for CD3 and for 45 min at RT for IRF4 and CCL18. Subsequently, tissues were rinsed in PBS-Saponin for 10 min and further treated with 3% bovine serum albumin (BSA) diluted in PBS-Saponin for 30 min at RT. The expression of CD3, IRF4 and CCL18 was investigated using CD3 polyclonal rabbit antibody (1 µg/ml, PBS-Saponin) from Dako Sweden AB (Stockholm, Sweden), IRF4 polyclonal rabbit antibody (0.5 µg/ml, PBS-Saponin) from Atlas antibodies (Stockholm, Sweden) and CCL18 polyclonal rabbit anti-human antibody (0.5 µg/ml, PBS-Saponin) from Sigma-Aldrich (St. Louis, MO, USA). Normal rabbit IgG from R&D systems (MN, USA) was used as negative control. After incubation with primary antibody, sections were blocked with 1% normal goat serum in PBS for 15 min. Afterwards, sections were incubated with a biotinylated secondary antibody provided in the Vectastain ABC-Elite Complex Kit (Vector labs, Burlingame, CA, USA) followed by application of the Elite ABC solution for 40 min at RT in the dark. Thereafter, sections were washed with PBS and the peroxidase activity was visualized with 0.3% (v/v) in DAB buffer containing 0.1% (v/v) H_2O_2. Finally, the slides were washed with distilled water, dehydrated through an ethanol series (70%, 95%, 99.9%) into xylene, mounted, and photographed using a light microscope. For CD3 stainings, the amount of positive cells was evaluated by three blinded observers, using a relative scale from 0 to 3, and statistical differences between periodontitis-affected and healthy biopsies were tested using the Wilcoxon signed-rank test.

RNA extraction

RNA was extracted from gingival biopsies using steel-bead matrix tubes and a tabletop Fast-Prep homogenizer by two sequential centrifugations for 20 s at speed 6.5 (Qbiogene, Irvie, CA, USA). The RNA was purified on RNeasy Spin Columns (Qiagen, Valencia, CA, USA), treated with DNAse H to ensure degradation of DNA, and thereafter eluated in RNase-free water. The average RNA yield was 15.6 µg. RNA quality was assessed using the RNA 6000 NanoLabChip Kit of the Bioanalyzer system from Agilent Technologies (Santa Clara, CA, USA).

Transcriptome sample preparation for sequencing

A total amount of 2–3 µg per sample was used as input material for the RNA sample preparations. All samples had RIN values above 8. The samples were bar-coded and prepared according to the protocol (Cat# RS-930-1001) from the manufacturer (Illumina, San Diego, CA, USA), as previously described by Stranneheim et al. [18]. All sample preparation reagents were taken from the Illumina mRNA Sample Preparation Kit or ordered from vendors specified in the mRNA sample preparation protocol, except for automation specific reagents: carboxylic acid beads used for precipitation; the ethanol and tetraethylene glycol (EtOH/TEG) and the Polyethylene Glycol and sodium chloride (PEG/NaCl) precipitation buffers.

Clustering and sequencing

The clustering of the bar-coded samples was performed on a cBot Cluster Generation System using an Illumina HiSeq Single Read Cluster Generation Kit according to the manufacturer's instructions. The library preparations were sequenced on an Illumina HiSeq 2000 as single-reads to 100 bp. Two sequencing runs were performed according to the manufacturer's instructions where two and three lanes were used in the first sequencing and

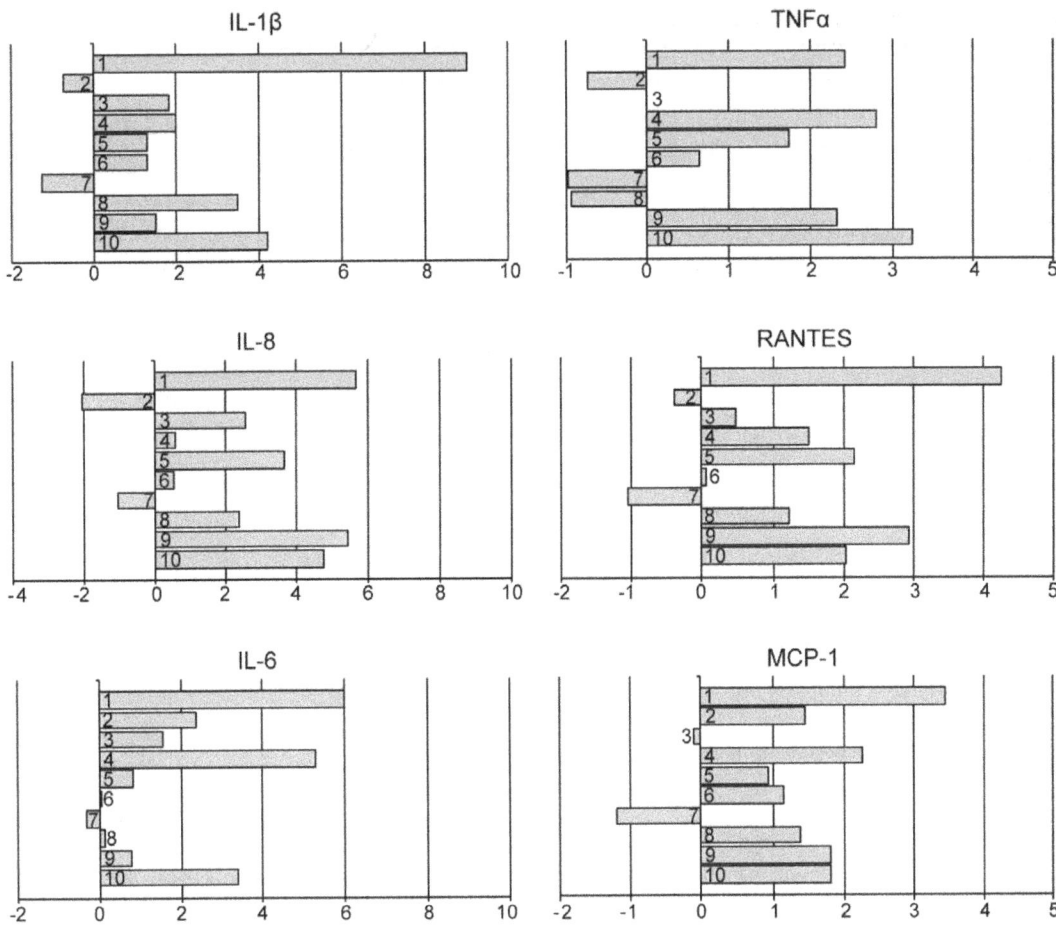

Figure 2. Expression of the inflammatory mediators in periodontitis-affected and healthy tissues obtained by RNA-seq. The bars show the expression (log$_2$ fold change) pattern based on RNA-Seq reads of IL-1β, IL-6, IL-8, TNFα, RANTES and MCP-1.

second sequencing run, respectively (Table S1). The runs generated a total of 402 million reads with an average of 15 million reads per sample that passed the Illumina Chastity filter; these reads were included in the study.

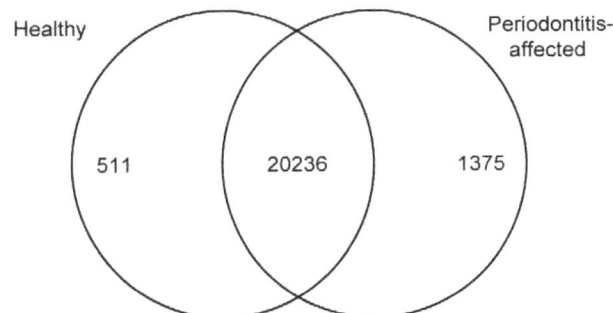

Figure 3. Venn diagram of mRNA transcripts. Venn diagram showing genes that were uniquely expressed in periodontitis-affected (1375) and healthy (511) gingival tissues. The intersection of the two circles refers to transcripts, which are expressed in both periodontitis-affected and healthy gingival tissues (20 236).

Sequence analysis

All sequences were aligned to the human genome reference hg19 with TopHat [19,20] version 1.1.4 and Samtools [21] version 0.1.8 using TopHat standard parameters except for parameters –solexa1.3-quals -p 8 –GTF Homo_sapiens.GRCh37.59.gtf. Annotations from Ensembl and RefSeq, downloaded from University of California, Santa Cruz (UCSC) Genome Browser, were used to assign features to genomic positions. Sequences aligned to the human genome were assigned to features and counted using HTSeq version 0.4.6 with parameters -m intersection-strict -s no -t exon. The R/Bioconductor package DESeq [22] was used to call differential gene expression on read counts generated by HTSeq and to perform hierarchical clustering of samples. All biological replicates for healthy and periodontitis-affected had R^2 (Spearman) correlation of gene expression (read counts) above 0.92.

Functional analyses of gene lists using WebGestalt

Analyses of gene categories and pathways was performed using the WEB-based Gene Set Analysis Toolkit v2 (WebGestalt) [23] with parameters: Id Type: Ensembl_gene_stable_id, Ref Set: Entrez Gene, Significance Level: $p<0.05$, Statistics Test: Hypergeometric, MTC: BH, Minimum: 2. KEGG analysis was used for pathway enrichment analysis and the Gene ontology (GO)

Table 2. Enriched regulated (KEGG) biological pathways among unique genes in periodontitis-affected tissues.

Pathway	Total genes in pathway	Unique genes in pathway[a]	Adj p value[b]
Neuroactive ligand-receptor interaction	256	19	8.18e-10
Cytokine-cytokine receptor interaction	267	18	6.75e-09
Chemokine signaling pathway	190	10	0.0004
Intestinal immune network for IgA production	50	5	0.0014
Alanine, aspartate and glutamate metabolism	31	5	0.0022
Tyrosine metabolism	46	4	0.0103
Calcium signaling pathway	178	7	0.0160
Hedgehog signaling pathway	56	4	0.0161
Systemic lupus erythematosus	140	6	0.0168
Glycine, serine and threonine metabolism	31	3	0.0196
Jak-STAT signaling pathway	155	6	0.0229
Vascular smooth muscle contraction	115	5	0.0271
Arhythmogenic right ventricular cardiomyopathy (ARVC)	76	4	0.0293

[a]Lists of uniquely expressed genes within the enriched pathways can be found in Table S1.
[b]adj p value indicates the significance of the enrichment, (adj $p < 0.05$).

category Biological process was used for the functional annotation analysis.

Results

Patients and gingival tissues

A total of 10 patients, six males and four females, with a mean age of 50 ± 8, were included in the study. For each patient, a total of four gingival biopsies of about the same size were obtained from periodontitis-affected and healthy gingiva, with two biopsies from each site. Bleeding status, probing depth and degree of inflammation in the gingival tissues for each of the two gingival sites was recorded (Table 1). To assess the degree of gingival inflammation in the periodontitis-affected and healthy tissues, histological and immunohistochemistry staining was performed using H&E and anti-CD3 (Fig. 1). Scoring of the degree of inflammatory cell infiltration, assessed by H&E staining, and the amount of CD3 positive cells showed significantly higher inflammation in tissue from periodontitis-affected sites ($p < 0.01$ for H&E and $p < 0.05$ for CD3; Table 1).

RNA-Sequencing

We sequenced cDNA from 10 periodontitis-affected and 10 healthy gingival tissues, with an average of 15 million reads of 100 bp in length per sample. A pairwise approach, where each periodontitis-affected biopsy had a healthy counterpart from the same individual, was used to eliminate the background noise of individual-specific gene transcription, enabling acquisition of more relevant data from the cohort. Aligning the sequence reads against the human genome yielded a median of 68% of uniquely aligned reads across all samples. The expression pattern, based on RNA-Seq reads, of well-known inflammatory mediators IL-1β, IL-6, IL-8, TNFα, Regulated upon Activation, Normal T-cell Expressed, and Secreted (RANTES) and Monocyte Chemotactic Protein-1 (MCP-1) were analyzed in all the tissue samples. The expression ($\log_2$ fold change) of these mediators was shown to be higher in the majority of the periodontitis-affected gingival tissue compared to healthy gingival tissue from the same patient (Fig. 2).

Table 3. Enriched regulated (KEGG) biological pathways among unique genes in healthy tissues.

Pathway	Total genes in pathway	Unique genes in pathway[a]	Adj p value[b]
Neuroactive ligand-receptor interaction	256	11	8.18e-10
Glycolysis/Gluconeogenesis	62	3	6.75e-09
Calcium signaling pathway	178	4	0.0004
Gap junction	90	3	0.0014
Pyruvate metabolism	40	2	0.0022
Tryptophan metabolism	40	2	0.0103

[a]Lists of uniquely expressed genes within the enriched pathways can be found in Table S1.
[b]adj p value indicates the significance of the enrichment, (adj $p < 0.05$).

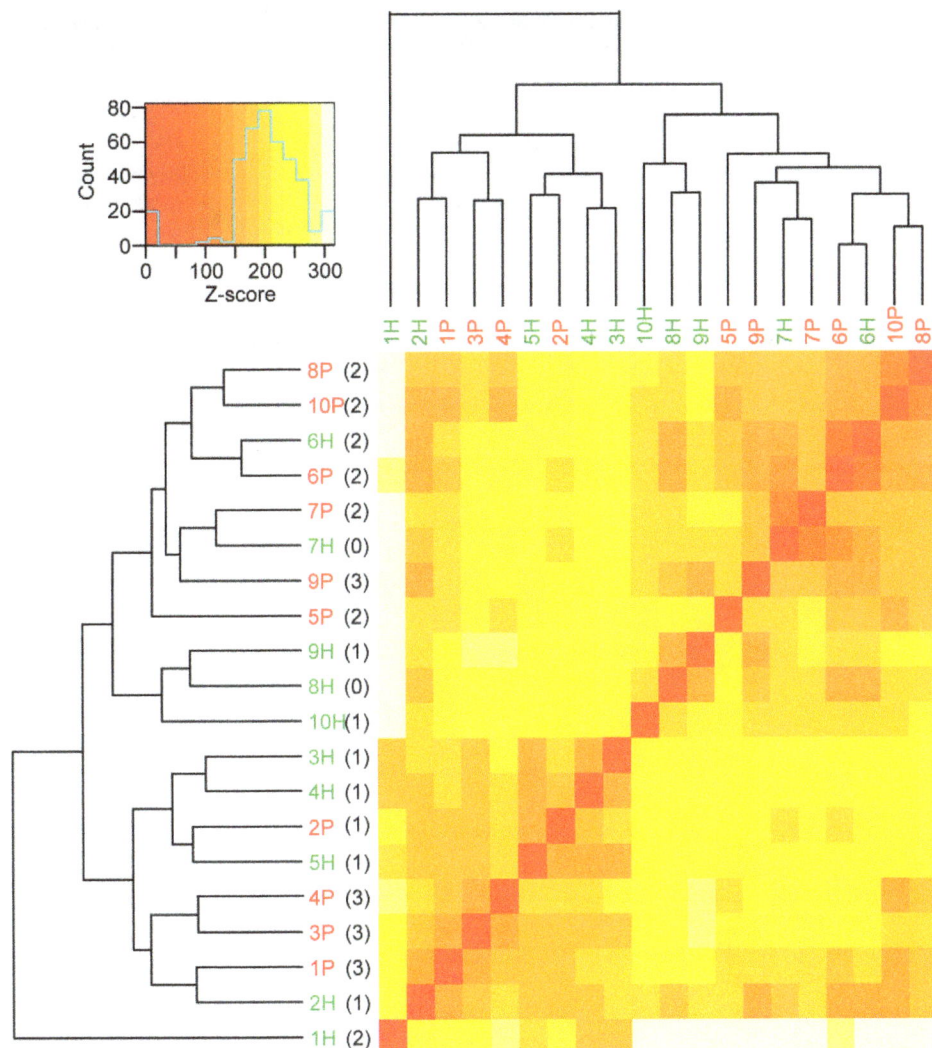

Figure 4. Clustering dendrogram and heatmap of periodontitis-affected and healthy biopsies. Clustering of all samples was based on gene transcripts with a median read above three times the background noise. The length of the branch between two biopsies and the colors of the heatmap correspond to degree of similarity between the gene expression profiles. Colors can be interpreted using the scale bar. Numbers in parentheses denote the inflammation scores of the biopsies after H&E histological evaluation.

Distribution of gene transcripts between periodontitis-affected and healthy gingival tissues

A total of 22 122 different mRNA transcripts were expressed in the periodontitis-affected and healthy gingival tissue samples. Among these transcripts, 1375 were unique to the periodontitis-affected tissue samples whereas 511 genes were uniquely transcribed in healthy gingival tissues (Fig. 3). KEGG enrichment analysis using WebGestalt [24] was performed among the unique genes for the periodontitis-affected and healthy tissues which revealed several regulated pathways indicative of inflammation for the periodontitis-affected condition (Table 2 and Table S1). In contrast, in the healthy gingival tissues, regulated pathways indicated a non-inflammatory profile among the unique genes, as demonstrated in Table 3 and Table S1.

Clustering of biopsies

Unsupervised hierarchical clustering was performed on all gene transcripts having a median read count above a cutoff level set to 0.3 read counts per feature, to exclude expression due to spurious transcription (Fig. 4). The gingival tissues from periodontitis-affected sites from different patients showed a more similar gene expression pattern than healthy gingival tissues from the same patient. Clustering according to individual, where the paired healthy and periodontitis-affected biopsies cluster together, was only observed for patient 6 and 7. However, the biopsies showed a general trend of clustering according to the degree of inflammation as assessed by H&E staining (Table 1), except for sample 7H, sample 2H and an outlier sample 1H, which clustered separately. There was also a trend of forming larger clusters depending on sequence run, but paired biopsies (periodontits-affected and healthy) from each patient were always analyzed in the same sequence run.

Differential gene expression between periodontitis-affected and healthy gingival tissues

Differential gene expression between periodontitis-affected and healthy gingival tissues was analyzed using read counts for each gene with the DeSeq package [22]. The analysis revealed a total of 453 significantly (adj $p<0.01$) differentially expressed genes. Additional analyses of genes expressed in periodontitis-affected

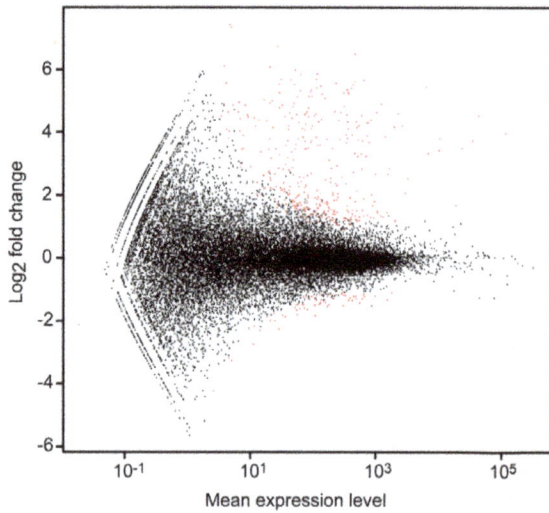

Figure 5. Volcano plot displaying differential expression. Differential gene expression (adj $p < 0.01$) between periodontitis-affected and healthy gingival tissues. The y axis corresponds to the $\log_2$ fold change value (M value), and the x axis displays the mean expression value.

gingiva, showed that 381 genes were upregulated, whereas 72 genes were shown to be down-regulated (Fig. 5, Table S2).

Gene Ontology enrichment analysis of differentially expressed genes

Investigation of functional associations of gene expression changes in the tissue samples was performed using WebGestalt. Gene ontology (GO) Biological process was used for enrichment analysis. Significant gene enrichments ($p < 0.05$) as well as their parent terms are demonstrated in Fig. 6. Several GO categories were over-represented among genes differentially expressed in periodontitis-affected versus healthy gingival tissues. The categories were mainly indicative of immune and inflammatory responses. Further enrichment analysis regarding Molecular function and Cellular components are provided in the supplementary data (Table S3).

Top 50 upregulated genes in periodontitis-affected gingival tissue

The top 50 significantly upregulated genes in periodontitis-affected gingival tissue with Unigene entry are displayed in Table 4 together with Ensemble ID, gene symbol, fold change, $\log_2$ fold

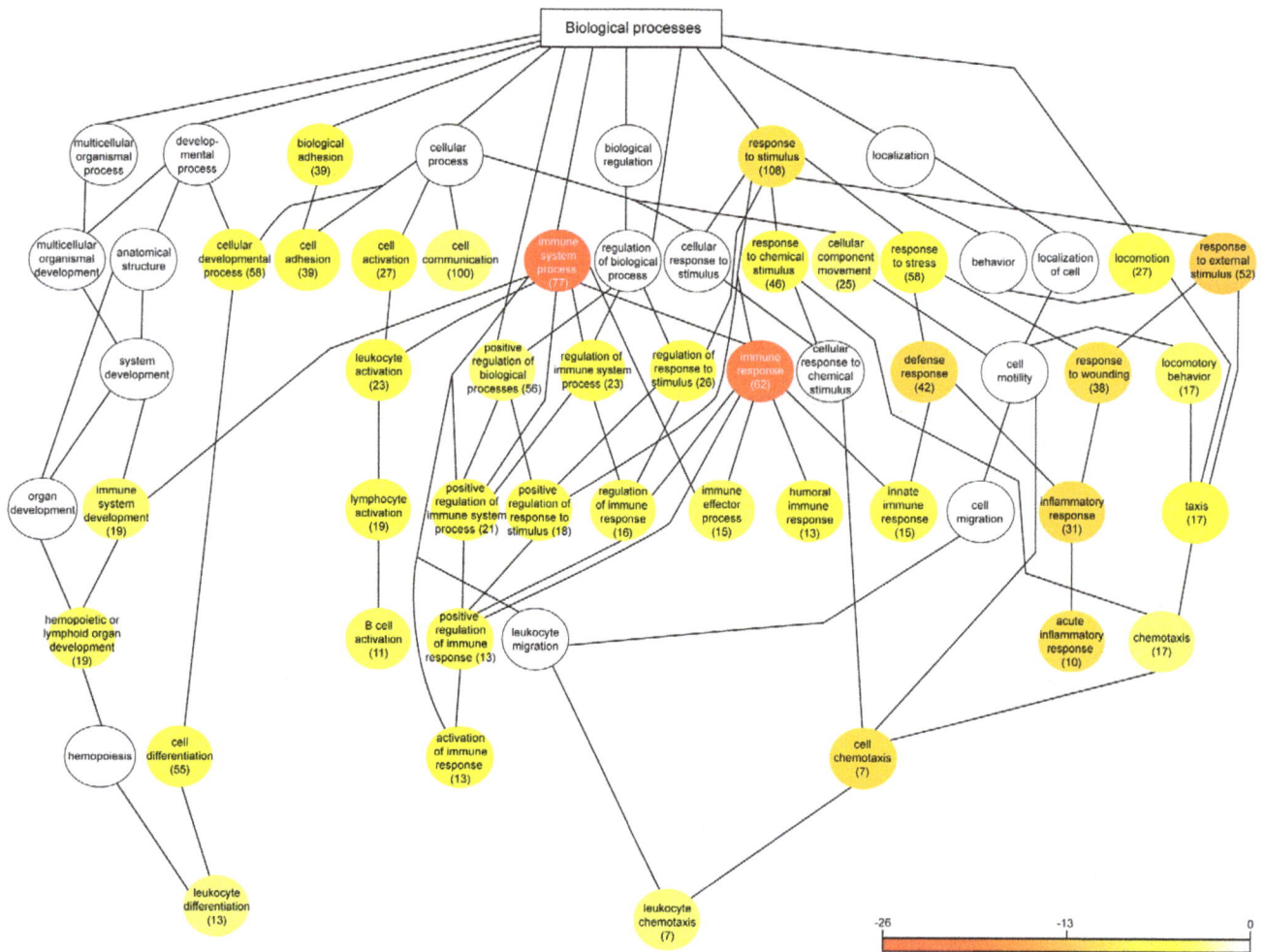

Figure 6. Gene ontology (GO) analysis of differentially expressed genes. All significant ($p < 0.05$) Biological processes (GO categories) and their parent terms are shown. The color of each node illustrates the significance and can be interpreted using the scale bar, which displays the p value. Each node is also marked with the number of significantly regulated genes mapped to the GO category.

Table 4. Top 50 upregulated genes in periodontitis-affected tissue with Unigene entry.

Ensemble ID	Gene symbol	Description	Fold change	Log$_2$ fold change	p value
ENSG00000188596	C12orf63	chromosome 12 open reading frame 63	69,15	6,11	9,54e-06
ENSG00000132704	FCRL2	Fc receptor-like 2	30,36	4,92	1,39e-10
ENSG00000143297	FCRL5	Fc receptor-like 5	25,24	4,66	5,24e-30
ENSG00000116748	AMPD1	adenosine monophosphate deaminase 1 (isoform M)	24,97	4,64	5,58e-05
ENSG00000187323	DCC	deleted in colorectal carcinoma	20,69	4,37	2,37e-09
ENSG00000137265	IRF4	interferon regulatory factor 4	20,10	4,33	1,50e-32
ENSG00000167077	MEI1	meiosis inhibitor 1	16,77	4,07	3,24e-16
ENSG00000101194	SLC17A9	solute carrier family 17, member 9	14,40	3,85	2,04e-14
ENSG00000122188	LAX1	lymphocyte transmembrane adaptor 1	14,28	3,84	3,83e-20
ENSG00000110777	POU2AF1	POU class 2 associating factor 1	14,12	3,82	9,81e-26
ENSG00000124256	ZBP1	Z-DNA binding protein 1	13,76	3,78	1,60e-14
ENSG00000170476	MGC29506	hypothetical protein MGC29506	13,33	3,74	1,20e-21
ENSG00000132185	FCRLA	Fc receptor-like A	12,18	3,61	2,47e-11
ENSG00000012223	LTF	lactotransferrin	12,09	3,61	8,54e-22
ENSG00000137673	MMP7	matrix metallopeptidase 7 (matrilysin, uterine)	11,37	3,51	8,33e-18
ENSG00000163534	FCRL1	Fc receptor-like 1	11,14	3,48	1,54e-05
ENSG00000177455	CD19	CD19 molecule	11,12	3,48	2,13e-08
ENSG00000061656	SPAG4	sperm associated antigen 4	11,09	3,47	1,62e-10
ENSG00000121895	TMEM156	transmembrane protein 156	11,00	3,46	2,35e-08
ENSG00000015413	DPEP1	dipeptidase 1 (renal)	10,93	3,45	8,81e-06
ENSG00000048462	TNFRSF17	tumor necrosis factor receptor superfamily, member 17	10,43	3,38	2,71e-08
ENSG00000169962	TAS1R3	taste receptor, type 1, member 3	10,42	3,38	2,28e-06
ENSG00000102096	PIM2	pim-2 oncogene	10,09	3,34	2,43e-23
ENSG00000183508	FAM46C	family with sequence similarity 46, member C	9,94	3,31	2,19e-24
ENSG00000168081	PNOC	prepronociceptin	9,75	3,29	1,83e-07
ENSG00000099958	DERL3	Der1-like domain family, member 3	9,45	3,24	2,26e-16
ENSG00000105369	CD79A	CD79a molecule, immunoglobulin-associated alpha	9,43	3,24	1,36e-18
ENSG00000189233	C8orf80	chromosome 8 open reading frame 80	9,03	3,17	2,42e-07
ENSG00000004468	CD38	CD38 molecule	8,75	3,13	7,57e-10
ENSG00000153789	FAM92B	family with sequence similarity 92, member B	8,21	3,04	2,95e-05
ENSG00000143603	KCNN3	potassium intermediate/small conductance calcium-activated channel, subfamily N, member 3	7,86	2,98	3,81e-07
ENSG00000007129	CEACAM21	carcinoembryonic antigen-related cell adhesion molecule 21	7,48	2,90	1,94e-05
ENSG00000170866	LILRA3	leukocyte immunoglobulin-like receptor, subfamily A (without TM domain), member 3	7,45	2,90	0,000111577
ENSG00000129988	LBP	lipopolysaccharide binding protein	7,33	2,87	7,78e-08
ENSG00000118308	LRMP	lymphoid-restricted membrane protein	7,24	2,86	7,08e-09
ENSG00000139193	CD27	CD27 molecule	7,21	2,85	4,63e-13
ENSG00000073849	ST6GAL1	ST6 beta-galactosamide alpha-2,6-sialyltranferase 1	7,11	2,83	4,37e-20
ENSG00000177272	KCNA3	potassium voltage-gated channel, shaker-related subfamily, member 3	7,07	2,82	4,64e-08
ENSG00000108405	P2RX1	purinergic receptor P2X, ligand-gated ion channel, 1	6,81	2,77	3,18e-05
ENSG00000026751	SLAMF7	SLAM family member 7	6,64	2,73	2,05e-16
ENSG00000124772	CPNE5	copine V	6,47	2,69	5,14e-10
ENSG00000132465	IGJ	immunoglobulin J polypeptide, linker protein for immunoglobulin alpha and mu polypeptides	6,41	2,68	6,97e-21
ENSG00000122224	LY9	lymphocyte antigen 9	6,39	2,68	1,71e-06
ENSG00000007312	CD79B	CD79b molecule, immunoglobulin-associated beta	6,28	2,65	1,89e-07

Table 4. Cont.

Ensemble ID	Gene symbol	Description	Fold change	Log$_2$ fold change	p value
ENSG00000134873	CLDN10	claudin 10	6,17	2,63	2,82e-06
ENSG00000172578	KLHL6	kelch-like 6 (Drosophila)	6,16	2,62	1,98e-11
ENSG00000196549	MME	membrane metallo-endopeptidase	6,01	2,59	2,29e-16
ENSG00000006074	CCL18	chemokine (C-C motif) ligand 18 (pulmonary and activation-regulated)	6,00	2,59	5,68e-10
ENSG00000173432	SAA1	serum amyloid A1	5,91	2,56	7,97e-10
ENSG00000159618	GPR114	G protein-coupled receptor 114	5,89	2,56	1,29e-05

change and p value. We investigated whether there were any available reports on the involvement of these genes in periodontitis or other chronic inflammatory conditions. Among the top 50 upregulated genes, we identified a number of candidate genes, which were not previously demonstrated to be involved in periodontitis but have been shown to be associated with other chronic conditions such as rheumatoid arthritis (RA). These candidate genes included FCRL5, adenosine monophosphate deaminase 1 (AMPD1), CCL18, tumor-necrosis factor receptor superfamily 17 (TNFRSF17) and leukocyte immunoglobin-like receptor, subfamily A (without TM domain) member 3 (LILRA3), and IRF4 which has shown to be involved in chronic inflammatory diseases such as RA and inflammatory bowel disease (IBD), (Table 5).

The protein expression of IRF4 and CCL18 in periodontitis-affected tissue

The expression of two of the top 50 differentially upregulated genes, IRF4 and CCL18 where further investigated at the protein level in gingival tissue samples from five additional patients with periodontitis. Immunohistochemical analysis showed that the transcription factor IRF4 and the chemokine CCL18 were expressed at the protein level in gingival tissue from patients with periodontitis (Fig. 7). IRF4 protein was expressed in cells including fibroblasts and inflammatory cells in the gingival connective tissue, as shown by morphology. For the chemokine CCL18, cellular staining of fibroblasts and inflammatory cells was observed, as well

as some diffuse extracellular staining, consistent with chemokine secretion.

Discussion

This study provides a novel quantitative comprehensive mapping of gene expression in gingival tissues from patients diagnosed with periodontitis, using RNA-Seq.

We first confirmed that the degree of inflammation was higher in periodontitis-affected gingival tissue compared to healthy tissues obtained from the same individual. Our results were based on immunohistological staining of CD3 positive cells, and further verified by RNA-Seq quantification of gene expression of the established inflammatory markers IL-1β, IL-6, IL-8, TNFα, RANTES and MCP-1. These inflammatory mediators have previously been reported to be elevated in patients with periodontitis [25,26,27].

Next, we performed unsupervised clustering of the gingival tissues to get an overview of the data generated from the RNA-Seq analysis. Cluster analysis revealed that the majority of periodontitis-affected clustered together and the majority of the healthy gingival tissues also clustered together, which is in line with our results regarding inflammation in the tissues. The degree of inflammation, rather than the individual, seemed to affect the clustering, indicating a common gene expression profile for periodontitis. Our results, based on the gene expression pattern of the inflammatory markers (IL-1β, IL-6, IL-8, TNFα, RANTES and MCP-1) and the immunohistochemical evaluation, confirmed

Table 5. Selected upregulated genes identified in periodontitis and involved in other chronic inflammatory diseases.

Ensemble ID	Gene symbol	Description	Fold change	Log$_2$ fold change	p value	Involvement in other diseases
ENSG00000143297	FCRL5	Fc receptor-like 5	25.24	4.66	5.98e-27	Rheumatoid arthritis (RA)
ENSG00000116748	AMPD1	adenosine monophosphate deaminase 1	24.97	4.64	0.0046	Rheumatoid arthritis (RA)
ENSG00000137265	IRF4	interferon regulatory factor 4	20.10	4.33	2.31e-29	Inflammatory Bowel Disease (IBD)
ENSG00000048462	TNFRSF17	tumor necrosis factor receptor superfamily, member 17	10.43	3.38	4.80e-06	Rheumatoid arthritis (RA)
ENSG00000170866	LILRA3	leukocyte immunoglobulin-like receptor, subfamily A (without TM domain), member 3	7.45	2.90	0.008037	Rheumatoid arthritis (RA)
ENSG00000006074	CCL18	chemokine (C-C motif) ligand 18 (pulmonary and activation-regulated	6.00	2.59	1.22e-07	Rheumatoid arthritis (RA)

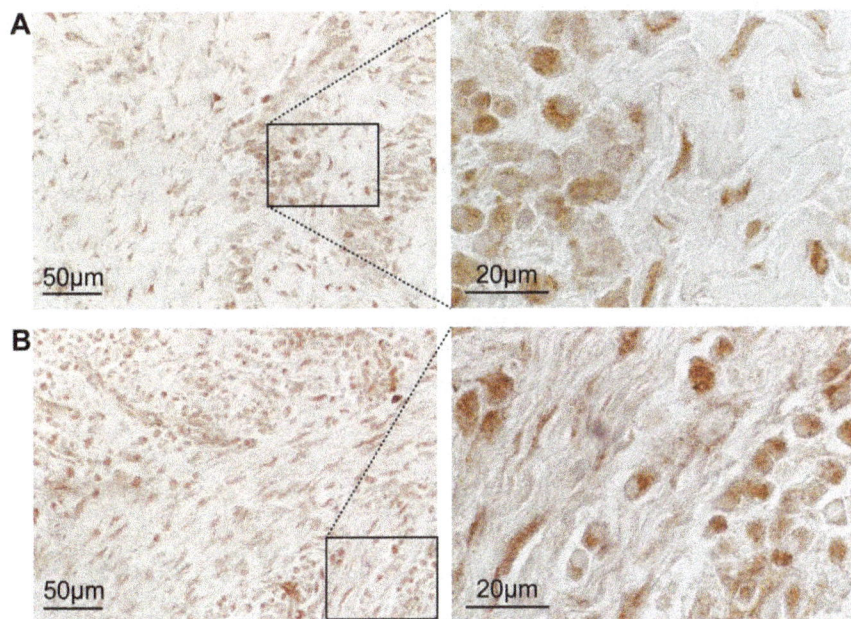

Figure 7. Immunohistochemical stainings of IRF4 and CCL18 in the connective tissue of periodontitis-affected gingival sections. A. Immunohistochemical staining of IRF4. B. Immunohistochemical staining of CCL18.

that the inflammation in periodontitis involves elevated levels of locally produced cytokines in the periodontium, as has been previously demonstrated [28]. However, cluster analysis revealed that three of the patients (patient no. 6, 7 and 2) deviated from the clustering pattern. For example, the healthy gingival tissue collected from patient 6 clustered with the periodontitis-affected tissue, which could be due to moderate inflammatory infiltration (H&E score 2) observed in the healthy gingival tissue. The clustering pattern in tissue from patient 7, where the healthy and diseased gingival tissue also clustered together, could be partly explained by the patient's history of osteoarthritis, which is a disease associated with elevated levels of circulating proinflammatory cytokines IL-6 and TNFα [29]. The cluster pattern for patient 2 differed from the rest of the patient group, which could be related to this patient undergoing investigation for the inflammatory disease sarcoidosis, and in turn might affect the systemic inflammatory response. Previous studies report that oral manifestations of sarcoidosis include aggressive destruction of the periodontium with rapid periodontal bone loss [30,31,32]. One of these studies also emphasizes the importance of patients diagnosed with sarcoidosis to be evaluated for other systemic involvements [31]. Thus, regarding our clustering pattern, it cannot be ruled out that general health differences might have some effect on the final outcome. However, the comparison of the gene expression profiles of all individuals should minimize potential interfering signals originating from single individuals affected with other diseases.

Our RNA-Seq analysis, investigating the gene expression profile in the gingival tissues showed that the genes were differentially distributed between healthy and periodontitis-affected samples. Enrichment analysis among uniquely expressed genes in the periodontitis-affected tissues showed regulated pathways indicative of inflammation, such as cytokine signaling, chemokine signaling and the JAK-STAT signaling pathway. Several cytokines such as interleukins, which are involved in periodontits, signal through the JAK-STAT signaling pathway [33]. On the other hand, in the healthy biopsies, pathways were indicative of non-inflammatory

processes that may be involved in the maintenance of the healthy gingival tissue. Future studies should also include investigation of genes within these pathways, which may contribute to understanding, prevention and treatment of periodontitis.

Differential gene expression analyses of periodontitis-affected vs. healthy gingival tissues showed the majority of differentially expressed genes to be upregulated in the periodontitis-affected tissues. Furthermore, GO enrichment analysis among these differentially expressed genes demonstrated that most of these genes were involved in immune and inflammatory processes. This is in line with the increased inflammatory response in the tissue, and also in accordance with our previous microarray studies on inflammatory-stimulated cell cultures reporting that gene expression profiles of TNFα-stimulated cells show an induction of inflammatory genes [34,35].

Up to date, RNA-Seq studies aimed to identify new genes involved in the pathogenesis of periodontits have not been reported. One *ab initio* study by Covani et al. [36] identified genes with potential roles in periodontitis, some of which have not previously been associated with the disease. However, the protein expression of these genes in periodontitis-affected tissues has not been confirmed. In our study we aimed to identify genes involved in the pathogenesis of periodontitis. Therefore, we further searched through the differentially expressed genes, focusing on the top 50 upregulated genes. Two of these 50 upregulated genes, IRF4 and CCL18, were also detected at the protein level in periodontitis affected-tissues, supporting these genes as novel finds in the pathogenesis of periodontitis. Furthermore, these two selected genes have been reported to be involved in other chronic inflammatory diseases such as RA. The transcription factor, IRF4, has been demonstrated to be involved in T-cell-dependent chronic inflammatory diseases such as IBD [37]. Mudter et al. 2011 reported a correlation between mRNA levels of IRF4 and production of cytokines such as IL-6 and IL-17 in the inflamed colon from patients with IBD, indicating that IRF4 is involved in the regulation of chronic mucosal inflammation [37]. In addition, the gene for CCL18 was upregulated in periodontitis-affected gingival tissues. This chemokine, expressed by macrophages, monocytes and dendritic cells, has been demonstrated to be increased in synovial tissue of RA patients [38]. It has also been suggested that blockage of CCL18 expression by anti-TNF-α antibodies identifies CCL18 as an additional target for anti-TNF-α therapy in patients with RA [39,40]. Studies are currently ongoing to investigate the expression of candidate genes novel for periodontitis in a larger cohort of patients with periodontitis and healthy controls, to be able to evaluate their impact and to further explore the possible therapeutic targeting of these genes. In addition, future studies will also be performed investigating the biological significance of the down-regulated genes in periodontitis.

In conclusion, we demonstrate for the first time, using RNA-seq, profile analysis of periodontitis revealing site-specific local variation in gene expression profiles of periodontitis-affected and healthy tissues obtained from patients diagnosed with periodontitis. Furthermore, we have identified differentially expressed novel genes in gingival tissue of periodontitis. Our findings provide a first step towards a quantitative comprehensive insight into the transcriptome of gingival tissue from patients with periodontitis, to enable identification of possible diagnostic markers of periodontitis as well as potential therapeutic targets.

Supporting Information

Table S1   Uniquely expressed genes within enriched pathways in periodontitis-affected and healthy gingival tissues.

Table S2   Full list of all significantly differentially expressed genes in periodontitis-affected and healthy gingival tissues.

Table S3   Gene Ontology enrichment analysis of differentially expressed genes.

Acknowledgments

We wish to thank Dr. Rachael Sugars for editing English-language and Nilminie Rathnayake for contributing to the collection of gingival biopsies.

Author Contributions

Conceived and designed the experiments: HD HS TB JL TYL. Performed the experiments: HD HS ML. Analyzed the data: HD HS TB JL TYL. Contributed reagents/materials/analysis tools: ML LJ JL TYL. Wrote the paper: HD HS TB ML LJ TYL.

References

1. Feng Z, Weinberg A (2006) Role of bacteria in health and disease of periodontal tissues. Periodontol 2000 40: 50–76.
2. Mahanonda R, Pichyangkul S (2007) Toll-like receptors and their role in periodontal health and disease. Periodontol 2000 43: 41–55.
3. Sorsa T, Tjaderhane L, Konttinen YT, Lauhio A, Salo T, et al. (2006) Matrix metalloproteinases: contribution to pathogenesis, diagnosis and treatment of periodontal inflammation. Ann Med 38: 306–321.
4. Papapanou PN, Abron A, Verbitsky M, Picolos D, Yang J, et al. (2004) Gene expression signatures in chronic and aggressive periodontitis: a pilot study. Eur J Oral Sci 112: 216–223.
5. Kim DM, Ramoni MF, Nevins M, Fiorellini JP (2006) The gene expression profile in refractory periodontitis patients. J Periodontol 77: 1043–1050.
6. Demmer RT, Behle JH, Wolf DL, Handfield M, Kebschull M, et al. (2008) Transcriptomes in healthy and diseased gingival tissues. J Periodontol 79: 2112–2124.
7. Beikler T, Peters U, Prior K, Eisenacher M, Flemmig TF (2008) Gene expression in periodontal tissues following treatment. BMC Med Genomics 1: 30.
8. Wang PL, Ohura K, Fujii T, Oido-Mori M, Kowashi Y, et al. (2003) DNA microarray analysis of human gingival fibroblasts from healthy and inflammatory gingival tissues. Biochem Biophys Res Commun 305: 970–973.
9. Kurashige Y, Saitoh M, Nishimura M, Noro D, Kaku T, et al. (2008) Profiling of differentially expressed genes in porcine epithelial cells derived from periodontal ligament and gingiva by DNA microarray. Arch Oral Biol 53: 437–442.
10. Steinberg T, Dannewitz B, Tomakidi P, Hoheisel JD, Mussig E, et al. (2006) Analysis of interleukin-1beta-modulated mRNA gene transcription in human gingival keratinocytes by epithelia-specific cDNA microarrays. J Periodontal Res 41: 426–446.
11. Schaefer AS, Richter GM, Nothnagel M, Manke T, Dommisch H, et al. (2010) A genome-wide association study identifies GLT6D1 as a susceptibility locus for periodontitis. Hum Mol Genet 19: 553–562.
12. Twine NA, Janitz K, Wilkins MR, Janitz M (2011) Whole transcriptome sequencing reveals gene expression and splicing differences in brain regions affected by Alzheimer's disease. PLoS One 6: e16266.
13. Richard H, Schulz MH, Sultan M, Nurnberger A, Schrinner S, et al. (2010) Prediction of alternative isoforms from exon expression levels in RNA-Seq experiments. Nucleic Acids Res 38: e112.
14. Sultan M, Schulz MH, Richard H, Magen A, Klingenhoff A, et al. (2008) A global view of gene activity and alternative splicing by deep sequencing of the human transcriptome. Science 321: 956–960.
15. Lang NP, Joss A, Orsanic T, Gusberti FA, Siegrist BE (1986) Bleeding on probing. A predictor for the progression of periodontal disease? J Clin Periodontol 13: 590–596.
16. Armitage GC (1996) Periodontal diseases: diagnosis. Ann Periodontol 1: 37–215.
17. Tu YK, Gilthorpe MS, Griffiths GS, Maddick IH, Eaton KA, et al. (2004) The application of multilevel modeling in the analysis of longitudinal periodontal data–part I: absolute levels of disease. J Periodontol 75: 127–136.
18. Stranneheim H, Werne B, Sherwood E, Lundeberg J (2011) Scalable transcriptome preparation for massive parallel sequencing. PLoS One 6: e21910.
19. Langmead B, Trapnell C, Pop M, Salzberg SL (2009) Ultrafast and memory-efficient alignment of short DNA sequences to the human genome. Genome Biol 10: R25.
20. Trapnell C, Pachter L, Salzberg SL (2009) TopHat: discovering splice junctions with RNA-Seq. Bioinformatics 25: 1105–1111.
21. Li H, Handsaker B, Wysoker A, Fennell T, Ruan J, et al. (2009) The Sequence Alignment/Map format and SAMtools. Bioinformatics 25: 2078–2079.
22. Anders S, Huber W (2010) Differential expression analysis for sequence count data. Genome Biol 11: R106.
23. Zhang B, Kirov S, Snoddy J (2005) WebGestalt: an integrated system for exploring gene sets in various biological contexts. Nucleic Acids Res 33: W741–748.
24. Web-based gene set analysis toolkit. Available: http://bioinfo.vanderbilt.edu/webgestalt. Accessed 2012 Aug 10.
25. Gamonal J, Acevedo A, Bascones A, Jorge O, Silva A (2000) Levels of interleukin-1 beta, -8, and -10 and RANTES in gingival crevicular fluid and cell populations in adult periodontitis patients and the effect of periodontal treatment. J Periodontol 71: 1535–1545.
26. Pradeep AR, Daisy H, Hadge P, Garg G, Thorat M (2009) Correlation of gingival crevicular fluid interleukin-18 and monocyte chemoattractant protein-1 levels in periodontal health and disease. J Periodontol 80: 1454–1461.
27. Passoja A, Puijola I, Knuuttila M, Niemela O, Karttunen R, et al. (2010) Serum levels of interleukin-10 and tumour necrosis factor-alpha in chronic periodontitis. J Clin Periodontol 37: 881–887.
28. Dasanayake AP (2010) Periodontal disease is related to local and systemic mediators of inflammation. J Evid Based Dent Pract 10: 246–247.
29. Stannus O, Jones G, Cicuttini F, Parameswaran V, Quinn S, et al. (2010) Circulating levels of IL-6 and TNF-alpha are associated with knee radiographic osteoarthritis and knee cartilage loss in older adults. Osteoarthritis Cartilage 18: 1441–1447.
30. Cohen C, Krutchkoff D, Eisenberg E (1981) Systemic sarcoidosis: report of two cases with oral lesions. J Oral Surg 39: 613–618.
31. Suresh L, Aguirre A, Buhite RJ, Radfar L (2004) Intraosseous sarcoidosis of the jaws mimicking aggressive periodontitis: a case report and literature review. J Periodontol 75: 478–482.
32. Moretti AJ, Fiocchi MF, Flaitz CM (2007) Sarcoidosis affecting the periodontium: a long-term follow-up case. J Periodontol 78: 2209–2215.
33. Hanada T, Yoshimura A (2002) Regulation of cytokine signaling and inflammation. Cytokine Growth Factor Rev 13: 413–421.
34. Davanian H, Bage T, Lindberg J, Lundeberg J, Concha HQ, et al. (2012) Signaling pathways involved in the regulation of TNFalpha-induced toll-like receptor 2 expression in human gingival fibroblasts. Cytokine 57: 406–416.
35. Bage T, Lindberg J, Lundeberg J, Modeer T, Yucel-Lindberg T (2010) Signal pathways JNK and NF-kappaB, identified by global gene expression profiling, are involved in regulation of TNFalpha-induced mPGES-1 and COX-2 expression in gingival fibroblasts. BMC Genomics 11: 241.
36. Covani U, Marconcini S, Giacomelli L, Sivozhelevov V, Barone A, et al. (2008) Bioinformatic prediction of leader genes in human periodontitis. J Periodontol 79: 1974–1983.

37. Mudter J, Yu J, Zufferey C, Brustle A, Wirtz S, et al. (2011) IRF4 regulates IL-17A promoter activity and controls RORgammat-dependent Th17 colitis in vivo. Inflamm Bowel Dis 17: 1343–1358.

38. Momohara S, Okamoto H, Iwamoto T, Mizumura T, Ikari K, et al. (2007) High CCL18/PARC expression in articular cartilage and synovial tissue of patients with rheumatoid arthritis. J Rheumatol 34: 266–271.

39. Haringman JJ, Smeets TJ, Reinders-Blankert P, Tak PP (2006) Chemokine and chemokine receptor expression in paired peripheral blood mononuclear cells and synovial tissue of patients with rheumatoid arthritis, osteoarthritis, and reactive arthritis. Ann Rheum Dis 65: 294–300.

40. Auer J, Blass M, Schulze-Koops H, Russwurm S, Nagel T, et al. (2007) Expression and regulation of CCL18 in synovial fluid neutrophils of patients with rheumatoid arthritis. Arthritis Res Ther 9: R94.

5

Baicalin Downregulates *Porphyromonas gingivalis* Lipopolysaccharide-Upregulated IL-6 and IL-8 Expression in Human Oral Keratinocytes by Negative Regulation of TLR Signaling

Wei Luo[1], Cun-Yu Wang[2], Lijian Jin[1]*

1 Faculty of Dentistry, The University of Hong Kong, Hong Kong SAR, China, **2** University of California Los Angeles, School of Dentistry, Los Angeles, California, United States of America

Abstract

Periodontal (gum) disease is one of the main global oral health burdens and severe periodontal disease (periodontitis) is a leading cause of tooth loss in adults globally. It also increases the risk of cardiovascular disease and diabetes mellitus. *Porphyromonas gingivalis* lipopolysaccharide (LPS) is a key virulent attribute that significantly contributes to periodontal pathogenesis. Baicalin is a flavonoid from *Scutellaria radix*, an herb commonly used in traditional Chinese medicine for treating inflammatory diseases. The present study examined the modulatory effect of baicalin on *P. gingivalis* LPS-induced expression of IL-6 and IL-8 in human oral keratinocytes (HOKs). Cells were pre-treated with baicalin (0–80 µM) for 24 h, and subsequently treated with *P. gingivalis* LPS at 10 µg/ml with or without baicalin for 3 h. IL-6 and IL-8 transcripts and proteins were detected by real-time polymerase chain reaction and enzyme-linked immunosorbent assay, respectively. The expression of nuclear factor-κB (NF-κB), p38 mitogen-activated protein kinase (MAPK) and c-Jun N-terminal kinase (JNK) proteins was analyzed by western blot. A panel of genes related to toll-like receptor (TLR) signaling was examined by PCR array. We found that baicalin significantly downregulated *P. gingivalis* LPS-stimulated expression of IL-6 and IL-8, and inhibited *P. gingivalis* LPS-activated NF-κB, p38 MAPK and JNK. Furthermore, baicalin markedly downregulated *P. gingivalis* LPS-induced expression of genes associated with TLR signaling. In conclusion, the present study shows that baicalin may significantly downregulate *P. gingivalis* LPS-upregulated expression of IL-6 and IL-8 in HOKs via negative regulation of TLR signaling.

Editor: Anne Wertheimer, University of Arizona, United States of America

Funding: This study was supported by the Hong Kong Research Grants Council (HKU766909M and HKU768411M to LJJ), and the Modern Dental Laboratory/HKU Endowment Fund to LJJ. The funders had no role in study design, data collection and analysis, decision to publish or preparation of the manuscript.

Competing Interests: The authors have declared that no competing interests exist.

* E-mail: ljjin@hkucc.hku.hk

Introduction

Periodontal disease is one of the main global oral health burdens and severe periodontal disease (periodontitis) is a major cause of tooth loss in adults globally [1]. Emerging evidence shows that it also increases the risk of some life-threating diseases like cardiovascular disease and diabetes mellitus [2–4]. Periodontitis is characterized by bacteria-induced, uncontrolled inflammatory destruction of tooth-supporting tissues and alveolar bone in susceptible individuals [5]. *Porphyromonas gingivalis* is a major periodontal pathogen and its lipopolysaccharide (LPS) is one of the key virulent attributes that significantly contributes to periodontal pathogenesis [6,7]. It can stimulate the host to produce a variety of pro-inflammatory cytokines like IL-6 and IL-8, thereby involving in the initiation and progression of periodontal disease [8–10].

Toll-like receptors (TLRs) are a family of pattern recognition receptors (PRRs) that recognize microbial components and mediate the activation of host response [11]. Microbial LPS utilizes TLR4 to activate nuclear factor-κB (NF-κB), p38 mitogen-activated protein kinase (MAPK) and c-Jun N-terminal kinase

(JNK), leading to the production of pro-inflammatory cytokines [11]. This process requires an initial recruitment of myeloid differentiation primary-response protein 88 (MyD88) to TLR4 [12–14]. In addition, there exists a TLR4-mediated MyD88-independent pathway that recruits toll/interleukin-1 receptor (TIR) domain-containing adaptor inducing interferon-β (TRIF) instead of recruitment of MyD88 to TLR4 in response to LPS, thereby activating the expression of interferon (IFN)-β and IFN-inducible genes like chemokine (C-X-C motif) ligand 10 (CXCL10) [15–18]. LPS is a TLR4 ligand and *P. gingivalis* LPS interacts with TLR4 to activate host response [19–21]. Nevertheless, it has been reported that *P. gingivalis* LPS could interact with TLR2 as well [22–24], due to the heterogeneity in lipid A structure of *P. gingivalis* LPS [8,25,26], and/or the contamination of LPS with some bioactive molecules like phosphorylated lipids and lipoproteins [27–29].

Recently, host modulatory therapy (HMT) has been proposed as a promising adjunct to conventional periodontal treatment [30,31]. Some examples of HMT in treatment of periodontitis include subantimicrobial dose of doxycycline, lipoxins and resolvin

E1 [32–34]. *Scutellariae radix* is an herb that has been used to treat inflammatory diseases in traditional Chinese medicine (TCM) since ancient times [35]. Baicalin is a flavonoid isolated from *Scutellaria radix* and it can suppress IL-8-induced metalloproteinase-8 (MMP-8) expression in human neutrophils [36]. In periodontal research, it has recently been shown that baicalin enables to inhibit the transcription of receptor activator of NF-κB ligand (RANKL) in human periodontal ligament cells, and reduces the loss of bone and collagens in rat models of periodontitis [37,38]. Furthermore, baicalin may inhibit IL-1β-induced MMP-1 expression and stimulate collagen-I production in human periodontal ligament cells [39].

In the present study, we found that baicalin significantly downregulated *P. gingivalis* LPS-upregulated expression of IL-6 and IL-8. Baicalin also inhibited *P. gingivalis* LPS-induced activation of NF-κB, p38 MAPK and JNK proteins, and markedly downregulated *P. gingivalis* LPS-induced expression of genes associated with TLR signaling, such as chemokine (C-C motif) ligand 2 (CCL2), granulocyte colony-stimulating factor (G-CSF or CSF3) and CXCL10.

Materials and Methods

Cell Culture

HOKs isolated from normal human oral mucosa (Sciencell, CA, USA) were cultured according to the manufacturer's instructions. Prior to cell culture, culture vessels were coated with poly-L-lysine (Sigma, MO, USA) at 2 µg/cm^2 at 37°C for 1 h. Cells were seeded at 5000 cells/cm^2 with the oral keratinocyte medium (Sciencell). The incubation condition was set at 37°C with an atmosphere of 5% CO_2 and 95% air. The medium was changed every two days for the first four days and daily thereafter until a monolayer was formed.

Preparation of *P. gingivalis* LPS and Baicalin

Lyophilized LPS from *P. gingivalis* with type II *fimA* (strain code TDC60) was kindly provided by Prof. Y. Abiko (Nihon University, Japan). The LPS was prepared using the hot phenol water method [40,41]. It was reconstituted in Dulbecco's phosphate-buffered saline (DPBS) to a concentration of 1.0 mg/ml, followed by filtration through a 0.2 µm cellulose acetate membrane filter (Millipore, MA, USA). Baicalin powder (solvent extracted with a purity >95% as tested by HPLC) was obtained from the Hong Kong Jockey Club Institute of Chinese Medicine, Hong Kong. It was dissolved in pure dimethyl sulfoxide (DMSO) (Sigma), and then diluted in DPBS to 1.0 mM and finally filtered for sterilization. Working solutions were made with fresh oral keratinocyte medium on the experiment day.

Total RNA Extraction and cDNA Synthesis

Total RNA was extracted using the RNeasy mini kit (Qiagen, CA, USA). Briefly, cells were lysed with the buffer RLT, and the lysate was applied to an RNeasy Mini spin column. After several rounds of washes using the buffer RW1 and RPE, total RNA was bound to the column and other cell components were efficiently washed away. At the end, total RNA was eluted in RNase-free water. To avoid the contamination of genomic DNA, on-column DNase digestion was performed during RNA purification. The concentration of purified RNA was quantified by measuring its 260 nm UV absorbance on a NanoDrop spectrophotometer (Thermo, MA, USA). The integrity of purified RNA was evaluated by checking the ratio of 28 S rRNA and 18 S rRNA bands on an agarose gel. cDNA was synthesized using the Quantitect Reverse Transcription Kit (Qiagen). In brief, 1.0 µg of total RNA was pre-

incubated with the gDNA Wipeout Buffer at 42°C for 2 min to remove any residual genomic DNA. The mixture was then incubated with the Quantiscript Reverse Transcriptase, Quantiscript RT Buffer and RT Primer Mix at 42°C for 30 min, followed by a termination step at 95°C for 5 min.

Real-time Polymerase Chain Reaction (PCR)

Each real-time PCR reaction mix contained 10.0 µl of the QuantiFast SYBR green master mix (Qiagen), 1.0 µl of cDNA template (5.0 ng), 1.0 µl of forward primer (10 µM), 1.0 µl of reverse primer (10 µM) and 7.0 µl of ultra-pure water. The reaction condition was set as follows: an initial activation at 95°C for 5 min, followed by 40 cycles at 95°C for 10 s and 60°C for 30 s. The primer sequences were: for IL-6, 5'-AATCAT-CACTGGTCTTTTGGAG (forward), 5'-GCATTTGTGGTTGGGTCA (reverse); and for IL-8, 5'-GA-CATACTCCAAACCTTTCCACC (forward), 5'-AACTTCTC-CACAACCCTCTGC (reverse); for β-actin (ACTB),5'-TTGGCAATGAGCGGTT (forward), 5'-AGTTGAAGG-TAGTTTCGTGGAT (reverse). All the primers were designed to amplify a region that lasts 100–250 base pairs long and contains at least one intron. They had passed our in-house amplification efficiency and specificity tests prior to usage. To check for nonspecific primer binding or co-amplification of residual genomic DNA, the melting curve was analyzed after each running. To detect foreign DNA contamination, a no-template control which contained all the reagents except the cDNA template was included in each running. Raw fluorescence data were analyzed by an Excel workbook called DART-PCR which automatically calculates threshold cycles, relative quantification values and amplification efficiencies [42].

Enzyme-linked Immunosorbent Assay (ELISA)

ELISA kits (R&D, MN, USA) were used to quantitatively determine the concentrations of IL-6 and IL-8 in culture supernatants. In brief, protein samples were pipetted into a microplate pre-coated with anti-IL-6 or anti-IL-8 antibodies and incubated at room temperature (RT) for 2 h. The plate was then washed three times with washing buffer to remove unbound samples. Subsequently, enzyme-linked polyclonal anti-IL-6 or anti-IL-8 antibodies were added and incubated at RT for 1 h. Following another three washes, a substrate solution was added and incubated at RT for 20 min. A blue color was then developed in direct proportion to the amount of the target cytokine in each well. Lastly, a stop solution was added to stop the color reaction. The absorbance was measured at 450 nm by a microplate reader (PerkinElmer, MA, USA).

Protein Extraction

Cytoplasmic and nuclear proteins were extracted using the NE-PER Nuclear and Cytoplasmic Extraction kit (Thermo). Two reagents, the Cytoplasmic Extraction Reagents I and II, were added to cell pellets to lyse cells. The cytoplasmic proteins released were collected by centrifugation. The remaining intact nuclei were lysed with the Nuclear Extraction Reagent and the nuclear proteins released were collected by centrifugation. The concentrations of fractionated proteins were measured by the BCA protein assay kit (Thermo).

Western Blot

Protein samples were separated on 10% SDS-polyacrylamide gels by electrophoresis and subsequently transferred to polyvinylidene difluoride membranes (Roche, IN, USA) by using the Mini-

A

B

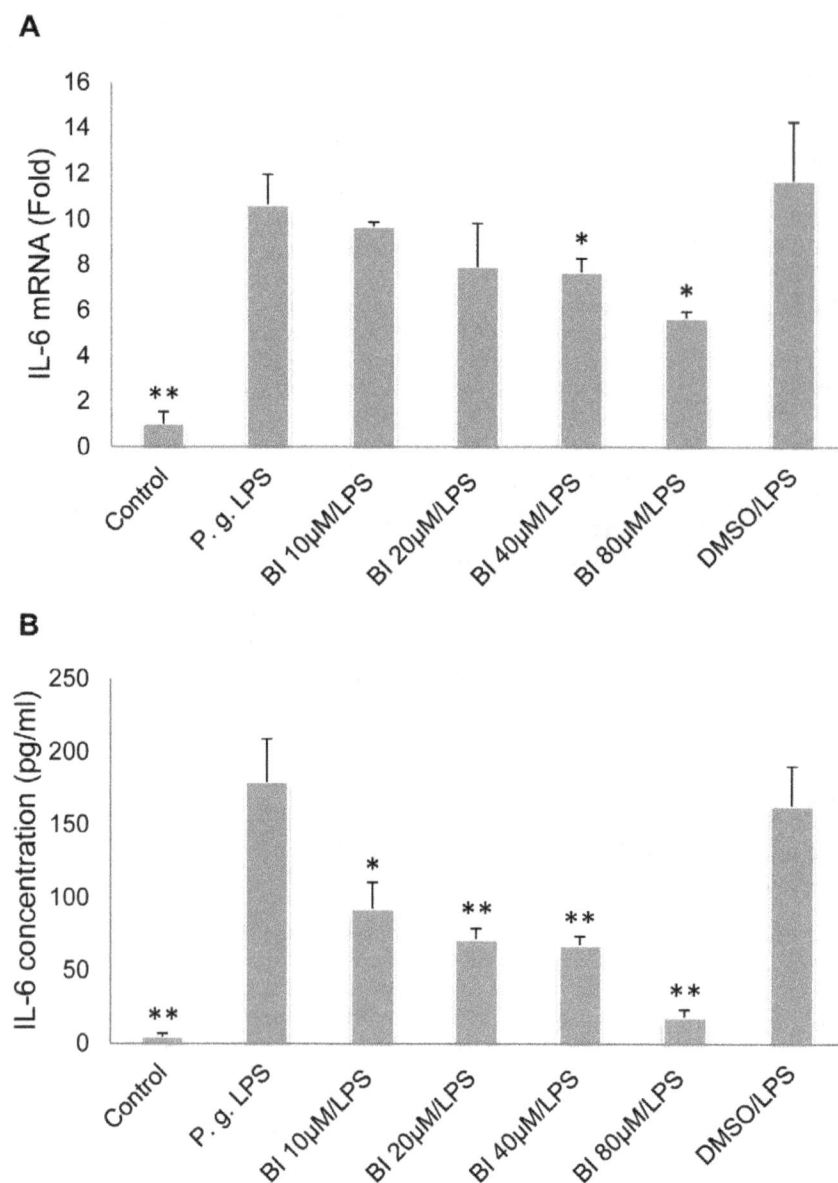

Figure 1. Baicalin significantly downregulates *P. gingivalis* **LPS-upregulated IL-6 expression. A**. Baicalin (BI) at 40 μM and 80 μM significantly downregulated *P. gingivalis* (*P.g.*) LPS-upregulated IL-6 mRNA expression. **B**. Baicalin at 10 μM, 20 μM, 40 μM, and 80 μM markedly downregulated *P.g.* LPS-upregulated IL-6 protein expression. Cells treated with culture media alone served as the blank control group, and those treated with *P.g.* LPS (10 μg/ml) alone represented the positive control group. Cells treated with 0.08% DMSO and *P.g.* LPS at 10 μg/ml served as the vehicle control group. Data of three independent experiments were depicted as relative fold change as compared with the blank control group (set as 1) (**A**), or presented as protein concentration (**B**). *$p < 0.05$ and **$p < 0.01$ as compared with the positive control group (*P.g.* LPS).

PROTEAN tetra electrophoresis system and Mini Trans-Blot transfer system (Bio-rad, CA, USA). Afterwards, the membranes were incubated with the Protein-Free T20 (TBS) Blocking Buffer (Thermo) at RT for 1 h and then probed with the primary antibodies (1:2000) at 4°C overnight with gentle agitation. On the next day, the membranes were washed and incubated with horseradish peroxidase (HRP)-conjugated secondary antibodies at RT for 1 h. They were then washed again and incubated with the SuperSignal West Pico Chemiluminescent Substrate (Thermo) for 5 min. The signals of antigen-antibody complexes were developed on X-ray films. The density of the developed bands was quantified by the ImageJ software. The rabbit monoclonal antibodies (mAbs) against human IκBα, phospho-IκBα (serine32), phospho-p38

MAPK (Thr180/Tyr182), phospho-JNK (Thr183/Tyr185) and α-tubulin were obtained from Cellsignaling (MA, USA). HRP-conjugated goat polyclonal antibodies against rabbit IgG were obtained from Thermo.

NF-κB p65 Transcription Factor Assay

A NF-κB p65 Transcription Factor Kit (Thermo) was used to measure the level of p65 transcription factor in nuclear protein samples. It contains a 96-well plate pre-coated with a biotinylated consensus DNA sequence which only binds p65. Briefly, nuclear protein samples were added to each well with binding buffer and incubated at RT for 1 h. The plate was then washed and incubated with primary anti-p65 antibody at RT for 1 h.

A

B

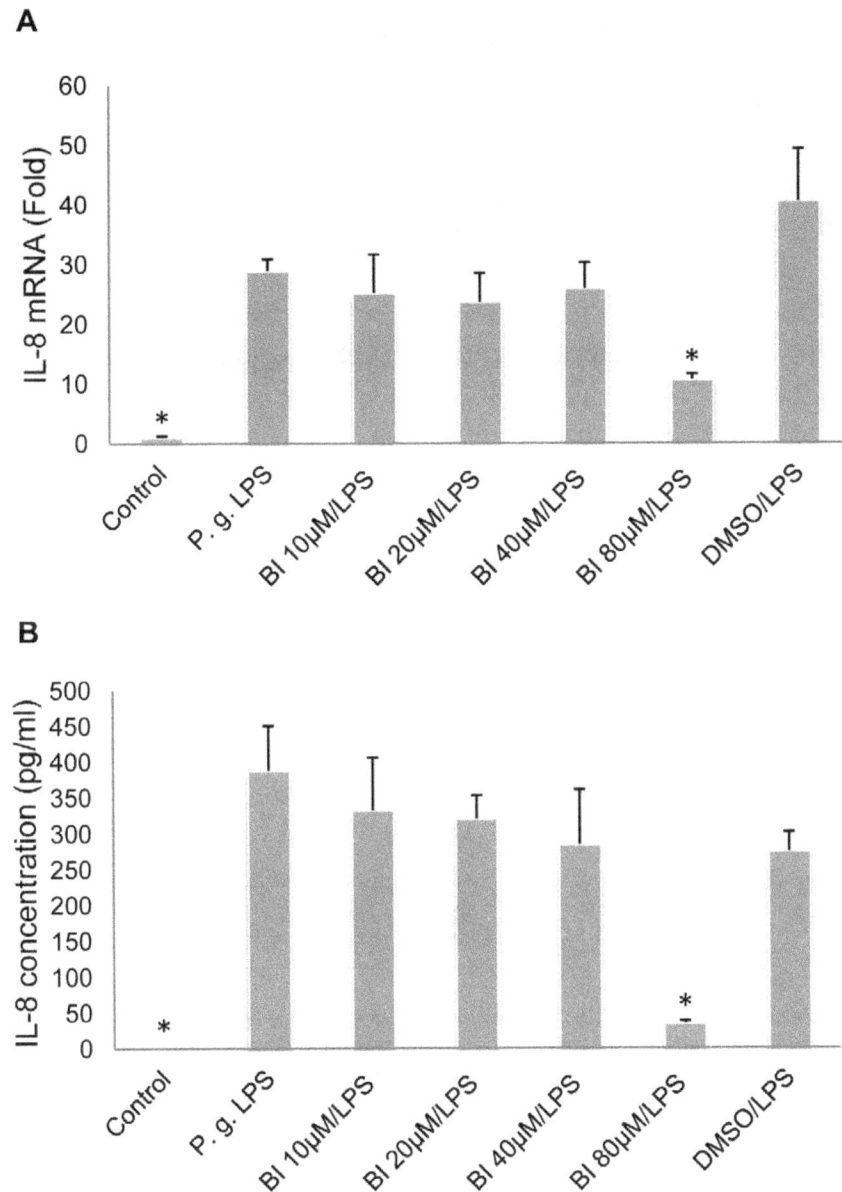

Figure 2. Baicalin significantly downregulates *P. gingivalis* **LPS-upregulated IL-8 expression. A**. Baicalin (BI) at 80 µM significantly downregulated *P. gingivalis* (*P.g.*) LPS-upregulated IL-8 mRNA expression. **B**. Baicalin at 80 µM significantly downregulated *P.g.* LPS-upregulated IL-8 protein expression. Cells treated with culture media alone served as the blank control group, and those treated with *P.g.* LPS (10 µg/ml) alone represented the positive control group. Cells treated with 0.08% DMSO and *P.g.* LPS at 10 µg/ml served as the vehicle control group. Data of three independent experiments were depicted as relative fold change as compared to the blank control group (set as 1) (**A**), or presented as protein concentration (**B**). *$p < 0.01$ as compared with the positive control group (*P.g.* LPS).

Following another around of washing, secondary HRP-conjugated antibodies were added to the plate and incubated at RT for 1 h. Lastly, a chemiluminescent substrate solution was added to the wells. The signal image was captured with a CCD camera and the signal intensity was measured by a multiplate reader.

PCR Array

A panel of 89 genes associated with TLR signal transduction was investigated simultaneously using the RT^2 Profiler^{TM} PCR Arrays (SAbiosciences, MD, USA). RNA samples were firstly reverse transcribed into cDNA templates by the RT^2 First Strand Kit (SAbiosciences). The diluted cDNA templates were subsequently mixed with the RT^2 qPCR Master Mix (SAbiosciences)

and H$_2$O. 25 µl of the mixture were loaded into each well of the array plate which contained pre-coated specific primers. The real-time PCR was performed as follows: an initial incubation at 95°C for 10 min, then 40 cycles at 95°C for 15 s and 60°C for 1 min. Data analysis was undertaken by using the SAbiosciences web-based PCR array data analysis software.

Statistical Analysis

All experiments were repeated three times. The data were presented as mean±SD and the statistical significance was evaluated by one way ANOVA using the SPSS 16.0 software. A *p*-value<0.05 was considered statistically significant.

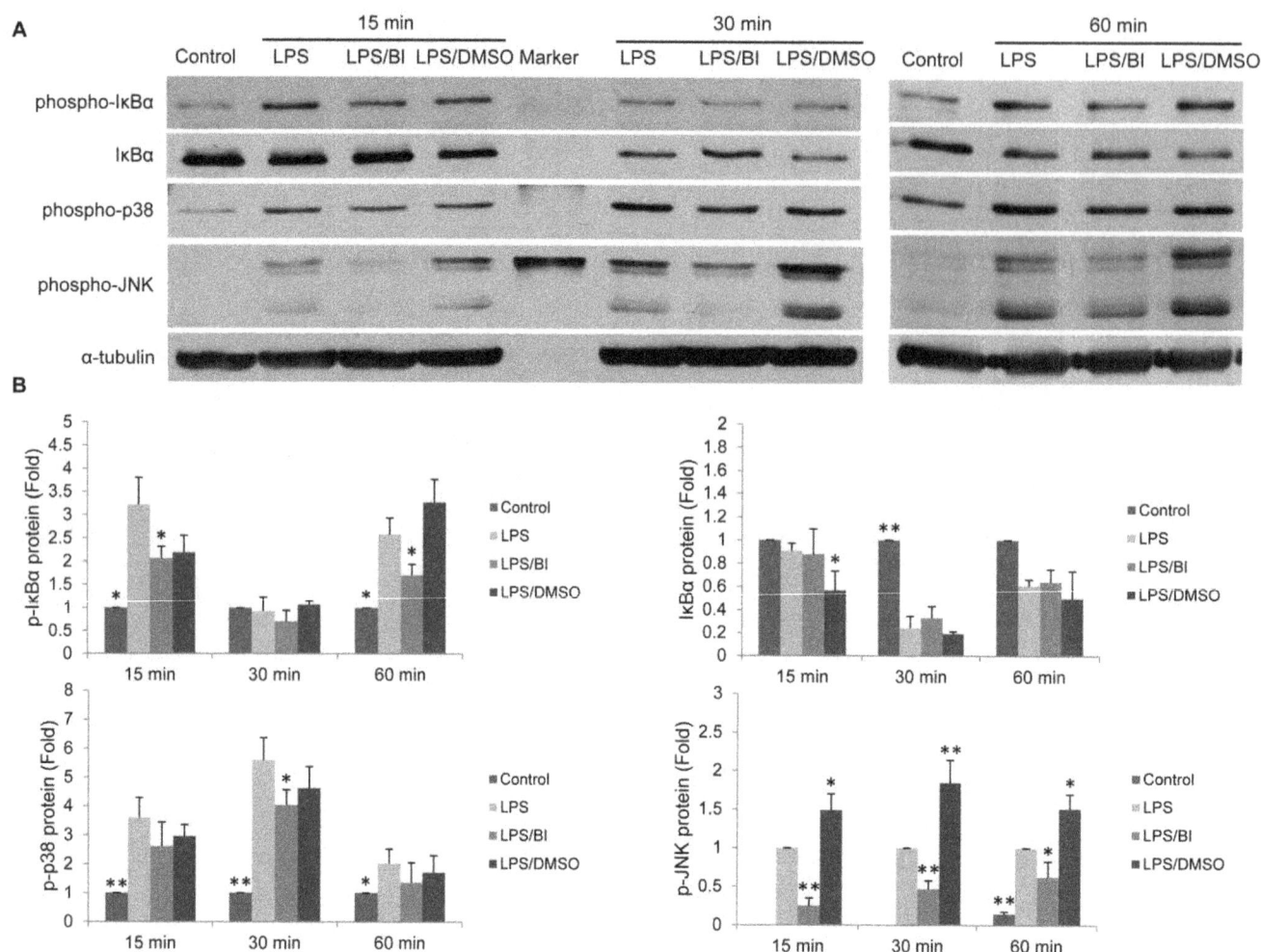

Figure 3. Baicalin inhibits *P. gingivalis* LPS-induced activation of NF-κB, p38 MAPK and JNK. A. The representative western blot experiment was performed by pooling cytoplasmic protein extracts equally from three independent experiments. 25 μg aliquots were loaded into each lane. The membrane was firstly probed with the rabbit anti-phospho-IκBα mAbs (1:2000), and sequentially stripped and re-probed with rabbit anti-phospho-p38 MAPK mAbs (1:2000), rabbit anti-phospho-JNK mAbs (1:2000), and rabbit anti-IκBα mAbs (1:2000). For loading control, the membrane was probed with rabbit anti-α-tubulin mAbs (1:4000). **B.** The densitometry analysis of the signals. Cells treated with culture media alone served as the blank control group, and those treated with *P. gingivalis* (*P.g.*) LPS (10 μg/ml) alone represented the positive control group. Cells treated with *P.g.* LPS at 10 μg/ml and 0.08% DMSO served as the vehicle control group. Data of three independent experiments were depicted as relative fold change as compared with the blank control group (set as 1). For the p-JNK protein, the positive control group (LPS) was set as 1 since the signals of the blank control group at 15 min and 30 min were undetectable. *$p<0.05$ and **$p<0.01$ as compared with the respective positive control group (LPS) at each time point. BI: baicalin.

Results

Baicalin Downregulated *P. gingivalis* LPS-upregulated Expression of IL-6 and IL-8

HOKs were pre-treated with baicalin (0–80 μM) for 24 h, and subsequently treated with fresh media containing *P. gingivalis* LPS (10 μg/ml) with or without baicalin (0–80 μM) for 3 h. The culture supernatants and total RNA were collected for ELISA and real-time PCR analyses, respectively. We discovered that baicalin at 40 μM and 80 μM significantly suppressed *P. gingivalis* LPS-upregulated IL-6 mRNA expression (Fig. 1A); and baicalin at 10 μM, 20 μM, 40 μM and 80 μM significantly downregulated *P. gingivalis* LPS-upregulated IL-6 protein expression (Fig. 1B). Baicalin at 80 μM also significantly suppressed *P. gingivalis* LPS-upregulated IL-8 mRNA and protein expression (Figs. 2A & 2B). As baicalin at 80 μM contained 0.08% DMSO, the observed downregulation could have been partially caused by DMSO. To

exclude this possibility, a vehicle control group was set up by treating cells firstly with 0.08% DMSO for 24 h, and then with *P. gingivalis* LPS (10 μg/ml) and 0.08% DMSO for 3 h. No DMSO-mediated inhibition on IL-6 or IL-8 expression was found (Figs. 1 and 2).

Baicalin Displayed Inhibitory Effect on *P. gingivalis* LPS-induced Activation of NF-κB, p38 MAPK and JNK

In resting cells, inactive NF-κB (p65/p50) is retained in the cytoplasm by an inhibitory protein called IκBα [43]. Upon stimulation, IκBα is ubiquitinated and degraded by 26 S proteasome, resulting in the translocation of NF-κB to the nucleus where it binds to the target genes and initiates gene transcription [43]. As NF-κB plays a central role in *P. gingivalis* LPS-mediated cell response and the expression of IL-6 and IL-8 is dependent on NF-κB signaling [44], we were interested to exam whether baicalin could have any inhibitory effects on *P. gingivalis* LPS-

A

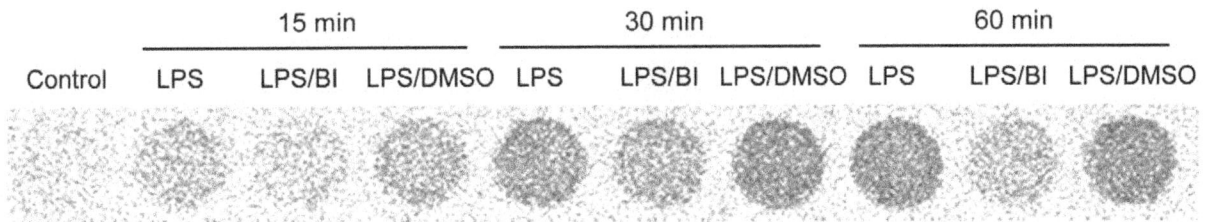

B

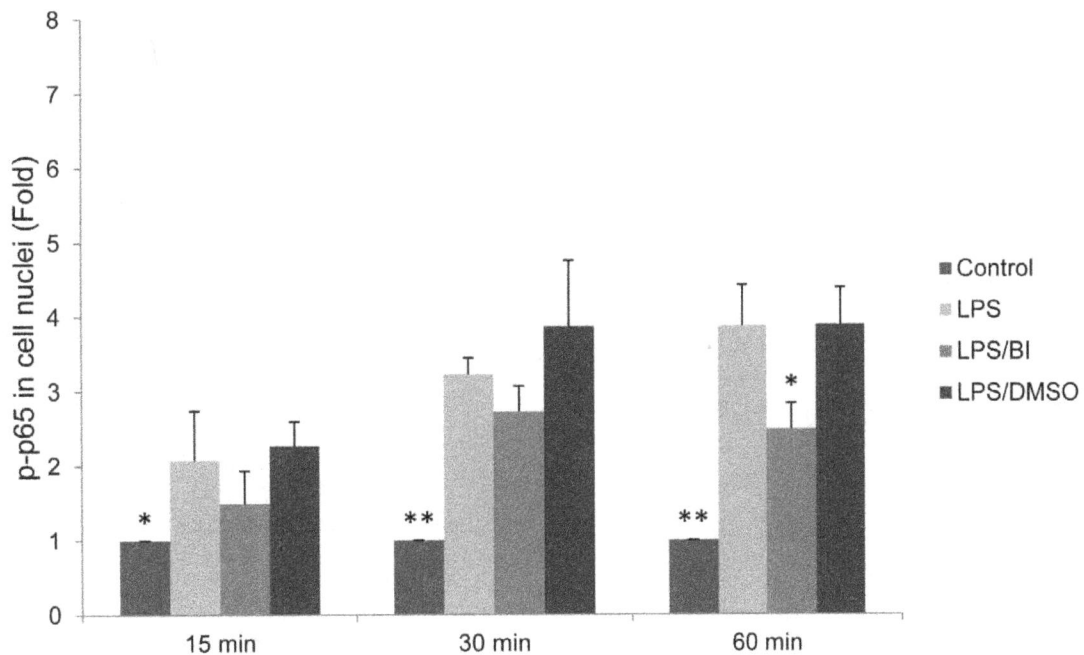

Figure 4. Baicalin suppresses _P. gingivalis_ LPS-induced nuclear translocation of p65. A. The representative experiment was performed by pooling nuclear protein extracts equally from three independent experiments. 2 µg aliquots were added to each well. The assay was carried out according to the manufacturer's instruction. **B.** The intensity analysis of the luminescent signals. Cells treated with culture media alone served as the blank control group, and those treated with _P. gingivalis_ (_P.g._) LPS (10 µg/ml) alone represented the positive control group. Cells treated with _P.g._ LPS at 10 µg/ml and 0.08% DMSO served as the vehicle control group. Data from three independent experiments were depicted as relative fold change as compared with the blank control groups (set as 1). *$p<0.05$ and **$p<0.01$ as compared with the respective positive control group (LPS) at each time point. BI: baicalin.

activated NF-κB. Cells were pre-treated with baicalin (80 µM) for 24 h, and thereafter treated with fresh media containing _P. gingivalis_ LPS (10 µg/ml) with or without baicalin (80 µM) for 15, 30, and 60 min. A vehicle control group was set up by treating cells firstly with 0.08% DMSO for 24 h, and then with _P. gingivalis_ LPS (10 µg/ml) and 0.08% DMSO for 15, 30, and 60 min. As shown in Fig. 3, baicalin significantly inhibited to different extents _P. gingivalis_ LPS-induced phosphorylation of IκBα, p38 MAPK and JNK which act as the downstream of TLR2/4 signaling pathways [45].

Baicalin Suppressed _P. gingivalis_ LPS-induced Nuclear Translocation of p65

The effect of baicalin on _P. gingivalis_ LPS-induced nuclear translocation of p65 was examined by using a p65 transcription factor kit. Cells were pre-treated with baicalin (80 µM) for 24 h, and then treated with fresh media containing _P. gingivalis_ LPS (10 µg/ml) with or without baicalin (80 µM) for 15, 30, and

60 min. Compared with _P. gingivalis_ LPS-treated samples, baicalin succeeded to suppress the amount of translocated p65 in the nuclear protein extracts at 60 min (Fig. 4).

Baicalin Modulated _P. gingivalis_ LPS-induced Expression of Genes Associated with TLR Signaling

Lastly, a PCR array assay was undertaken to profile the expression of genes associated with TLR signaling. Cells were pre-treated with baicalin (80 µM) or culture media for 24 h, and then treated with fresh media containing _P. gingivalis_ LPS (10 µg/ml) with or without baicalin (80 µM) for 3 h. The total RNA was purified and reverse transcribed into cDNA templates. The templates used in PCR array were pooled equally from three independent experiments. Compared with the _P. gingivalis_ LPS-treated cells, the expression of CCL2, CSF2, CSF3, CXCL10, IL-8, V-fos FBJ murine osteosarcoma viral oncogene homolog (FOS) and interferon, beta 1, fibroblast (IFNB1) was significantly downregulated over two folds in baicalin/_P. gingivalis_ LPS treated

Table 1. The fold change in the expression of genes in baicalin/*P. gingivalis* LPS-treated cells (test) with reference to the *P. gingivalis* LPS-treated cells (control).

Wells	Genes	Fold Change	Wells	Genes	Fold Change
A01	BTK	1.04	B01	ELK1	1.37
A02	CASP8	1.11	B02	FADD	1.86
A03	**CCL2**	**0.13**	*B03*	*FOS*	*0.46*
A04	CD14	0.67	B04	HMGB1	1.65
A05	*CD80*	*2.30*	B05	HRAS	1.22
A06	CD86	1.00	B06	HSPA1A	1.66
A07	CHUK	1.21	B07	HSPD1	1.52
A08	CLEC4E	0.80	B08	IFNA1	1.44
A09	*CSF2*	*0.49*	*B09*	*IFNB1*	*0.41*
A10	**CSF3**	**0.21**	B10	IFNG	1.04
A11	**CXCL10**	**0.17**	B11	IKBKB	1.08
A12	EIF2AK2	0.91	B12	IL10	1.04
C01	IL12A	0.96	D01	CD180	0.60
C02	IL1A	0.77	D02	LY86	1.04
C03	IL1B	0.72	D03	LY96	1.07
C04	IL2	1.04	D04	MAP2K3	1.13
C05	IL6	0.55	D05	MAP2K4	1.19
C06	*IL8*	*0.34*	D06	MAP3K1	1.42
C07	*IRAK1*	*2.39*	D07	MAP3K7	1.40
C08	IRAK2	0.64	D08	MAP3K7IP1	1.43
C09	IRF1	1.23	D09	MAP4K4	1.08
C10	IRF3	1.14	D10	MAPK8	1.16
C11	*JUN*	*2.06*	D11	MAPK8IP3	1.95
C12	LTA	1.21	D12	MYD88	1.26
E01	NFKB1	0.70	F01	RIPK2	1.28
E02	NFKB2	1.54	*F02*	*SARM1*	*2.57*
E03	NFKBIA	0.81	*F03*	*SIGIRR*	*2.72*
E04	NFKBIL1	1.35	F04	ECSIT	1.98
E05	NFRKB	1.84	F05	TBK1	1.07
E06	NR2C2	1.30	F06	TICAM2	1.58
E07	PELI1	1.27	*F07*	*TIRAP*	*2.90*
E08	PPARA	1.98	*F08*	*TLR1*	*2.14*
E09	PRKRA	1.28	F09	TLR10	1.20
E10	PTGS2	0.66	F10	TLR2	0.78
E11	REL	1.32	F11	TLR3	0.88
E12	RELA	1.54	F12	TLR4	1.04
G01	TLR5	0.72	H01	B2M	0.70
G02	*TLR6*	*2.34*	H02	HPRT1	0.96
G03	TLR7	1.04	H03	RPL13A	1.27
G04	TLR8	1.04	H04	GAPDH	0.97
G05	TLR9	0.73	H05	ACTB	1.21
G06	TNF	0.84			
G07	TNFRSF1A	1.06			
G08	TOLLIP	1.16			
G09	TRAF6	1.35			
G10	TICAM1	0.96			
G11	UBE2N	1.20			

The genes downregulated over four folds are highlighted in bold, and those up or downregulated two to four folds are highlighted in italics.

cells (Table 1). Notably, CCL2, CSF3 and CXCL10 were markedly downregulated over four folds. On the other hand, other genes including cluster of differentiation 80 (CD80), interleukin-1 receptor-associated kinase 1 (IRAK1), jun proto-oncogene (JUN), TLR6, Ubiquitin-conjugating enzyme E2 variant 1 (UBE2V1), sterile α and TIR motif–containing 1 (SARM1), single Ig IL-1-related receptor (SIGIRR), TIR domain containing adaptor protein (TIRAP) and TLR1 were significantly upregulated over two folds in baicalin/LPS-treated cells (Table 1).

Discussion

Periodontal disease results essentially from the consequence of a disrupted immuno-inflammatory homeostasis of bacteria-host interactions [5]. In susceptible individuals, when host response fails to limit and resolve early infection timely, cytokine expression may become dysregulated and destructive to tissues [46,47]. As IL-6 is a stimulator of bone resorption and IL-8 is a potent neutrophil chemoattractant and activator [48,49], prolonged and excessive production of these pro-inflammatory cytokines could contribute to periodontal tissue damage. Our present study shows that baicalin could significantly downregulate *P. gingivalis* LPS-upregulated production of IL-6 and IL-8 in HOKs. This observation goes in line with the concept of host modulatory therapy, suggesting that baicalin could potentially be used for modulation of host response in treatment of periodontal disease.

The present study also reveals that baicalin may inhibit *P. gingivalis* LPS-induced activation of NF-κB, p38 MAPK and JNK. Due to their involvements in a variety of human diseases, NF-κB, p38 MAPK and JNK have become therapeutic targets and several NF-κB inhibitors have been discovered, such as sulindac [50], IKK inhibitor [51,52] and resveratrol [53]. It has been shown that SD828, a p38 MAPK antagonist, could suppress LPS-induced alveolar bone loss in periodontitis rats [54], and JNK inhibitors like CEP-1347 and AS601245 exhibit protective effects on neurons [55,56]. In the present study, the exact mechanism of baicalin-induced inhibition of *P. gingivalis* LPS-upregulated expression of IL-6 and IL-8 in HOKs remains to be further elucidated. While it could be speculated that the inhibition observed could have been exerted directly on IKK, p38 MAPK and JNK; or on the upstream kinases such as transforming-growth-factor-β-activated kinase 1 (TAK1) (kinase of IKK and p38/JNK MAPK) [57–59], interleukin-1 receptor-associated kinase 1 (IRAK1) (kinase of TAK1), or IRAK4 (kinase of IRAK1) [60–62].

According to the PCR array results, CCL2 [63], CSF3 [64,65] and CXCL10 [66] were greatly downregulated over four folds by baicalin treatment. The transcription of CCL2 and CSF3 is regulated by NF-κB [67,68]. In response to LPS, CXCL10 is induced in a TLR4-mediated MyD88-independent pathway [15,69,70]. The exact reasons that baicalin could downregulate both LPS-induced MyD88-dependent and MyD88-independent genes remain unclear. The possible mechanisms are as follows: i) baicalin might enable to interfere with the binding of *P. gingivalis* LPS to TLR4; ii) it could inhibit multiple downstream kinases of TLR4 signaling, such as IKK, TAK1 and TANK-binding kinase 1 (TBK1) (kinase of IRF3) [71]; iii) as the optimal transcription of CXCL10 requires a coordinated binding of activated IRF3 and NF-κB to the promoter region [15,69], baicalin-mediated inhibition of NF-κB could have interfered with the expression of CXCL10. Further study is warranted to clarify these points.

Over the last three decades, the growing knowledge of periodontal pathogenesis has appreciated the crucial role of host response in the initiation and development of periodontal disease. Recently, TLR signaling has become an attractive target of host modulation therapy due to its central role in activating immuno-imflammatory response in the development of periodontitis [72]. To date, a number of negative regulatory strategies for over-activated TLR signaling have been proposed, such as natural/synthetic antagonists [73,74], BB-loop peptides [75], miRNA [76] and kinase inhibitors [77]. Here, we report for the first time that baicalin can significantly downregulate *P. gingivalis* LPS-upregu-lated IL-6 and IL-8 expression in HOKs, through negative regulation of TLR signaling. Based on these findings, baicalin may potentially serve as a host response modulator in the control of periodontal disease by negative regulation of TLR signaling. Further clinical study is warranted to investigate the effectiveness

of baicalin as a potential adjunct in treatment of patients with inflammatory diseases like periodontal disease.

Acknowledgments

We are grateful to Prof. Y. Abiko (Nihon University, Japan) for providing *P. gingivalis* LPS in the study.

Author Contributions

Conceived and designed the experiments: LJJ WL CYW. Performed the experiments: WL. Analyzed the data: WL LJJ CYW. Contributed reagents/materials/analysis tools: LJJ CYW. Wrote the paper: WL LJJ.

References

1. Jin LJ, Armitage GC, Klinge B, Lang NP, Tonetti M, et al. (2011) Global oral health inequalities: Task group-periodontal disease. Adv Dent Res 23: 221–226.
2. Parahitiyawa NB, Jin LJ, Leung WK, Yam WC, Samaranayake LP (2009) Microbiology of odontogenic bacteraemia: beyond endocarditis. Clin Microbiol Rev 22: 46–64.
3. Li X, Tse HF, Jin LJ (2011) Novel endothelial biomarkers: implications for periodontal disease and CVD. J Dent Res 90: 1062–1069.
4. Lalla E, Papapanou PN (2011) Diabetes mellitus and periodontitis: a tale of two common interrelated diseases. Nat Rev Endocrinol 7: 738–748.
5. Darveau RP (2010) Periodontitis: a polymicrobial disruption of host homeostasis. Nat Rev Microbiol 8: 481–490.
6. Yilmaz O (2008) The chronicles of Porphyromonas gingivalis: the microbium, the human oral epithelium and their interplay. Microbiology 154: 2897–2903.
7. Jain S, Darveau RP (2010) Contribution of Porphyromonas gingivalis lipopolysaccharide to periodontitis. Periodontol 2000 54: 53–70.
8. Herath TDK, Wang Y, Seneviratne CJ, Lu Q, Darveau RP, et al. (2011) Porphyromonas gingivalis lipopolysaccharide lipid A heterogeneity differentially modulates the expression of IL-6 and IL-8 in human gingival fibroblasts. J Clin Periodontol 38: 694–701.
9. Souza PP, Palmqvist P, Lundgren I, Lie A, Costa-Neto CM, et al. (2010) Stimulation of IL-6 cytokines in fibroblasts by toll-like receptors 2. J Periodontal Res 89: 802–807.
10. Seo T, Cha S, Kim TI, Lee JS, Woo KM (2012) Porphyromonas gingivalis-derived lipopolysaccharide-mediated activation of MAPK signaling regulates inflammatory response and differentiation in human periodontal ligament fibroblasts. J Microbiol 50: 311–319.
11. Akira S, Takeda K (2004) Toll-like receptor signalling. Nat Rev Immunol 4: 499–511.
12. Wesche H, Henzel WJ, Shillinglaw W, Li S, Cao Z (1997) MyD88: an adapter that recruits IRAK to the IL-1 receptor complex. Immunity 7: 837–847.
13. Medzhitov R, Preston-Hurlburt P, Kopp E, Stadlen A, Chen C, et al. (1998) MyD88 is an adaptor protein in the hToll/IL-1 receptor family signaling pathways. Mol Cell 2: 253–258.
14. Kawai T, Adachi O, Ogawa T, Takeda K, Akira S (1999) Unresponsiveness of MyD88-deficient mice to endotoxin. Immunity 11: 115–122.
15. Kawai T, Takeuchi O, Fujita T, Inoue J, Mühlradt PF, et al. (2001) Lipopolysaccharide stimulates the MyD88-independent pathway and results in activation of IFN-regulatory factor 3 and the expression of a subset of lipopolysaccharide-inducible genes. J Immunol 167: 5887–5894.
16. Hoshino K, Kaisho T, Iwabe T, Takeuchi O, Akira S (2002) Differential involvement of IFN-β in Toll-like receptor stimulated dendritic cell activation. Int Immunol 14: 1225–1231.
17. Yamamoto M, Sato S, Hemmi H, Hoshino K, Kaisho T, et al. (2003) Role of adaptor TRIF in the MyD88-independent Toll-like receptor signaling pathway. Science 301: 640–643.
18. Sakaguchi S, Negishi H, Asagiri M, Nakajima C, Mizutani T, et al. (2003) Essential role of IRF-3 in lipopolysaccharide-induced interferon-beta gene expression and endotoxin shock. Biochem Biophys Res Commun 306: 860–866.
19. Poltorak A, He X, Smirnova I, Liu MY, Van Huffel C, et al. (1998) Defective LPS signaling in C3H/HeJ and C57BL/10ScCr mice: mutations in Tlr4 gene. Science 282: 2085–2088.
20. Ogawa T, Asai Y, Hashimoto M, Takeuchi O, Kurita T, et al. (2002) Cell activation by Porphyromonas gingivalis lipid A molecule through Toll-like receptor 4- and myeloid differentiation factor 88-dependent signaling pathway. Int Immunol 14: 1325–1332.
21. Sawada N, Ogawa T, Asai Y, Makimura Y, Sugiyama A (2007) Toll-like receptor 4-dependent recognition of structurally different forms of chemically synthesized lipid As of Porphyromonas gingivalis. Clin Exp Immunol 148: 529–536.
22. Hirschfeld M, Weis JJ, Toshchakov V, Salkowski CA, Cody MJ, et al. (2001) Signaling by toll-like receptor 2 and 4 agonists results in differential gene expression in murine macrophages. Infect Immun 69: 1477–1482.
23. Yoshimura A, Kaneko T, Kato Y, Golenbock DT, Hara Y (2002) Lipopolysaccharides from periodontopathic bacteria Porphyromonas gingivalis

and Capnocytophaga ochracea are antagonists for human toll-like receptor 4. Infect Immun 70: 218–225.
24. Burns E, Bachrach G, Shapira L, Nussbaum G (2006) Cutting edge: TLR2 is required for the innate response to Porphyromonas gingivalis: activation leads to bacterial persistence and TLR2 deficiency attenuates induced alveolar bone resorption. J Immunol 177: 8296–8300.
25. Netea MG, van Deuren M, Kullberg BJ, Cavaillon JM, Van der Meer JW (2002) Does the shape of lipid A determine the interaction of LPS with Toll-like receptors? Trends Immunol 23: 135–139.
26. Darveau RP, Pham TT, Lemley K, Reife RA, Bainbridge BW, et al. (2004) Porphyromonas gingivalis lipopolysaccharide contains multiple lipid A species that functionally interact with both toll-like receptors 2 and 4. Infect Immun 72: 5041–5051.
27. Hirschfeld M, Ma Y, Weis JH, Vogel SN, Weis JJ (2000) Cutting edge: repurification of lipopolysaccharide eliminates signaling through both human and murine Toll-like receptor 2. J Immunol 165: 618–622.
28. Ogawa T, Asai Y, Makimura Y, Tamai R (2007) Chemical structure and immunobiological activity of Porphyromonas gingivalis lipid A. Front Biosci 12: 3795–3812.
29. Kumada H, Haishima Y, Watanabe K, Hasegawa C, Tsuchiya T, et al. (2008) Biological properties of the native and synthetic lipid A of Porphyromonas gingivalis lipopolysaccharide. Oral Microbiol Immunol 23: 60–69.
30. Oringer RJ, Research Science, and Therapy Committee of the American Academy of Periodontology (2002) Modulation of the host response in periodontal therapy. J Periodontol 73: 460–470.
31. Bhatavadekar NB, Williams RC (2009) Modulation of the host inflammatory response in periodontal disease management: exciting new directions. Int Dent J 59: 305–308.
32. Serhan CN, Jain A, Marleau S, Clish C, Kantarci A, et al. (2003) Reduced inflammation and tissue damage in transgenic rabbits overexpressing 15-lipoxygenase and endogenous anti-inflammatory lipid mediators. J Immunol 171: 6856–6865.
33. Preshaw PM, Hefti AF, Jepsen S, Etienne D, Walker C, et al. (2004) Subantimicrobial dose doxycycline as adjunctive treatment for periodontitis. A review. J Clin Periodontol 31: 697–707.
34. Hasturk H, Kantarci A, Goguet-Surmenian E, Blackwood A, Andry C, et al. (2007) Resolvin E1 regulates inflammation at the cellular and tissue level and restores tissue homeostasis in vivo. J Immunol 179: 7021–7029.
35. Ikemoto S, Sugimura K, Yoshida N, Yasumoto R, Wada S, et al. (2000) Antitumor effects of Scutellariae radix and its components baicalein, baicalin, and wogonin on bladder cancer cell lines. Urology 55: 951–955.
36. Zhu G, Li C, Cao Z (2007) Inhibitory effect of flavonoid baicalin on degranulation of human polymorphonuclear leukocytes induced by interleu-kin-8: potential role in periodontal diseases. J Ethnopharmacol 109: 325–330.
37. Wang GF, Wu ZF, Wan L, Wang QT, Chen FM (2006) Influence of baicalin on the expression of receptor activator of nuclear factor-kappaB ligand in cultured human periodontal ligament cells. Pharmacology 77: 71–77.
38. Cai X, Li C, Du G, Cao Z (2008) Protective effects of baicalin on the ligature-induced periodontitis in rats. J Periodontal Res 43: 14–21.
39. Cao Z, Li C, Zhu G (2010) Inhibitory effects of baicalin on IL-1beta-induced MMP-1/TIMP-1 and its stimulated effect on collagen-I production in human periodontal ligament cells. Eur J Pharmacoly 641: 1–6.
40. Koga T, Nishihara T, Fujiwara T, Nisizawa T, Okahashi N, et al. (1985) Biochemical and immunobiological properties of lipopolysaccharide (LPS) from Bacteroides gingivalis and comparison with LPS from Escherichia coli. Infect Immun 47: 638–647.
41. Maruyama M, Hayakawa M, Zhang L, Shibata Y, Abiko Y (2009) Monoclonal antibodies produced against lipopolysaccharide from fimA Type II Porphy-omonas gingivalis. Hybridoma 28: 431–434.
42. Peirson SN, Butler JN, Foster RG (2003) Experimental validation of novel and conventional approaches to quantitative real-time PCR data analysis. Nucleic Acids Res 31: 73–80.
43. Karin M, Ben-Neriah Y (2000) Phosphorylation meets ubiquitination: the control of NF-kB activity. Annu Rev Immunol 18: 621–663.

44. Carayol N, Chen J, Yang F, Jin T, Jin LJ, et al. (2006) A Dominant Function of IKK/NF-kB Signaling in Global Lipopolysaccharide-induced Gene Expression. J Biol Chem 281: 31142–31151.

45. Chang L, Karin M (2001) Mammalian MAP kinase signalling cascades. Nature 410: 37–40.

46. Garlet GP (2010) Destructive and protective roles of cytokines in periodontitis: a re-appraisal from host defense and tissue destruction viewpoints. J Dent Res 89: 1349–1363.

47. Liu YC, Lerner UH, Teng YT (2010) Cytokine responses against periodontal infection: protective and destructive roles. Periodontol 2000 52: 163–120.

48. Baggiolini M, Walz A, Kunkel SL (1989) Neutrophil-activating peptide- 1/ interleukin-8, a novel cytokine that activates neutrophils. J Clin Invest 84: 1045–1049.

49. Palmqvist P, Persson E, Conaway HH, Lerner UH (2002) IL-6, leukemia inhibitory factor, and oncostatin M stimulate bone resorption and regulate the expression of receptor activator of NF-kappa B ligand, osteoprotegerin, and receptor activator of NF-kappa B in mouse calvariae. J Immunol 169: 3353–3362.

50. Berman KS, Verma UN, Harburg G, Minna JD, Cobb MH, et al. (2002) Sulindac enhances tumor necrosis factor-α-mediated apoptosis of lung cancer cell lines by inhibition of nuclear factor-κB. Clin Cancer Res 8: 354–360.

51. Burke JR, Pattoli MA, Gregor KR, Brassil PJ, MacMaster JF, et al. (2003) BMS-345541 is a highly selective inhibitor of IκB kinase that binds at an allosteric site of the enzyme and blocks NF-κB-dependent transcription in mice. J Biol Chem 278: 1450–1456.

52. Kishore N, Sommers C, Mathialagan S, Guzova J, Yao M, et al. (2003) A selective IKK-2 inhibitor blocks NF-κBdependent gene expression in IL-1β stimulated synovial fibroblasts. J Biol Chem 278: 32861–32871.

53. Park HJ, Jeong SK, Kim SR, Bae SK, Kim WS, et al. (2009) Resveratrol inhibits Porphyromonas gingivalis lipopolysaccharideinduced endothelial adhesion molecule expression by suppressing NF-kappaB activation. Arch Pharm Res 32: 583–591.

54. Rogers JE, Li F, Coatney DD, Otremba J, Kriegl JM, et al. (2007) A p38 mitogen-activated protein kinase inhibitor arrests active alveolar bone loss in a rat periodontitis model. J Periodontol 78: 1992–1998.

55. Saporito MS, Brown EM, Miller MS, Carswell S (1999) CEP-1347/KT-7515, an inhibitor of c-jun N-terminal kinase activation, attenuates the 1-methyl-4-phenyl tetrahydropyridine-mediated loss of nigrostriatal dopaminergic neurons In vivo. J Pharmacol Exp Ther 288: 421–427.

56. Carboni S, Hiver A, Szyndralewiez C, Gaillard P, Gotteland JP, et al. (2004) AS601245 (1,3-benzothiazol-2-yl (2-[[2-(3-pyridinyl) ethyl] amino]-4 pyrimidinyl) acetonitrile): a c-Jun NH2-terminal protein kinase inhibitor with neuroprotective properties. J Pharmacol Exp Ther 310: 25–32.

57. Yamaguchi K, Shirakabe K, Shibuya H, Irie K, Oishi I, et al. (1995) Identification of a member of the MAPKKK family as a potential mediator of TGF-beta signal transduction. Science 270: 2008–2011.

58. Lee J, Mira-Arbibe L, Ulevitch RJ (2000) TAK1 regulates multiple protein kinase cascades activated by bacterial lipopolysaccharide. J Leukoc Biol 68: 909–915.

59. Wang C, Deng L, Hong M, Akkaraju GR, Inoue J, et al. (2001) TAK1 is a ubiquitin-dependent kinase of MKK and IKK. Nature 412: 346–351.

60. Cao Z, Henzel WJ, Gao X (1996) IRAK: a kinase associated with the interleukin-1 receptor. Science 271: 1128–1131.

61. Li S, Strelow A, Fontana EJ, Wesche H (2002) IRAK-4: a novel member of the IRAK family with the properties of an IRAK-kinase. Proc Natl Acad Sci USA 99: 5567–5572.

62. Janssens S, Beyaert R (2003) Functional diversity and regulation of different interleukin-1 receptor-associated kinase (IRAK) family members. Mol Cell 11: 293–302.

63. Deshmane SL, Kremlev S, Amini S, Sawaya BE (2009) Monocyte chemoattractant protein-1 (MCP-1): an overview. J Interferon Cytokine Res 29: 313–326.

64. Demetri GD, Griffin JD (1991) Granulocyte colony-stimulating factor and its receptor. Blood 78: 2791–2808.

65. Lieschke GJ, Grail D, Hodgson G, Metcalf D, Stanley E, et al. (1994) Mice lacking granulocyte colony-stimulating factor have chronic neutropenia, granulocyte and macrophage progenitor cell deficiency, and impaired neutrophil mobilization. Blood 84: 1737–1746.

66. Liu M, Guo S, Hibbert JM, Jain V, Singh N, et al. (2011) CXCL10/IP-10 in infectious diseases pathogenesis and potential therapeutic implications. Cytokine Growth Factor Rev 22: 121–130.

67. Ueda A, Ishigatsubo Y, Okubo T, Yoshimura T (1997) Transcriptional regulation of the human monocyte chemoattractant protein-1 gene. Cooperation of two NF-kappaB sites and NF-kappaB/Rel subunit specificity. J Biol Chem 272: 31092–31099.

68. Campbell IK, van Nieuwenhuijze A, Segura E, O'Donnell K, Coghill E, et al. (2011) Differentiation of inflammatory dendritic cells is mediated by NF-κB1-dependent GM-CSF production in CD4 T cells. J Immunol 186: 5468–5477.

69. Doyle S, Vaidya S, O'Connell R, Dadgostar H, Dempsey P, et al. (2002) IRF3 mediates a TLR3/TLR4-specific antiviral gene program. Immunity 17: 251–263.

70. Toshchakov V, Jones BW, Perera PY, Thomas K, Cody MJ, et al. (2003) TLR4, but not TLR2, mediates IFN-beta-induced STAT1alpha/beta-dependent gene expression in macrophages. Nat Immunol 3: 392–398.

71. Fitzgerald KA, McWhirter SM, Faia KL, Rowe DC, Latz E, et al. (2003) IKKε and TBK1 are essential components of the IRF3 signaling pathway. Nature Immunol 4: 491–496.

72. Hajishengallis G (2009) Toll gates to periodontal host modulation and vaccine therapy. Periodontol 2000 51: 181–207.

73. Macagno A, Molteni M, Rinaldi A, Bertoni F, Lanzavecchia A, et al. (2006) A cyanobacterial LPS antagonist prevents endotoxin shock and blocks sustained TLR4 stimulation required for cytokine expression. J Exp Med 203: 1481–1492.

74. Kim HM, Park BS, Kim JI, Kim SE, Lee J, et al. (2007) Crystal structure of the TLR4-MD-2 complex with bound endotoxin antagonist Eritoran. Cell 130: 906–917.

75. Toshchakov VY, Fenton MJ, Vogel SN (2007) Cutting edge: differential inhibition of TLR signaling pathways by cell permeable peptides representing BB loops of TLRs. J Immunol 178: 2655–2660.

76. Benakanakere MR, Li Q, Eskan MA, Singh AV, Zhao J, et al. (2009) Modulation of TLR2 protein expression by miR-105 in human oral keratinocytes. J Biol Chem 284: 23107–23115.

77. Dominguez C, Powers DA, Tamayo N (2005) p38 MAP kinase inhibitors: many are made, but few are chosen. Curr Opin Drug Discov Devel 8: 421–430.

6

Porphyromonas gingivalis Peptidylarginine Deiminase, a Key Contributor in the Pathogenesis of Experimental Periodontal Disease and Experimental Arthritis

Neville Gully[1], Richard Bright[1], Victor Marino[1], Ceilidh Marchant[1], Melissa Cantley[2], David Haynes[2], Catherine Butler[3], Stuart Dashper[3], Eric Reynolds[3], Mark Bartold[1]*

1 Colgate Australian Clinical Dental Research, School of Dentistry, University of Adelaide, Adelaide, South Australia, Australia, 2 Discipline of Anatomy and Pathology, School of Medical Sciences, University of Adelaide, Adelaide, South Australia, Australia, 3 Oral Health Collaborative Research Centre, Melbourne Dental School, The University of Melbourne, Melbourne, Victoria, Australia

Abstract

Objectives: To investigate the suggested role of *Porphyromonas gingivalis* peptidylarginine deiminase (PAD) in the relationship between the aetiology of periodontal disease and experimentally induced arthritis and the possible association between these two conditions.

Methods: A genetically modified PAD-deficient strain of *P. gingivalis* W50 was produced. The effect of this strain, compared to the wild type, in an established murine model for experimental periodontitis and experimental arthritis was assessed. Experimental periodontitis was induced following oral inoculation with the PAD-deficient and wild type strains of *P. gingivalis*. Experimental arthritis was induced via the collagen antibody induction process and was monitored by assessment of paw swelling and micro-CT analysis of the radio-carpal joints. Experimental periodontitis was monitored by micro CT scans of the mandible and histological assessment of the periodontal tissues around the mandibular molars. Serum levels of anti-citrullinated protein antibodies (ACPA) and *P. gingivalis* were assessed by ELISA.

Results: The development of experimental periodontitis was significantly reduced in the presence of the PAD-deficient *P. gingivalis* strain. When experimental arthritis was induced in the presence of the PAD-deficient strain there was less paw swelling, less erosive bone damage to the joints and reduced serum ACPA levels when compared to the wild type *P. gingivalis* inoculated group.

Conclusion: This study has demonstrated that a PAD-deficient strain of *P. gingivalis* was associated with significantly reduced periodontal inflammation. In addition the extent of experimental arthritis was significantly reduced in animals exposed to prior induction of periodontal disease through oral inoculation of the PAD-deficient strain versus the wild type. This adds further evidence to the potential role for *P. gingivalis* and its PAD in the pathogenesis of periodontitis and exacerbation of arthritis. Further studies are now needed to elucidate the mechanisms which drive these processes.

Editor: Özlem Yilmaz, University of Florida, United States of America

Funding: This study was supported in part by research grants from the Australian Dental Research Fund (ADRF 56/2010) and the National Health & Medical Council of Australia (NHMRC 1023747). The funders had no role in study design, data collection and analysis, decision to publish, or preparation of the manuscript.

Competing Interests: The authors have declared that no competing interests exist.

* Email: mark.bartold@adelaide.edu.au

Introduction

The endogenous microbes inhabiting humans often interact in complex ways with their hosts. Changes in the local environment can lead to qualitative and/or quantitative changes in commensal microbial communities that, if left unchecked, can result in disease. Chronic periodontitis is a common inflammatory condition affecting the tissues surrounding teeth. A prolonged, uncontrolled inflammatory response to the sub-gingival microbial load may lead to loss of periodontal ligament attachment and the adjacent alveolar bone [1]. In recent years periodontitis has been linked to the development of other disorders, such as coronary heart disease, diabetes mellitus and low birth weight [2]. While these associations are largely based on epidemiological evidence and for most there is currently no apparent common underlying cause, dysregulation of the inflammatory response seems to be a common underlying feature [3]. Two of the most prevalent chronic inflammatory conditions affecting humans that share many common features, including destruction of both fibrous connective tissue and bone, osteoclast activation and many common risk factors, are periodontitis and rheumatoid arthritis (RA) [4,5].

While elevated microbial load is an important factor in the initiation of periodontitis, it is the increase in proportion of specific microbial pathogens that is likely to be the crucial factor in the subsequent progression of this condition [6]. Periodontitis, particularly in its more severe form, has been linked to a biofilm that contains a consortium of oral pathogens that includes the Gram negative anaerobe *Porphyromonas gingivalis*. [7,8]. *P. gingivalis* expresses a peptidylarginine deiminase (PAD) known as PPAD, an enzyme that modifies peptidylarginine residues to citrulline and is unique in this regard amongst prokaryotes [9]. PPAD is not evolutionarily related to the mammalian PADs that catalyse the same reaction, which is the modification of the guanidino group of arginine residues to produce peptidyl-citrulline and ammonia. While citrullination mediated by host PADs is generally considered a fundamental process (e.g apoptosis), it is also associated with inflammation in mammals [10].

When investigating potential common causal links between periodontitis and RA, the ability of *P. gingivalis* to citrullinate peptides is noteworthy as auto-antibodies against citrullinated peptides are highly specific and sensitive in RA diagnosis [11]. Post-translationally modified peptides and proteins containing citrulline can exhibit altered epitopes compared to those that are unmodified [12]. Accordingly, citrullination has been reported to trigger an auto-immune response [11,13] via modified self-proteins and peptides perceived as foreign by the immune system [14]. While citrullinated peptides may be involved in the pathogenesis of RA the nature of their role is unclear and the contributions of host or prokaryote PADs to citrullination is unknown.

It has been proposed that the increased levels of *P. gingivalis* in patients suffering from chronic periodontitis might influence the development of RA, via PPAD promotion of peptide citrullination, thus explaining the over representation of patients presenting with periodontitis suffering from RA [15–17].

Therefore the aims of this investigation were to construct a PAD-deficient *P. gingivalis* strain and compare the onset and severity of arthritis and periodontitis in a mouse model in the presence of either the wild type or PAD-negative strain.

Materials and Methods

Ethics

Approval for the use of BALB/c mice in this study was obtained from the University of Adelaide, Animal Ethics Committee (Project N° M-2012-183R). The animals were housed in the University of Adelaide PC2 Animal holding facility (OGTR certification No 2067/2008). Approval to culture and prepare inoculates of the genetically modified *P. gingivalis* strain ECR527 was granted by the Institutional Biosafety Committee of the University of Adelaide (Approval No: IBC Dealing ID 10890). The animals were assessed daily for a number of general health parameters including dull/ruffled coat, a change in temperament, reduced food/water intake or a reluctance to move and body weight recorded.

Bacterial Strains and Culture Conditions

P. gingivalis strain W50 (wild type) was obtained from the culture collection of the Oral Health CRC, Melbourne Dental School, University of Melbourne. A PAD-deficient strain (ECR527) was derived from W50 for this study. *P. gingivalis* strains were routinely maintained on Horse Blood Agar (HBA) plates and antibiotic selection of 10 µg/mL erythromycin when appropriate. *E. coli* alpha-select gold cells (Bioline, London, UK) were grown at 37°C in Luria Bertani (LB) Broth or maintained on LB agar with 100 µg/mL ampicillin when harbouring pGEM-TEasy plasmids (Promega, Madison, WI, USA).

DNA Analysis and Manipulations

Oligonucleotide primers used in this study are listed in Table 1. Genomic DNA from *P. gingivalis* strains was prepared using the DNeasy Blood and Tissue kit (Qiagen) and plasmid DNA was extracted from *E. coli* using the QIAprep spin miniprep kit (Qiagen, Venlo, Netherlands). DNA was sequenced by Applied Genetics Diagnostics, The University of Melbourne.

RT-PCR

RNA was isolated using a NucleoSpin RNA II Total RNA Isolation kit (Macherey-Nagel, Duren, Germany) and cDNA was generated using a SuperScrip III Reverse Transcriptase First-Strand Synthesis SuperMix for qRT-PCR kit with random hexamers (Life Technologies, California, USA), both according to the manufacturer's instructions. BIOTAQ Red DNA Polymerase (Bioline, London, UK) was then used to PCR from the following templates: 125 ng of cDNA, 125 ng RNA that was not reverse transcribed, milliQ H_2O and 13 ng W50 genomic DNA in 50 µL reactions with gene-specific primer pairs (Table 1) for 30 cycles in a G-Storm GS1 thermal cycler (Gene Works, Adelaide, Australia). The expected product size from each primer pair was 682 bp for PG1424-RT-Fwd and PG1423-RT-Rev; and 1181 bp from PG1424-RT-Fwd and PG1422-RT-Rev. DNA was electrophoresed at 80 V for 40 min using a 1.0% agarose gel prepared with tris-acetate buffer (40 mM tris-acetate, 1 mM EDTA, pH 8).

Construction of *P. gingivalis* PAD-deficient Strain ECR527

The recombination cassette for deletion of the *pad* gene consisted of 972 bp upstream of the *PG1424* (*pad*) ORF which encompassed *PG1426*, followed by the *ermF* gene encoding erythromycin resistance in *P. gingivalis*, followed by 741 bp downstream of the *PG1424* ORF which encompassed *PG1423*. This recombination cassette resulted in replacement of *PG1424* with *ermF* and was constructed from three separate PCR products that were spliced together using gene splicing by overlap extension PCRs (SOE PCR) to form the final cassette. SOE PCRs were performed essentially as previously described [18]. The PCR products that flanked the PG1424 ORF were amplified from W50 genomic DNA: *PG1426* (primers PG1426-Fwd and ErmF-PG1426-Rev) and *PG1423* (primers ErmF-PG1423-Fwd and PG1423-Rev). The *ermF* gene was amplified from pVA2198 [19] with primers PG1426-ErmF-Fwd and PG1423-ErmF-Rev. All PCRs were performed with Herculase II DNA Polymerase (Stratagene, La Jolla, Ca, USA) except for the final SOE PCR which was amplified with Platinum Taq DNA Polymerase High Fidelity (Life Technologies, California, USA). PCR products were purified using the NucleoSpin Extract II purification kit (Macherey Nagel, Duren, Germany) according to manufacturer's instructions. The final PCR product was ligated with pGEM-TEasy and transformed into *E. coli* alpha-select gold competent cells (Bioline) by heat shock according to manufacturer's instructions. The resulting plasmid was sequenced to confirm the fidelity of the recombination cassette then it was linearised and 200 ng electroporated into *P. gingivalis* W50 in a 0.1 cm gap cuvette at 1.8 kV, 200 Ohms resistance. The resulting PAD-deficient strain was named ECR527.

Measurement of PAD Activity

A colorimetric microtitre plate assay for the determination of enzymatic deimination of the substrate N-α-benzoyl-L-arginine ethyl ester (BAEE) was performed as previously described [20,21]. Briefly, cells from three biological replicate cultures each of *P. gingivalis* W50 and ECR527 (OD_{650} 1.1–1.3) were washed and

Table 1. Oligonucleotide primers used in this study.

Oligonucleotide Primer	Sequence (5′-3′)[a]	Purpose
PG1424-RT-Fwd	ATCGAAGCAGATGTCGTCTCAT	RT PCR
PG1423-RT-Rev	TACGAAACCAATGCTCAGATTTTG	RT PCR
PG1422-RT-Rev	ATAGTTGGATGCGAGAGAAGGA	RT PCR
PG1426-Fwd	GAAGCACGTAATAAGGACAATGAC	*pad* recombination cassette
ErmF-PG1426-Rev	ACGGGCAATTTCTTTTTTGTCATTGTTTGATATGTTTTATGATGTTATGAA	*pad* recombination cassette
PG1426-ErmF-Fwd	TTCATAACATCATAAAACATATCAAACAATGACAAAAAAGAAATTGCCCGT	*pad* recombination cassette
PG1423-ErmF-Rev	GTATTCTCAAATAAGGGGCCTTACGAAGGATGAAATTTTTCAGG	*pad* recombination cassette
ErmF-PG1423-Fwd	CCTGAAAAATTTCATCCTTCGTAAGGCCCCTTATTTGAGAATAC	*pad* recombination cassette
PG1423-Rev	CATCGACGATGATATCTCCTGT	*pad* recombination cassette

[a]Underlined sequence of SOE primers indicates the part of the primer that is not complementary to the target sequence, but provides complementarity with a second PCR product for splicing.

resuspended in 0.2 M Tris-HCl (pH 8), 1 mM EDTA, 1 μM flavin mononucleotide and 10 mM cysteine. A 10 μL aliquot of BAEE (30 mM) was added to 50 μL cells (1×10^8 cfu) and incubated at 37°C for 30 min before addition of 200 μL of detection reagent. The detection reagent was assembled daily from its two components with one part A (0.5% diacetyl monoxime and 0.01% thiosemicarbazide) added to two parts B (0.25 mg of $FeCl_3$/mL in 24.5% sulphuric acid and 17% phosphoric acid). The reaction plate was heated at 105°C for 25 min, then cooled and optically measured at 490 nm using a Bio-Tek Powerwave

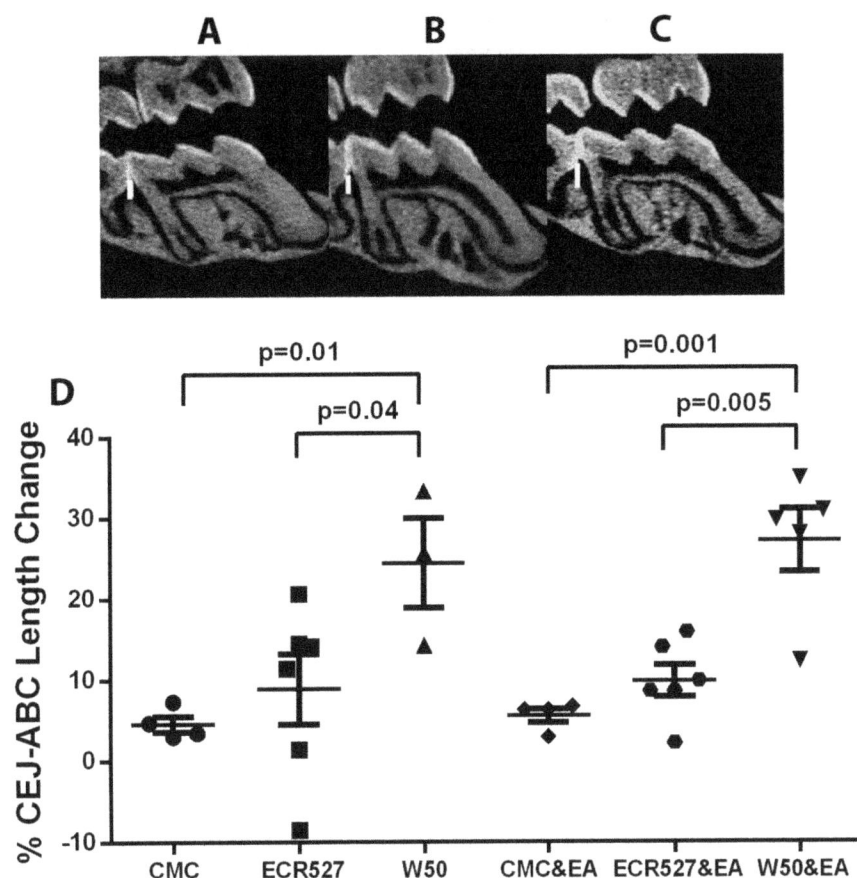

Figure 1. Micro CT appearance and analysis of periodontal bone loss. A. Micro CT of mouse jaw for CMC control group. B. Micro CT of mouse jaw for ECR527 & EA group. C. Micro CT of mouse jaw W50 & EA group. D. Measurements of bone changes in the jaw were calculated by measuring the cemento-enamel junction-alveolar bone crest on three slices for each mouse using CTAn sagital sections. Data represent mean (± SEM). The number of animals in each group was 6 and measurements were performed in triplicate. Statistical analysis was done by one way ANOVA and Tukey multiple comparisons. White bars represent CEJ/ABC distance measurements. *Abbreviations:* CMC = carboxymethyl cellulose; ECR527 = PAD-deficient *P. gingivalis*; W50 = wild type *P. Gingivalis*; EA = experimental arthritis

Table 2. Recovery of viable *P. gingivalis* from oral swabs after final inoculation.

Group	Recovery 0 hr	Recovery 6 hr	Recovery 24 hr	PPAD activity
Control	−	−	−	−
Wild-type (W50)	+	+	+	*
PAD-deficient (ECR527)	+	+	+	−

(+) Viable wild type (W50) and PAD-deficient (ECR527) *P. gingivalis strains* W50 and ECR527 were recovered from the gingiva of each group of mice inoculated separately with each strain at the three time points assayed. The colonies in both groups were black pigmented with gram negative staining organisms.
(−) No viable organisms were recovered from the control group receiving the vehicle (2% CMC).
(*) PPAD activity was only demonstrated in the group of mice where *P. gingivalis* W50 was recovered from gingival swabs.

spectrophotometer (Biotek Instruments, Winooski, VT, USA). A standard curve was generated using 0–400 µM L-citrulline using the same method to quantify citrulline in samples.

Animal Groupings

Thirty six female BALB/c mice between 6 and 8 weeks old were acquired from the Laboratory Animal Services (LAS) of the University of Adelaide. Six experimental groups each containing six mice were used. All groups received oral inoculations for the duration of the study and three groups in addition to the inoculations were induced with experimental arthritis (EA) using a mouse monoclonal antibody against type II collagen (Arthrogen-CIA Arthritogenic Monoclonal Antibody, Chondrex Inc., Redwood, WA, USA).

Group 1: Control: 2% Carboxylmethylcellulose (CMC) (Sigma, St Louis, MO, USA)

Group 2: PPAD⁻: PAD-deficient *P. gingivalis* (ECR527)

Group 3: PPAD⁺: Wild type *P. gingivalis* (W50)

Group 4: Control + EA: 2% CMC with induced EA

Group 5: PPAD⁻ + EA: PAD-deficient *P. gingivalis* (ECR527) with induced EA

Group 6: PPAD⁺ + EA: Wild type *P. gingivalis* (W50) with induced EA

Induction of Experimental Periodontitis by Oral Inoculation

The preparation of the inocula and the inoculation protocol to induce an experimental periodontitis in female BALB/c mice has been previously described [22]. All mice were inoculated with either wild type *P. gingivalis* (Groups 3 and 6) or PAD-deficient *P. gingivalis* (Groups 2 and 5). The control groups (Groups 1 and 4)

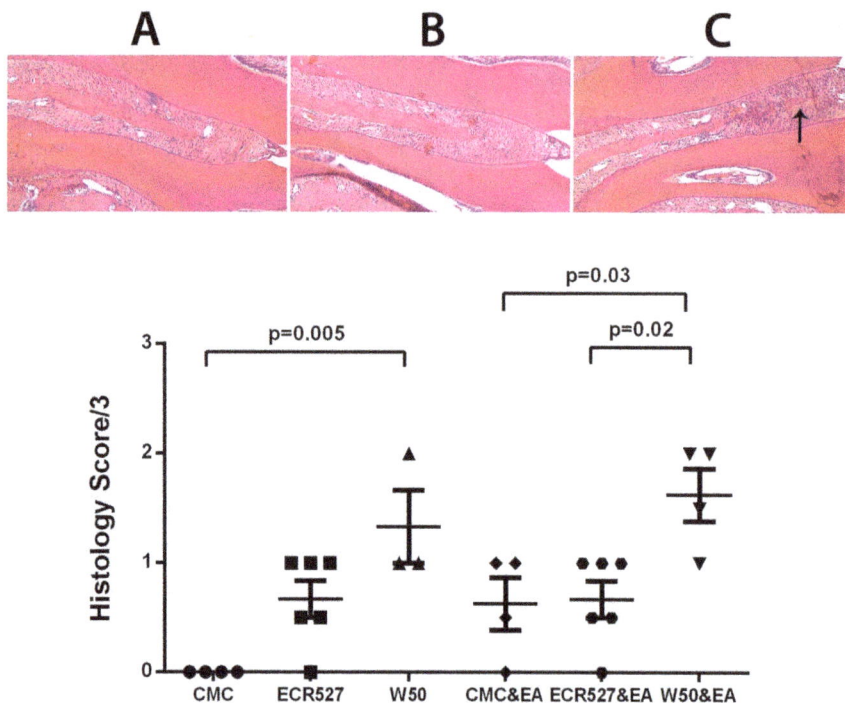

Figure 2. Histological analysis of maxillary periodontal tissues. A. Histology of mouse jaw for CMC control group at day 63. B. Histology of mouse jaw for ECR527 & EA group at day 63. C. Histology of mouse jaw for W50 & EA group at day 63. Arrow indicates increased inflammatory reaction in supra-crestal alveolar bone gingival tissue. D. Histological scores (mean ± SEM) for the presence of osteoclasts and evidence of bone erosion around the first and second upper molars for all groups in the study. Original magnification of A–C = 100X. The number of animals in each group was 6 and measurements were performed in triplicate. Statistical analysis was done by one way ANOVA and Tukey multiple comparisons. *Abbreviations:* CMC = carboxymethyl cellulose; ECR527 = PAD-deficient *P. gingivalis*; W50 = wild type *P. Gingivalis*; EA = experimental arthritis.

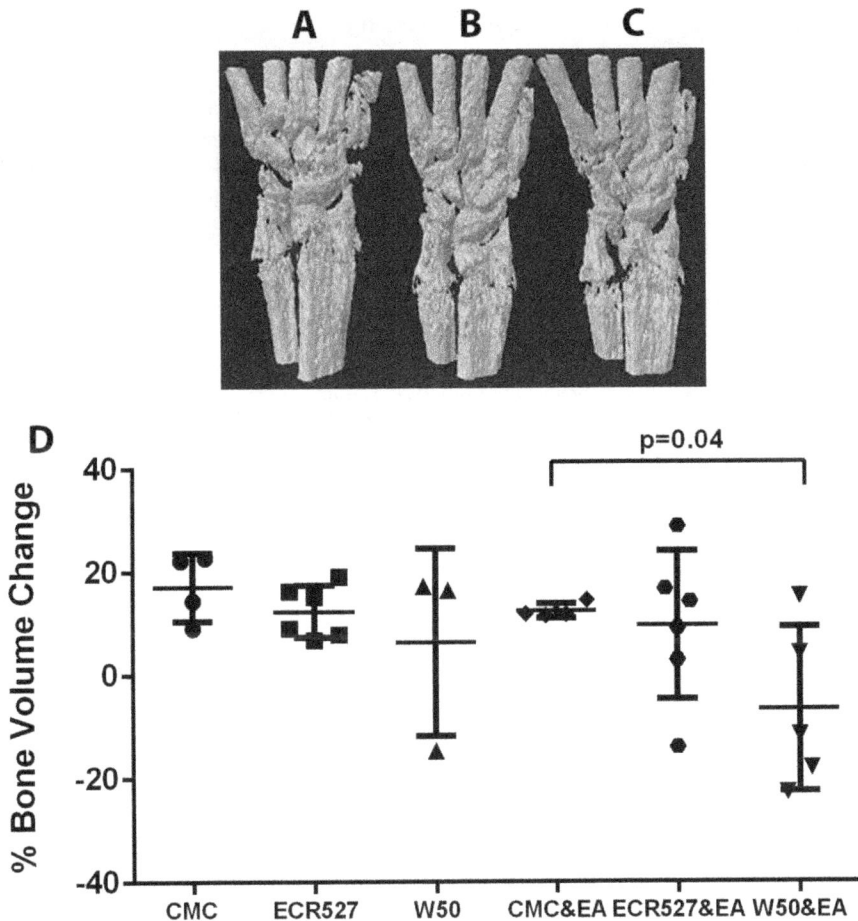

Figure 3. Micro CT appearance and analysis of bone erosion in front paw radio-carpal joint. A. Micro CT appearance of paw for CMC control group at day 63. B. Micro CT appearance of paw for ECR527 & EA group at day 63. C. Micro CT appearance of paw for W50 & EA group at day 63. D. The front paws (left and right combined), were processed to determine bone loss/growth between the two scanned time points in the radio-carpal joint. Data represent mean (± SEM). The number of animals in each group was 6 and measurements were performed in duplicate. Statistical analysis was done by one way ANOVA and Bonferroni multiple comparisons. *Abbreviations:* CMC = carboxymethyl cellulose; ECR527 = PAD-deficient *P. gingivalis*; W50 = wild type *P. Gingivalis*; EA = experimental arthritis

were inoculated with the suspension vehicle for *P. gingivalis* strains, 2% CMC. PPAD activity for both strains was assessed prior to the preparation of each inoculum using the colorimetric method described above. Animals were inoculated over two intensive sequences, each comprising four inoculations over an eight day period. The first sequence commenced two days after the mice had completed 7 days of antibiotic treatment of 1 mg/mL kanamycin (Sigma, St. Louis, MO, USA) in deionised water *ad libitum*. The inoculation sequences were separated by a period of two weeks and during this period mice were inoculated twice a week. Following the second intensive inoculation sequence all mice continued to be inoculated twice a week for the remainder of the experimental period. All animal inoculations were performed by experienced professional staff within a Class II Biological safety cabinet and PC2 animal holding facility.

Induction of Collagen Antibody-induced Arthritis - Experimental Arthritis

Experimental arthritis (EA) was induced in Groups 4–6 by intravenous tail vein injection with 1.5 mg of a mouse monoclonal antibody against type II collagen (Arthrogen-CIA Arthritogenic Monoclonal Antibody, Chondrex Inc., Redwood, WA, USA).

This procedure was performed two days after completion of the second intensive inoculation sequence (day 44). To aid in the induction of EA a dose of 5 μg of lipopolysaccharide (LPS) was intraperitoneally administered three days after the antibody exposure, as described previously [23].

Visual Scoring of Paw Swelling

Front and rear paws were visually assessed and scored each day by two experienced observers to assess swelling and inflammation. Two different scales were used to assess paw changes throughout the experiment. Firstly each inflamed toe or knuckle received a score of 1 and a fully inflamed swollen wrist/ankle a score of 5. Each assessed paw received a score between 0–15 and the total score per mouse was 0–60 [24]. The second system employed a scoring system whereby each paw was allocated a score from zero to four according to the level of inflammation and swelling to make a total score of 16 for each animal. 0 = normal paw, 1 = mild but definite redness and swelling of the wrist/ankle, 2 = moderate swelling and redness of the wrist/ankle with digit involvement, 3 = severe swelling and redness of the paw with digit involvement and 4 = maximum inflammation the entire paw, with multiple digit involvement.

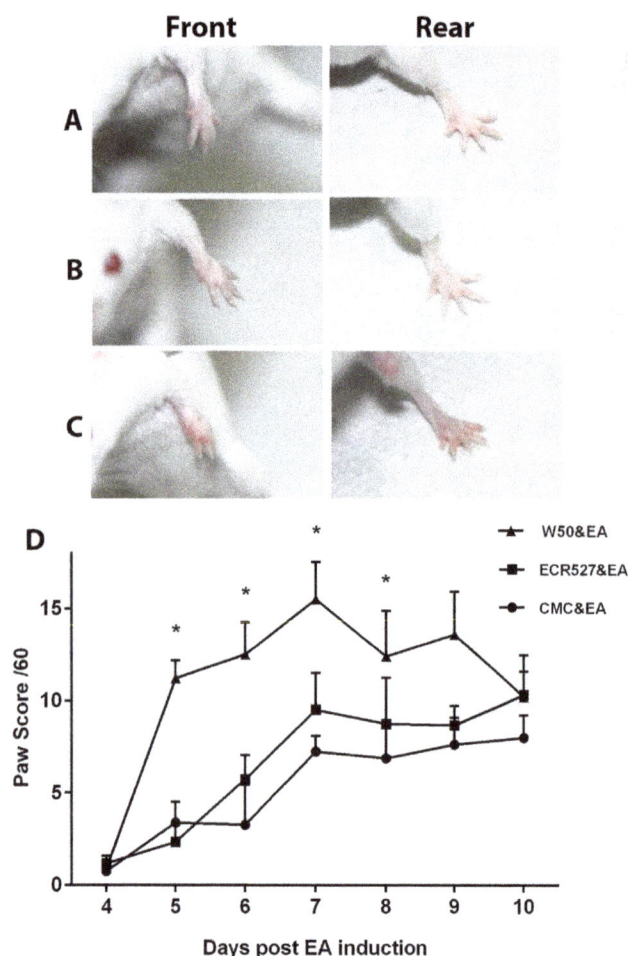

Figure 4. Visual appearance and scoring of paw swelling. A. Appearance of front and rear paws for CMC control group at day 7 post EA induction. B. Appearance of front and rear paws for ECR527 & EA group at day 7 post EA induction. C. Appearance of front and rear paws for W50 & EA group at day 7 post EA induction. D. Total paw score grade out of a 60 including front and back paws. Data represent mean (± SEM). The number of animals in each group was 6 and measurements were performed once daily per animal Statistical analysis was done by two way ANOVA and Tukey multiple comparisons. Raw data for data points are shown in Figure S1. *Abbreviations:* CMC = carboxymethyl cellulose; ECR527 = PAD-deficient *P. gingivalis*; W50 = wild type *P. Gingivalis*; EA = experimental arthritis

Live Animal Micro-computed Tomography

Mice were scanned using the Skyscan 1076 High Resolution live animal computed tomography (micro CT) (SkyScan, Bruker, Belgium) to determine changes in bone volume in the radio-carpal joint and cemento-enamel junction to the alveolar bone crest (CEJ-ABC) length in the jaws. The scanning width was set to 35 mm with a resolution of 9 μm. Detailed specifications for micro CT imaging have previously been published [22]. Animals were anaesthetised prior to scanning with a mixture of ketamine and xylazine and positioned on a polystyrene foam holder then placed within an enclosed container with a HEPA filter at the ends. The container was placed in the 3 cm carbon fibre bed of the micro CT scanner. Mice were scanned before the induction of experimental inflammatory disease to obtain baseline measurements and again at the completion of the study (10 days post experimental arthritis induction).

Micro-CT Data Processing

Scans were reconstructed using Skyscan NRECON software (Version 1.6.6.0). Settings used; smoothing = 1, ring artefact = 15, beam hardening = 30% and misalignment compensation was adjusted manually using the DataViewer program (Skyscan, Bruker, Belgium). The BMP files created were opened in CT Analyser (Version 1.12.0.0+) to create a volume of interest. To realign images and save the appropriate plane for either the radio-carpal joint or determining the CEJ-ABC distance, DataViewer (Version 1.4.4 64-bit) was used. Transaxial images were saved for the bone volume determinations in the radio-carpal joint, and sagittal images for the CEJ-ABC distance. The images were then opened in CTAnalyser to measure bone volume or CEJ-ABC distance. The histogram settings were set at 100 and 255 to measure both the bone volume in the radio-carpal joint and CEJ-ABC junction distance. The bone volume was calculated in a set number (200) 9 μm slices above and below a standard reference point set within the radiocarpal joint. The CEJ-ABC distance was measured between the second and third molars on three slices for each mouse [22,25].

Serum Collection

Approximately 100 μL of blood was collected from cheek puncture bleeds at the commencement of the study (Time = 0) and at 6 weeks. Cardiac puncture was used at the conclusion of the study (week 9). Blood was allowed to clot for 1 hour at room temperature, centrifuged at 1000 *g* for 20 min at room temperature and the serum removed and dispensed into aliquots and stored prior to analysis at −80°C.

ELISA Assays

An anti-CCP kit (AXIS-Shield, Dundee, Scotland) was modified and used to assess levels of anti-CCP antibodies in mouse sera. Week 9 serum was diluted 1:200 and analysed according to the manufacturer's instructions by substitution of an anti-mouse horseradish peroxidase-conjugated secondary to detect mouse IgG (Cell Signalling Technology, Boston, MA, USA).

Antibodies to wild type *P. gingivalis* were detected by coating Costar Maxisorp 96 well plates (Corning, Tewksbury, MA, USA) with 1×10^8 formalin fixed cells in 50 mM bicarbonate buffer, pH 9.4, overnight at 4°C. Wells were washed 3 times in PBS/0.05% Tween-20 (PBS-T) and blocked with 5% skim milk in PBS-T for 1 hr at room temperature followed by three washes of PBS-T. An antibody against *P. gingivalis* purchased from the Developmental Studies Hybridoma Bank (Iowa City, IA, USA) was used as a control and to produce a standard curve. Mouse serum samples from time (day 0, 6 weeks and 9 weeks) were diluted 1:100, added to wells in duplicate and incubated at room temperature for 2 hrs. Wells were washed three times and incubated with a mouse horseradish peroxidase-conjugated secondary antibody (1:10000) (Cell Signalling Technology, Boston, MA, USA) for 45 minutes at room temperature. After the final washes the substrate reagent was prepared (R&D, Minneapolis, MN, USA) and added to wells. The colour reaction was stopped with 2 M H_2SO_4 and the plate read at 450 nm on the Power-wave plate reader using dedicated KC4 microplate data analysis software (Biotek Instruments, Winooski, VT, USA).

Histological Evaluation

At the conclusion of the study (day 63) mice were euthanized by CO_2 inhalation. All paws and heads were retrieved from each mouse and placed into 10% buffered formalin for two days. Following fixation, the specimens were rinsed thoroughly in

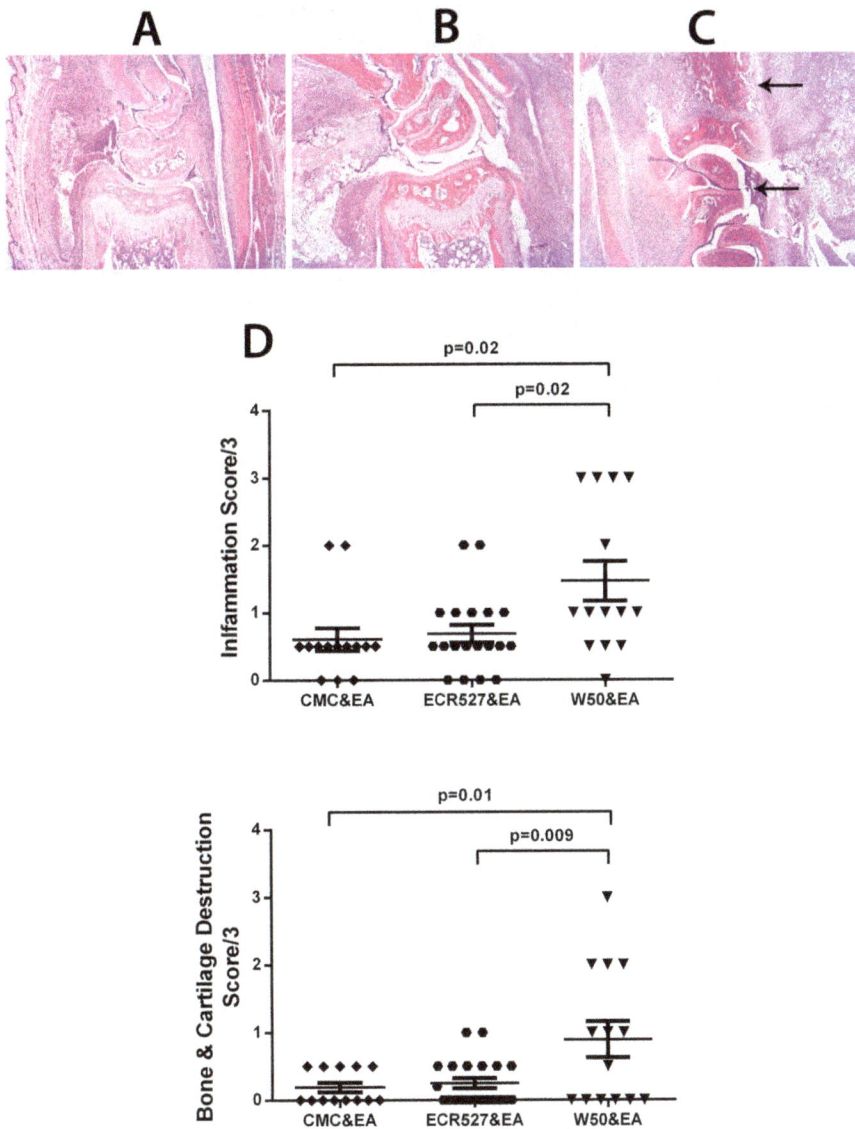

Figure 5. Histological assessment of joint inflammation. A. Histology of the radio-carpal joint for CMC control group at day 63. B. Histology of the radio-carpal joint for ECR527 & EA group at day 63. C. Histology of the radio-carpal joint for W50 & EA group at day 63. Arows indicate increased inflamaotry reaction in joint. D. Histological scores (mean ± SEM) for (a) inflammation and (b) bone and cartilage destruction for both front and rear paws combined. Original magnification of A–C = 100X. The number of animals in each group was 6 and measurements were performed in triplicate. Statistical analysis was done by One way ANOVA and Bonferroni multiple comparisons. *Abbreviations:* CMC = carboxymethyl cellulose; ECR527 = PAD-deficient *P. gingivalis*; W50 = wild type *P. Gingivalis*; EA = experimental arthritis

physiological buffered saline (PBS) and then decalcified in 10% EDTA for 14 days with regular replacement of the solution over this period. Complete decalcification was confirmed by digital radiography and specimens paraffin embedded and sectioned at a thickness of 7 μm. Sections were stained with haematoxylin and eosin for histological analysis. Slides were viewed using a Leica DM1000 microscope and imaged with a connected Leica DFC450 Camera system (Leica Microsystems, Wetzlar, Germany). The front and rear paws were assessed for inflammatory changes, bone and cartilage destruction and pannus formation. A point scale (0–3) was used to score the severity of inflammatory changes based on the number and type of inflammatory cells, (0 = normal tissue, 0–5% inflammatory cells; 1 = mild inflammation 5–25% inflammatory cells; 2 = moderate inflammation 25–50% inflammatory cells; 3 = severe inflammation >50% inflammatory cells). Bone and

cartilage destruction was assessed in a similar fashion (0 = normal, 1 = mild cartilage destruction, 2 = evidence of bone and cartilage destruction, 3 = severe bone and cartilage destruction. Pannus formation in the joint was also noted. The periodontium of the maxillary molars was assessed for inflammation with interdental papilla reduction, and presence of osteoclasts with bone erosion particularly between the first and second molars. The severity of each parameter was scored separately on a scale from 0 to 3 (0 = normal, 1 = mild effect, 2 = moderate effect, 3 = severe effect). The sections assessed and selected for each mouse were all at the level where the distal root of the first molar and proximal root of the second molar was clearly visible [23].

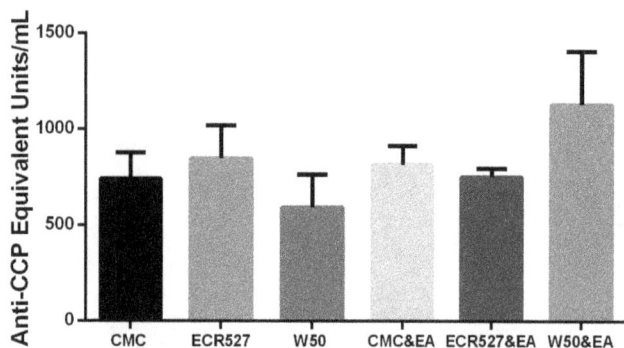

Figure 6. Serum anti-CCP antibody levels. The mean (± SEM) titre of anti-CCP antibodies detected in the sera of mice at week 9 from each of the 6 treatment groups. Raw data for data points are shown in Figure S2. The number in each group was 6 and measurements were performed in duplicate. Statistical analysis was done by one way ANOVA and Tukey multiple comparisons. *Abbreviations:* CMC = carboxymethyl cellulose; ECR527 = PAD-deficient *P. gingivalis*; W50 = wild type *P. Gingivalis*; EA = experimental arthritis

Recovery of *P. gingivalis* from the Oral Cavity

Three groups of six mice were inoculated with either 2% CMC (vehicle control), wild type *P. gingivalis* or PAD-deficient *P. gingivalis*. The inoculation sequence employed was identical to that of Groups 1–3 described previously. At 0, 6 and 24 hrs after the final inoculation sequence the animals gingivae were swabbed using periodontal strips and these were used to inoculate Brain Heart Infusion Broth. Broth cultures were gown under anaerobic conditions for seven days and an inoculum from each culture spread onto anaerobic blood agar plates. Following seven days of

anaerobic incubation a typical black-pigmented colony from each group was Gram stained and assayed for PPAD activity.

Statistical Analysis

The data collected from all surviving mice in this study was analysed by one-way ANOVA. When the global test was statistically significant ($p<0.05$), post hoc comparisons were performed using the Tukey or Bonferroni's Multiple Comparison, 95% confidence level. Unpaired t-tests were also used for 2 group comparisons. All testing was carried out with Graph Pad Prism 6 as the statistical analysis package. Significance levels were set at $p<0.05$ for all tests.

Results

Construction of PAD-deficient *P. gingivalis* Strain (ECR527)

Peptidylarginine deiminase is encoded on the wild type *P. gingivalis* genome at locus PG1424. It is predicted by MicrobesOnline [26] to be the first gene in a 3 gene operon with PG1423 and PG1422, which we have confirmed in *P. gingivalis* W50 using reverse transcription PCR. The RT-PCR products corresponded to the predicted sizes of 682 bp for the primer pair specific for PG1424/PG1423 and 1181 bp for the primer pair specific for PG1424/PG1422 (data not shown). A recombination cassette was constructed using gene splicing by Overlap Extension PCRs where the open reading frame of the *ermF* gene, which confers erythromycin resistance was inserted in place of the PG1424 ORF, so that *ermF* would be expressed from the PG1424 promoter. Replacement of the PG1424 ORF with the *ermF* ORF was successfully achieved in *P. gingivalis* strain W50 with the resulting mutant (ECR527) noticeably slower to pigment than wild type W50. Loss of PPAD activity by the PAD-deficient *P. gingivalis*

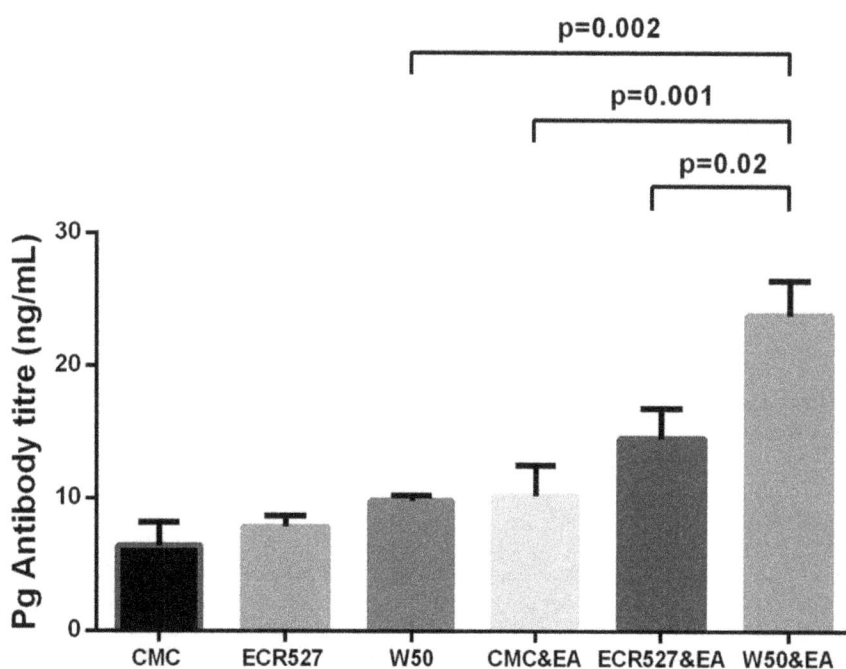

Figure 7. Serum anti-*P. gingivalis* levels. The mean (± SEM) titre of anti-*P.gingivalis* detected in the sera of mice over 9 week time course. Raw data for data points are shown in Figure S3. The number in each group was 6 and measurements were performed in duplicate. Statistical analysis was done by one way ANOVA and Tukey multiple comparisons. *Abbreviations:* CMC = carboxymethyl cellulose; ECR527 = PAD-deficient *P. gingivalis*; W50 = wild type *P. Gingivalis*; EA = experimental arthritis

was confirmed biologically by loss of the ability of ECR527 cultures to deiminate the substrate BAEE whereas 1×10^8 cfu of wild type *P. gingivalis* produced 20.4 ± 0.8 nmol N-α-benzoylcitrulline ethyl ester in 30 min from 300 nmol BAEE.

Post Inoculation Recovery of *P. gingivalis* from Gingiva

Following incubation, black-pigmented colonies of Gram negative bacteria were observed on blood agar plates from the swabs obtained at 0, 6 and 24 hours post final inoculation with wild type *P. gingivalis* W50 and PAD-deficient *P. gingivalis*. However no growth was observed from swabs of animals inoculated with 2% CMC vehicle control. PPAD activity was positive only for bacteria recovered from animals exposed to W50 (Table 2).

Micro-CT Analysis of Periodontal Bone Loss

To determine the effect of PPAD on the periodontium, bone loss in the jaws of the mice, the cemento-enamel junction to alveolar bone crest (CEJ-ABC) length was measured in all 6 groups (Figure 1). No significant difference between PAD-deficient *P. gingivalis* and the CMC vehicle control was observed. However a significant increase in CEJ-ABC distance reflecting increased bone loss was observed between wild type P. *gingivalis* and CMC vehicle control ($p = 0.01$) and wild type *P. gingivalis* with experimental arthritis and CMC vehicle control with experimental arthritis ($p = 0.001$). Furthermore, there was significantly higher bone loss between wild type *P. gingivalis* W50 and PAD-deficient *P. gingivalis* ($p = 0.04$) over wild type *P. gingivalis* with experimental arthritis and PAD-deficient *P. gingivalis* with experimental arthritis ($p = 0.005$).

Histological Analysis of Maxillary Periodontal Tissues

Histological assessment of the periodontal tissue around the first and second maxillary molars demonstrated a statistically significant number of osteoclasts and evidence of bone resorption in the experimental arthritis groups where the difference between the PAD-deficient *P. gingivalis* and the CMC groups were also significantly different to the wild type *P. gingivalis* group ($p = 0.03$ and $p = 0.02$ respectively; Figure 2). There was no statistical difference seen between the non-experimental arthritis groups and the experimental arthritis group which had CMC or PAD-deficient *P. gingivalis* inoculations. Interestingly, the control group with induced experimental arthritis showed evidence of bone resorption which was not seen in the CMC group where there was no induced experimental arthritis.

Micro-CT Analysis of Bone Erosion in Front Paw Radio-carpal Joint

Animals were micro-CT scanned and the radio-carpal joints of both paws (combined) were analysed for changes in bone volume over time. The W50 group with EA showed significantly lower bone volume change reflecting increased bone loss, than the CMC with experimental arthritis group in the radio-carpal joint ($p < 0.04$) (Figure 3). Other group comparisons were not significant.

Visual Scoring of Paw Swelling

Front and rear paws of all mice induced with experimental arthritis were scored daily for swelling and inflammation. There was no significant difference between the control (CMC inoculated group) and the group inoculated with PAD-deficient *P. gingivalis* for the onset of disease and maximum paw score at the height of the disease (day 6–7). However this was not the case for the group that received wild type *P. gingivalis*. There was a rapid onset with swelling and inflammation evident at day 4 and continued for the next 3 days with paw scores significantly higher ($p < 0.0001$) than those of the CMC and PAD-deficient *P. gingivalis* groups (Figure 4).

Histological Assessment of Joint Inflammation

Histological assessment of the sections of inflamed paws in the experimental arthritis group of animals confirmed the observations from the clinical paw scores that the level of inflammation and cartilage and bone destruction was significantly higher in the group inoculated with wild type control groups ($p = 0.02$ and 0.01 respectively). A significant difference was also noted between the wild type *P. gingivalis* and PAD-deficient strain for inflammation and bone/cartilage destruction ($p = 0.02$ and $p = 0.009$ respectively). No differences were observed between the PAD-deficient strain and the CMC control groups (Figure 5). There was no paw inflammation observed in groups that did not undergo experimental arthritis induction.

Serum anti-CCP Antibody Levels

Control mice (inoculated with CMC) demonstrated a background level of anti-CCP antibodies (ACPA). Similar levels were demonstrated in the groups inoculated with wild type *P. gingivalis* and PAD-deficient *P. gingivalis* strains. There was no significant increases in anti-CCP titre in the CMC and *P. gingivalis* ECR527 inoculated groups compared to the groups with no EA. Only mice induced with EA and with pre-existing periodontitis induced by *P. gingivalis* W50 demonstrated a trend towards an increase in anti-CCP antibodies, but this was not significant (Figure 6).

Serum anti-*P. gingivalis* Levels

Mice developed antibodies to *P. gingivalis* over the course of the experiment. Antibody titres increased significantly following induction of experimental arthritis at week 9 in all groups. However those inoculated with wild type *P. gingivalis* produced a higher titre than experimental arthritis alone ($p = 0.001$) and experimental arthritis plus PAD-deficient *P. gingivalis*. ($p = 0.02$) (Figure 7)

Discussion

Of the many hypotheses proposed for a linking mechanism between periodontal disease and RA, the role of citrullination and production of anti-cyclic citrullinated antibodies is of particular interest [15,27]. Citrullination is a common post-translational modification based on the conversion of arginine into citrulline. It occurs frequently in various tissues of the body, particularly at sites of inflammation, and is initiated by peptidylarginine deiminases (PADs). A key concept in the pathogenesis of RA is the preclinical phase which precedes the clinical manifestation of RA [28]. This concept is predicated on the identification of serum autoantibodies years before the development of RA. Indeed there is good evidence to suggest that the immunological conflict often predates the onset of RA by several years. A key component in this process is the production of anti-citrullinated protein antibodies [10]. The production of citrullinated proteins and anti-citrullinated protein antibodies at extra-articular sites prior to the development of RA is well documented [10]. It has been proposed that the inflamed periodontal tissues may be one such site [29].

A number of animal models of experimental arthritis have been studied, each presenting certain advantages and disadvantages [30]. The model chosen for this study, collagen antibody induced arthritis, is characterized by macrophage and polymorphonuclear leukocyte infiltrate within the joints. In this model the anti-collagen antibody is adoptively transferred and therefore it does not rely on specific B- and T-cell responses for disease to ensue.

Nonetheless the development of arthritis in the CAIA model is similar to other models with regards to the inflammatory cytokine response and pannus formation within the affected joints [31,32].

While the role of anti-citrullinated protein antibodies in the pathogenesis of rheumatoid arthritis has been controversial, there is good evidence to support a pathogenic role for these antibodies in the development of both experimental arthritis and human rheumatoid arthritis. [33,34]. While not studied in as much detail as other experimental arthritis models, anti-citrullinated protein antibodies have been suggested to play a role in the severity of disease in the collagen antibody induced arthritis model of experimental arthritis [35,36]. To date there have been no reports concerning an anti-citrullinated protein antibody response in experimental periodontitis. In this regard the present study is significant since it reports that mice with experimental periodontitis and subsequent induction of experimental arthritis demonstrated a trend (not significant) towards an increase in anti-citrullinated protein antibody titre. The precise role that anti-citrullinated protein antibodies play in this process await further investigation.

Shortly after P. gingivalis was shown to be the only prokaryote to produce a peptidylarginine deiminase (PPAD) a hypothesis was presented in which the ability of this organism to citrullinate proteins through secretion of PPAD could be one mechanism whereby anti-citrullinated protein antibodies could develop and result in an exaggerated antibody response with subsequent joint inflammation and development of rheumatoid arthritis [9,15].

To explore this concept further we constructed a knock-out P. gingivalis strain deficient in PPAD expression (ECR527) with view to examining the role of PPAD in the development of both experimental periodontitis and arthritis. We have recently completed sequencing of the PAD-deficient P. gingivalis on our in-house ion torrent and found no secondary mutations, indicating that the experimental results were solely due to the deletion of pad from P. gingivalis (unpublished data).

There is only one other report in the literature that has used a PAD-deficient P. gingivalis strain in a experimental arthritis model [37]. However, our study complements and extends this earlier study [37] by investigating experimental periodontitis in addition to experimental arthritis and a combination of both. This is an important extension of the earlier study [37] which investigated the effect of subcutaneous inoculation of P. gingivalis on experimental arthritis only. Furthermore we demonstrated that both the wild type and PAD-deficient strain of P. gingivalis survived in the oral cavity after oral inoculation. Recent observations indicate that experimental periodontitis can only progress in the presence of a biofilm containing viable P. gingivalis [38]. In this study we used P. gingivalis W50 as it is highly virulent in murine periodontitis models [39–45].

With regards to the induction of experimental periodontitis it was noteworthy that oral inoculation with the PAD-deficient strain resulted in a significantly reduced amount of periodontal bone loss compared to oral inoculation with the wild type P. gingivalis. The reasons for this response are as yet unclear and require further investigation but this finding does implicate a role for PAD in the pathogenesis of periodontitis.

When periodontitis was first induced followed by induction of experimental arthritis studies it was noted that inoculation with the PAD-deficient P. gingivalis strain resulted in reduced severity and onset of arthritis. This is in agreement with a previous study in which it was noted that inoculation with PAD-deficient strain of P. gingivalis resulted in reduced severity of collagen-induced experimental arthritis [37].

In recent years the concepts of molecular mimicry and posttranslational modification of proteins in auto-immune reactions such as RA have been actively debated [28,46]. Interestingly, P. gingivalis appears as a likely agent involved in these processes. For example, cross reactivity of antibodies to P. gingivalis heat shock protein (HSP 60) and host-derived heat shock protein in the pathogenesis of RA has been documented [47]. Another case for molecular mimicry involving P. gingivalis has been made whereby antibodies against citrullinated human α-enolase cross react with citrullinated P. gingivalis enolase [27]. Similarly, the ability of P. gingivalis to produce PPAD which can citrullinate host proteins and lead to an early anti-citrullinated protein antibody response has also implicated this bacterium in the pathogenesis of RA [37]. While antibodies to PPAD have been detected in the sera of mice injected with P. gingivalis, the titre is very low and this reaction probably does not contribute to the process of P. gingivalis-induced exacerbation of experimental arthritis [37]. In the present study, when periodontitis was induced the anti-citrullinated protein antibody serum levels for control and PAD-deficient strains were similar. However, following induction of experimental arthritis the anti-citrullinated protein antibody titres were elevated only for the wild type strain and not for the controls or PAD-deficient strains. This implies a synergistic role for PPAD in the development of experimental arthritis. This observation is in line with those from a study using a different model of collagen-induced experimental arthritis [37].

The emerging data now significantly implicate local citrullination within inflamed periodontal tissues as having the potential to be an extra-articular source of citrullination and production of anti-citrullinated protein antibodies. To date, smoking has been considered a major risk factor in the pathogenesis of RA whereby smoking leads to citrullination within the lung and a priming anti-citrullinated protein antibody response which leads to exacerbation of the anti-citrullinated protein antibody response and associated tissue destruction within inflamed joints. In light of recent observations of the presence of inflammation-associated citrullination, presence of PAD-2 and PAD-4 in gingival tissues [28,48] as well as PPAD in serum [49] now provides good evidence for another important extra-articular source for citrullination and anti-citrullinated protein antibody production to occur years in advance of the development of the clinical signs and symptoms of RA. In this regard it is significant that individuals with untreated RA who are non-smokers but presenting with chronic periodontitis have a significantly high level of anti-citrullinated protein antibody titres [50].

In conclusion this study has demonstrated that PPAD appears to be a significant factor in the development of experimental periodontitis and exacerbation of experimental arthritis. Interpretation of these findings must be made in the context that the animal models used do not completely reflect the complexities of human dises for both periodontitis and rheumatoid arthrits.

Nonetheless these findings adds further evidence for a potentail role of P. gingivalis in the pathogenesis and exacerbation of arthritis. Further studies are now needed to elucidate the mechanisms which drive these processes.

Supporting Information

Figure S1 Raw data used for determination of data points in Figure 4.

Figure S2 Raw data used for determination of data points in Figure 6.

Figure S3 Raw data used for determination of data points in Figure 7.

Data S1

Acknowledgments

The authors wish to thank Ruth Williams from Adelaide Microscopy for her expert assistance with the Skyscan1076 live animal microCT scanner and Associate Professor Renato Morona from the School of Molecular and Biomedical Science for the use of his PC2 laboratory facilities to grow and maintain the genetically modified *P. gingivalis* strain ECR527.

Author Contributions

Conceived and designed the experiments: NG RB VM CM MC DRH CAB SD ECR PMB. Performed the experiments: NG RB VM CM MC CAB SD. Analyzed the data: NG RB VM CM MC DRH CAB SD ECR PMB. Contributed reagents/materials/analysis tools: NG RB VM CM MC DRH CAB SD ECR PMB. Wrote the paper: NG RB VM CM MC DRH CAB SD ECR PMB. Research Funding: NG DRH CAB PMB. Manuscript revision and submission: NG RB VM CM MC DRH CAB SD ECR PMB.

References

1. Page RC, Offenbacher S, Schroeder HE, Seymour GJ, Kornman KS (1997) Advances in the pathogenesis of periodontitis: summary of developments, clinical implications and future directions. Periodontol 2000 14: 216–48.
2. Linden GJ, Lyons A, Scannapieco FA (2013) Periodontal systemic associations: review of the evidence. J Clin Periodontol 40 Suppl 14: S8–19.
3. Kornman KS (2009) A Call to Action. J Periodontol 80: 1019–1020.
4. de Pablo P, Chapple IL, Buckley CD, Dietrich T (2009) Periodontitis in systemic rheumatic diseases. Nat Rev Rheumatol 5: 218–224.
5. Bartold PM, Marshall RI, Haynes DR (2005) Periodontitis and rheumatoid arthritis: a review. J Periodontol 76 (11 Suppl): 2066–2074.
6. Byrne SJ, Dashper SG, Darby IB, Adams GG, Hoffmann B, et al. (2009) Progression of chronic periodontitis can be predicted by the levels of *Porphyromonas gingivalis* and *Treponema denticola* in subgingival plaque. Oral Microbiol Immunol 24: 469–477.
7. Shiloah J, Patters MR, Waring MB (2000) The prevalence of pathogenic periodontal microflora in healthy young adult smokers. J Periodontol 71: 562–567.
8. van Winkelhoff AJ, Loos BG, van der Reijden WA, van der Velden U (2002) *Porphyromonas gingivalis, Bacteroides forsythus* and other putative periodontal pathogens in subjects with and without periodontal destruction. J Clin Periodontol 29: 1023–1028.
9. McGraw WT, Potempa J, Farley D, Travis J (1999) Purification, characterization, and sequence analysis of a potential virulence factor from *Porphyromonas gingivalis*, peptidylarginine deiminase. Infect Immun 67: 3248–3256.
10. Holers VM (2013) Autoimmunity to citrullinated proteins and the initiation of rheumatoid arthritis. Curr Op Immunol 25: 728–735.
11. Schellekens GA, de Jong BA, van den Hoogen FH, van de Putte LB, van Venrooij WJ (1998) Citrulline is an essential constituent of antigenic determinants recognized by rheumatoid arthritis-specific autoantibodies. J Clin Invest 101: 273–281.
12. Masson-Bessiere C, Sebbag M, Girbal-Neuhauser E, Nogueira L, Vincent C, et al. (2001) The major synovial targets of the rheumatoid arthritis-specific antifilaggrin autoantibodies are deiminated forms of the alpha- and beta-chains of fibrin. J Immunol 166: 4177–4184.
13. Girbal-Neuhauser E, Durieux JJ, Arnaud M, Dalbon P, Sebbag M, et al. (1999) The epitopes targeted by the rheumatoid arthritis-associated antifilaggrin autoantibodies are posttranslationally generated on various sites of (pro)filaggrin by deimination of arginine residues. J Immunol 162: 585–594.
14. Doyle HA, Mamula MJ (2002) Posttranslational protein modifications: new flavors in the menu of autoantigens. Curr Opin Rheumatol 14: 244–249.
15. Rosenstein ED, Greenwald RA, Kushner IJ, Weissmann G (2004) Hypothesis: the humoral immune response to oral bacteria provides a stimulus for the development of rheumatoid arthritis. Inflammation 28: 311–318.
16. Wegner N, Lundberg K, Kinloch A, Fisher B, Malmström V, et al. (2010) Autoimmunity to specific citrullinated proteins gives the first clues to the etiology of rheumatoid arthritis. Immunol Rev 233: 34–54.
17. Wegner N, Wait R, Sroka A, Eick S, Nguyen KA, et al. (2010) Peptidylarginine deiminase from *Porphyromonas gingivalis* citrullinates human fibrinogen and alpha-enolase: implications for autoimmunity in rheumatoid arthritis. Arthritis Rheum 62: 2662–2672.
18. Horton RM (1995) PCR-mediated recombination and mutagenesis. SOEing together tailor-made genes. Mol Biotechnol 3: 93–99.
19. Fletcher HM, Schenkein HA, Morgan RM, Bailey KA, Berry CR, et al. (1995) Virulence of a *Porphyromonas gingivalis* W83 mutant defective in the *prtH* gene. Infect Immun 63: 1521–1528.
20. Knipp M, Vasak M (2000) A colorimetric 96-well microtiter plate assay for the determination of enzymatically formed citrulline. Anal Biochem 286: 257–264.
21. Abdullah SN, Farmer EA, Spargo L, Logan R, Gully N (2013) *Porphyromonas gingivalis* peptidylarginine deiminase substrate specificity. Anaerobe 23: 102–108.
22. Cantley MD, Bartold PM, Marino V, Reid RC, Fairlie DP, et al. (2009) The use of live-animal micro-computed tomography to determine the effect of a novel phospholipase A2 inhibitor on alveolar bone loss in an in vivo mouse model of periodontitis. J Periodontal Res 44: 317–322.
23. Cantley MD, Haynes DR, Marino V, Bartold PM (2011) Pre-existing periodontitis exacerbates experimental arthritis in a mouse model. J Clin Periodontol. 38: 532–541.
24. Nandakumar KS, Andrén M, Martinsson P, Bajtner E, Hellström S, et al. (2003) Induction of arthritis by single monoclonal IgG anti-collagen type II antibodies and enhancement of arthritis in mice lacking inhibitory FcgammaRIIB. Eur J Immunol 33: 2269–2277.
25. Park CH, Abramson ZR, Taba M Jr, Jin Q, Chang J, et al. (2007) Three-dimensional micro-computed tomographic imaging of alveolar bone in experimental bone loss or repair. J Periodontol 78: 273–281.
26. Dehal PS, Joachimiak MP, Price MN, Bates JT, Baumohl JK, et al. (2010) MicrobesOnline: an integrated portal for comparative and functional genomics. Nucleic Acids Res 38 (Database issue): D396–400.
27. Lundberg K, Wegner N, Yucel-Lindberg T, Venables PJ (2010) Periodontitis in RA-the citrullinated enolase connection. Nat Rev Rheumatol 6: 727–730.
28. Demoruelle MK, Deane KD, Holers VM (2014) When and where does inflammation begin in rheumatoid arthritis. Curr Opin Rheumatol 26: 64–71.
29. Harvey GP, Fitzsimmons TR, Dhamarpatni AA, Marchant C, Haynes DR, et al. (2013) Expression of peptidylarginine deiminase-2 and -4, citrullinated proteins and anti-citrullinated protein antibodies in human gingiva. J Periodontal Res 48: 252–261.
30. Asquith DL, Miller AM, McInnes IB, Liew FY (2009) Animal models of rheumatoid arthritis. Eur J Immunol. 39: 2040–2044.
31. Nandakumar KS, Svensson L, Holmdahl R (2003) Collagen type II-specific monoclonal antibody-induced arthritis in mice: description of the disease and the influence of age, sex, and genes. Am J Pathol 163: 1827–1837.
32. Nandakumar KS, Holmdahl R (2006) Antibody-induced arthritis: disease mechanisms and genes involved at the effector phase of arthritis. Arthritis Res Ther 2006; 8: 223–234.
33. Klareskog L, Rönnelid J, Lundberg K, Padyukov L, Alfredsson L (2008) Immunity to citrullinated proteins in rheumatoid arthritis. Annu Rev Immunol 26: 651–675.
34. Thiele GM, Duryee MJ, Dusad A, Hunter CD, Lacy JP, et al. (2012) Citrullinated mouse collagen administered to DBA/1J mice in the absence of adjuvant initiates arthritis. Int Immunopharmacol 13: 424–431.
35. Kuhn KA, Kulik L, Tomooka B, Braschler KJ, Arend WP, et al. (2006) Antibodies against citrullinated proteins enhance tissue injury in experimental autoimmune arthritis. J Clin Invest 116: 961–973.
36. Willis VC, Gizinski AM, Banda NK, Causey CP, Knuckley B, et al. (2011) N-α-benzoyl-N5-(2-chloro-1-iminoethyl)-L-ornithine amide, a protein arginine deiminase inhibitor, reduces the severity of murine collagen-induced arthritis. J Immunol 186: 4396–4404.
37. Maresz KJ, Hellvard A, Sroka A, Adamowicz K, Bielecka E, et al. (2013) *Porphyromonas gingivalis* facilitates the development and progression of destructive arthritis through its unique bacterial peptidylarginine deiminase (PAD). PLoS Pathog 9: e1003627.
38. Dashper S, O'Brien-Simpson N, Liu SW, Paolini R, Mitchell H, et al. (2014) Oxantel disrupts polymicrobial biofilm development of periodontal pathogens. Antimicrob Agents Chemother. 58: 378–85. doi:10.1128/AAC.01375-13. Epub 2013 Oct 28.
39. Bird PS, Gemmell E, Polak B, Paton RG, Sosroseno W, et al. (1995). Protective immunity to *Porphyromonas gingivalis* infection in a murine model. J. Periodontol 66: 351–362.
40. Kesavalu L, Holt SC, Ebersole JL (1998) Virulence of a polymicrobic complex, *Treponema denticola* and *Porphyromonas gingivalis*, in a murine model. Oral Microbiol Immunol 13: 373–377.
41. O'Brien-Simpson NM, Paolini RA, Hoffmann B, Slakeski N, Dashper SG, et al. (2001) Role of RgpA, RgpB, and Kgp proteinases in virulence of *Porphyromonas gingivalis* W50 in a murine lesion model. Infect. Immun 69: 7527–7534.
42. Pathirana RD, O'Brien-Simpson NM, Veith PD, Riley PF, Reynolds EC(2006) Characterization of proteinase-adhesin complexes of *Porphyromonas gingivalis*. Microbiology 152: 2381–2394.
43. O'Brien-Simpson NM, Pathirana RD, Paolini RA, Chen YY, Veith PD, et al. (2005) An immune response directed to proteinase and adhesin functional epitopes protects against Porphyromonas gingivalis-induced periodontal bone loss. J Immunol 175: 3980–3989.
44. Orth RK, O'Brien-Simpson NM, Dashper SG, Reynolds EC (2011) Synergistic virulence of *Treponema denticola* and *Porphyromonas gingivalis* in a murine periodontitis model. Molecular Oral Microbiology 26: 229–240.

45. Rajapakse PS, O'Brien-Simpson NM, Slakeski N, Hoffmann B, Reynolds EC (2002) Immunization with the RgpA-Kgp proteinase-adhesin complexes of Porphyromonas gingivalis protects against periodontal bone loss in the rat periodontitis model. Infect Immun 70: 2480–2424

46. Wegner N, Wait R, Venables PJ (2009) Evolutionarily conserved antigens in autoimmune disease: implications for an infective aetiology. Int J Biochem Cell Biol 41: 390–397.

47. Jeong E, Lee J-Y, Kim S-J, Choi J (2012) Predominant immunoreactivity of *Porphyromonas gingivalis* heat shock protein in autoimmune disease. J Periodont Res 47: 811–816.

48. Nesse W, Westra J, van der Wal JE, Abbas F, Nicholas AP, et al. (2012) The periodontium of periodontitis patients contains citrullinated proteins which may play a role in ACPA (anti-citrullinated protein antibody) formation. J Clin Periodontol 39: 599–607.

49. Quirke AM, Lugli EB, Wegner N, Hamilton BC, Charles P, et al. (2014) Heightened immune response to autocitrullinated *Porphyromonas gingivalis* peptidylarginine deiminase: a potential mechanism for breaching immunologic tolerance in rheumatoid arthritis. Ann Rheum Dis 73: 263–269.

50. Potikuri D, Dannana KC, Kanchinadam S, Agrawal S, Kancharla A, et al. (2012) Periodontal disease is significantly higher in non-smoking treatment-naïve rheumatoid arthritis patients: results from a case-control study. Ann Rheum Dis 71: 1541–1544.

7

Experimental Gingivitis Induces Systemic Inflammatory Markers in Young Healthy Individuals

Jörg Eberhard[1][*][●], Karsten Grote[2][●], Maren Luchtefeld[2], Wieland Heuer[1], Harald Schuett[2], Dimitar Divchev[2], Ralph Scherer[3], Ruth Schmitz-Streit[5], Daniela Langfeldt[5], Nico Stumpp[1], Ingmar Staufenbiel[4], Bernhard Schieffer[2][●], Meike Stiesch[1][●]

1 Department of Prosthetic Dentistry and Biomaterials Science, Hannover Medical School, Hannover, Germany, 2 Department of Cardiology and Angiology, Hannover Medical School, Hannover, Germany, 3 Department of Medical Statistics, Hannover Medical School, Hannover, Germany, 4 Department of Operative Dentistry and Periodontology, Hannover Medical School, Hannover, Germany, 5 Institute for Microbiology, Christian-Albrechts-University Kiel, Kiel, Germany

Abstract

Objectives: We here investigated whether experimental gingivitis enhances systemic markers of inflammation which are also known as surrogate markers of atherosclerotic plaque development.

Background: Gingivitis is a low-level oral infection induced by bacterial deposits with a high prevalence within Western populations. A potential link between the more severe oral disease periodontitis and cardiovascular disease has already been shown.

Methods: 37 non-smoking young volunteers with no inflammatory disease or any cardiovascular risk factors participated in this single-subject interventional study with an intra-individual control. Intentionally experimental oral inflammation was induced by the interruption of oral hygiene for 21 days, followed by a 21-days resolving phase after reinitiation of oral hygiene. Primary outcome measures at baseline, day 21 and 42 were concentrations of hsCRP, IL-6, and MCP-1, as well as adhesion capacity and oxLDL uptake of isolated blood monocytes.

Results: The partial cessation of oral hygiene procedures was followed by the significant increase of gingival bleeding (34.0%, $P < 0.0001$). This local inflammation was associated with a systemic increase in hsCRP (0.24 mg/L, $P = 0.038$), IL-6 (12.52 ng/L, $P = 0.0002$) and MCP-1 (9.10 ng/l, $P = 0.124$) in peripheral blood samples between baseline and day 21, which decreased at day 42. Monocytes showed an enhanced adherence to endothelial cells and increased foam cell formation after oxLDL uptake ($P < 0.050$) at day 21 of gingivitis.

Conclusions: Bacterial-induced gingival low-level inflammation induced a systemic increase in inflammatory markers. Dental hygiene almost completely reversed this experimental inflammatory process, suggesting that appropriate dental prophylaxis may also limit systemic markers of inflammation in subjects with natural gingivitis. International Clinical Trials Register Platform of the World Health Organization, registry number: DRKS00003366, URL: http://apps.who.int/trialsearch/Default.aspx.

Editor: Hugo ten Cate, Maastricht University Medical Center, The Netherlands

Funding: This study was in part supported by the Deutsche Forschungsgemeinschaft DFG, Bonn, Germany (Eb 223/5-1). The authors acknowledge funding of the publication costs by the Deutsche Forschungsgemeinschaft. The funders had no role in study design, data collection and analysis, decision to publish, or preparation of the manuscript.

Competing Interests: The authors have declared that no competing interests exist.

* E-mail: eberhard.joerg@mh-hannover.de

● These authors contributed equally to this work.

Introduction

Gingivitis and periodontitis are two distinct chronic inflammatory processes belonging to the spectrum of periodontal diseases of the oral cavity affecting the tooth supporting tissues in response to bacterial accumulation. In contrast to periodontitis, gingivitis is initiated only after a few days of inadequate oral hygiene procedures by local plaque deposits adjacent to the highly vascularised gingival tissues. Gingivitis is a superficial inflamma-tory affection and is not destructive towards the surrounding connective and bone tissues and completely declines with the initiation of adequate oral hygiene procedures. In gingivitis bleeding of the gums may occur even after gentle mechanical stimulation in severe cases or following tooth brushing and chewing [1]. In contrast, in susceptible subjects periodontitis is characterized by the irreversible loss of bone and periodontal ligament that is if untreated followed by tooth loss [2]. In addition to various epidemiological studies demonstrating a potential link between periodontitis and cardiovascular diseases [3] it has been demonstrated that the treatment of patients suffering from periodontitis reduces acute parameters of atherosclerosis and improves endothelial function [4,5]. Equivalent data are not available for gingivitis, although the prevalence of moderate to severe periodontitis in western populations is 3% to 46% whereas gingivitis affects almost all individuals [6,7,8].

Inflammatory processes play a pivotal role in the pathogenesis of atherosclerosis and mediate the development of the disease, from initial leukocyte recruitment to sudden plaque rupture and subsequent myocardial infarction with often fatal outcome [9,10]. Several systemic inflammatory markers have been identified as independent risk factors for cardiovascular diseases. The ability to measure levels of these inflammatory markers in the systemic circulation has provoked interest in their development as biomarkers or surrogate markers for potential use in risk assessment [11,12]. In this regard, the acute phase reactant C-reactive protein (CRP) is a potential predictor of future atherosclerotic vascular disease, whereas cytokines and chemo-kines such as interleukin (IL)-6 or monocyte chemoattractant protein-1 (MCP-1, also known as CCL2) are established mediators of the chronic inflammatory process within the vascular wall in various experimental models (6–9). Activation of blood monocytes represents an early and crucial event in the development of atherosclerosis. Activated monocytes are prone to adhere more likely at inflamed sites of the endothelium to invade the arterial wall. Subsequently, they differentiate into foam cells in order to initiate atherosclerotic plaque growth. In this regard, chronic systemic inflammation has been shown to be linked to adverse cardiovascular outcomes [10]. Systemic or local infection may provide an additional inflammatory stimulus that could accelerate atherogenesis. However, the pathophysiological pathways between chronic extravascular infections and atherosclerosis remain unclear [3].

Although gingivitis is a highly prevalent chronic bacterial disease in susceptible children, adults and the elderly, persisting for decades in subjects, and is an essential precursor of periodontitis limited data are available today addressing detrimental systemic effects of gingivitis. Systemic effects of experimental or natural gingivitis have been rarely investigated and the existing studies did not show correlations between gingivitis and systemic levels of pro-inflammatory mediators or surrogate markers of atherosclerosis [13]. Recently, studies using broad-range frequency techniques using 454 pyrosequencing of 16S rRNA genes identified bacteria associated with gingivitis in atherosclerotic plaques and potentially highlight a mechanism by which low-level gingival inflammation may also affect cardiovascular diseases [14].

We now report the results of an intervention study using a single-subject design with an intra-individual control. Experimentally induced gingivitis in young, healthy volunteers was initiated by termination of oral hygiene and resolved after restart of oral hygiene to determine the effects and causal association of this highly prevalent chronic inflammatory oral disease on circulating inflammatory markers which in some studies have been suggested as surrogate markers of atherosclerotic plaque development.

Methods

Study Design

Over a period of 42 days, it was our goal to evaluate the effects of oral hygiene cessation and restart on surrogate markers of atherosclerotic plaque development and activation of blood monocytes in young healthy individuals (Fig. 1). Oral hygiene

cessation was selected as the intervention for the present study because of the high reproducibility of the following inflammatory responses in the gingival tissues. This model was introduced by Löe et al. as the "Experimental Gingivitis Model" in 1965 [15]. The primary outcome was the in-group differences between baseline and day 21 in clinical, laboratory and experimental parameters of inflammation during the study. Participants were selected according to the following inclusion criteria: (1) 20–30 years of age, (2) non-smokers, (3) no clinical signs of gingival inflammation (redness, swelling, bleeding) at ≥90% sites observed, (4) no probing pocket depth >3 mm at any site and (5) no alveolar bone loss. Exclusion criteria were: (1) presence of systemic diseases (e.g., diabetes mellitus or cardiovascular, kidney, liver or lung disease) (2) pregnancy or breastfeeding, (3) history of drug abuse, (4) allergic diathesis, (5) medications, in particular currently ingestion of non-steroidal or steroidal anti-inflammatory drugs, analgesic or antibiotics within 3 months before entering the study, (6) untreated carious lesions and/or insufficient restorations, implants, crowns at teeth in the maxillary right quadrant and (7) mouth breathing. All participants gave written informed consent. The study was performed in accordance with the Helsinki Declaration, approved by the ethical Committee of Hannover Medical School and registered at the International Clinical Trials Register Platform of the World Health Organization (http://apps. who.int/trialsearch/Default.aspx, ID: DRKS00003366).

Volunteers, which were addressed by public announcement in the Hannover area, who met the inclusion criteria were scheduled for a dental and periodontal screening appointment and full medical and dental histories were collected. All participants had a college degree. After inclusion in the study, all participants received a professional scaling and polishing of all tooth surfaces to remove supra- and subgingival plaque, stain and calculus 14 days prior to the start of the experimental gingivitis phase. The intervention was initiated at baseline when all participants refrained from any oral hygiene at seven upper teeth of the right maxilla. This model of limited inflammation has been described previously and was used as a model for an inflammatory status in the oral cavity that may represent a inflammatory condition affecting the majority of cases in the general population [16]. The subjects were clinically examined and 20 ml peripheral venous blood was sampled at baseline as well as on day 21 (experimental gingivitis) and at the follow-up appointment 21 days after termination and 42 days after initiation of the experimental gingivitis phase. Professional tooth cleaning and topical fluoride application was applied at day 21 of the experimental gingivitis phase (Fig. 1). Hereby at day 21 the intervention was terminated and during the following 21 days rigorous oral hygiene procedures were applied in order that the subjects served as their own control.

Periodontal Clinical Examination

Periodontal data were recorded by three experienced and calibrated dentists at baseline and day 21. The data included the presence or absence of supragingival dental plaque using a modification of the Silness-Löe plaque index (PI) at the buccal and oral sites of the selected teeth and the observable inflammatory changes of the gingival tissues by the gingival index (GI) at four sites per tooth [17,18]. The volume of the gingival crevicular fluid (GCF) was determined after gentle drying of the tooth for ten seconds followed by insertion of a filter paper strip (Periopaper, Pro Flow Incorporated) for 30 seconds into the gingival sulcus at four sites of the upper right first premolar. The GCF was measured with a calibrated Periotron 6000 gingival fluid meter (Pro Flow Incorporated) and expressed in Periotron units (PU). Gingival bleeding on probing was also recorded (BOP) with a

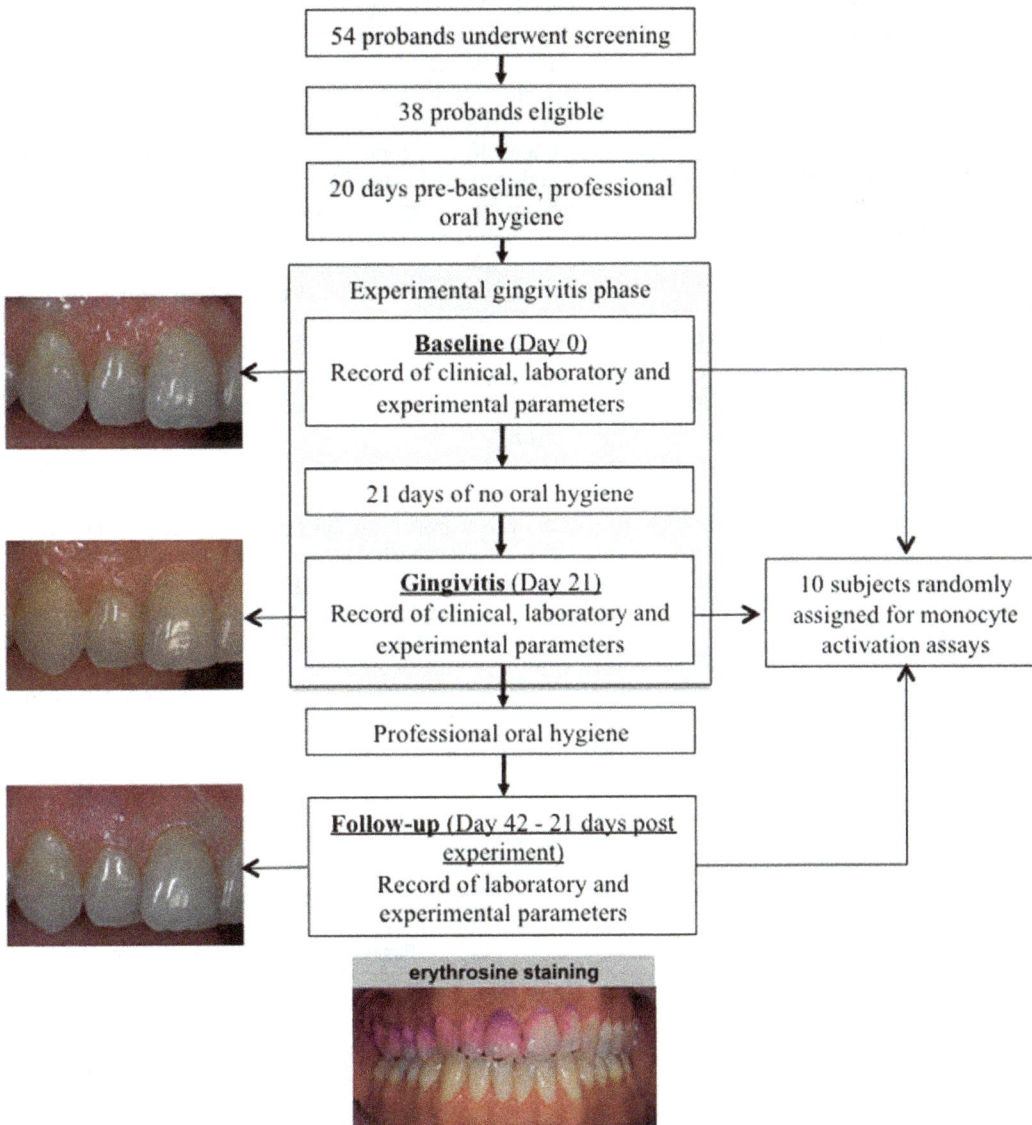

Figure 1. Flowchart of the study design from screening to follow-up. After a baseline visit, eligible volunteers were scheduled for intensive professional tooth cleaning and oral hygiene instructions to remove all biofilm deposits before starting the experimental gingivitis phase. After 21-days of cessation from any oral hygiene procedures in the upper right maxilla massive bacterial biofilms has been formed on the selected tooth hard substances, which are visible to the naked eye as yellowish plaques. Plaque covering of the tooth was routinely documented after erythrosine staining. The professional removal of all bacterial deposits and the restart of oral homecare terminated the experimental gingivitis phase. At baseline, day 21 (gingivitis) and 21 days after completion of the experimental gingivitis phase (follow-up) blood samples were obtained for serum parameters and monocyte activation assays.

pressure-calibrated probe (TPS probe, Vivacare) at four sites of all selected tooth sites: mesio-buccal, disto-buccal, mesio-oral and disto-oral. All measurements were recorded at four identical sites per tooth. The averaged scores for supragingival plaque and gingival inflammation (the sum of indexed scores divided by the total number of recorded sites), the amount of gingival crevicular fluid (the sum of the Periotron units per tooth divided by the number of sites) and the score for gingival bleeding on probing (the number of sites with gingival bleeding divided by the total number of sites, multiplied by 100) were calculated for each subject.

Species-specific Detection of Bacteria in Plaque Samples

Supragingival plaque was collected with sterile paper strips (VDW) at day 21 from all participants at the upper teeth of the right maxilla. Total genomic DNA was isolated using the QIAamp DNA Mini kit (Qiagen) according to the manufacturer's protocol for Gram-positive bacteria, but including a mechanical disruption step with a Precellys 24 bead mill (Bertin Technologies) prior to the first step of the protocol. Total genomic DNA was used as template for PCR-based detection of ten representative bacterial species commonly found in supragingival plaque samples belonging to different complexes according to Socransky et al. and Haffajee et al. [19,20]. The 'red complex', comprising of *Porphyromonas gingivalis*, *Tannerella forsythia*, and *Treponema denticola*, has been identified as the 'disease-related' complex. For supragingival plaque it has been shown that members of the red and orange complexes (e.g. *Fusobacterium nucleatum*) were most frequently associated with inflamed sites [19]. In the remaining clusters (purple, green and yellow) were moderately pathogenic species, including initial and early colonizers. The species-specific primers for the selected microorganisms are listed in table 1. All PCR reactions were performed on a TProfessional thermocycler (Biometra) in a total reaction volume of 20 μl. The reaction mix contained 2 μl of genomic DNA as template, 200 nM of each specific primer, 1x PCR buffer (including 1.5 mM magnesium chloride; Qiagen), 1.5 U HotStar Taq polymerase (Qiagen), 200 mM of each dNTP (Roth) and PCR-grade water (Roche). The thermal cycling protocol for each primer set was as follows: Initial denaturation at 95°C for 15 min; 40 amplification cycles consisting of denaturation at 94°C for 30 s, annealing at 55°–68°C for 45 s, elongation at 72°C for 1 min; final extension at 72°C for 10 min. 5 μl of each amplification reaction were analyzed by 1% agarose gel electrophoresis. A clear single band of expected size (table 1) was evaluated as positive detection signal and respective PCR products were subsequently sequenced.

Cardiovascular and Laboratory Assessment

Carotid intima-media thickness (IMT) was assessed at baseline and at day 42 by B-mode duplex sonography using a 10.5-MHz linear transducer. IMT was measured at the common carotid artery approximately 10 mm proximal to the bifurcation. The mean values from both sides are reported. Non-invasive blood pressure measurement was performed at baseline and at day 42 in seated position by Riva-Rocci/Korotkow's method. A standard 2D-Doppler transthoracic echocardiogram was performed at baseline and at day 21. Left ventricular function was assessed

qualitatively. Valvular status was quantified by color and continuous-wave Doppler flow.

Serum and plasma samples were obtained at baseline, day 21 of the experimental gingivitis phase and at the follow-up re-evaluation at day 42. All samples were collected between 7.45 and 8.30 a.m. after a period of at least eight hours of fasting. Blood counts and measurements of lipid levels were done by standard laboratory testing. Serum concentrations of hsCRP were determined by immunonephelometry (detection limit 0.23 mg/L, Cardiophase hsCRP, Siemens). Serum levels of IL-6 (detection limit 0.70 pg/mL) and MCP-1 (detection limit 5.0 pg/mL) were measured by enzyme-linked immunosorbent assay (Quantikine HS, R&D Systems) with the help of a plate reader (μQuant; Bio-Tek Instruments).

Cell Culture

Human endothelial cells (human umbilical vein endothelial cells = HUVECs) were obtained from Lonza. Cells were cultured in endothelial cell growth medium (EGM-2; Lonza) supplemented with 2% FCS and growth factors and cultured on gelatin coated cell culture plates. Cells between passage 2 and 4 were used for experiments. Human leukocytes were isolated from the blood of the subjects. Erythrocytes were removed by hemolysis (155 mM NH_4Cl, 10 mM $KHCO_3$, 0.01% ethylenediaminetetraacetic acid; for 10 min) and cells were resuspended in X-vivo 15 medium (Lonza). Monocytic cells were enriched by plastic adherence over night, non-adherent cells were removed.

Table 1. Species-specific primers used to identify ten different bacterial species in plaque samples of experimental gingivitis at day 21 of the study.

Bacterial species	Primer	Annealing temperature	Expected amplicon size (bp)	Reference
Prevotella intermedia	F: 5'-CGTGGACCAAAGATTCATCGGTGGA-3'	64°C	259	[40]
	R: 5'-CCGCTTTACTCCCCAACAAA-3'			
Fusobacterium nucleatum	F: 5'-AGAGTTTGATCCTGGCTCAG-3'	60°C	360	[41]
	R: 5'-GTCATCGTGCACACAGAATTGCTG-3'			
Streptococcus oralis	F: 5'-TCCCGGTCAGCAAACTCCAGCC-3'	66°C	374	[42]
	R: 5'-GCAACCTTTGGATTTGCAAC-3'			
Streptococcus sanguinis	F: 5'-GGATAGTGGCTCAGGGCAGCCAGTT-3'	70°C	313	[42]
	R: 5'-GAACAGTTGCTGGACTTGCTTGTC-3'			
Capnocytophaga sputigena	F: 5'-AGAGTTTGATCCTGGCTCAG-3'	55°C	185	[43]
	R: 5'-GATGCCGCTCCTATATACCATTAGG-3'			
Eikenella corrodens	F: 5'-CTAATACCGCATACGTCCTAAG-3'	60°C	688	[44]
	R: 5'-CTACTAAGCAATCAAGTTGCCC-3'			
Tannerella forsythia	F: 5'-GCGTATGTAACCTGCCCGCA-3'	60°C	641	[44]
	R: 5'-TGCTTCAGTGTCAGTTATACCT-3'			
Porphyromonas gingivalis	F: 5'-AGGCAGCTTGCCATACTGCG-3'	60°C	404	[44]
	R: 5'-ACTGTTAGCAACTACCGATGT-3'			
Treponema denticola	F: 5'-TAATACCGAATGTGCTCATTTACAT-3'	60°C	316	[44]
	R: 5'-TCAAAGAAGCATTCCCTCTTCTTCTTA-3'			
Veillonella parvula	F: 5'-GAAGCATTGGAAGCGAAAGTTTCG-3'	57°C	623	[45]
	R: 5'-GTGTAACAAGGGAGTACGGACC-3'			
Aggregatibacter actinomycetemcomitans	F: 5'-TAGCCCTGGTGCCCGAAGC-3'	68°C	557	[46]
	R: 5'-CATCGCTGGTTGGTTACCCTCTG-3'			

Cell Adhesion

50,000 monocytes/well were seeded on a confluent monolayer of HUVECs in a 96-well plate in EGM-2 medium (Lonza). Adhesion was carried out for two hours at 37°C and 5% CO_2. Non-adherent cells were removed by 2 washing steps with PBS. Adherent cells were visualized per well in triplicates using a cell culture microscope (CKX31; Olympus) and captured with a digital camera (C-5060; Olympus). Adherent monocytes on a monolayer of endothelial cells were quantified using computer-assisted image analysis software (ImageJ 1.43 h, NIH).

Foam Cell Formation

50,000 monocytes/well were seeded in a 96-well plate in X-vivo 15 medium (Lonza) and monocyte-derived macrophages were obtained by plastic adherence for 4 days. Macrophages were stimulated for 4 hours with oxLDL (10 µg/ml). After treatment, cells were washed twice with PBS, fixed with formalin and dehydrated with 2-propandiol. Cellular lipids were stained with oil red O (Sigma) for 30 minutes. Oil red O-stained cells were visualized in three randomly chosen microscopic fields per well using a cell culture microscope (CKX31; Olympus) and captured with a digital camera (C-5060; Olympus). Percentage of Oil red O-positive cells was quantified using computer-assisted image analysis software (ImageJ 1.43 h, NIH).

Statistical Analysis

The statistical analysis was conducted with the statistical programming language R for the hypothesis testing and for the construction of graphs. The local two-sided Type-I-errors were set to 5% resulting in an explorative data analysis. In all comparisons of baseline values against gingivitis status and gingivitis status against follow-up, two-sided Wilcoxon signed-rank tests for paired samples were used. The exact P-values and exact confidence intervals were calculated for the monocytes adhesion assays and foam cell formations. Due to the exploratory character of the study all P-values were not adjusted for multiplicity. Results are presented as median differences with two-sided 95% confidence intervals as well as corresponding two-sided P-values. Post-hoc power calculations were based on the two-sample t test for paired data using a two-sided significance level of 0.05. The estimators for the mean differences and standard deviations were calculated from the present data.

Results

Subjects Characteristics

52 individuals were screened at the Hannover Medical School of Dentistry; of those 38 met the inclusion criteria and 37 subjects completed the clinical trial (Fig. 1). First subject in was 1st March 2010, last subject out was 28 July 2010. One volunteer showed clinical signs of congenital heart valve insufficiency and was withdrawn from the study. 37 non-smoking young and healthy volunteers (mean age 23.35 ± 3.64 years) were enrolled in this study free of any traditional risk factor or inflammatory disease. The baseline characteristics of the subjects are presented in table 2.

As safety parameter and as marker of pre-existing atherosclerosis, the intima-media thickness of the left and right common carotid artery was determined. At baseline and after 42 days no differences were found (baseline: 0.55 ± 0.16 mm, 21 days: 0.54 ± 0.18 mm, $P=0.160$). Neither blood pressure nor serum cholesterol fraction showed significant differences when baseline was compared to day 21. Moreover, echocardiographical assessment of left ventricular function and valvular status was performed at baseline and at day 21 and showed no differences within the individuals.

Markers of Experimental Gingivitis

All volunteers developed experimental gingivitis as determined by all recorded parameters. The cessation of oral hygiene for 21 days in the upper right maxilla was followed by the accumulation of bacterial deposits on the tooth surfaces adjacent to the gingival tissues surrounding the teeth (absolute difference 2.04 PI, 95% CI, 1.91 to 2.17; $P<0.0001$) and is depicted in Figure 2A. This plaque formation was followed by the induction of inflammatory changes of the gingival tissues that became obvious by redness and swelling of the marginal gingiva categorized by the Gingival Index (absolute difference -1.29 GI, 95% CI, 1.11 to 1.40; $P<0.0001$, Fig. 2B). The accumulating inflammatory processes in the marginal gingival tissues between baseline and day 21 were associated with an increased volume of the gingival sulcus fluid (absolute difference 33.20 PU, 95% CI, 25.13 to 40.12; $P<0.0001$, Fig. 2C) and increased frequencies of bleeding on probing (absolute difference 34.00%, 95% CI, 28.00 to 39.00%; $P<0.0001$, Fig 2D).

Verification of Bacterial Plaque Composition

Aiming to identify ten bacterial species belonging to different clusters introduced by Haffajee et al. [19] and commonly found in sub- or supragingival plaque a species-specific PCR amplification was performed. We identified bacteria belonging to the red-complex in low detection frequencies within the study population of 37 subjects, *Porphyromonas gingivalis* (0.0%), *Tanerella forsythus* (13.5%) and *Treponema pallidum* (0.0%). Whereas *Fusobacterium nucleatum* (orange complex) was detected in every plaque sample from all test persons (100.0%). *Veilonella parvula* (purple complex) was observed in 97.3%, *C. sputigena* (green complex) in 94.1%, *E. corrodens* (green complex) in 88.6% and *S. sanguinis* (yellow complex) in 65.7% of all samples (Fig. 3). In summary, we could detect seven from ten representative bacterial species commonly found in plaque samples in high frequency across the whole group of participants. Whereas species from the red-complex associated with periodontitis, were absent or in low frequency.

Surrogate Markers of Atherosclerosis

Analysis of plasma samples revealed enhanced levels of circulating markers of inflammation when experimental gingivitis was induced. First of all, hsCRP mean difference was found to be significantly elevated under experimental gingivitis conditions 0.24 mg/L, 95% CI 0.01 to 1.20; $P=0.038$ (Fig. 4A). At follow-up, hsCRP levels tended to decline but were still slightly enhanced (median difference -0.02 mg/lL, 95% CI 0.28 to 0.71; $P=0.927$. Likewise, we observed enhanced circulating levels of the inflammatory mediators for IL-6 (Median difference 12.52 ng/l, 95% CI 1.25 to 43.85; $P=0.0002$) and MCP-1 (Median difference 9.10 ng/l, 95% CI -3.70 to 28.65; $P=0.124$) (Fig. 4B and C) between baseline and gingivitis, which both returned to baseline levels at the follow-up appointment (Median difference for IL-6 -12.51 ng/l, 95% CI -44.65 to -1.36; $P=0.001$ and median difference for MCP-1 -12.10 ng/l, 95% CI -27.00 to 0.50; $P=0.057$). Compared to baseline blood leukocyte and monocyte cell counts were increased upon experimental gingivitis (median differences 0.45×10^9/L, 95% CI -0.049 to 0.949, $P=0.0001$, respectively 0.010×10^9/L, 95% CI 0.099 to 0.150, $P=0.068$) and did not yet decline back to baseline levels at follow-up (mean differences for leukocytes 0.15×10^9/L, 95% CI -0.499 to 0.700,

Table 2. Baseline characteristics of the patients.

Characteristic	Study Group	Reference intervals*
	(N = 37)	(Male/Female)
Age - yr	23.4±3.6	
Male/Female sex - no. (%)	6/31 (16.2/83.8)	
Smoking status - no. (%)		
Never smoked	31 (83.8)	
Former Smoker[¶]	6 (16.2)	
Current smoker	0 (0)	
Family history of cardiovascular disease - no. (%)	3 (8.1)	
Race or ethnic group - no. (%)[§]		
White	31 (83.8)	
Asian	6 (16.2)	
Black	0 (0)	
Body-mass index[§§]	22.9±4.5	18.5–24.9
Blood pressure - mm Hg		
Systolic	124.0±12.0	<140
Diastolic	81.0±8.8	<90
Cholesterol fractions Male/Female (SD) - mmol/l		
S-cholesterol	5.9±1.8/6.2±2.1	3.3–6.2/3.3–6.2
S-HDL-cholesterol	1.8±0.3/2.4±0.8	>1.0/>1.2
S-LDL-cholesterol	4.0±1.4/4.0±1.4	1.8–4.5/1.7–4.2
Haemogram		
haemoglobin - g/dl	13.2±1.4	12.0–17.5
erythrocyte count - $\times 10^{12}$/liter	4.6±0.5	4.0–5.9
thrombocyte count - $\times 10^{9}$/liter	261.5±55.9	150.0–450.0
neutrophile count - $\times 10^{9}$/liter	5.8±0.8	1.1–8.8
eosinophile count - $\times 10^{9}$/liter	0.2±0.1	<0.5
basophile count - $\times 10^{9}$/liter	0.5±0.3	0.0–1.0
haematocrit - %	41.3±3.2	36.0–50.4

[¶]Smoking was terminated at least 12 months prior to the start of the study.
[§]Race was self-reported.
[§§]Body-mass index is defined as the weight in kilograms divided by the square of the hight in meters.
*All parameters fall within the reference intervals or are designated as "normal".

$P = 0.404$, and for monocytes 0.000×10^9/L, 95% CI -0.049 to 0.100, $P = 0.591$ (Fig. 4D, E).

Monycyte Activation Assays

Monocytes were isolated from the blood of ten randomly assigned study participants and subsequently subjected to ex vivo cell culture assays verifying monocyte activation. Of note, experimentally induced gingivitis led to significantly enhanced adherence of monocytes on endothelial cells (Fig. 5A) as well as to augmented oxLDL-uptake and foam cell formation (Fig. 5B). Both processes returned to baseline levels at day 42. Of note, monocyte activation is known to be crucially involved in the development of atherosclerosis and thereby fundamental to the etiology of coronary artery disease.

A post-hoc power analysis using observed mean differences and SDs demonstrated that this study had more than 80% power to detect differences between baseline and gingivitis for all parameters, except for MCP-1 (11% power), hsCRP (62% power) and Leucocyte counts (55% power).

Discussion

The present interventional study showed that even in healthy young individuals, experimentally induced gingivitis as low-level extravascular oral bacterial infection lead to an acute systemic inflammation with enhanced systemic levels of CRP, IL-6, MCP-1 and activated monocytes known as markers and mediators of vascular atherosclerotic disease. This inflammatory process seems to be almost completely reversible by appropriate dental hygiene.

Gingivitis is a chronic local infection affecting the tooth surrounding tissues, caused by bacteria of the dental plaque (e.g. *Streptococcus oralis*, *Veilonella ssp.* etc.) and is accompanied by a local inflammatory response of the host. The oral inflammatory response is, in contrast to periodontitis, limited to the soft gingival tissues not affecting the bone. Moreover, gingivitis differs from periodontitis with respect to its microbial composition and inflammatory responses [21]. In consequence, it was not expected at the beginning of the study to observe systemic effects from gingivitis, although they have already been shown for periodontitis [5]. Recently, Wahaidi et al. [13] was not able to show an

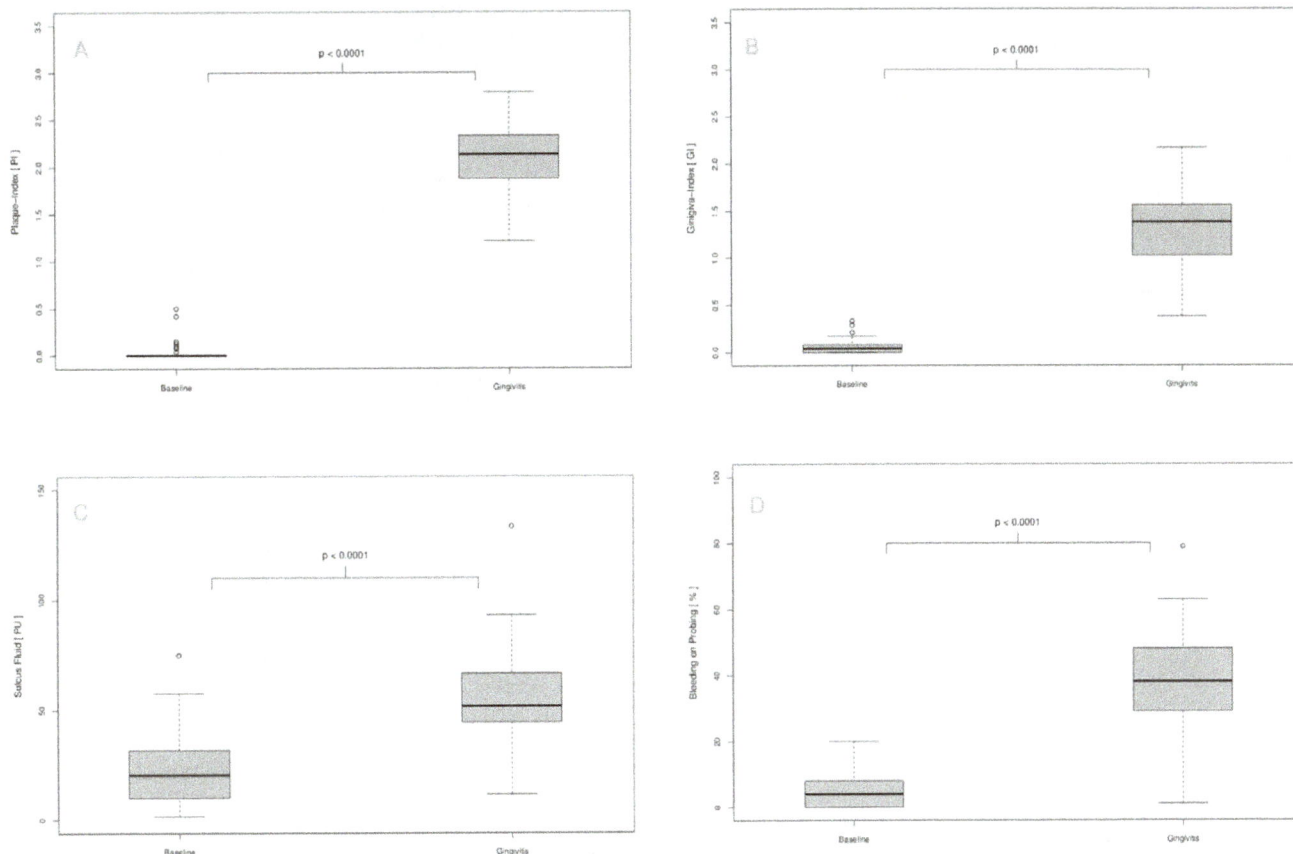

Figure 2. Characterization of oral clinical parameters at baseline and after 21 days of experimental gingivitis. The box-plots illustrate the plaque accumulation on tooth hard-substances during the 21-days non-brushing period followed by the progression of three selected clinical inflammatory parameters documenting the inflammatory status of the gingival tissues. The time interval and clinical observations are characteristic for an inflammatory lesion denoted as gingivitis.

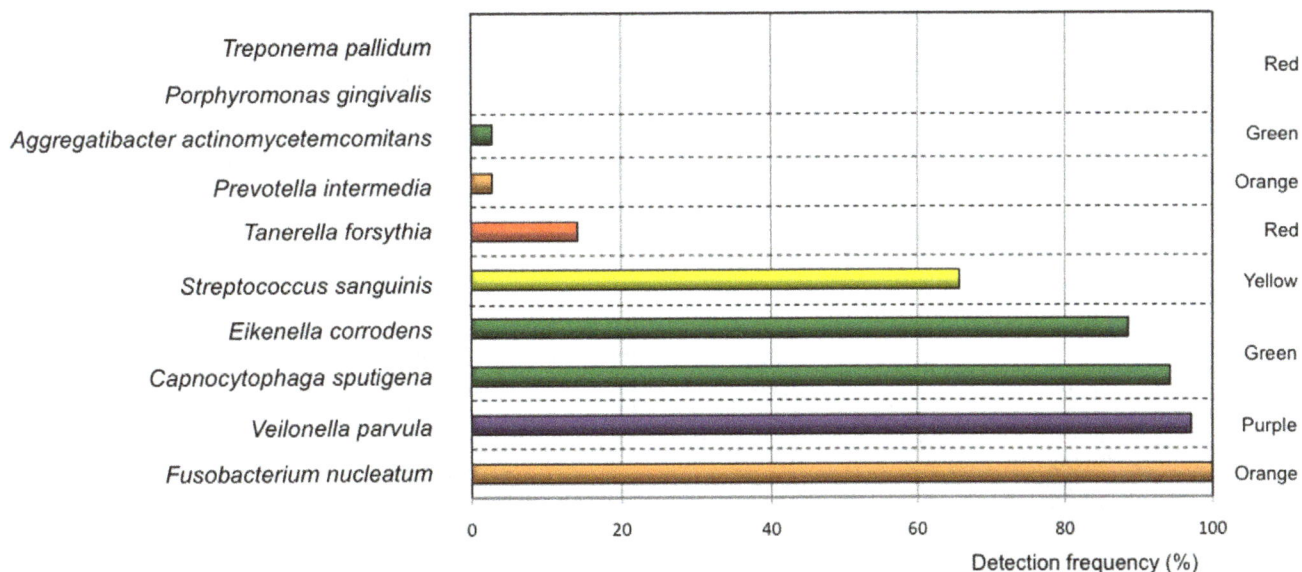

Figure 3. Species-specific detection of bacteria in 21-day old dental biofilms. The box-plots represent the PCR-based detection frequency of ten representative bacterial species within the study population of 37 subjects. The colors of the bars comply with the color codes of the bacterial complexes introduced by Socransky et al. [20].

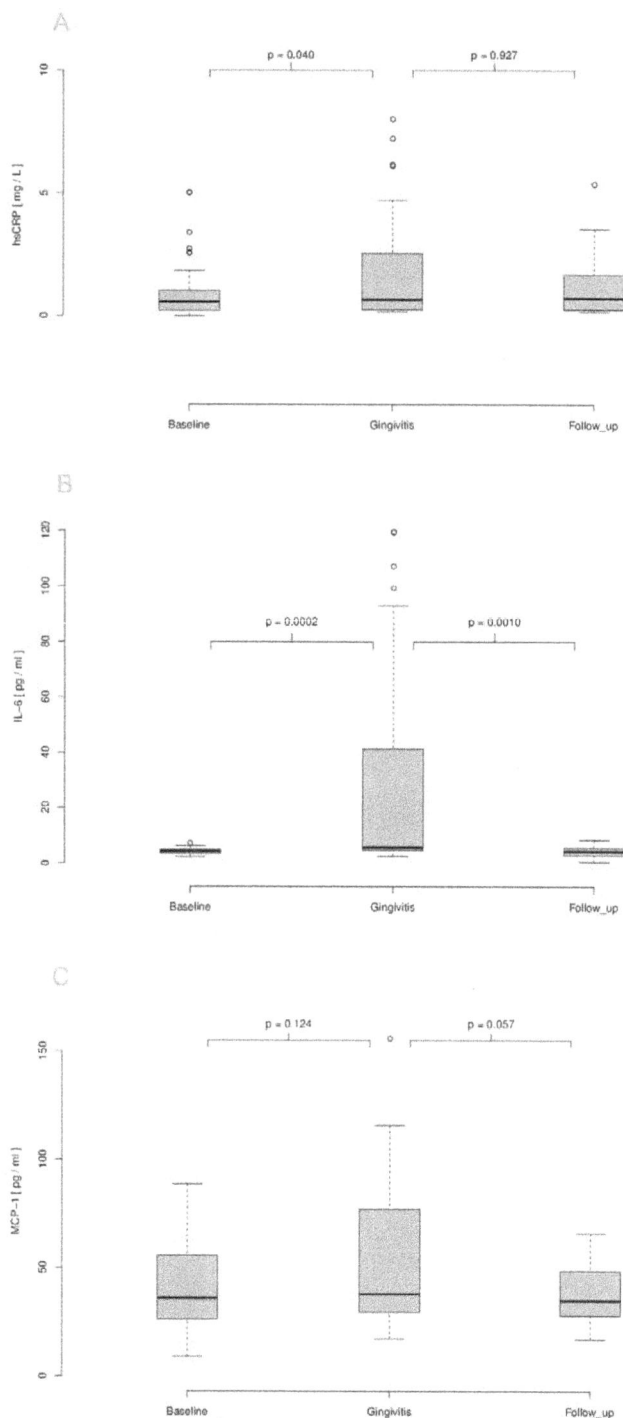

Figure 4. Characterization of serum parameters of inflammation at baseline, experimental gingivitis and follow-up. (A) Serum of participants was analyzed for hsCRP by immunonephelometrie. Plasma of participants was analyzed for IL-6 (B) and MCP-1 (C) by ELISA. Serums of participants were analyzed for leucocyte (D) and monocyte (E) cell counts by flow cytometry. P-values were calculated using two-sided Wilcoxon signed-rank tests for paired samples.

between serum CRP levels and the degree of gingivitis. In contrast, elevated levels of serum IL-6 were found in patients suffering from type 2 diabetes and natural gingivitis compared to patients with diabetes and healthy gingival conditions [23]. The different observations between these studies and the present study may be explained at least in part by the young healthy participants of the present study, which do not have any traditional risk factors for cardiovascular diseases. In addition, a very sensitive method for the detection of CRP in serum was used.

Most likely, the observed gingival inflammatory processes, which was induced in the present study affect approximately 75% of Western populations [1]. In contrast to periodontitis, gingivitis affects children, adults and elderly in nearly equal ratios [8]. Clinically, this inflammatory process becomes obvious by bleeding during brushing the teeth, normally on a limited number of teeth. For the present study this clinical appearance was tried to mimick by inducing the inflammatory processes also just on a limited number of teeth, here seven, during a 21-days plaque accumulation phase. The inflammatory reactions of the gingival tissues are only mild and clinically nearly inconspicuous to the untrained eye. We studied well-characterized young healthy volunteers that yet did not show any traditional risk factor for cardiovascular diseases. Thus, we are assured that the observed systemic changes are a consequence of the local gingival inflammatory processes. However, the participants did not respond equally and showed inter-individual differences regarding the amount of dental plaque load, clinical signs of inflammation and serum markers of inflammation.

To further address the oral inflammatory status, we analyzed the presence of ten different species belonging to variable complexes according to Haffajee et al. [19], in which potential pathogens spread across different clusters. Bacterial species predominantly associated with subgingival lesions of destructive periodontitis were if at all in very low numbers present in the developing supragingival plaques of the present study [24,25]. Only *Fusobacterium nucleatum*, a so called 'bridge-bacterium' between health and disease, could be detected in high frequency in all plaque samples. Generally periopathogens, namely *Porphyromonas gingivalis*, are in the focus of research aimed to identify pathological mechanisms between periodontitis and systemic diseases [26]. The present study demonstrated that systemic effects could also be induced by low-level gingival inflammation and by bacterial plaques that do not harbour traditional periopathogens like *Porphyromonas gingivalis*. Hence, the present study is the first report that demonstrates adverse effects of local experimentally induced gingival inflammation on circulating serum levels of CRP, IL-6 and MCP-1 and activation of monocytes. These results demonstrated an enhanced systemic inflammatory status of the subjects during the course of the study. Future experiments are warranted to evaluate if natural gingivitis also enhances systemic inflammatory markers and the risk for atherosclerotic diseases. Elevated CRP, IL-6 and MCP-1 serum levels could serve as a direct marker of the inflammatory activity in the subjects' gingiva. The serum concentrations of hsCRP and IL-6 during the state of gingivitis reached levels, which were previously shown to be associated with high cardiovascular event rate i.e. myocardial infarction [27,28]. The broad concordance between clinical markers of gingival inflammation and systemic inflammatory markers and monocyte activation suggests a relationship between the local and systemic recations. Only one epidemiological study has been published aimed to identify associations between gingival inflammation and angina pectoris, however, the reported results are critical due to various confounding factors and unpredictable outcomes of self-reported data sampling [29]. For the present study the clinical parameters

association of experimental gingivitis and systemic CRP and IL-6 levels in a population of healthy adults aged 18 to 30 years. These experiments were in accordance with a study of natural gingivitis by Wohlfeil et al. [22]. This group also showed no correlation

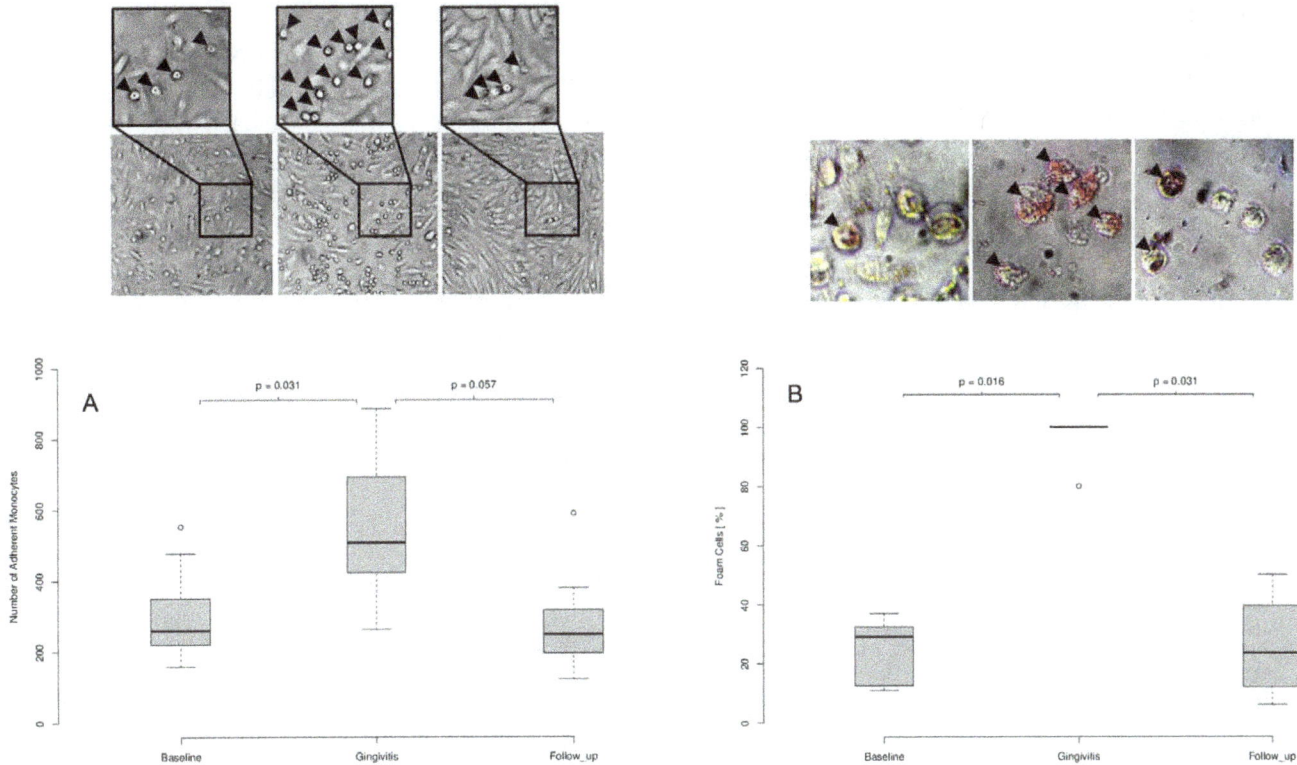

Figure 5. Monocyte adhesion assays and foam cell formation at baseline, gingivitis and follow-up. Blood monocytes were isolated from the blood of the volunteers at baseline (day 0), gingivitis (day 21) and follow-up (day 42) and subjected to ex vivo activation assays. (A) Number of adherent monocytes on cultured endothelial cells (HUVECs). Arrowheads in the enlarged picture detail indicate adherent monocytes. (B) Percentage foam cell formation after stimulation with oxLDL (10 µg/ml). Arrowheads indicate oil red O-positive foam cells. Representative pictures are shown. *P*-values were calculated using two-sided Wilcoxon signed-rank tests for paired samples.

of experimental gingivitis were not followed after day 21 of the experimental gingivitis phase, because multiple studies have shown that the clinical signs of gingivitis decline within seven days after the re-initiation of oral hygiene procedures in a group of subjects highly familiar with oral hygiene [30,31].

A potential limitation of this study is the sample size of 37 volunteers. However, the single-subject design with the subject as its own control is highly sensitive to detect individual differences. The here presented findings with young healthy individuals could not be generalized since elder subjects have an overall higher risk burden. Nevertheless, we especially have chosen young healthy subjects with no cardiovascular risk factors, to study systemic effects of experimental gingivitis. Thus, this approach offers the best prospect to uncover a potential relationship between local oral inflammation in gingivitis and systemic effects on surrogate markers of atherosclerosis. Definitely, larger randomised multi-center trials with elder subjects are necessary to investigate the hypothesis whether oral low-level gingivitis increases the risk for atherosclerosis or even enhances cardiovascular events.

The mechanisms by which local inflammatory processes of the oral cavity affect systemic conditions remain largely unknown and future experimental studies are warranted. Gingivitis involves bacterial infection with a range of Gram-positive and Gram-negative bacteria that invade the superficial gingival tissues [32]. During progression of the gingival disease, the epithelium becomes ulcerated to expose the underlying connective tissues and blood capillaries and facilitates entry of biofilm organisms or their products (e.g. bacterial heat-shock proteins) to the circulation during eating or tooth brushing [33]. Pathogens which have

entered the bloodstream can directly invade blood vessel walls and atherosclerotic plaques [34,35,36]. Finally both, local oral infection and circulating infection products lead to an increase in the levels of circulating cytokines, chemokines and acute phase proteins, which are known to be associated with an increased cardiovascular event rate. The present study is the first report that demonstrated elevated serum levels of CRP, IL-6 and MCP-1 in the course of experimental gingivitis. Of interest, even gingival tissues were found to synthesize CRP [37]. Other inflammatory diseases, such as lupus erythematosus and rheumatoid arthritis are also associated with an increased cardiovascular risk supporting a mechanistic link between local extravascular inflammation and cardiovascular diseases [38,39].

It will be a task for future studies to identify the mechanisms that may account for the observed individual levels of local and systemic host responses. The potential confirmation that natural gingival inflammatory processes are an extravascular stimuli for systemic inflammation and atherogenesis will have great public health implications.

Author Contributions

Conceived and designed the experiments: JE KG BS MS. Performed the experiments: JE ML WH DD HS RSS DL NS IS. Analyzed the data: JE KG RS BS MS. Contributed reagents/materials/analysis tools: JE KG ML RS RSS DL BS MS. Wrote the paper: JE KG ML BS MS.

References

1. Kebschull M, Demmer RT, Papapanou PN (2010) "Gum bug, leave my heart alone!"–epidemiologic and mechanistic evidence linking periodontal infections and atherosclerosis. J Dent Res 89: 879–902.

2. Pihlstrom BL, Michalowicz BS, Johnson NW (2005) Periodontal diseases. Lancet 366: 1809–1820.

3. Lockhart PB, Bolger AF, Papapanou PN, Osinbowale O, Trevisan M, et al. (2012) Periodontal disease and atherosclerotic vascular disease: does the evidence support an independent association?: a scientific statement from the American Heart Association. Circulation 125: 2520–2544.

4. Elter JR, Hinderliter AL, Offenbacher S, Beck JD, Caughey M, et al. (2006) The effects of periodontal therapy on vascular endothelial function: a pilot trial. Am Heart J 151: 47.

5. Tonetti MS, D'Aiuto F, Nibali L, Donald A, Storry C, et al. (2007) Treatment of periodontitis and endothelial function. N Engl J Med 356: 911–920.

6. Demmer RT, Papapanou PN (2010) Epidemiologic patterns of chronic and aggressive periodontitis. Periodontol 2000 53: 28–44.

7. Ericsson JS, Abrahamsson KH, Ostberg AL, Hellstrom MK, Jonsson K, et al. (2009) Periodontal health status in Swedish adolescents: an epidemiological, cross-sectional study. Swed Dent J 33: 131–139.

8. Li Y, Lee S, Hujoel P, Su M, Zhang W, et al. (2010) Prevalence and severity of gingivitis in American adults. Am J Dent 23: 9–13.

9. Hansson GK (2005) Inflammation, atherosclerosis, and coronary artery disease. N Engl J Med 352: 1685–1695.

10. Libby P, Ridker PM, Hansson GK (2011) Progress and challenges in translating the biology of atherosclerosis. Nature 473: 317–325.

11. Uno K, Nicholls SJ (2010) Biomarkers of inflammation and oxidative stress in atherosclerosis. Biomark Med 4: 361–373.

12. Drakopoulou M, Toutouzas K, Stefanadi E, Tsiamis E, Tousoulis D, et al. (2009) Association of inflammatory markers with angiographic severity and extent of coronary artery disease. Atherosclerosis 206: 335–339.

13. Wahaidi VY, Kowolik MJ, Eckert GJ, Galli DM (2011) Endotoxemia and the host systemic response during experimental gingivitis. J Clin Periodontol 38: 412–417.

14. Koren O, Spor A, Felin J, Fak F, Stombaugh J, et al. (2011) Human oral, gut, and plaque microbiota in patients with atherosclerosis. Proc Natl Acad Sci U S A 108 Suppl 1: 4592–4598.

15. Loe H, Theilade E, Jensen SB (1965) Experimental Gingivitis in Man. J Periodontol 36: 177–187.

16. Slawik S, Staufenbiel I, Schilke R, Nicksch S, Weinspach K, et al. (2011) Probiotics affect the clinical inflammatory parameters of experimental gingivitis in humans. Eur J Clin Nutr 65: 857–863.

17. Silness J, Löe H (1964) Periodontal Disease in Pregnancy. II. Correlation between Oral Hygiene and Periodontal Condition. Acta Odontol Scand 22: 121–135.

18. Löe H, Silness J (1963) Periodontal Disease in Pregnancy. I. Prevalence and Severity. Acta Odontol Scand 21: 533–551.

19. Haffajee AD, Socransky SS, Patel MR, Song X (2008) Microbial complexes in supragingival plaque. Oral Microbiol Immunol 23: 196–205.

20. Socransky SS, Haffajee AD, Cugini MA, Smith C, Kent RL Jr (1998) Microbial complexes in subgingival plaque. J Clin Periodontol 25: 134–144.

21. Honda T, Domon H, Okui T, Kajita K, Amanuma R, et al. (2006) Balance of inflammatory response in stable gingivitis and progressive periodontitis lesions. Clin Exp Immunol 144: 35–40.

22. Wohlfeil M, Wehner J, Schacher B, Oremek GM, Sauer-Eppel H, et al. (2009) Degree of gingivitis correlates to systemic inflammation parameters. Clin Chim Acta 401: 105–109.

23. Andriankaja OM, Barros SP, Moss K, Panagakos FS, DeVizio W, et al. (2009) Levels of serum interleukin (IL)-6 and gingival crevicular fluid of IL-1beta and prostaglandin E(2) among non-smoking subjects with gingivitis and type 2 diabetes. J Periodontol 80: 307–316.

24. Zee KY, Samaranayake LP, Attstrom R (1996) Predominant cultivable supragingival plaque in Chinese "rapid" and "slow" plaque formers. J Clin Periodontol 23: 1025–1031.

25. Haffajee AD, Teles RP, Patel MR, Song X, Veiga N, et al. (2009) Factors affecting human supragingival biofilm composition. I. Plaque mass. J Periodontal Res 44: 511–519.

26. Gaetti-Jardim E Jr, Marcelino SL, Feitosa AC, Romito GA, Avila-Campos MJ (2009) Quantitative detection of periodontopathic bacteria in atherosclerotic plaques from coronary arteries. J Med Microbiol 58: 1568–1575.

27. Ridker PM, Rifai N, Stampfer MJ, Hennekens CH (2000) Plasma concentration of interleukin-6 and the risk of future myocardial infarction among apparently healthy men. Circulation 101: 1767–1772.

28. Ridker PM, Hennekens CH, Buring JE, Rifai N (2000) C-reactive protein and other markers of inflammation in the prediction of cardiovascular disease in women. N Engl J Med 342: 836–843.

29. Ylostalo PV, Jarvelin MR, Laitinen J, Knuuttila ML (2006) Gingivitis, dental caries and tooth loss: risk factors for cardiovascular diseases or indicators of elevated health risks. J Clin Periodontol 33: 92–101.

30. Eberhard J, Reimers N, Dommisch H, Hacker J, Freitag S, et al. (2005) The effect of the topical administration of bioactive glass on inflammatory markers of human experimental gingivitis. Biomaterials 26: 1545–1551.

31. Eberhard J, Jepsen S, Albers HK, Acil Y (2000) Quantitation of arachidonic acid metabolites in small tissue biopsies by reversed-phase high-performance liquid chromatography. Anal Biochem 280: 258–263.

32. Saglie FR, Pertuiset JH, Rezende MT, Sabet MS, Raoufi D, et al. (1987) Bacterial invasion in experimental gingivitis in man. J Periodontol 58: 837–846.

33. Forner L, Larsen T, Kilian M, Holmstrup P (2006) Incidence of bacteremia after chewing, tooth brushing and scaling in individuals with periodontal inflammation. J Clin Periodontol 33: 401–407.

34. Elkaim R, Dahan M, Kocgozlu L, Werner S, Kanter D, et al. (2008) Prevalence of periodontal pathogens in subgingival lesions, atherosclerotic plaques and healthy blood vessels: a preliminary study. J Periodontal Res 43: 224–231.

35. Chiu B (1999) Multiple infections in carotid atherosclerotic plaques. Am Heart J 138: S534–536.

36. Libby P, Egan D, Skarlatos S (1997) Roles of infectious agents in atherosclerosis and restenosis: an assessment of the evidence and need for future research. Circulation 96: 4095–4103.

37. Lu Q, Jin L (2010) Human gingiva is another site of C-reactive protein formation. J Clin Periodontol 37: 789–796.

38. de Groot L, Posthumus MD, Kallenberg CG, Bijl M (2010) Risk factors and early detection of atherosclerosis in rheumatoid arthritis. Eur J Clin Invest 40: 835–842.

39. Boucelma M, Haddoum F, Chaudet H, Kaplanski G, Mazouni-Brahimi N, et al. (2011) Cardiovascular risk and lupus disease. Int Angiol 30: 18–24.

40. Baumgartner JC, Watkins BJ, Bae KS, Xia T (1999) Association of black-pigmented bacteria with endodontic infections. J Endod 25: 413–415.

41. Conrads G, Gharbia SE, Gulabivala K, Lampert F, Shah HN (1997) The use of a 16s rDNA directed PCR for the detection of endodontopathogenic bacteria. J Endod 23: 433–438.

42. Hoshino T, Kawaguchi M, Shimizu N, Hoshino N, Ooshima T, et al. (2004) PCR detection and identification of oral streptococci in saliva samples using gtf genes. Diagn Microbiol Infect Dis 48: 195–199.

43. Conrads G, Mutters R, Fischer J, Brauner A, Lütticken R, et al. (1996) PCR reaction and dot-blot hybridization to monitor the distribution of oral pathogens within plaque samples of periodontally healthy individuals. J Periodontol 67: 994–1003.

44. Ashimoto A, Chen C, Bakker I, Slots J (1996) Polymerase chain reaction detection of 8 putative periodontal pathogens in subgingival plaque of gingivitis and advanced periodontitis lesions. Oral Microbiol Immunol 11: 266–273.

45. Igarashi E, Kamaguchi A, Fujita M, Miyakawa H, Nakazawa F (2009) Identification of oral species of the genus Veillonella by polymerase chain reaction. Oral Microbiol Immunol 24: 310–313.

46. Kim SG, Kim SH, Kim MK, Kim HS, Kook JK (2005) Identification of Actinobacillus actinomycetemcomitans using species-specific 16S rDNA primers. J Microbiol 43: 209–212.

8

A Phage Display Selected 7-mer Peptide Inhibitor of the *Tannerella forsythia* Metalloprotease-Like Enzyme Karilysin Can Be Truncated to Ser-Trp-Phe-Pro

Peter Durand Skottrup[1]*, Grete Sørensen[1], Miroslaw Ksiazek[2], Jan Potempa[2,3], Erik Riise[1]

1 Biomolecular Interaction Group, Department of Drug Design and Pharmacology, Faculty of Health and Medical Sciences, University of Copenhagen, Copenhagen, Denmark, 2 Department of Microbiology, Faculty of Biochemistry, Biophysics and Biotechnology, Jagiellonian University, Krakow, Poland, 3 Oral Health and Systemic Diseases Research Group, University of Louisville, School of Dentistry, Louisville, Kentucky, United States of America

Abstract

Tannerella forsythia is a gram-negative bacteria, which is strongly associated with the development of periodontal disease. Karilysin is a newly identified metalloprotease-like enzyme, that is secreted from *T. forsythia*. Karilysin modulates the host immune response and is therefore considered a likely drug target. In this study peptides were selected towards the catalytic domain from Karilysin (Kly18) by phage display. The peptides were linear with low micromolar binding affinities. The two best binders (peptide14 and peptide15), shared the consensus sequence XWFPXXXGGG. A peptide15 fusion with Maltose Binding protein (MBP) was produced with peptide15 fused to the N-terminus of MBP. The peptide15-MBP was expressed in *E. coli* and the purified fusion-protein was used to verify Kly18 specific binding. Chemically synthesised peptide15 (SWFPLRSGGG) could inhibit the enzymatic activity of both Kly18 and intact Karilysin (Kly48). Furthermore, peptide15 could slow down the autoprocessing of intact Kly48 to Kly18. The WFP motif was important for inhibition and a truncation study further demonstrated that the N-terminal serine was also essential for Kly18 inhibition. The SWFP peptide had a Ki value in the low micromolar range, which was similar to the intact peptide15. In conclusion SWFP is the first reported inhibitor of Karilysin and can be used as a valuable tool in structure-function studies of Karilysin.

Editor: Richard C. Willson, University of Houston, United States of America

Funding: This work was supported by the Lundbeck Foundation [grant number R54-A5291 to PDS]; the National Institutes of Health [Grant number DE 09761, United States of America to JP]; National Science Center [2011/01/B/NZ6/00268, Kraków, Poland to JP]; the European Community [FP7-HEALTH-2010-261460 "Gums&Joints" to JP]; the Foundation for Polish Science [TEAM project DPS/424–329/10 to JP]; the Faculty of Biochemistry, Biophysics and Biotechnology of the Jagiellonian University (FBB&B-UJ) [project no. K/DSC/000361 to MK]; and structural funds from the European Union [POIG.02.01.00-12-064/08 to FBB&B-UJ]. The funders had no role in study design, data collection and analysis, decision to publish, or preparation of the manuscript.

Competing Interests: The authors have declared that no competing interests exist.

* E-mail: pds@farma.ku.dk

Introduction

Periodontitis is a serious bacterial infection-driven inflammatory disease affecting the periodontium, i.e., the tissues that surround and support the teeth. The 'red complex' is a term used for the three bacterial taxa that are considered the major periodontopathogens (*Treponema denticola*, *Porphyromonas gingivalis* and *Tannerella forsythia*) that lead to disease development [1]. These pathogens all produce high levels of extracellular proteolytic activity [2–8], which contributes to the periodontitis symptoms; loss of attachment between the tooth and the gingiva, which is due to bone degradation and weakening of the soft tissues surrounding the root of a tooth. This ultimately leads to formation of deep periodontal pockets and teeth loss [9]. Furthermore, accumulating evidence suggests that severe forms of periodontitis contribute to development of the systemic diseases, stroke, diabetes and rheumatoid arthritis [10–14]. Current periodontitis therapies are based upon mechanical removal of supra- and subgingival bacterial plaque from the tooth surface in conjunction with the use of antibiotics. Unfortunately, this treatment is not always fully effective, and focus was therefore directed towards development of protease inhibitors as an alternative weapon towards the period-

ontopathogen effects. In fact, a factor Xa inhibitor could inhibit the *P. gingivalis* gingipain proteases RgpA and RgpB and was bactericidal towards *P. gingivalis* [15]. Furthermore, chlorhexidine and benzamidine were used successfully to inhibit *P. gingivalis* gingipains [16,17]. Furthermore, doxycycline could inhibit protease activity from *P. gingivalis* and *T. denticola* [18].

T. forsythia is a gram-negative bacteria, which secrete proteases that act as virulence factors (PrtH, a cysteine protease and BspA, a trypsin-like protease). PrtH displays hemolysin activity and one study suggested that BspA mediates *T. forsythia* attachment to fibronectin and fibrinogen [19–21]. Karilysin, a newly identified metalloprotease isolated from *T. forsythia* [6] is secreted as a 472-residue protein and has the following composition; a 20-residue signal sequence, a 14-residue pro-peptide, an 18 kDa catalytic peptidase domain and a 30 kDa C-terminal domain of unknown function. The full length enzyme could be recombinantly expressed but the enzyme matured through sequential autolysis, by first generating a fully active 48 kDa variant, followed by formation of the catalytic domain (named Kly18) [6,22]. Kly18 structural analysis demonstrated a similarity to mammalian matrix metalloproteinases (MMPs) [22]. MMPs are a separate family within the 'metzincin' clan of MPs and participate in turnover of extracellular-matrix components and selective activation/inactivation of other proteins and enzymes. The MMP activity is tightly regulated, however uncontrolled MMP-proteolysis can occur, leading to tissue destruction, apoptosis and inflammation [23]. Metalloproteases derived from microbial pathogens were documented as important virulence factors contributing to evasion of antimicrobial mechanisms of the innate immune system [24].

Only limited information is available on the biology of Karilysin. Recent data demonstrated that Karilysin can inactivate the antimicrobial peptide LL-37 by proteolytic cleavage [7]. This suggests that Karilysin can contribute to evasion of the human immune response. This hypothesis has been further substantiated by recent findings that Karilysin-expressing *T. forsythia* isolates inhibits all pathways of the complement system by Karilysin-mediated degradation of complement system proteins (mannose-binding lectin, ficolin-2, ficolin-3, C4 and C5) [25]. For these reasons Karilysin is considered a potential target for therapeutic intervention but no Karilysin inhibitors currently exist.

In this study phage display was used to identify a peptide that specifically bound Karilysin and efficiently inhibited the proteolytic activity of Karilysin.

Materials and Methods

Miscellaneous Reagents

Karilysin catalytic domain (Kly18) and intact Kly48 were produced as previously described [6]. Active human MMP-3 catalytic domain, Bovine Serum Albumine (BSA), LB-medium and FITC-Casein were from Sigma-Aldrich. Maltose-binding protein (MBP) was from ProSpec-Tany TechnoGene Ltd. Peroxidase conjugated mouse anti-M13 phage monoclonal antibody, LMW (Low Molecular Weight)-SDS Marker and 1 ml MBPTrap HP columns were from GE-Healthcare. Peptide phage libraries (7-mer and 7-mer cysteine-constrained), pMAL-pIII vector, M13KE insert extension primer (NEB #E8101), −96 gIII sequencing primer (NEB #S1259), monoclonal anti-MBP HRP-conjugate, *EagI* and *Acc65I* were from New England Biolabs. Maxisorp microtiter plates and black fluorescence non-surface treated plates were both from NUNC. OPD-tablets (*o*-Phenylenediamine dihydrochloride) were from DAKO. All peptides were synthesised by Genscript. T4-DNA ligase was from Invitrogen. QIAquick gel extraction kit was from QIAgen. Ampicillin was from Calbiochem. Isopropyl β-D-thiogalactoside (IPTG) was from VWR.

Biopanning

Phage libraries displaying seven amino acids in random sequence order at the N-terminal end of protein III were used for affinity selection of peptide binders towards Kly18. Both a linear and a constrained version of the peptide library were used for the selection. Microtiter plates were coated at 4°C for 16 hours with purified Kly18 at 0.66 μM using 100 μl per well. These plates were subsequently washed in PBS (20 mM sodium phosphate, 150 mM NaCl, pH 7.4) supplemented with 0.05% Tween-20 (PBS-T) and then blocked with 4% BSA in PBS for 2 h at room temperature. Bacteriophage at 10^{11} pfu/100 μl were used for each panning round. The constrained and linear libraries were mixed and panned together as a mixture in PBS supplemented with 0.1% Tween20, pH = 7.4. After incubation for one hour at room temperature plates were washed ten times with PBS-T (0.1% Tween20) and bound peptide-phage were eluted with glycine/HCl, pH = 2.2 for 10 min. followed by neutralisation with Tris-base, pH = 9.0. Eluted phage were used to infect exponentially growing TG1 cells overnight at 37°C. The following day peptide-phage were precipitated from the cell supernatant with phage

precipitation buffer (20% (w/v) PEG6000), 2.5 M NaCl) and redissolved in PBS as described [26]. After four rounds of panning, single clones were isolated and tested for Kly18 binding in phage ELISA (see below). Single stranded DNA was extracted from positive clones according to [27] and the DNA was sequenced in the region corresponding to the random peptide region.

Phage ELISA

Kly18 wells were coated and blocked as above. The following washes and incubations were performed at room temperature. After blocking, the plates were washed three times in PBS-T and one hundred μl solutions of the individual phage clones diluted 1:1 in 4% BSA/PBS were added in a concentration of 1×10^{10} pfu/ml and further incubated for one hour. Wells were washed ten times with PBS-T and next 100 μl of peroxidase conjugated mouse anti-M13 monoclonal antibody diluted 1/1000 in 2% BSA/PBS, pH = 7.4 was added and incubated for one hour. The plates were washed ten times and detection was carried out by adding 100 μl of an OPD solution (1 OPD-tablet dissolved in 3 ml H_2O and 5 μl 30% H_2O_2). The reaction was stopped by adding 100 μl of 1 M H_2SO_4 and absorbance values (*A*) were measured at 490 nm using an immunorcader (Emax).

Estimation of Peptide-phage Binding Affinity by the Use of Inhibition ELISA

Nunc Maxisorp plates were coated with Kly18 and blocked as described earlier. Titration curves of each clone revealed the phage concentration that gave half-maximum response, and this concentration was used for the individual inhibition assays. The inhibition assay was performed essentially as described previously [28]. Briefly, the individual phage clones were incubated with decreasing concentrations of Kly18 in 4% skimmed milk/PBS for 1 hour with extensive mixing. The mix was added to Kly18 coated and blocked wells and the unbound free phage were allowed to bind for 1 hour. Wells were washed with PBS-T five times and developed as above. The absorbance values were measured at 490 nm after 30 min of incubation at 22°C. Absorbance values determined at each Kly18 concentration (*A*) were divided by the absorbance measured in the presence of zero Kly18 (A_0), thereby yielding normalized values (A/A_0). These values were plotted against the Kly18 concentration to construct the inhibition curve. Curve fitting revealed the Kly18 concentration required for 50% inhibition (I_{50}) as described previously [28]. The assay was performed in triplicate.

Subcloning, Expression and Purification of the Maltose Binding Protein-peptide15 Fusion Protein

Peptide15 phage single stranded DNA was isolated as above and 25 ng of DNA was used as template for amplification of the peptide15 DNA by PCR using the M13KE insert extension primer and the −96 gIII sequencing primer. The programme used was 25 cycles of 95°C for 30 sec., 55°C for 30 sec. and 72°C for 30 sec. The PCR product was isolated as a single DNA band after agarose gel electrophoresis and digested with *Acc65I* and *EagI1*. The peptide15 DNA with flanking sequences was again purified after agarose gel electrophoresis. The peptide15 DNA was subcloned into *Acc65I*/*EagI* digested pMAL-pIII vector by T4-DNA ligase and transformed into chemocompetent TG1 cells. Clones were amplified, sequenced and preserved as glycerol stocks. A MBP-peptide15 clone was used for fusion-protein production by expansion in LB-medium (supplemented with 10 mM $MgCl_2$, 0.2% glucose and 1 mM ampicillin) and when $OD_{600} = 0.6$ was reached the culture was induced with 1 mM IPTG for 3 hours at

A

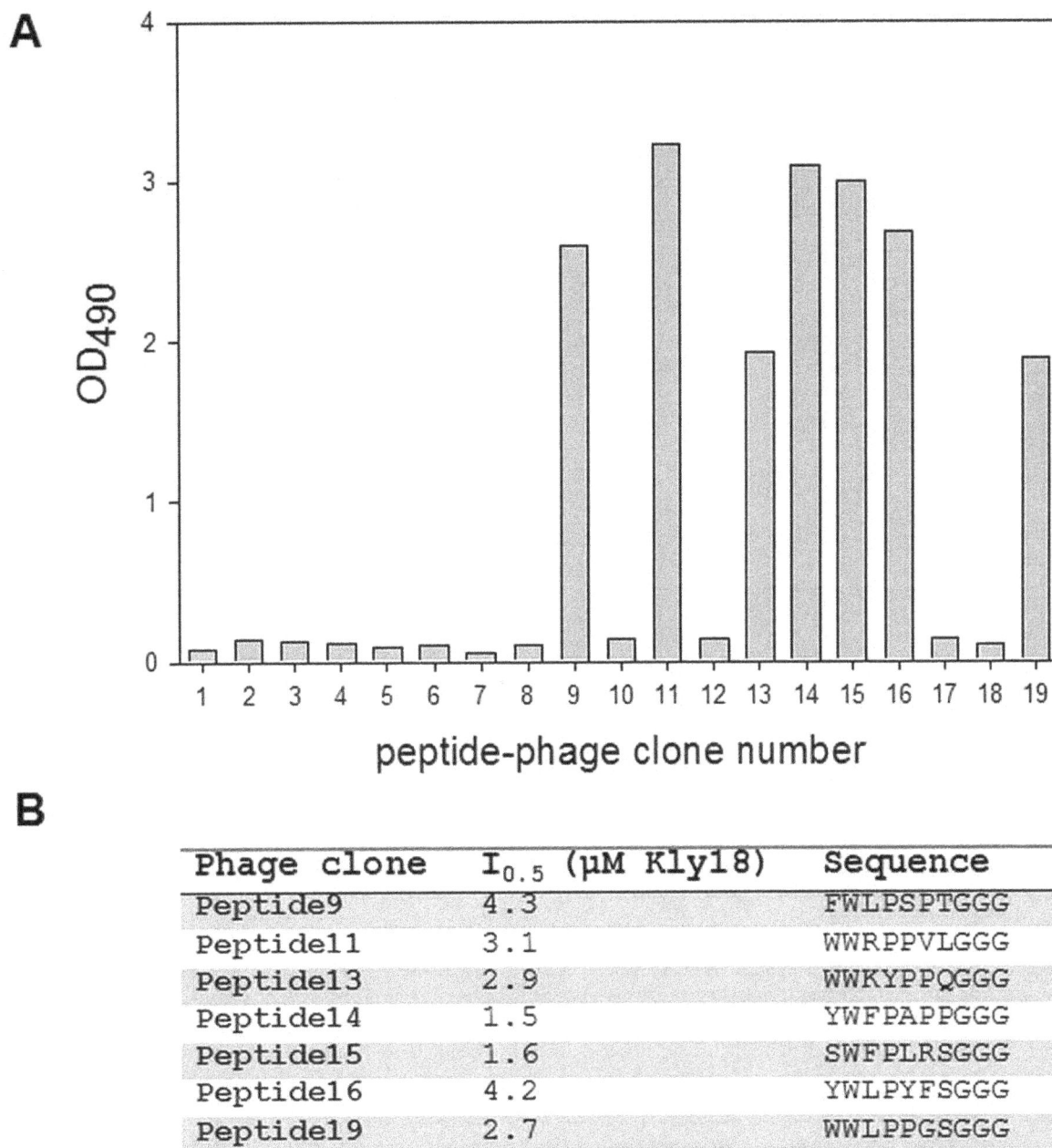

B

Phage clone	$I_{0.5}$ (µM Kly18)	Sequence
Peptide9	4.3	FWLPSPTGGG
Peptide11	3.1	WWRPPVLGGG
Peptide13	2.9	WWKYPPQGGG
Peptide14	1.5	YWFPAPPGGG
Peptide15	1.6	SWFPLRSGGG
Peptide16	4.2	YWLPYFSGGG
Peptide19	2.7	WWLPPGSGGG

Figure 1. Phage ELISA test of nineteen selected clones after four panning rounds, peptide sequences and estimated apparent afffinity. A) Optical density responses detected after the binding of peptide-phage to immobilized Kly18 are shown. Background binding to BSA has been subtracted for each clone. Clones with signals above 0.5 were deemed positive and further sequenced. B) Peptide-phage clones were tested in inhibition ELISA for estimation of affinity. All clones (except clone 13) shared the WXP motif.

30°C. The periplasmic fraction was isolated according to [29] and extensively dialysed into buffer A (20 mM Tris-HCl, 200 mM NaCl, 1 mM EDTA, pH 7.4). The dialysed fraction was applied to a 1 ml MBPTrap HP column at a flow rate of 1 ml/min and following extensive column wash with buffer A, MBP-peptide15 was eluted with 100% buffer B (20 mM Tris-HCl, 200 mM NaCl, 1 mM EDTA, 10 mM Maltose, pH 7.4). After dialysis into PBS, MBP-peptide15 purity was confirmed by SDS-PAGE.

Kly18 Detection by MBP-peptide15 ELISA

Kly18 and human MMP-3 catalytic domains were coated at the concentration of 0.66 µM. Blank wells were included for background determination. All wells were blocked in 4% BSA/PBS for 1 hour. After wash with PBS-T (5 times), MBP-peptide15 in 2% BSA/PBS diluted to 25 µg/ml was incubated for one hour with shaking. After wash with PBS-T (5 times), a monoclonal anti-MBP HRP-conjugate was added diluted 1:5000 in 2% BSA/PBS. Wells were washed ten times in PBS-T and developed with OPD substrate as above. To demonstrate that binding to Kly18 was mediated by peptide15 and not by MBP itself, control ELISA experiments were performed using MBP instead of MBP-peptide15.

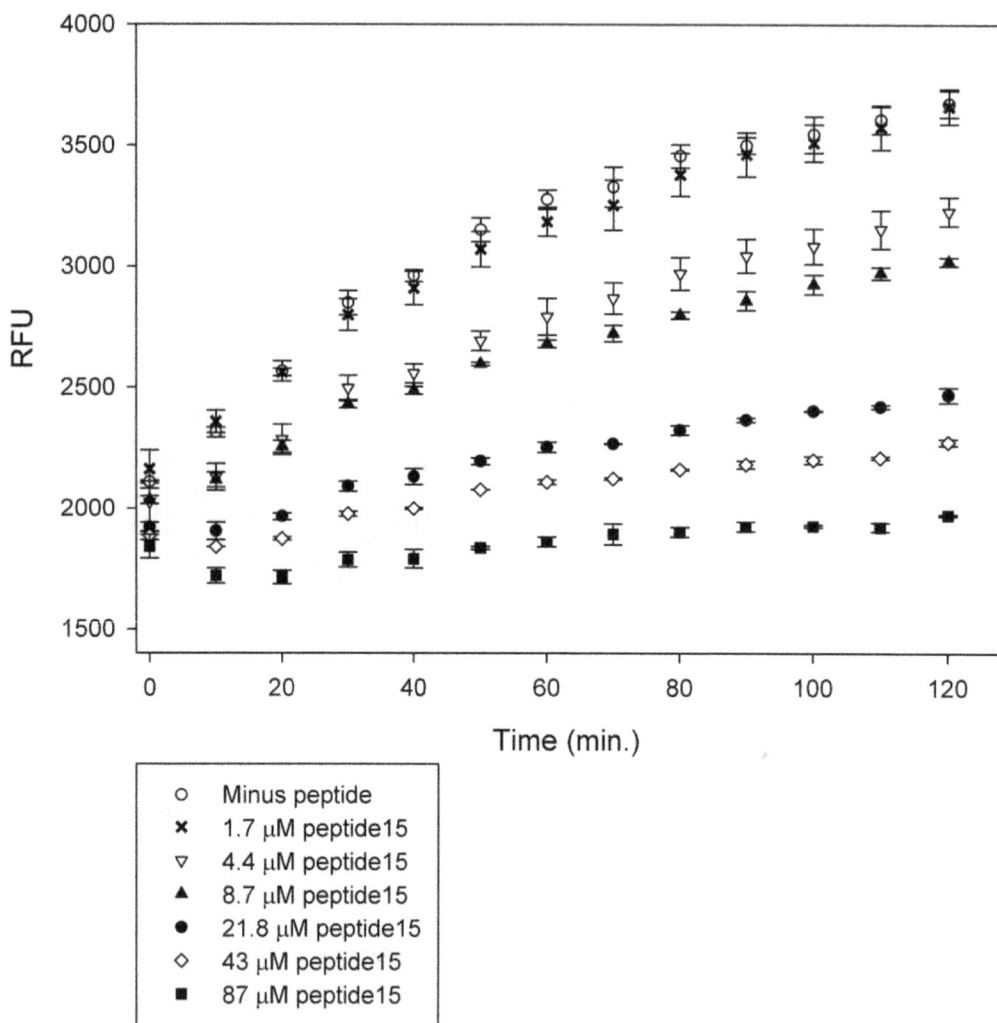

Figure 2. Peptide15 inhibits the proteolytic activity of Kly18. Peptide15 was pre-incubated with Kly18 in varying concentrations followed by addition of the substrate FITC-casein. The peptide15 inhibitory effect was seen as a decrease in Relative Fluorescence Units (RFU) in a dose-response manner. Error bars represent standard deviations between three experiments.

Assay for Monitoring Peptide15 Inhibitory Activity towards Kly18

Kly18 and Kly48 protease activities were monitored essentially as described [6]. One hundred μl working volumes were used in black untreated polypropylene microtitre plates and FITC-casein was used as the substrate. Assays were performed at 37°C using 500 nM of Kly18 (or Kly48) in assay buffer (100 mM Tris-HCl, 5mM $CaCl_2$, pH 8.0), at a FITC-casein concentration of 25 μg/ml. Released fluorescence was measured using a micro-titer plate reader at excitation/emission wavelengths of 485/538 nm. Peptides were dissolved in Milli Q water and added in varying molarities. The assay setup was as follows; Kly18 (or Kly48) was diluted in assay buffer together with peptide, followed by 30 minutes incubation on a vertical shaker at 22°C. Then FITC-casein was added and fluorescence formation was monitored at 37°C for 90 minutes with measurements every ten minutes. For estimation of inhibition constants (Ki) for peptide inhibition of Kly18, a fixed amount of Kly18 (500 nM as above) was incubated with varying concentrations of FITC-casein (5–25 μg/ml) in the presence of varying amounts of Kly18 peptide inhibitor (0–10 μM). Enzyme velocities were plotted, curves fitted and

determination of Ki was performed using GraphPad Prism 5.04 using the macro for competitive inhibitor.

Assay for Monitoring the Effect of Peptide15 on the Auto-processing of Kly48

Karilysin (Kly48) at 13 μM was incubated at 37°C in 50 mM Tris-HCl, 2.5 mM $CaCl_2$, 0.02% NaN_3 pH 8.0 alone or in the presence of the peptide SWFPL at 455 μM. At different time points samples were withdrawn and the Kly48 autocatalytic processing was monitored by SDS-PAGE using 10% gels and the Tris-HCl/Tricine buffer system [30]. Gels were stained with 0.1% Coomassie Brilliant Blue R-250 in 10% acetic acid followed by destaining. Samples were run alongside a Low Molecular Weight SDS-PAGE Marker.

Results and Discussion

Isolation of Kly18 Binding Peptide-phage

Peptide phage display is an excellent tool for fast identification of lead structures that can be further modified as protease inhibitors [31]. In the present study 7-mer peptide libraries were

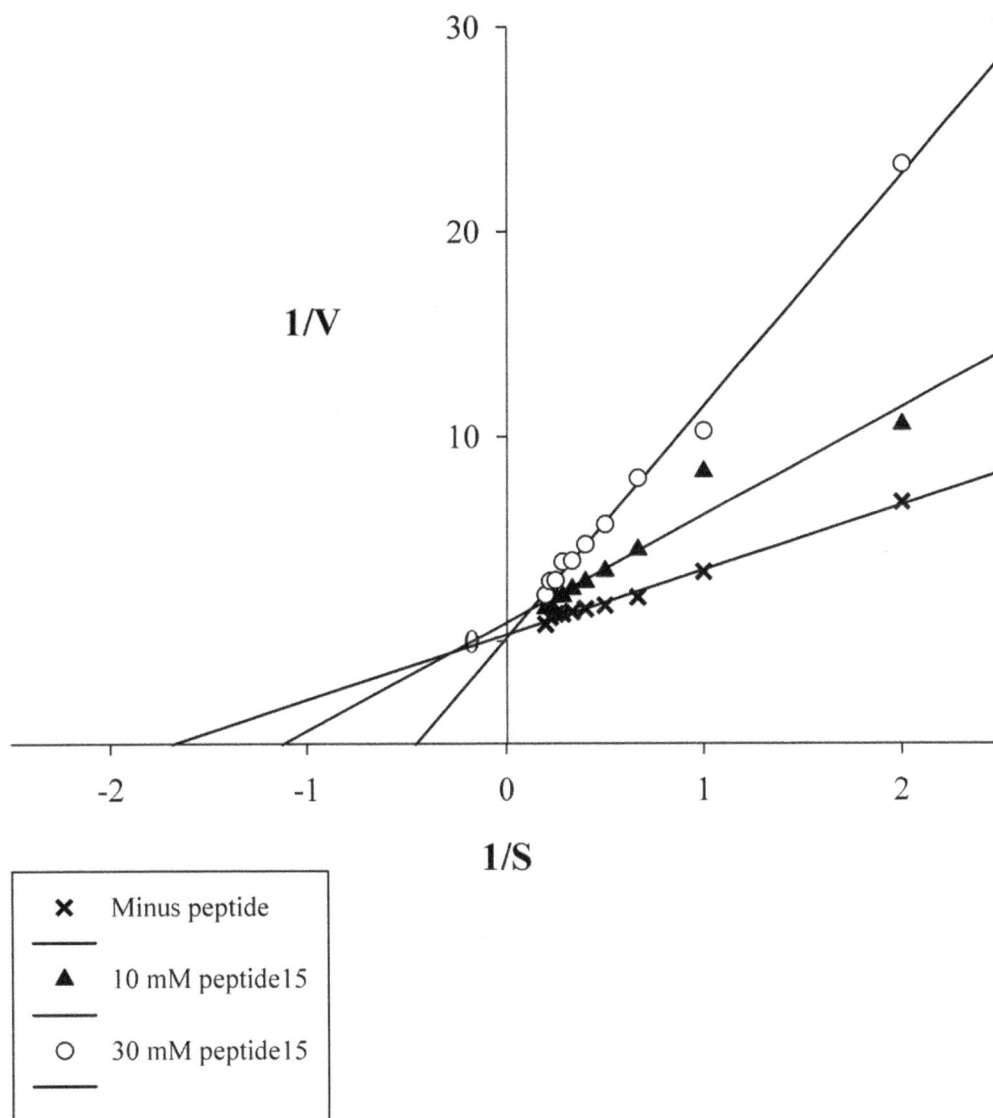

Figure 3. Peptide15 displays the characteristics of a competitive inhibitor. Shown are 1/V-1/S plot of peptide15 inhibition of Kly18. Kly18 was pre-incubated with fixed concentrations of peptide15 (10 μM and 30 μM) for 30 minutes, followed by incubation with varying concentrations of FITC-casein (5–50 μg/ml). As seen from the Lineweaver-Burke plot the Y-intercept is approximately the same for un-inhibited Kly18 as Kly18 inhibited with 10 μM and 30 μM, respectively. This suggested that peptide15 was a competitive inhibitor of Kly18. Linear regression lines were made using SigmaPlot 11.0. Data represent mean values from three experiments per substrate concentration.

used for bio-panning against the catalytic domain from Karilysin (Kly18). A cyclic 7-mer disulfide-constrained library (ACX₇CGGGS) and a linear 7-mer library (X₇GGGS) were mixed and used for selection on Kly18. Both libraries were fused to the N-terminal of protein III and displayed on phage. After four bio-panning rounds against surface-immobilized Kly18 a large enrichment in Kly18 binding phage was observed (>500 compared to the BSA control, data not shown). Nineteen clones were amplified and phage ELISA revealed seven Kly18-binders, peptide-phage 9,11,13,14,15,16,19 (Figure 1A). All seven peptide-phage displayed apparent affinities in the low micromolar range (Figure 1B). Only linear binders were isolated suggesting that the linear binders were of higher affinity than any potential cyclic peptides present in the library. In bio-panning experiments against other protein targets, we have used the same approach of mixing linear and cyclic libraries, but in these cases we isolated

constrained peptides as well as linear peptides (unpublished). This suggested that we could exclude the possibility of a higher growth rate of the linear peptide library as the reason why we only isolated linear binders. All identified Kly18-binding peptide-phage (except peptide13) had the WXP motif, clearly demonstrating that these amino acids are important for Kly18 binding (Figure 1B). Interestingly, no peptides were found with the WXP motif in position 1–3 and all the peptides had the WXP peptide motif placed in position 2–4, thereby suggesting that an amino acid is essential in position one prior to the WXP motif for structural stability. Furthermore, it was evident that the X-position in the Kly18-binding motif was dependent upon basic amino acids (arginine/lysine) or bulky hydrophobic residues (leucine/phenyl-alanine) (Figure 1B). A decision was made to further focus on peptide15 (SWFPLRSGGGS).

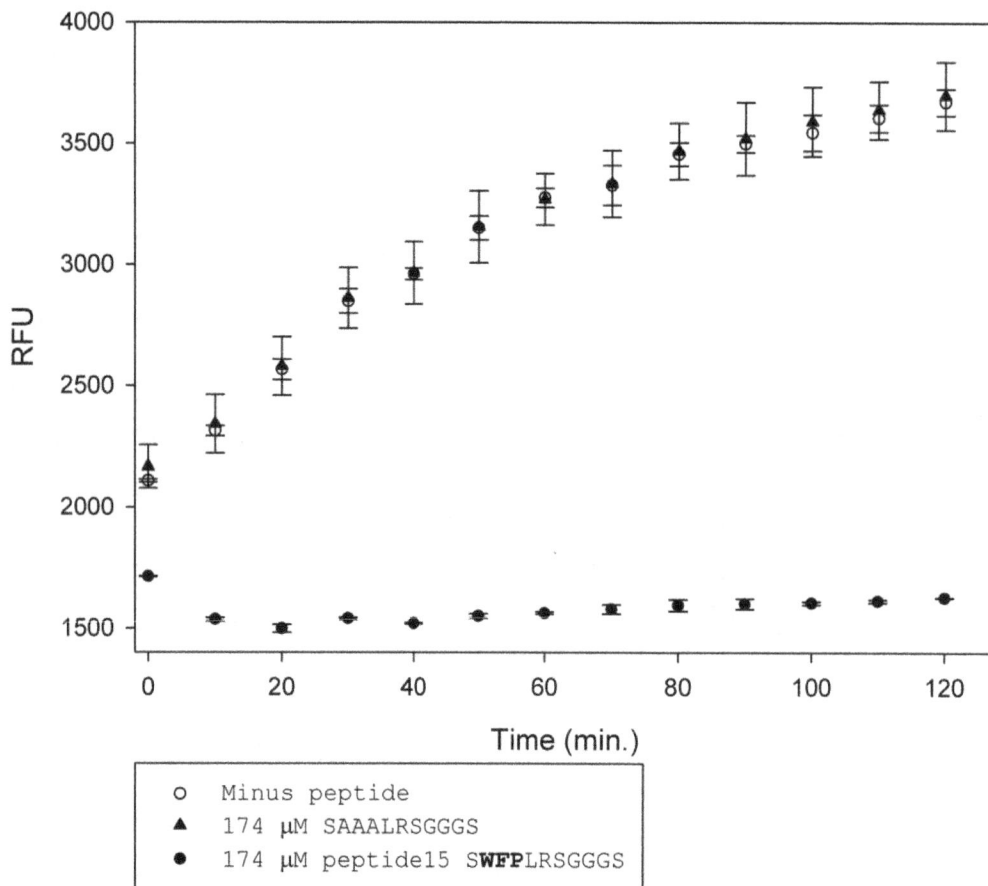

Figure 4. The WFP peptide motif is reponsible for Kly18 binding and inhibition. Pre-incubation of Kly18 with peptide15, (NH_2)-SWFPLRSGGGS-$(CONH_2)$, and a control peptide (NH_2)-SAAALRSGGGS-$(CONH_2)$, demonstrated that Kly18 inhibition could only be achieved with peptide15. Therefore, we concluded that the WFP motif was not only important for Kly18 binding but also for Kly18 inhibition. Error bars represent standard deviations between two experiments.

Free Soluble Peptide15 Inhibits Kly18 Proteolytic Activity

Peptide15 was chemically synthesised for activity testing. Initially, the peptide was synthesised in its entirety, mimicking all of the sequence displayed on phage. The peptide15 N-terminal was free during panning, however the C-terminal was fused to the phage. Consequently, peptide15 did not have a free negatively charged carboxylate at its C-terminal during panning. Therefore, in order to limit an effect of a C-terminal carboxylate, peptide15 was synthesised with a C-terminal amidation to block any unwanted C-terminal effects. The peptide15 synthesised was therefore (NH_2)-SWFPLRSGGGS-$(CONH_2)$. The Kly18 proteolytic activity was monitored with FITC-casein as the substrate and peptide15 inhibited Kly18-mediated FITC-casein cleavage in a dose-response manner (Figure 2). Furthermore, peptide15 displayed the characteristics of a competitive inhibitor as shown from a $1/V$-$1/S$ plot of peptide15 inhibition of Kly18. As seen from the Lineweaver-Burke plot the Y-intercept is approximately the same for un-inhibited Kly18 as Kly18 inhibited with 10 µM peptide15 and 30 µM peptide15, respectively (Figure 3). This suggested that peptide15 was a competitive inhibitor of Kly18.

To investigate the importance of the peptide15 WFP motif for Kly18 inhibition a control peptide was chemically synthesised with the WFP motif replaced by a triple alanine, (NH_2)-SAAALRSGGGS-$(CONH_2)$. Even in a very high dose (174 µM) the control peptide had a curve similar to that of Kly18 with no

peptide present, thereby demonstrating that the WFP motif was crucial for inhibition of Kly18 (Figure 4).

Peptide15 Truncation Study and Comparative Kinetic Analysis

Peptide15 was synthesised in its entirety, including the linker sequence attached to the phage (GGGS) and the question arose if the amino acids flanking the WFP motif were necessary for Kly18 inhibition. To answer this, fifteen truncation variants of peptide15 were designed, termed 15-1 to 15–16 and the peptide15 lead structure was named 15-0 (Table 1). Peptide version 15-9 (WFPLRSGGGS) was too hydrophobic for synthesis but all others could be produced. Initially all peptide versions were screened in a relatively high single concentration (87 µM) to reveal if omission of single amino acid residues displayed dramatic effects on Kly18 inhibition. The peptide15 truncated version (NH_2)-SWFP-$(CONH_2)$ retained efficient inhibitory potency but the peptide (NH_2)-WFP-$(CONH_2)$ was completely inactive towards Kly18 (Figure 5). The data clearly demonstrated that the serine in position 1 was crucial for inhibition of Kly18 as all peptide versions lacking this serine (15-8,15-10,15-11,15-12,15-13,15-14,15-15) lost most or all of their Kly18 inhibition capacity (Figure 5). Therefore, the Kly18 inhibiting peptide motif was expanded to (NH_2)-SWFP-$(CONH_2)$. A possible explanation is that in absence of serine the presence of a charged amino group attached directly to the

Table 1. Peptides used in the truncation study.

Name	Sequence
15-0	(NH_2)-SWFPLRSGGGS-$(CONH_2)$
15-1	(NH_2)-SWFPLRSGGG-$(CONH_2)$
15-2	(NH_2)-SWFPLRSGG-$(CONH_2)$
15-3	(NH_2)-SWFPLRSG-$(CONH_2)$
15-4	(NH_2)-SWFPLRS-$(CONH_2)$
15-5	(NH_2)-SWFPLR-$(CONH_2)$
15-6	(NH_2)-SWFPL-$(CONH_2)$
15-7	(NH_2)-SWFP-$(CONH_2)$
15-8	(NH_2)-WFP-$(CONH_2)$
15-9*	(NH_2)-WFPLRSGGGS-$(CONH_2)$
15-10	(NH_2)-WFPLRSGGG-$(CONH_2)$
15-11	(NH_2)-WFPLRSGG-$(CONH_2)$
15-12	(NH_2)-WFPLRSG-$(CONH_2)$
15-13	(NH_2)-WFPLRS-$(CONH_2)$
15-14	(NH_2)-WFPLR-$(CONH_2)$
15-15	(NH_2)-WFPL-$(CONH_2)$
15-16	(NH_2)-SWAPLRSGGGS-$(CONH_2)$

Shown are all possible truncation combinations of peptide15, while still retaining the WFP motif. Each structure is given a number. The peptide15 lead structure has the number 15-0. Structure 15-9 was too hydrophobic for synthesis.

tryptophan of the (NH_2)-WFP-$(CONH_2)$ motif could interfere with the binding and inhibitory mechanism of the peptide. Interestingly, full length peptide15 with an alanine substitution in position 3 (15-16), (NH_2)-SWAPLRSGGGS-$(CONH_2)$, was also inactive towards Kly18 (Figure 5). This demonstrated that the phenylalanine was also crucial for the inhibitory activity of peptide15.

Detailed kinetic analysis of peptides 15-0.,15-5., 15-6. and 15-7. revealed similar Ki values in the low micromolar area (Figure 6). This demonstrated that peptide15 can be truncated to the tetra-peptide (NH_2)-SWFP-$(CONH_2)$ without compromising inhibitory potency.

Peptide15 (SWFPL) Inhibits the Proteolytic Activity of Intact Karylysin (Kly48) and Delays the Auto-processing of Kly48 to Kly18

We next wanted to test if the inhibitory effect of peptide15 on Kly18 could be reproduced on intact Karilysin (Kly48). The experiment was performed essentially as described for Kly18 and the results demonstrated a clear dose-response inhibition of Kly48 by (NH_2)-SWFPL-$(CONH_2)$ (Figure 7A). Kly48 is unstable and auto-processes itself into Kly38 and Kly18 over time. Consequently, it was important to establish if SWFPL could modulate the Kly48 auto-processing. As seen from the SDS-PAGE gels in Figure 7B and 7C, (NH_2)-SWFPL-$(CONH_2)$ inhibited the auto-processesing efficiently and even after 48 hours there was still a considerable amount of Kly48 present. Taken together these two studies confirmed that peptide15 inhibited the proteolytic activity of Kly48 and this dataset strongly suggested that it may be possible to use peptide15 to lock Karilysin in the intact Kly48 form, and

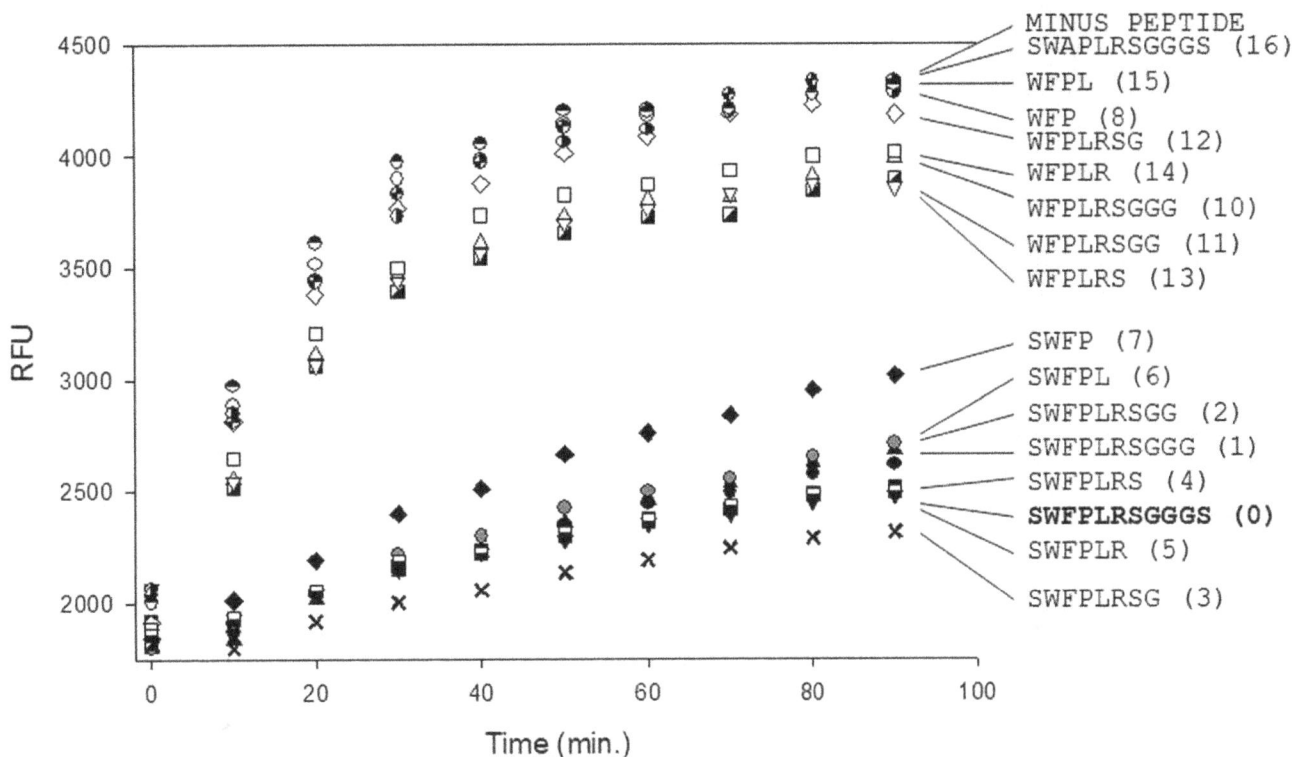

Figure 5. Screening of truncated peptides demonstrates that a tetra-peptide version of peptide15 can inhibit Kly18. Different length versions of peptide15 were tested for Kly18 inhibitory activity. All peptides were screened in a relatively high single concentration (87 µM) to reveal if omission of single amino acid residues displayed dramatic effects on Kly18 inhibition. The data demonstrated that peptide15 can be limited to (NH_2)-SWFP-$(CONH_2)$ (structure 15-7) and still inhibit Kly18.

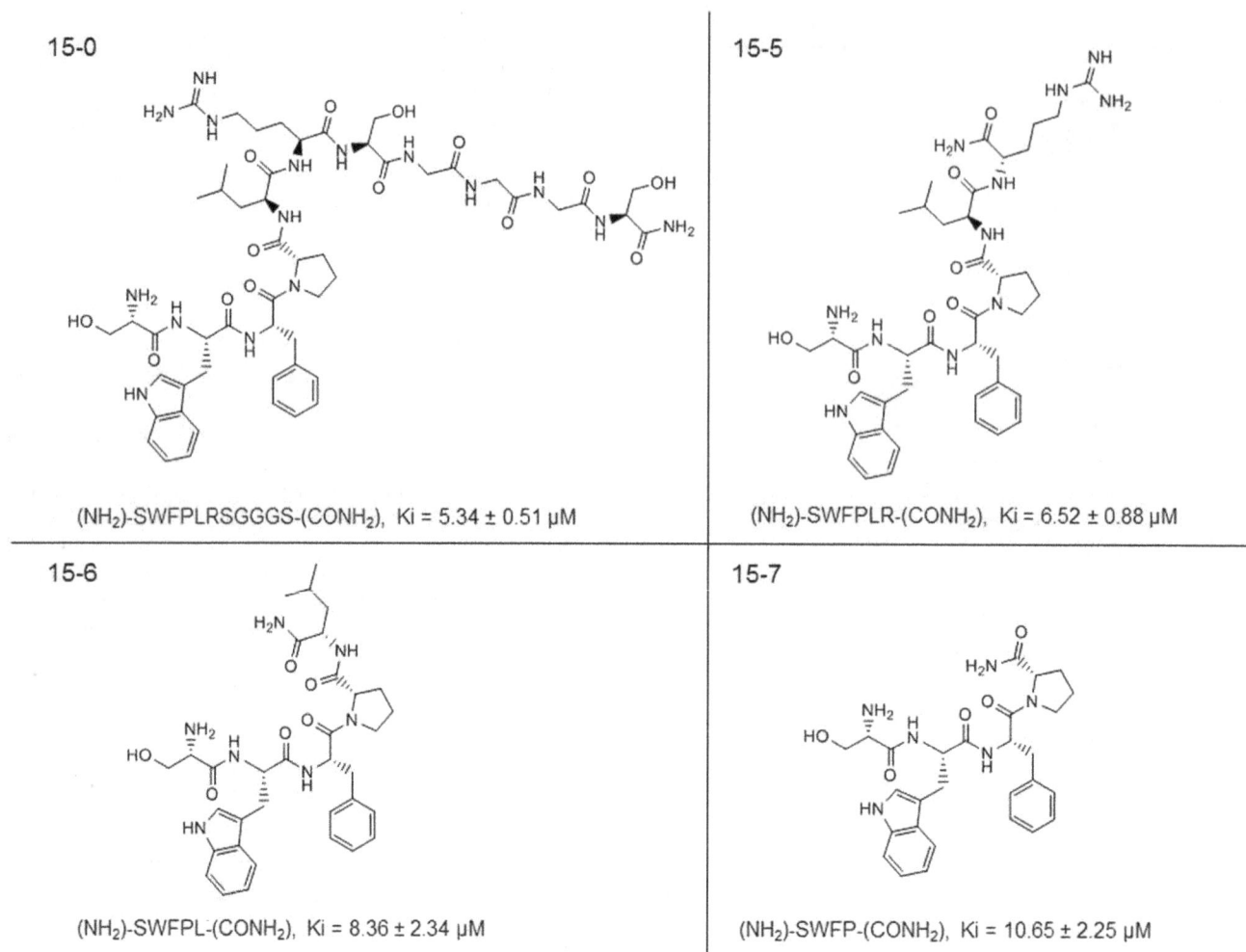

15-0

(NH₂)-SWFPLRSGGGS-(CONH₂), Ki = 5.34 ± 0.51 μM

15-5

(NH₂)-SWFPLR-(CONH₂), Ki = 6.52 ± 0.88 μM

15-6

(NH₂)-SWFPL-(CONH₂), Ki = 8.36 ± 2.34 μM

15-7

(NH₂)-SWFP-(CONH₂), Ki = 10.65 ± 2.25 μM

Figure 6. The tetrapeptide displays a Ki value similar to that of the peptide 15 lead structure. Shown are chemdraw structure models of the peptide versions 15-0, 15-5, 15-6 and 15-7. All truncated versions of peptide15 and intact peptide15 had low micromolar Ki values.

use that complex for crystallisation trials. This could reveal the structure of the intact enzyme.

Expression of MBP-peptide15 Fusion Construct and Specificity Test

In figure 8 a structural alignment of Kly18 and the catalytic domain of human MMP-3 is shown and as is the case with most human MMP's (MMP-1, MMP-7-14), Kly18 and human MMP-3 are structurally similar [22]. It was therefore important to establish if peptide15 was a general binder of MMP catalytic domains. To develop a probe for cross-reactivity tests, peptide15 was expressed as a MBP N-terminal fusion protein and purified in a simple one-step purification strategy. Purity was judged to be greater than 90% by SDS-PAGE (data not shown) and the MBP-peptide15 was used in ELISA to test cross-reactivity towards human MMP-3. MBP-peptide15 bound Kly18 but not MMP-3, thereby underlining peptide15 specificity (figure 9A). By performing a control ELISA experiment using MBP instead of MBP-peptide15, we could confirm that the binding observed was due to the specific interaction between peptide15 and Kly18 (Figure 9B).

As MMP catalytic domains are highly similar it is a challenge to find specific peptides. This was demonstrated in a recent study, which identified a cyclic MMP-9-binding peptide

(CTTHWGFTLC) by phage display with high affinity. However, this peptide also had high affinity for MMP-2 [32]. Peptide phage display has also been used to identify substrate specificity of individual MMPs and by using a 15-mer peptide library Deng and co-workers demonstrated that collagenase 3/MMP-13 has a preference towards the peptide sequence GPLGMRGL. But three other MMPs (stromelysin-1/MMP-3, gelatinase B/MMP-9 and collagenase 1/MMP-1) had lower activity towards the isolated peptide substrate [33]. Furthermore, a recent study demonstrated that a unique MMP-11 substrate peptide could be isolated by phage display, which explained why MMP-11 does not have any activity towards substrates specific for other MMPs [34]. Consequently, one could argue that the peptide15 mode of action is that of a substrate competitive inhibitor. This is especially relevant due to the fact that the exact peptide sequence needed for Kly18 substrate cleavage is yet to be fully elucidated [6]. To explore this possibility peptide15 was incubated with or without a large excess of Kly18 and the mixture was analyzed by liquid chromatography mass spectrometry. The results demonstrated that peptide15 could not be cleaved by Kly18 as the mass peak m/z = 1149, corresponding to (NH₂)-SWFPLRSGGGS-(CONH₂), was found in both preparations and no cleavage products were found (data not shown).

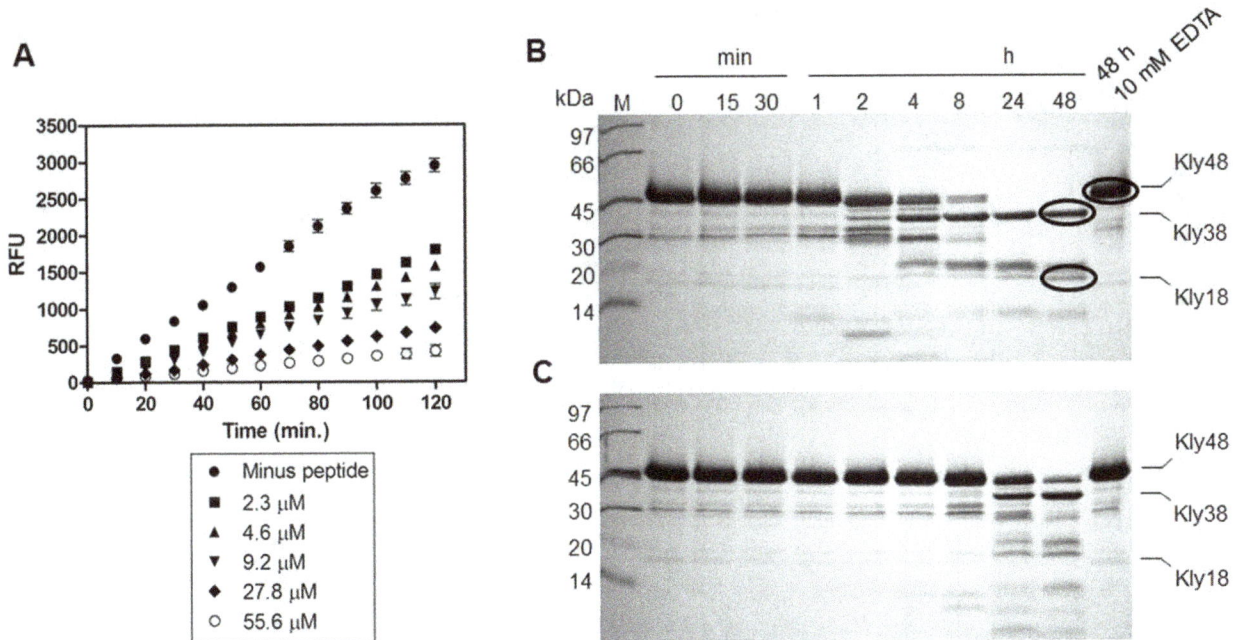

Figure 7. SWFPL inhibits the proteolytic activity of intact Karilysin (Kly48) and delays the auto-processing of Kly48 to Kly18. A) Kly48 was pre-incubated with SWFPL in varying concentrations (2.3 μM to 55.6 μM) followed by addition of the substrate FITC-casein. The SWFPL inhibitory effect was seen as a decrease in Relative Fluorescence Units (RFU) in a dose-response manner. Error bars represent standard deviations between three experiments. B+C) Intact Karilysin (Kly48) at 13 μM was incubated alone (B) or with the peptide inhibitor (C) at 455 μM. At indicated time points samples were withdrawn for SDS-PAGE analysis. It is clear that SWFPL inhibited the time-dependent autoprocessing of Kly48 to Kly38 and Kly18. Even after 48 hours a significant amount of Kly48 was still present.

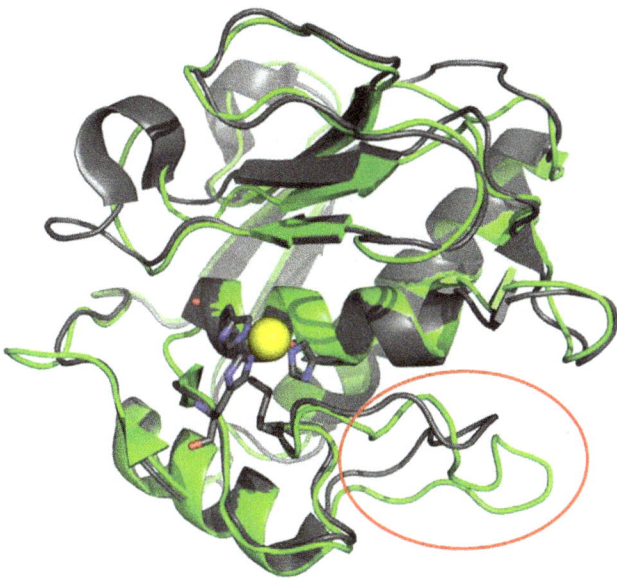

Figure 8. Structural alignment of the catalytic domains from Karilysin (Kly18) and human Matrix Metalloprotease-3 (MMP-3). MMP-3 is seen in green and Kly18 is seen in grey. The figure was prepared using Pymol (DeLano Scientific LLC) and the coordinate files 1CQR (MMP-3) and 2XS3 (Kly18). The structure alignment was performed using the 'align' function in PyMol. The Kly18 was structurally similar to MMP-3 as well as other mammalian MMP's (MMP-1 to 3, MMP-7 to MMP-14, MMP-16 and MMP-20) (Cerda-Costa et al. 2011). The figure displays the zinc (yellow sphere) that is coordinated by the three active site histidines (H155, H159 and H165). The specificity loop is indicated with a red circle.

The development of MMP inhibitors is highly relevant, due to the involvement of MMPs in several pathologies [23]. Some candidate molecules act by blocking the MMP-active sites via binding to the catalytic Zn^{2+} through chelators such as hydroxamate [23]. These approaches have been successful for MMP inhibition. However, the inhibitors have a broad specificity towards other MMPs due to very similar active site geometries of matrix metalloproteinases [23]. An alternative approach to specific MMP inhibitor design is to utilize larger molecules, such as peptides, that interact with the active site as well as exosites unique to individual MMPs [35]. Kly18 contains the metzincin MMP 3-histidine zinc-binding motif (HEXXHXXGXXH) and Kly18 was previously inhibited by small molecules chelators (EDTA, 1,10-phenanthroline) similar to mammalian MMPs [6]. Furthermore, the active site of the Kly18 structure had the classical MMP composition with small deviations in the specificity loop (seen as a red circle in Figure 8) [22]. As peptide15 binds exclusively to Kly18 and at the same time inhibits the enzyme, peptide15 may act by a combined effect of active site targeting and specificity loop exosite interaction. However, detailed structural analysis of Kly18-peptide15 co-crystals will provide final proof on the inhibition mechanism.

Conclusions

Periodontitis is a devastating disease of great discomfort to affected patients. Furthermore, recent findings link periodontitis to inflammatory diseases like rheumatoid arthritis, thereby further underlining the importance of disease treatment and containment [36]. Inhibitors of the periodontopathogen-derived proteases by small molecules, peptides or antibodies represent a rational approach to disease management. Inhibitors toward the most relevant proteases, of which Karilysin could be one, might be

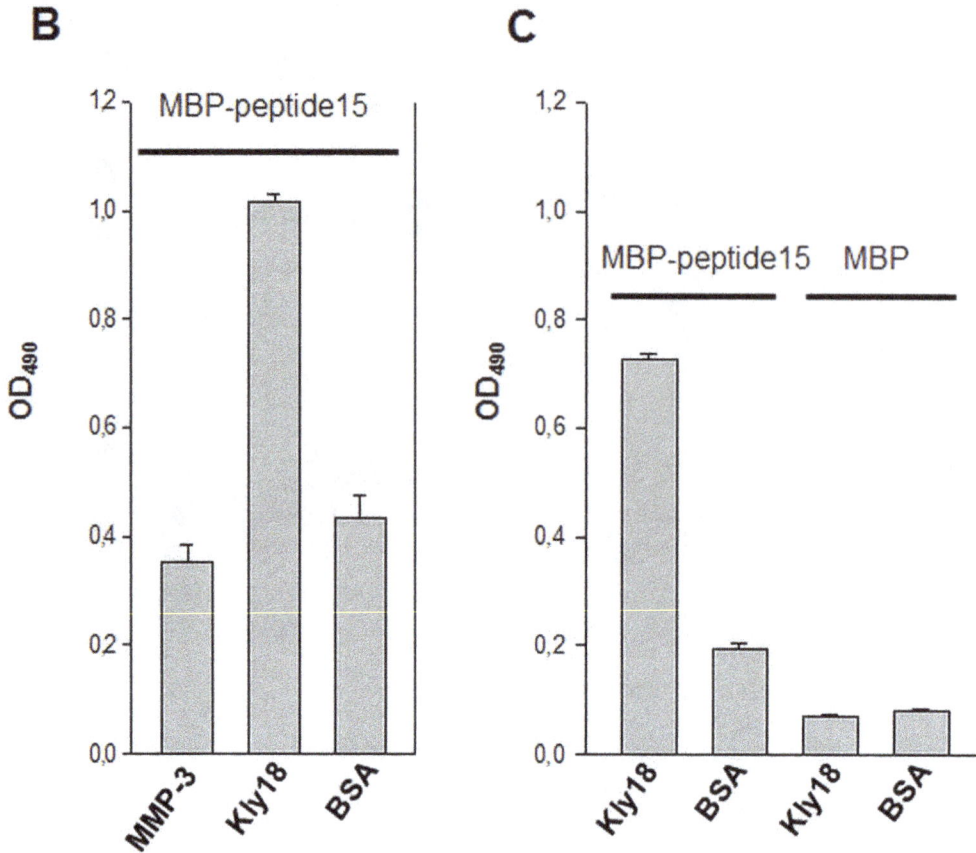

Figure 9. Peptide15-MBP is specific for Kly18. A) The peptide15-MBP fusion protein interacted exclusively with Kly18, thereby demonstrating that peptide15 was specific for Kly18. **B)** To demonstrate that binding to Kly18 was mediated by peptide15 and not by MBP itself, control experiments were performed using MBP instead of MBP-peptide15. Error bars represent standard deviations between three experiments.

applied as a combination therapy in the fight against the periodontopathogens of the 'red complex'. These inhibitors could be formulated in existing media, such as mouth wash, tooth paste or even chewing gum.

In this study, the first inhibitor of Karilysin was identified and characterized. The results supplied us with a detailed understanding of which amino acid residues were important for the inhibitory function of peptide15. The peptide will be a valuable probe in structure-function studies of Karilysin and detailed co-crystallisa-tion studies can reveal the underlying molecular mechanism for the inhibition. From co-crystallisation structural data it may be possible to design peptidomimetics with improved Ki-values.

Author Contributions

Conceived and designed the experiments: PDS JP ER. Performed the experiments: PDS GS MK. Analyzed the data: PDS MK JP ER. Wrote the paper: PDS JP ER.

References

1. Socransky SS, Haffajee AD, Cugini MA, Smith C, Kent RL (1998) Microbial complexes in subgingival plaque. Journal of Clinical Periodontology 25: 134–144.

2. Byrne DP, Wawrzonek K, Jaworska A, Birss AJ, Potempa J, et al. (2009) Role of the cysteine protease interpain A of Prevotella intermedia in breakdown and release of haem from haemoglobin. Biochem J 425: 257–264.

3. Carlisle MD, Srikantha RN, Brogden KA (2009) Degradation of human alpha- and beta-defensins by culture supernatants of Porphyromonas gingivalis strain 381. J Innate Immun 1: 118–122.

4. Fitzpatrick RE, Aprico A, Wijeyewickrema LC, Pagel CN, Wong DM, et al. (2009) High molecular weight gingipains from Porphyromonas gingivalis induce cytokine responses from human macrophage-like cells via a nonproteolytic mechanism. J Innate Immun 1: 109–117.

5. Ishihara K, Wawrzonek K, Shaw LN, Inagaki S, Miyamoto M, et al. (2010) Dentipain, a Streptococcus pyogenes IdeS protease homolog, is a novel virulence factor of Treponema denticola. Biol Chem 391: 1047–1055.

6. Karim AY, Kulczycka M, Kantyka T, Dubin G, Jabaiah A, et al. (2010) A novel matrix metalloprotease-like enzyme (karilysin) of the periodontal pathogen Tannerella forsythia ATCC 43037. Biological Chemistry 391: 105–117.

7. Koziel J, Karim AY, Przybyszewska K, Ksiazek M, Rapala-Kozik M, et al. (2010) Proteolytic inactivation of LL-37 by karilysin, a novel virulence mechanism of Tannerella forsythia. J Innate Immun 2: 288–293.

8. Monteiro AC, Scovino A, Raposo S, Gaze VM, Cruz C, et al. (2009) Kinin danger signals proteolytically released by gingipain induce Fimbriae-specific IFN-gamma- and IL-17-producing T cells in mice infected intramucosally with Porphyromonas gingivalis. J Immunol 183: 3700–3711.

9. Imamura T (2003) the role of gingipains in the pathogenesis of periodontal disease. Journal of periodontology 74: 111–118.

10. Behle JH, Papapanou PN (2006) Periodontal infections and atherosclerotic vascular disease: an update. Int Dent J 56: 256–262.

11. Jordan RC (2004) Diagnosis of periodontal manifestations of systemic diseases. Periodontol 2000 34: 217–229.

12. Persson GR (2006) What has ageing to do with periodontal health and disease? International dental journal 56: 240–249.

13. Pihlstrom BL, Michalowicz BS, Johnson NW (2005) Periodontal diseases. Lancet 366: 1809–1820.

14. Wegner N, Wait R, Sroka A, Eick S, Nguyen KA, et al. (2010) Peptidylarginine deiminase from Porphyromonas gingivalis citrullinates human fibrinogen and

alpha-enolase: implications for autoimmunity in rheumatoid arthritis. Arthritis Rheum 62: 2662–2672.

15. Matsushita K, Imamura T, Tancharoen S, Tatsuyama S, Tomikawa M, et al. (2006) Selective inhibition of Porphyromonas gingivalis growth by a factor Xa inhibitor, DX-9065a. Journal of Periodontal Research 41: 171–176.

16. Cronan CA, Potempa J, Travis J, Mayo JA (2006) Inhibition of Porphyromonas gingivalis proteinases (gingipains) by chlorhexidine: synergistic effect of Zn(II). Oral Microbiol Immunol 21: 212–217.

17. Krauser JA, Potempa J, Travis J, Powers JC (2002) Inhibition of arginine gingipains (RgpB and HRgpA) with benzamidine inhibitors: zinc increases inhibitory potency. Biological Chemistry 383: 1193–1198.

18. Grenier D, Plamondon P, Sorsa T, Lee HM, McNamara T, et al. (2002) Inhibition of proteolytic, serpinolytic, and progelatinase-b activation activities of periodontopathogens by doxycycline and the non-antimicrobial chemically modified tetracycline derivatives. J Periodontol 73: 79–85.

19. Grenier D (1995) Characterization of the trypsin-like activity of Bacteroides forsythus. Microbiology 141: 921–926.

20. Saito T, Ishihara K, Kato T, Okuda K (1997) Cloning, expression, and sequencing of a protease gene from Bacteroides forsythus ATCC 43037 in Escherichia coli. Infect Immun 65: 4888–4891.

21. Sharma A, Sojar HT, Glurich I, Honma K, Kuramitsu HK, et al. (1998) Cloning, expression, and sequencing of a cell surface antigen containing a leucine-rich repeat motif from Bacteroides forsythus ATCC 43037. Infect Immun 66: 5703–5710.

22. Cerda-Costa N, Guevara T, Karim AY, Ksiazek M, Nguyen KA, et al. (2011) The structure of the catalytic domain of Tannerella forsythia karilysin reveals it is a bacterial xenologue of animal matrix metalloproteinases. Mol Microbiol 79: 119–132.

23. Overall CM, Lopez-Otin C (2002) Strategies for MMP inhibition in cancer: innovations for the post-trial era. Nat Rev Cancer 2: 657–672.

24. Potempa J, Pike RN (2009) Corruption of Innate Immunity by Bacterial Proteases. Journal of Innate Immunity 1: 70–87.

25. Jusko M, Potempa J, Karim AY, Ksiazek M, Riesbeck K, et al. (2012) A metalloproteinase karilysin present in the majority of Tannerella forsythia isolates inhibits all pathways of the complement system. Journal of immunology 188 in press.

26. Skottrup PD, Leonard P, Kaczmarek JZ, Veillard F, Enghild JJ, et al. (2011) Diagnostic evaluation of a nanobody with picomolar affinity toward the protease RgpB from Porphyromonas gingivalis. Anal Biochem 415: 158–167.

27. Sambrook J, Fritsch EF, Maniatis T (1989) Molecular Cloning: A Laboratory Manual.

28. Rath S, Stanley CM, Steward MW (1988) An inhibition enzyme-immunoassay for estimating relative antibody-affinity and affinity heterogeneity. Journal of Immunological Methods 106: 245–249.

29. Johansen LK, Albrechtsen B, Andersen HW, Engberg J (1995) pFab60: A new, efficient vector for expression of antibody Fab fragments displayed on phage. Protein Engineering 8: 1063–1067.

30. Schagger H, von Jagow G (1987) Tricine-sodium dodecyl sulfate-polyacrylamide gel electrophoresis for the separation of proteins in the range from 1 to 100 kDa. Anal Biochem 166: 368–379.

31. Nixon AE (2002) Phage display as a tool for protease ligand discovery. Curr Pharm Biotechnol 3: 1–12.

32. Koivunen E, Arap W, Valtanen H, Rainisalo A, Medina OP, et al. (1999) Tumor targeting with a selective gelatinase inhibitor. Nat Biotechnol 17: 768–774.

33. Deng SJ, Bickett DM, Mitchell JL, Lambert MH, Blackburn RK, et al. (2000) Substrate specificity of human collagenase 3 assessed using a phage-displayed peptide library. J Biol Chem 275: 31422–31427.

34. Pan W, Arnone M, Kendall M, Grafstrom RH, Seitz SP, et al. (2003) Identification of peptide substrates for human MMP-11 (stromelysin-3) using phage display. J Biol Chem 278: 27820–27827.

35. Jani M, Tordai H, Trexler M, Banyai L, Patthy L (2005) Hydroxamate-based peptide inhibitors of matrix metalloprotease 2. Biochimie 87: 385–392.

36. Detert J, Pischon N, Burmester GR, Buttgereit F (2010) The association between rheumatoid arthritis and periodontal disease. Arthritis Res Ther 12: 218.

9

Association between *MMP-1* g.-1607dupG Polymorphism and Periodontitis Susceptibility

Dandan Li[1♦], Qi Cai[1♦], Lan Ma[1,2], Meilin Wang[1,2], Junqing Ma[1], Weibing Zhang[1], Yongchu Pan[1]*, Lin Wang[1]*

1 Institute of Stomatology, Nanjing Medical University, Nanjing, China, 2 Department of Epidemiology, Nanjing Medical University, Nanjing, China

Abstract

Background: Matrix metalloproteinase-1 (MMP-1) plays an important role during the destruction of periodontal tissue. Although multiple studies had focused on the association between *MMP-1 g.-1607dupG* and periodontitis susceptibility, the results remained inconclusive. The purpose of this meta-analysis was to explore its role in the development of periodontitis.

Methods: Retrieved studies from Pubmed, Web of Science, Medline and Google Scholar Search regarding *MMP-1 g.-1607dupG* and periodontitis susceptibility were included into the final analysis with definite selection and exclusion criteria. Overall and stratified analyses based on disease type, severity, ethnicity and smoking status were performed. Odds ratio (OR) and 95% confidence interval (CI) were used to evaluate the association between *MMP-1 g.-1607dupG* and periodontitis susceptibility, while Q test and Egger's test were adopted respectively to assess heterogeneity among studies and publication bias.

Results: A total of 1580 periodontitis cases and 1386 controls in 11 case-control studies were included in the meta-analysis. The pooled results showed significant association between periodontitis susceptibility and *MMP-1 g.-1607dupG* polymorphism in homozygote (2G/2G versus 1G/1G, OR = 1.50, 95% CI = 1.02–2.20) and dominant model analysis (2G/2G+2G/1G versus 1G/1G, OR = 1.28, 95% CI = 1.04–1.57). For subgroups by type of periodontitis, increased risk of chronic periodontitis was observed on heterozygote (2G/1G versus 1G/1G, OR = 2.01, 95% CI = 1.58–2.56) and dominant model (OR = 1.27, 95% CI = 1.03–1.57). Furthermore, similar association was also detected in severe chronic periodontitis (2G/2G versus 1G/1G, OR = 2.15, 95% CI = 1.35–3.43; 2G/2G+2G/1G versus 1G/1G, OR = 1.64, 95% CI = 1.12–2.39; 2G/2G versus 2G/1G+1G/1G, OR = 1.86, 95% CI = 1.31–2.64).

Conclusions: Our meta-analysis demonstrated that *MMP-1 g.-1607dupG* polymorphism was associated with chronic periodontitis, especially the severity of the disease condition.

Editor: Balraj Mittal, Sanjay Gandhi Medical Institute, India

Funding: This study was supported in part by the National Natural Science Foundation of China (30973361, 81170981 and 81000457), Natural Science Foundation of JiangSu Province (81000457), Natural Science Foundation for Colleges and Universities in JiangSu Province (10kJB320004), Project of State Key Laboratory of Oral Diseases (SKLODSCU2009KF05) and Project Funded by the Priority Academic Program Development of JiangSu Higher Education Institutions (PAPD). The funders had no role in study design,data collection and analysis,decision to publish,or preparation of the manuscript.

Competing Interests: The authors have declared that no competing interests exist.

* E-mail: nydwlktz@gmail.com (LW); 393774987@qq.com (YP)

♦ These authors contributed equally to this work.

Introduction

Periodontitis are of the most common oral diseases around the world with high prevalence of 10%–15% [1], constituted by two major types: chronic periodontitis (CP) and aggressive periodontitis (AgP). As kinds of inflammatory diseases, they could not only cause great periodontium damage by interaction between pathogens challenge and host immunological reaction [2,3], but also contribute to tooth loosening and loss. Furthermore, their potential adverse effects on systemic health [4], such as adverse pregnancy outcome [5], diabetes mellitus [6], cardiovascular disease [7,8] and some other general diseases [9,10], should also be paid much attention to.

Matrix metalloproteinases (MMPs), a series of proteolytic enzymes responsible for the degradation of extracellular matrix

and basement membranes in the beginning and developing courses of a wide range of diseases [11–13], have been verified to be involved in the pathogenesis of periodontitis [14,15]. Among them, MMP-1 is the most abundant component of the periodontal tissue matrix [16,17], regulating the degradation of native interstitial collagens [18]. It is worth noting that fibrillar collagens types I and III, the predominant types of interstitial collagens in periodontium which are resistant to most proteinases, can be degraded by MMP-1 [19]. Consequently, tissue inhibitors of metalloproteinases (TIMPs) have been used as the hypurgia for human periodontitis to control MMP-mediated extracellular matrix breakdown [16].

Owing to the important role of MMP-1 in the pathogenesis of periodontitis, a variety of molecular epidemiological studies have been conducted to explore the association between *MMP-1* polymorphisms and the susceptibility of periodontitis. The guanine addition at the -1607 position, the substitution of guanine for adenine at position -519 as well as the adenine to thymidine mutation at position -442 of the *MMP-1* gene promoter were supposed to be the functional polymorphisms associated with periodontitis. However, polymorphism at position -1607 (*MMP-1 g.-1607dupG*, rs1799750) was the most extensive studied locus. During the past few years, various studies from different ethnic groups were conducted to test its relevance with periodontitis susceptibility. Nevertheless, these results still remained inconsistent, which warranted us to perform a meta-analysis to further clarify its role in the pathogenesis of periodontitis.

Methods

Search Strategy and Data Extraction

To systematically retrieve all the case-control studies related to the association between *MMP-1 g.-1607dupG* and periodontitis risks, databases of PubMed, Web of Science, Medline and Google Scholar Search were searched (by May 30, 2012) with the key words "periodontitis", "*MMP-1*" (or "matrix metalloproteinase-1") and "polymorphism" (or "variant"). The references of all identified publications were manually searched for additional studies. In the search results, only English articles were taken in. All selected studies complied with the two main criteria: (1) independent case-control study evaluating the association between *MMP-1* polymorphism and periodontitis susceptibility; (2) the number or frequency of genotype given in detail. Studies with insufficient information (e.g. neither the frequency nor the number of genotype was given) were excluded. Two investigators (Li and Pan) independently extracted the data and reached a consensus in order to minimize the bias and improve the reliability. Then information including the first author's name, year of publication, country of origin, ethnicity, type of periodontitis, source of control, number of cases and health controls, genotyping method, Hardy-Weinberg Equilibrium among controls and the main result of each publication was picked up. Different ethnic descents were classified as Caucasian, Asian or Mixed (derived from an admixture of different ethnic groups).

Statistical Analysis

Hardy-Weinberg equilibrium of the genotype distributions among controls were estimated by a goodness-of-fit χ^2 test. The association between *MMP-1 g.-1607dupG* and susceptibility of periodontitis was estimated by odds ratio (OR) and 95% confidence interval (CI). In addition to the overall analysis, stratified analyses based on disease type, severity, ethnicity and smoking status were performed respectively. The 2G/2G+2G/1G versus 1G/1G and 2G/2G versus 2G/1G+1G/1G comparison were estimated to assume dominant and recessive effects of the variant 2G allele respectively. The statistical significance of pooled ORs was determined by Z test. Q test based on *P* and I^2 value was used to assess heterogeneity among studies. I^2 was a value that could describe the percentage of variation across studies. The bigger I^2 value, the stronger heterogeneity is. *P*>0.05 for the Q-test indicated no significant heterogeneity across studies, and the fixed-effects model (the Mantel-Haenszel method) was applied; if not, the random-effects model was used (the DerSimonian and Laird method) [20].

Publication bias was evaluated with the linear regression asymmetry test by Egger et al [21]. *P*<0.05 was used as an indication for the presence of potential publication bias. All analyses were done with STATA software (version 11; StataCorp

LP, College Station, TX, USA), and the *P* values were all two-sided.

Results

Characteristics of Studies

11 relevant papers with 1580 cases and 1386 controls about *MMP-1 g.-1607dupG* polymorphism were recruited and put into the final meta-analyses [22–32] (Figure 1). All studies were case-control studies, including nine studies [22,23,26–32] for CP, one study [25] for AgP and one [24] for both. There were four studies of Asian descent [24–26,31], four studies of European descent [22,23,28,29] and three studies of mixed ethnicity descent [27,30,32]. The distribution of genotypes in the controls was not in agreement with HWE for three studies [28,30,31]. (Table 1).

There were only 2 studies for *MMP-1*-519 A/G, neither found any relationship with periodontitis [23,28]. Meanwhile, *MMP1*-422 A/T was only mentioned in one literature [23] (Table 1). Therefore, meta-analyses for the latter two SNPs were not performed in the present study.

Overall Analysis

In general, the *MMP-1* -1607 2G/2G homozygote was significantly associated with an increased risk of periodontitis compared with wild-type homozygote (1G/1G) (OR = 1.50, 95% CI = 1.02–2.20). Significant association was also found in the dominant genetic model (OR = 1.28, 95%CI = 1.04–1.57), but neither in recessive model (OR = 1.31, 95%CI = 0.95–1.79) nor in heterozygote comparison (OR = 1.23, 95%CI = 0.98–1.53).

Stratified Analysis by Type of Disease

Appreciable differences were identified in the etiology feature between CP and AgP [33], implicating that there might be different genetic mechanism between them. Subgroup analysis showed that individuals were more susceptible to CP (OR = 1.27, 95% CI = 1.03–1.57) rather than AgP (OR = 1.14, 95% CI = 0.56–2.32) under the dominant model (Figure 2). The significantly elevated risk of CP was also observed in heterozygote comparison (OR = 2.01, 95% CI = 1.58–2.56) (Table 2).

Stratified Analysis by Severity

As showed in Table 2, significant association between the variation and severe CP was found in almost all types of comparisons. However, no significant relationship was found in moderate periodontitis (Table 2).

Stratified Analysis by Ethnicity and Smoking Status

No significant association was found in Asians or Caucasians under any genetic model when analyzing the association between *MMP-1 g.-1607dupG* and CP by ethnicity. Similar effects were also observed in stratified analysis by smoking status.

Heterogeneity Analysis

Heterogeneity among studies was observed in *MMP-1 g.-1607dupG* recessive model (I^2 = 57.3%, *P* = 0.012) and homozygote comparison (I^2 = 53.3%, *P* = 0.023). Z test of subgroup analysis indicated that type of periodontitis (P_z = 0.024) and smoking condition (P_z = 0.048) may be the main source of heterogeneity by homozygote comparison.

Sensitive Analysis

There are three of the 11 studies at variance with Hardy-Weinberg Equilibrium [28,30,31]. Among them, the study of Loo

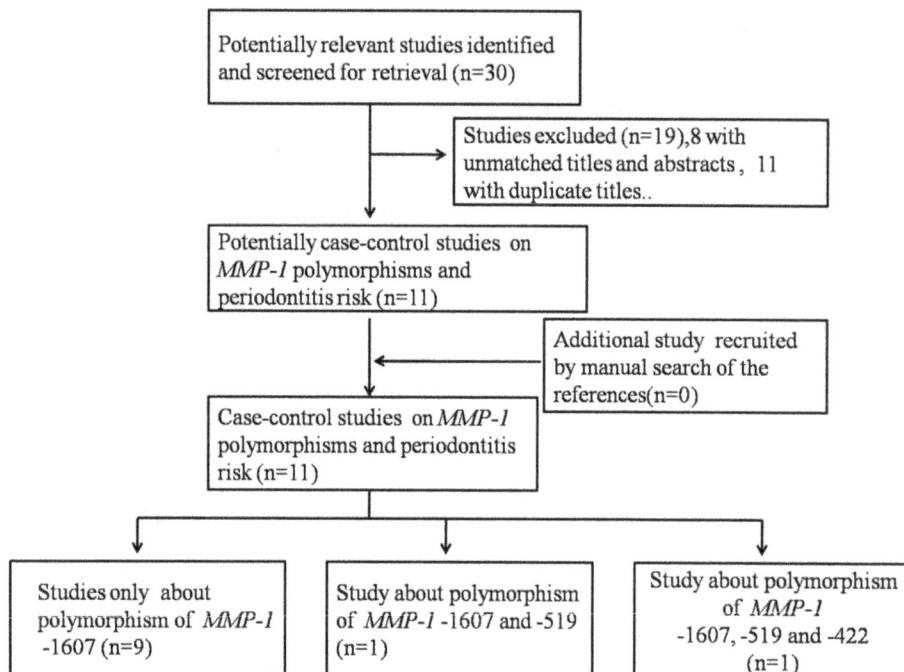

Figure 1. Studies identification diagram.

et al. [31] was found to be the major source of heterogeneity by sensitive analysis (Figure 3), and heterogeneity was effectively removed after excluding this study under the dominant model ($I^2 = 30.9\%$, $P = 0.162$). In addition, the pooled ORs and 95% CI

Table 1. Relevant literatures concerning relationships between *MMP-1* polymorphisms and periodontitis.

Author	Year	Country	Ethnicity	Type of disease	Source of control	Sample size of case/control	genotyping methods	HWE among controls	Result
MMP1 -1607dupG									
de Souza [22]	2003	Brazil	Caucasian	CP	HB	50/37	PCR-RFLP	0.87	+[a]
Holla [23]	2004	Czech	Caucasian	CP	PB	133/196	PCR-RFLP	0.52	+[a]
Itagaki [24]	2004	Japan	Asian	AgP	HB	37/142	Taqman	0.47	−
				CP	HB	205/142	Taqman	0.47	−
Cao [25]	2005	China	Asian	AgP	HB	40/52	PCR-RFLP	0.77	+
Cao [26]	2006	China	Asian	CP	HB	60/50	PCR-RFLP	0.99	+[b]
Astolfi [27]	2006	Brazil	Mixed	CP	PB	114/109	PCR-RFLP	0.68	−
Pirhan [28]	2008	Turkey	Caucasian	CP	HB	101/97	PCR-RFLP	0.009	−
Ustun [29]	2008	Turkey	Caucasian	CP	HB	126/54	PCR-RFLP	0.75	−
Repeke [30]	2009	Brazil	Mix	CP	PB	178/190	PCR-RFLP	0.0005	−
Loo [31]	2011	China	Asian	CP	PB	280/250	PCR-RFLP	1.36E−39	+
Luczyszyn [32]	2012	Brazil	Mix	CP	HB	60/67	PCR-RFLP	0.07	−
MMP1 -519 A>G									
Holla [23]	2004	Czech	Caucasian	CP	PB	133/196	PCR-RFLP	0.52	−
Pirhan [28]	2008	Turkey	Caucasian	CP	HB	102/97	PCR-RFLP	0.009	−
MMP1 -422 A>T									
Holla [23]	2004	Czech	Caucasian	CP	PB	133/196	PCR-RFLP	0.52	+[c]

+The significant relevance between *MMP-1* polymorphism and the risk of periodontitis was picked up in this article.
−No association between MMP-1 polymorphism and the risk of periodontitis was picked up in this article.
[a]only association with severe chronic periodontitis in non-smoking population.
[b]only association with severe chronic periodontitis.
[c]only association with severe chronic periodontitis in smoking population.

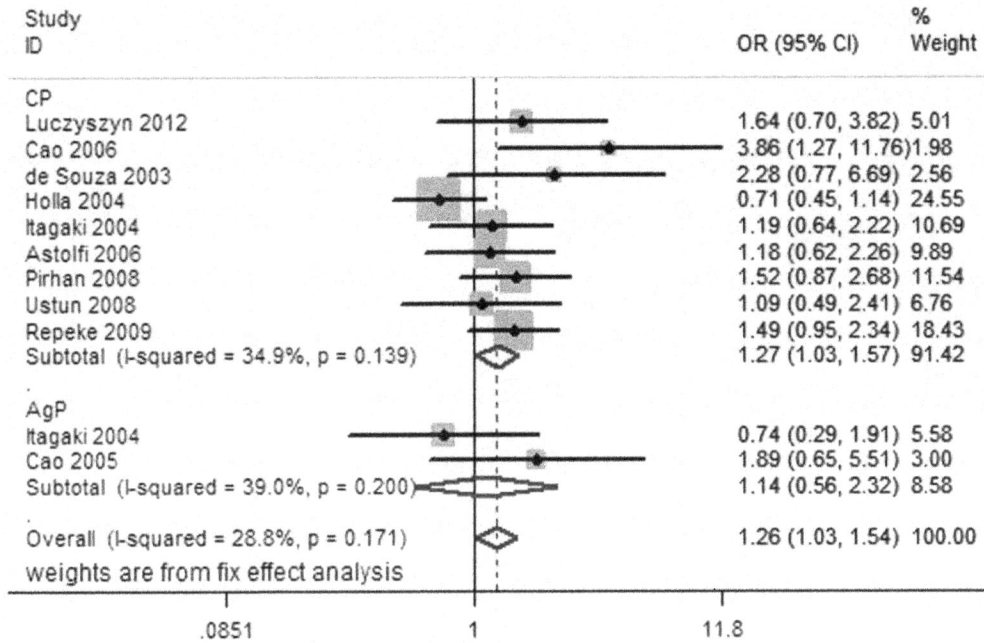

Figure 2. Forest plot of periodontitis risk associated with *MMP-1 g.-1607dupG* **by type of disease under dominant model (2G/2G+1G/2G vs. 1G/1G).** Fixed-effects model was used.

Table 2. Meta-analysis for *MMP-1 g.-1607dupG* polymorphism and periodontitis risk.

Variables	N^a	2G/2G versus 1G/1G		2G/1G versus 1G/1G		2G/2G+2G/1G versus 1G/1G		2G/2G versus 2G/1G+1G/1G		2G versus 1G	
		OR (95%CI)	P^b	OR (95%CI)	P^b	OR (95%CI)	P^b	OR (95%CI)	P^b	OR (95%CI)	P^b
Total	10	**1.50 (1.02-2.20)**	0.023	1.23 (0.98-1.53)	0.522	**1.28 (1.04-1.57)**	0.162	1.31 (0.95-1.79)	0.012	**1.28 (1.03-1.59)**	0.040
Type of disease											
CP	9	1.41 (0.96-2.07)	0.040	**2.01 (1.58-2.56)**	0.368	**1.27 (1.03-1.57)**	0.139	1.17 (0.96-1.43)	0.059	1.23 (0.99-1.51)	0.012
AgP	2	1.54 (0.28-8.55)	0.031	1.30 (0.59-2.84)	0.222	1.14 (0.56-2.32)	0.200	1.64 (0.35-7.70)	0.008	1.34 (0.48-3.73)	0.010
Severity of CP											
moderate	4	1.31 (0.74-2.32)	0.312	1.25 (0.73-2.16)	0.531	1.29 (0.77-2.15)	0.409	1.14 (0.76-1.70)	0.559	1.14 (0.87-1.51)	0.306
Severe	5	**2.15 (1.35-3.43)**	0.191	1.35 (0.89-2.05)	0.753	**1.64 (1.12-2.39)**	0.444	**1.86 (1.31-2.64)**	0.187	**1.38 (1.16-1.65)**	0.101
Ethnicity^c											
Caucasian	4	1.22 (0.59-2.51)	0.047	1.06 (0.75-1.48)	0.363	1.06 (0.78-1.45)	0.099	1.01 (0.71-1.44)	0.160	1.04 (0.86-1.25)	0.058
Asian	2	2.79 (0.56-13.98)	0.020	1.31 (0.74-2.32)	0.242	1.61 (0.95-2.73)	0.071	2.01 (0.72-5.61)	0.027	1.75 (0.77-3.95)	0.011
Mixed	3	1.33 (0.89-1.98)	0.976	**1.48 (1.03-2.14)**	0.474	**1.42 (1.01-1.99)**	0.793	1.05 (0.77-1.45)	0.472	1.20 (0.95-1.50)	0.094
Smoking status^c											
Smoking	3	1.14 (0.43-3.02)	0.222	1.12 (0.54-2.34)	0.976	1.12 (0.55-2.29)	0.682	1.19 (0.53-2.65)	0.140	1.19 (0.81-1.76)	0.415
non-smoking	7	1.36 (0.80-2.32)	0.012	1.17 (0.89-1.54)	0.497	1.25 (0.84-1.87)	0.046	1.20 (0.96-1.50)	0.014	1.21 (0.90-1.65)	0.001

^{a}Number of comparisons.
^{b}P value of Q-test for heterogeneity test. Random-effects model was used when P value for heterogeneity test <0.05; otherwise, fix-effects model was used.
^{c}AgP individuals are not included.

under the dominant model in overall comparison was obviously influenced (OR = 1.28, 95% CI = 1.04–1.57). (Before excluding, OR = 1.10, 95% CI = 0.60–2.03). The other two studies were reserved because they did not substantially affect the heterogeneity and the results (Figure 3). Then the statistical process was limited to ten articles left.

Publication Bias Analysis

Egger's test was conducted to assess the publication bias of the included studies. No publication bias was found in any genetic models. (t = −1.46, P = 0.183 for 2G/2G+2G/1G versus 1G/1G).

Discussion

Since 2003, there have been 11 studies focusing on the relationship between the SNP at position -1607 of *MMP-1* and periodontitis susceptibility. De Souza et al. found that subjects carrying -1607 2G allele tended to be more susceptible to severe CP in non-smoking Brazilian subjects [22]. Similar results were then observed in Czech [23] and Chinese subjects [26]. Elevated risk of CP and AgP was also found in 2G carriers of Asian origins by Loo [31] and Cao [25] et al. The other studies, however, obtained negative results [24,27,28–30,32]. In sum, the definite role of *MMP-1 g.-1607dupG* in the development of periodontitis remains controversy.

By recruiting all of the above studies, we conducted the current meta-analysis and finally found that this variant could contribute to increased risk of periodontitis. In stratified analysis by type of disease, its association with susceptibility of CP rather than AgP was observed. Furthermore, its association with elevated risk of severe CP was also obtained. However, we did not find any meaningful associations in stratified analysis by ethnic and smoking status, both of which were considered to be the relevant factors of periodontitis.

MMP-1, playing a crucial role in paradentium destruction, was suggested to be an important risk factor of CP. It was previously demonstrated that 2G allele instead of 1G allel at *MMP-1* -1607 created a new 5'-GGA-3' core recognition sequence for members of the erythroblast transformation specific family as the binding site, causing increased transcriptional activity, systemically accelerate *MMP-1* gene transcription and protein over-expression, expounding the molecular basis of a anabatic matrix degradation. [34]. In addition, some scholars demonstrated that *MMP1*-1607 2G allele was associated with increased MMP-1 mRNA expression in vivo [30]. Therefore, it was biologically plausible that individuals carrying *MMP1*-1607 2G allele were associated with over-expression of MMP-1, consequently contributing to more susceptibility to CP.

On the other hand, lack of association with AgP was found in the current study, not only implicating that MMP-1 might not been entirely activated in the pathogenesis of AgP, but also providing further evidence that AgP was different from CP in some aspects. Some scholars considered that AgP and CP shared some susceptibility genes, but not all [35]. Similarly, effect of some genetic variants had also been proved to be different [36] or even contract [37] on CP and AgP. Therefore, the role MMP-1 played in the development of AgP, if any, may not be as important as it did in CP. However, the negative association should be carefully interpreted because of the limited sample size.

Several limitations should be addressed. Firstly, the sample size is still a formidable problem. Based on the current sample size, we only had 63% power at a 0.05 or smaller with level to detect an OR of 1.2 or greater and 0.83 or smaller with an exposure frequency of 30%. Secondly, gene-environment interactions which may modulate the periodontitis susceptibility were limited owing to the lack of the origin data in the including studies.

Stated thus, our meta-analysis suggested that *MMP-1 g.-1607dupG* contribute to the elevated risk of CP. Further studies

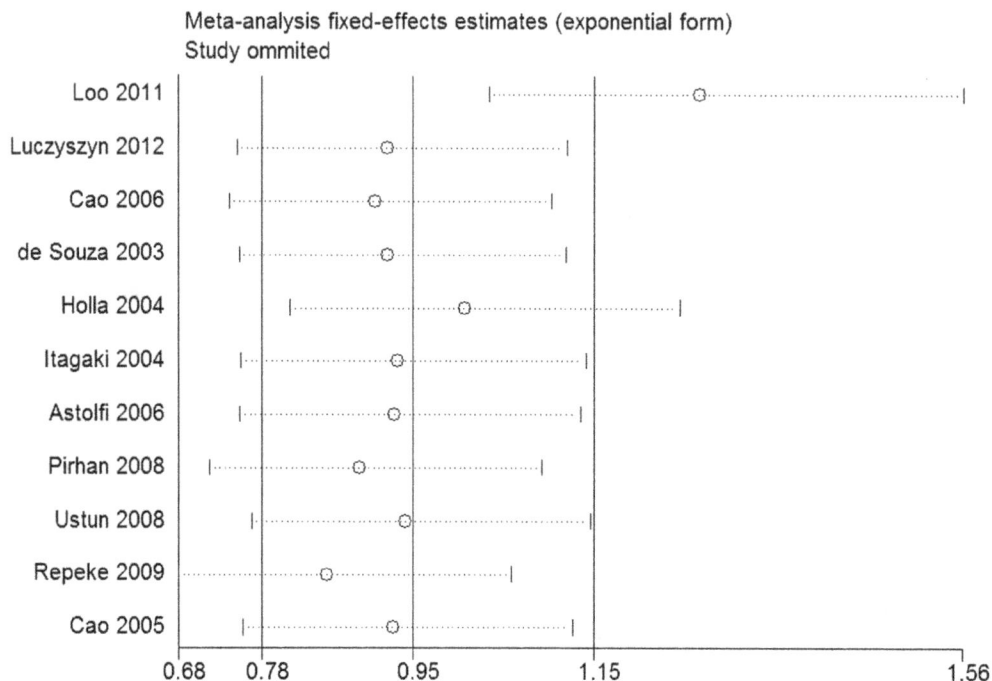

Figure 3. The result of sensitive analysis under the dominant model (2G/2G+1G/2G vs. 1G/1G). Fix effect model was used.

with large sample size and detailed information are needed to validate these results.

References

1. Albandar JM, Rams TE (2002) Global epidemiology of periodontal diseases: an overview. Periodontol 2000 29: 7–10.
2. Page RC, Offenbacher S, Schroeder HE, Seymour GJ, Kornman KS (1997) Advances in the pathogenesis of periodontitis: summary of developments, clinical implications and future directions. Periodontol 2000 14: 216–248.
3. Silva N, Dutzan N, Hernandez M, Dezerega A, Rivera O, et al. (2008) Characterization of progressive periodontal lesions in chronic periodontitis patients: levels of chemokines, cytokines, matrix metalloproteinase-13, periodontal pathogens and inflammatory cells. J Clin Periodontol 35: 206–214.
4. Mealey BL (1999) Influence of periodontal infections on systemic health. Periodontol 2000 21: 197–209.
5. Dasanayake AP, Russell S, Boyd D, Madianos PN, Forster T, et al. (2003) Preterm low birth weight and periodontal disease among African Americans. Dental Clinics of North America 47: 115.
6. Mealey BL, Rethman MP (2003) Periodontal disease and diabetes mellitus. Bidirectional relationship. Dent Today 22: 107–113.
7. Desvarieux M, Demmer RT, Rundek T, Boden-Albala B, Jacobs DR, et al. (2003) Relationship between periodontal disease, tooth loss, and carotid artery plaque. Stroke 34: 2120–2125.
8. Yamazaki K, Honda T, Oda T, Ueki-Maruyama K, Nakajima T, et al. (2005) Effect of periodontal treatment on the C-reactive protein and proinflammatory cytokine levels in Japanese periodontitis patients. Journal of periodontal research 40: 53–58.
9. Scannapieco F, Rethman M (2003) The relationship between periodontal diseases and respiratory diseases. Dentistry today 22: 79.
10. Contreras A, Slots J (2001) Typing of herpes simplex virus from human periodontium. Oral microbiology and immunology 16: 63–64.
11. Ravanti L, Kahari VM (2000) Matrix metalloproteinases in wound repair (review). Int J Mol Med 6: 391–407.
12. Nagase H, Woessner JF, Jr. (1999) Matrix metalloproteinases. J Biol Chem 274: 21491–21494.
13. Birkedal-Hansen H, Moore WG, Bodden MK, Windsor LJ, Birkedal-Hansen B, et al. (1993) Matrix metalloproteinases: a review. Crit Rev Oral Biol Med 4: 197–250.
14. Lee W, Aitken S, Sodek J, McCulloch C (1995) Evidence of a direct relationship between neutrophil collagenase activity and periodontal tissue destruction in vivo: role of active enzyme in human periodontitis. Journal of periodontal research 30: 23–33.
15. Sorsa T, Tjaderhane L, Salo T (2004) Matrix metalloproteinases (MMPs) in oral diseases. Oral Dis 10: 311–318.
16. Verstappen J, Von den Hoff J (2006) Tissue inhibitors of metalloproteinases (TIMPs): their biological functions and involvement in oral disease. Journal of dental research 85: 1074–1084.
17. Hannas AR, Pereira JC, Granjeiro JM, Tjaderhane L (2007) The role of matrix metalloproteinases in the oral environment. Acta Odontol Scand 65: 1–13.
18. Ejeil AL, Igondjo-Tchen S, Ghomrasseni S, Pellat B, Godeau G, et al. (2003) Expression of matrix metalloproteinases (MMPs) and tissue inhibitors of metalloproteinases (TIMPs) in healthy and diseased human gingiva. Journal of periodontology 74: 188–195.
19. Visse R, Nagase H (2003) Matrix metalloproteinases and tissue inhibitors of metalloproteinases. Circulation research 92: 827–839.
20. DerSimonian R, Laird N (1986) Meta-analysis in clinical trials. Control Clin Trials 7: 177–188.
21. Egger M, Davey Smith G, Schneider M, Minder C (1997) Bias in meta-analysis detected by a simple, graphical test. BMJ 315: 629–634.
22. de Souza AP, Trevilatto PC, Scarel-Caminaga RM, Brito RB, Line SR (2003) MMP-1 promoter polymorphism: association with chronic periodontitis severity in a Brazilian population. J Clin Periodontol 30: 154–158.
23. Izakovičová Hollá L, Jurajda M, Fassmann A, Dvorakova N, Znojil V, et al. (2004) Genetic variations in the matrix metalloproteinase-1 promoter and risk of susceptibility and/or severity of chronic periodontitis in the Czech population. Journal of clinical periodontology 31: 685–690.
24. Itagaki M, Kubota T, Tai H, Shimada Y, Morozumi T, et al. (2004) Matrix metalloproteinase-1 and -3 gene promoter polymorphisms in Japanese patients with periodontitis. J Clin Periodontol 31: 764–769.
25. Cao Z, Li C, Jin L, Corbet EF (2005) Association of matrix metalloproteinase-1 promoter polymorphism with generalized aggressive periodontitis in a Chinese population. J Periodontal Res 40: 427–431.
26. Cao Z, Li C, Zhu G (2006) MMP-1 promoter gene polymorphism and susceptibility to chronic periodontitis in a Chinese population. Tissue Antigens 68: 38–43.
27. Astolfi CM, Shinohara AL, da Silva RA, Santos MC, Line SR, et al. (2006) Genetic polymorphisms in the MMP-1 and MMP-3 gene may contribute to chronic periodontitis in a Brazilian population. J Clin Periodontol 33: 699–703.
28. Pirhan D, Atilla G, Emingil G, Sorsa T, Tervahartiala T, et al. (2008) Effect of MMP-1 promoter polymorphisms on GCF MMP-1 levels and outcome of periodontal therapy in patients with severe chronic periodontitis. J Clin Periodontol 35: 862–870.
29. Ustun K, Alptekin NO, Hakki SS, Hakki EE (2008) Investigation of matrix metalloproteinase-1-1607 1G/2G polymorphism in a Turkish population with periodontitis. J Clin Periodontol 35: 1013–1019.
30. Repeke CE, Trombone AP, Ferreira SB, Jr., Cardoso CR, Silveira EM, et al. (2009) Strong and persistent microbial and inflammatory stimuli overcome the genetic predisposition to higher matrix metalloproteinase-1 (MMP-1) expression: a mechanistic explanation for the lack of association of MMP1–1607 single-nucleotide polymorphism genotypes with MMP-1 expression in chronic periodontitis lesions. J Clin Periodontol 36: 726–738.
31. Loo WTY, Wang M, Jin L, Cheung MNB, Li G (2011) Association of matrix metalloproteinase (MMP-1, MMP-3 and MMP-9) and cyclooxygenase-2 gene polymorphisms and their proteins with chronic periodontitis. Archives of Oral Biology.
32. Luczyszyn SM, de Souza CM, Braosi AP, Dirschnabel AJ, Claudino M, et al. (2012) Analysis of the association of an MMP1 promoter polymorphism and transcript levels with chronic periodontitis and end-stage renal disease in a Brazilian population. Arch Oral Biol.
33. Benoist HM, Seck-Diallo A, Diouf A, Yabbre S, Sembene M, et al. (2011) Profile of chronic and aggressive periodontitis among Senegalese. J Periodontal Implant Sci 41: 279–284.
34. Rutter JL, Mitchell TI, Buttice G, Meyers J, Gusella JF, et al. (1998) A single nucleotide polymorphism in the matrix metalloproteinase-1 promoter creates an Ets binding site and augments transcription. Cancer Res 58: 5321–5325.
35. Yoshie H, Kobayashi T, Tai H, Galicia JC (2007) The role of genetic polymorphisms in periodontitis. Periodontology 2000 43: 102–132.
36. Deng H, Liu F, Pan Y, Jin X, Wang H, et al. (2011) BsmI, TaqI, ApaI, and FokI polymorphisms in the vitamin D receptor gene and periodontitis: a meta-analysis of 15 studies including 1338 cases and 1302 controls. J Clin Periodontol 38: 199–207.
37. Ding C, Zhao L, Sun Y, Li L, Xu Y (2012) Interleukin-1 receptor antagonist polymorphism (rs2234663) and periodontitis susceptibility: A meta-analysis. Arch Oral Biol 57: 585–593.

Author Contributions

Conceived and designed the experiments: YP LW. Performed the experiments: DL QC. Analyzed the data: JM WZ. Contributed reagents/materials/analysis tools: LM MW. Wrote the paper: YP LW.

10

Deep Sequencing of the Oral Microbiome Reveals Signatures of Periodontal Disease

Bo Liu[1,2,9], Lina L. Faller[3,9], Niels Klitgord[3,9], Varun Mazumdar[3,9], Mohammad Ghodsi[1,2], Daniel D. Sommer[1], Theodore R. Gibbons[1,4], Todd J. Treangen[1,10], Yi-Chien Chang[3], Shan Li[5], O. Colin Stine[5], Hatice Hasturk[8], Simon Kasif[3,7,9], Daniel Segrè[3,6,7]*, Mihai Pop[1,2,4]*, Salomon Amar[3,11]*

1 Center for Bioinformatics and Computational Biology, University of Maryland, College Park, Maryland, United States of America, 2 Department of Computer Science, University of Maryland, College Park, Maryland, United States of America, 3 Bioinformatics Program, Boston University, Boston, Massachusetts, United States of America, 4 Biological Sciences Graduate Program, University of Maryland, College Park, Maryland, United States of America, 5 Department of Epidemiology and Public Health, University of Maryland School of Medicine, Baltimore, Maryland, United States of America, 6 Department of Biology, Boston University, Boston, Massachusetts, United States of America, 7 Department of Biomedical Engineering, Boston University, Boston, Massachusetts, United States of America, 8 The Forysth Institute, Department of Periodontology, Cambridge, Massachusetts, United States of America, 9 Children's Informatics Program, Harvard-Massachusetts Institute of Technology Division of Health Sciences and Technology, Boston, Massachusetts, United States of America, 10 The McKusick-Nathans Institute for Genetic Medicine, The Johns Hopkins University School of Medicine, Baltimore, Maryland, United States of America, 11 Center for Anti-Inflammatory Therapeutics; Boston University Goldman School of Dental Medicine, Boston, Massachusetts, United States of America

Abstract

The oral microbiome, the complex ecosystem of microbes inhabiting the human mouth, harbors several thousands of bacterial types. The proliferation of pathogenic bacteria within the mouth gives rise to periodontitis, an inflammatory disease known to also constitute a risk factor for cardiovascular disease. While much is known about individual species associated with pathogenesis, the system-level mechanisms underlying the transition from health to disease are still poorly understood. Through the sequencing of the 16S rRNA gene and of whole community DNA we provide a glimpse at the global genetic, metabolic, and ecological changes associated with periodontitis in 15 subgingival plaque samples, four from each of two periodontitis patients, and the remaining samples from three healthy individuals. We also demonstrate the power of whole-metagenome sequencing approaches in characterizing the genomes of key players in the oral microbiome, including an unculturable TM7 organism. We reveal the disease microbiome to be enriched in virulence factors, and adapted to a parasitic lifestyle that takes advantage of the disrupted host homeostasis. Furthermore, diseased samples share a common structure that was not found in completely healthy samples, suggesting that the disease state may occupy a narrow region within the space of possible configurations of the oral microbiome. Our pilot study demonstrates the power of high-throughput sequencing as a tool for understanding the role of the oral microbiome in periodontal disease. Despite a modest level of sequencing (~2 lanes Illumina 76 bp PE) and high human DNA contamination (up to ~90%) we were able to partially reconstruct several oral microbes and to preliminarily characterize some systems-level differences between the healthy and diseased oral microbiomes.

Editor: Sarah K. Highlander, Baylor College of Medicine, United States of America

Funding: SA and HA were supported by National Institutes of Health (NIH)-National Institute of Dental and Craniofacial Research grants R01DE015345, and R01DE014079. MP, DDS, TJT, BL and TG were supported in part by the NIH grant R01-HG-04885, the National Science Foundation grant IIS-0812111 to MP, and by the Bill and Melinda Gates Foundation (PI Jim Nataro) subcontract to MP. DS, LF, VM and NK were partially supported by NIH grant RC2-GM-092602-01. The work of YC, SK, DS, LF, VM at Boston University was also supported in part by GO grant from National Institute of General Medical Sciences (1RC2GM092602-01 to COMBREX). The funders had no role in study design, data collection and analysis, decision to publish, or preparation of the manuscript.

Competing Interests: The authors have declared that no competing interests exist.

* E-mail: dsegre@bu.edu (DS); mpop@umiacs.umd.edu (MP); samar@bu.edu (SA)

9 These authors contributed equally to this work.

Introduction

Understanding the role of microbial communities in human health is emerging as one of the most important and fascinating biomedical challenges of our times [1,2,3,4]. Our body harbors an enormous amount of microbial cells, estimated to exceed the number of human cells by an order of magnitude [5]. These microbes are organized into complex communities specifically adapted to inhabit different niches of the human body, such as the skin, and the respiratory, gastrointestinal, and urogenital tracts. Such ecosystems carry a broad range of functions indispensable for

the wellbeing of the host [6]. At the same time, the rise of pathogens within such communities, causing infection and inflammation, constitutes an ongoing challenge in biomedical research. This is especially true in light of the slow rate at which new antibiotics are discovered [7], and the increase in the number of microbes that can resist treatment [8,9]. In contrast to the traditional view of individual pathogens being responsible for disease onset, recent microbial ecosystem diversity analyses seem to point to a new perspective in which the transition from health to disease is attributed to a shift in the global balance of the microbial flora rather than to the specific appearance of individual pathogens [10,11,12,13]. However, the mechanisms that underlie the connection between disease or infection and the dynamics of the host-associated ecosystems are still poorly understood.

In this work, we focus on the role of the oral microbial ecosystem in periodontal disease. Periodontal disease is the most common infectious disease affecting tooth-supporting structures. Left untreated, periodontitis can lead to, or aggravate existing systemic conditions such as cardiovascular disease, diabetes, pulmonary diseases, and obesity [14,15,16]. In dentistry, understanding the changes in the oral microbiome that foretell the early stages of periodontitis and dental caries, the most prevalent chronic oral diseases, may allow the better diagnosis and treatment before the appearance of the telltale clinical manifestations of these diseases (such as tissue damage in periodontal pockets or dental hard tissue loss). The emergence and evolution of antibiotic resistance in periodontal pathogens has affected the therapeutic success rates for this disease [17,18]. New approaches are urgently needed to help regain control over periodontal disease, and microbiome studies offer a promising new angle of attack. Unraveling the complex interactions that define the oral microbiome is a fundamental, but complex component of this endeavor.

Recent developments in systems biology make it possible to perform quantitative modeling of genome-scale metabolic networks for individual microbial species [19,20] and have been recently extended to explore small microbial consortia [21,22], possibly paving the way for future quantitative studies of the microbiome. However, at the ecosystem level, current modeling efforts and quantitative analyses are heavily limited by the unavailability of relevant data. Towards this goal, increasingly accessible metagenomic sequencing approaches hold the promise to enable a global systemic view of the human oral microbiome [1,4,23]. Recent advances in sequencing technology are enabling scientists to generate billions of nucleotide bases at a fraction of the cost per base of traditional methods [24]. This deep sequencing has revealed an unexpectedly high diversity of the human oral microbiome: dental plaque pooled from 98 healthy adults comprised about 10,000 microbial phylotypes [25] - an order of magnitude higher than the previously reported 700 oral microbial phylotypes as identified by cultivation or traditional cloning and sequencing [26,27]. The total diversity of the global oral microbiome can be estimated to be around 25,000 phylotypes [25]. To date, however, we do not know how many of these microbes contribute to periodontal disease, what metabolic functions are key players in the transition from health to disease, or how common or exclusive are the oral microbiomes of unrelated healthy individuals.

Here we combine the collection of whole-community sequencing data with a number of computational analyses to provide a snapshot of the microbial component of periodontal disease at a high resolution. Specifically, we collected subgingival plaque samples from healthy and periodontally affected patients and subjected them to 16S rDNA analysis and deep sequencing in order to explore their microbiome. Our analyses reveal a number of trends in genomic diversity and biological function enrichment during disease that allow us to formulate a novel hypothesis on the nature of periodontal disease. We also demonstrate the power of high-throughput sequencing approaches by reconstructing an unculturable member of the TM7 group, complementing an initial analysis that relied on single cell genomic approaches. We also characterize several regions of variation within one of the dominant members of the oral cavity, *Actinomyces naeslundii*. This paper describes a genomic and metabolic examination of the differences between the healthy and diseased periodontal microbiome.

Results and Discussion

A Deep Look at the Oral Microbiome in Health and Disease

Current knowledge of the composition and functional spectrum of the human oral microbiome is limited by the difficulty to culture the majority of microbes that populate the oral cavity. We used deep sequencing technology to overcome this limitation, and produce a substantial genomic data set for the human microbiome under health and periodontal disease conditions. Specifically, we generated 16S rDNA data from five subjects (3 periodontally healthy [H] and 2 chronic periodontitis [P] patients, Table 1). In addition, a total of 495,195 16S rDNA sequences were generated with the 454 FLX sequencing technology, yielding an average of ~30,000 sequences per sample after removing low-quality sequences (roughly 3-times more sequences per sample than generated in a recent survey of oral microbes [28]). A total of 272,709,876 sequence reads were generated using the Illumina GAII platform, 76 bp, paired-end run (mean library size 207 bp) from the whole metagenome of four of the above-mentioned subjects (H1, H2, P1, and P2; Table 1). The low quality nucleotides were trimmed from all sequences and fragments matching to the human genome reference (NCBI release GRCh37.p1) were removed from further analysis. The level of human DNA contamination varied between different samples averaging ~87% of the sample, i.e. the oral microbiome represents just one eighth of the entire dataset or a total of 33,681,771 (12.4%) sequences (Table 1). This level of contamination is consistent with that observed in other studies, such as the Human Microbiome Project (manuscript in preparation). Despite the moderate yield (in terms of fraction of microbial sequences in the data-set) our results show that valuable biological insights can be derived from the data, thus indicating that informative and clinically relevant whole-metagenomic analyses of the oral microbiota can be conducted in a cost-effective manner.

Beyond the Taxonomical View of Periodontitis

The standard view of periodontitis, largely based on traditional microbiological approaches, associates the disease with the rise and damaging action of a small set of well-characterized pathogens. A first question we wanted to address using our data is whether, and to what extent, this traditional view still holds from the vantage point of metagenomic sequencing. Taxonomic profiling of the samples, whether derived from targeted 16S rRNA sequencing or from whole-metagenomic data (WGS) (Methods and Figure 1) reveals a community dominated, on average, by the bacterial phyla Firmicutes, Actinobacteria, Bacteroidetes, Fusobacteria and Proteobacteria, consistent with previous studies [28,29]. Together, these groups account for 80–95% of the entire oral microbiome. At the genus level we identify a total of 55 distinct genera in the 16S rDNA data and 58 distinct genera in the WGS data that are present at an abundance of 0.1% or higher (an additional 73 and 62 rare genera can be found in the 16S rDNA and WGS data, respectively). The most abundant genera comprise previously characterized oral bacteria: *Actinomyces*, *Prevotella*, *Streptococcus*, *Fusobacterium*, *Leptotrichia*, *Corynebacterium*, *Veillonella*, *Rothia*, *Capnocytophaga*, *Selenomonas*, *Treponema*, and TM7 genera 1 and 5.

The TM7 division was prevalent in our samples (11 out of 15 samples contain this division at >2% abundance), averaging 5.7% (standard deviation 7.2) of the entire population in the 16S rDNA data (WGS-based estimates also range ~6%), and up to 26.8% in sample P11. This division was statistically enriched in diseased samples (p< = 0.05, Metastats [30], Figure 1). TM7 is a novel

Table 1. Summary of sample information including high-quality read counts, taxonomic assignment of most abundant genus in each sample, and level of human contamination.

Phenotype	Subject (Tooth)	Clinical	16S rDNA		Dominant genus	Shotgun		Human DNA	Dominant genus
			# Reads	Sample		# Reads	Sample		
Periodontal disease	1(14)	advanced	51,056	P11	*Prevotella*	9.7M	P1	68.86%	*Prevotella*
	1(19)	moderate	20,149	P12	*Fusobacterium*				
	1(30)	moderate	41,355	P13	*Prevotella*				
	2(30)	moderate	46,444	P21	*Prevotella*	4.9M	P2	81.98%	*Prevotella*
Healthy	3(1)	healthy	23,702	H11	*Streptococcus*	12.4M	H1	60.61%	*Streptococcus*
	3(2)	healthy	44,869	H12	*Peptostreptococcus*				
	3(3)	healthy	32,405	H13	*Streptococcus*				
	3(4)	healthy	56,116	H14	*Leptotrichia*				
	4(3)	healthy	6,205	H21	*Streptococcus*	6.7M	H2	89.78%	*Actinomyces*
	4(14)	healthy	35,356	H22	*Actinomyces*				
	4(19)	healthy	14,110	H23	*Neisseria*				
	4(30)	healthy	25,662	H24	*Actinomyces*				
	5(3)	early	12,295	H31	*Fusobacterium*	NA	NA	NA	NA
	5(19)	healthy	30,891	H32	*Kingella*				
	5(30)	healthy	12,605	H33	*Actinomyces*				

The clinical labels represent: 'healthy' – healthy periodontal pocket; 'early' – early periodontal disease (bleeding under probing but no attachment loss), 'moderate' – moderate periodontal disease; 'advanced' – advanced periodontal disease. For a description of the clinical parameters used to make these determinations see Materials and Methods. The absence of metagenomic data from subject 5 is indicated with 'NA' in the appropriate cells.

candidate bacterial division with no cultivated representatives, and previous studies have shown microbes from this division to be commonly found in the human oral flora but at relatively low abundance, generally around 1% of the population [31,32], though abundances as high as 8% were previously reported [6]. The high abundance of TM7 microbes present in our samples, and their correlation with periodontal disease, indicate that the prevalence of this poorly studied bacterial division within the oral cavity, and its role in disease, have yet to be fully appreciated.

When comparing healthy and diseased samples we observe a shift in the composition of the oral microbiota (Figure 1 and Table S1), supporting the well characterized transition (p value$<10^{-15}$ using Fisher's exact test) from a gram-positive dominated community in the healthy samples, to a gram-negative dominated community in periodontal disease [12]. On one hand, our findings recapitulate prior results that indicate that the gram-negative genera *Selenomonas* [33,34], *Prevotella* [35], *Treponema* [36], *Tannerella* [36], *Haemophilus* [37] and *Catonella* [38] are significantly enriched in periodontal disease. Further, we have found a set of gram-positive genera that are significantly enriched in healthy samples: *Streptococcus, Actinomyces,* and *Granulicatella*. Surprisingly, however, neither *Fusobacterium*, nor *Porphyromonas* were found to be significantly more abundant in the periodontal disease samples, despite being previously implicated in this disease [12,39]. This is likely due to the high variance in the abundance of these organisms across our samples, as well as the small sample size which affects our statistical power.

Clustering analysis (Figure 1) reveals sample H31 (a control) to have a microbiota most similar to the diseased samples. This observation prompted a careful analysis of the clinical data collected during sampling. The data revealed some symptoms of mild periodontal disease (such as bleeding at probing time, see Materials and Methods for more details) that were not found in any of the other healthy samples, indicating that the microbiota may shift into a disease state before the full clinical symptoms of the disease are apparent. Also note that the diseased samples (including H31) cluster together tightly while the healthy samples are more widely distributed. This phenomenon is discussed in more detail below.

Taxonomic enrichment, however, cannot fully explain the etiology of periodontal disease. All organisms that exhibit an enrichment in either healthy or diseased samples are present in all the samples, irrespective of disease status, i.e. the mere presence of pathogens in the periodontal pocket is not sufficient to trigger periodontitis. The disease might be correlated with the presence of specific virulence factors within the genomes of particular pathogens, or might be initiated once the abundance of one or more pathogens crosses a specific threshold. The mechanisms that keep pathogenic bacteria 'in check' during health but allow them to bloom during disease are not yet understood. These observations support our suggestion that a full understanding of periodontal disease requires whole-genome and whole-system analyses.

Metabolism, Virulence Factors and Drug and Metal Resistance as Disease Signatures

In addition to providing a taxonomic overview, our metagenomic sequencing data contain high-resolution functional information. We annotated the function of genes identified in the assembled whole-metagenome data according to the KEGG Orthology, and used the resulting data to compare the functional potential of the oral microbiome in health and disease. The metabolic profiles of healthy and diseased samples differ in a number of important ways (Figure 2). The diseased microbiome is enriched in metabolic functions that are consistent with a parasitic

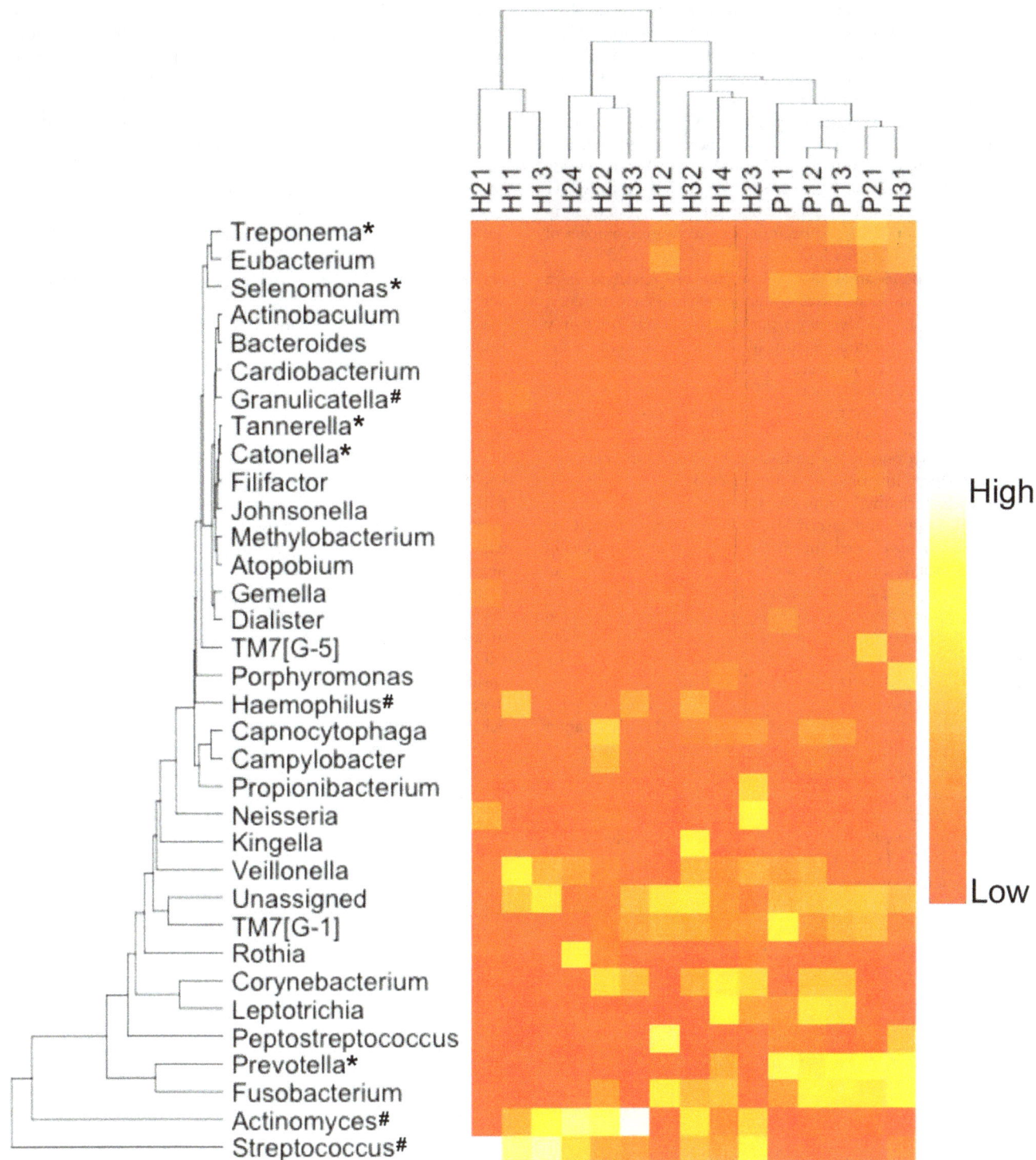

Figure 1. Relative abundance of genera in the samples estimated from 16S rDNA sequencing. * - genus significantly enriched in cases; ˆ - genus significantly enriched in controls (p< = 0.05, Metastats [30]). Only genera with >1% abundance in at least one sample were included. Colors reflect relative abundance from low (red) to high (white). Sample H31 (control) clusters together with the diseased samples, consistent with clinical observations of early symptoms of periodontal disease.

lifestyle made possible by the availability of nutrients derived from the degradation of host tissue and from bacterial cells destroyed by the host immune response (Table S2 for the statistical significance of enrichment of individual processes). Among these are functions for fatty acid metabolism and acetyl-coenzyme A degradation,

aromatic amino acid degradation, ferrodoxin oxidation, and energy-coupling factor (ECF) class transporters. The periodontal pocket has been previously shown to be enriched for such nutrients in patients with periodontitis [40]. Several of these metabolic functions have also been associated with an intracellular lifestyle (e.g. fatty acid metabolism [41]), or with anaerobic metabolism (e.g. ferrodoxin oxidation, and acetyl-CoA degradation), high-lighting the diversity of survival strategies employed by the microbes inhabiting the periodontal pocket during disease. Also enriched in disease are a number of virulence factors such as the presence of conjugative transposons, type IV secretion systems, and the biosynthesis of toxic factors (e.g. acetone, butanol, and ethanol biosynthesis), as well as the Lipid-A of lipopolysaccharide (LPS) biosynthesis. LPS is a group of molecules known to trigger host immune response and inflammation and their enrichment in disease provides a possible explanation for the systemic impact of periodontitis on the human host.

Finally, the periodontal disease samples are enriched in a number of functions related to drug and metal resistance (mercury, cobalt-zinc-cadmium). Mercury resistance has been previously characterized as a common feature of oral bacteria, even in the absence of mercury-containing amalgam, and is frequently associated with antibiotic resistance [42]. The role drug resistance plays in disease is, however, unclear as antibiotic resistance factors are present in both healthy and diseased samples.

Comparatively, only a few pathways are significantly enriched in the healthy microbiome (or depleted in the diseased microbiome), including pathways for fatty acid biosynthesis, purine metabolism, and glycerol-3-phosphate metabolism. Certain fatty acids have been shown to have a protective role in periodontal health [43,44,45] and it is possible that some of these are synthesized by the healthy microbiota. However, most of what is known about the role of fatty acids in periodontal health is based on nutritional studies and the contribution of the oral microbiota has yet to be characterized. Glycerol-3-phosphate is a lipid metabolite that has been shown to occur in higher concentration in periodontal disease samples [46]. Our study hints that a possible explanation for this observation is a decrease in the ability of the disease microbiome to metabolize this compound. Also enriched are genes related to homoserine metabolism, possibly related to quorum sensing functions within the healthy microbiome, as homoserine lactones are frequently used as quorum sensing molecules in oral bacteria [47]. The enrichment, within our healthy samples, of the reactions downstream of homo-serine lactone pathway may indicate a fully functioning quorum sensing system, allowing for the communication between organisms that is the hallmark of a healthy biofilm system. In poly-microbial biofilms it has been shown that mutants lacking quorum-sensing molecules, while able to construct biofilms, are unable to obtain the correct structure and thickness [48,49]. The depletion of pathways related to quorum sensing in our diseased samples may indicate a possible cause of disease progression due to the inability of the healthy microbiome to maintain a protective biofilm.

A Systems Level Perspective on Oral Disease

The functional characterization reported above suggests that, beyond the taxonomic details, one can identify ecosystem-level signatures of periodontal disease consistent with its clinical manifestations. However, from the above analysis, it is still not clear whether these signatures reflect isolated instances of disease-related molecular processes, or fit into a coherent picture of the disease as a predictably different state of the whole oral microbial flora. We addressed this question by performing additional analyses at different levels of resolution, and found that a major systemic change seems to be identifiable between the healthy and diseased microbiomes. The diseased samples harbor a more diverse microbial community (as measured by the Shannon

diversity index, Figure 3A), yet clustering analysis at the taxonomic level (Figure 1, Figure 3B) and in terms of enzyme content (Figure 3C), as well as pairwise comparisons of individual healthy and diseased samples based on tetramer (subsequences of length 4) frequencies (Figure 3D), all indicate that disease samples are more similar to each other than the healthy samples. In other words, the diseased state appears to be associated with a constrained and predictable region in the space of all possible states a microbiome can take. Thus, although the periodontal disease microbiomes are more diverse in terms of community structure, that structure is quite similar across different patients. In contrast, the healthy microbiome in any individual patient has relatively lower taxonomic diversity, but its exact composition differs significantly across patients.

Combined with the metabolic analyses described above, these results suggest that some systems-level changes may be associated with periodontal disease and the transition between health and disease. Microbial consortia in healthy individuals (Figure 4A) may rely on a highly diverse and rapidly changing supply of nutrients, as well as on good availability of oxygen for respiration. The relative paucity of enriched pathways in our healthy case analysis may reflect the diversity of metabolic pathways represented in the community. This is also supported by the clustering analysis of 16S rDNA data (Figure 3B) and of enzyme frequency data (Figure 3C), which show that the healthy data points do not tend to cluster together (Figure 4A, bottom left inset), and is consistent with a community with a lower taxonomic diversity (Figure 3A). On the contrary, the metabolic functions present in the microbial flora associated with periodontal disease (Figure 4B) seem to display a significant enrichment in specific metabolic pathways, compatible with an oxygen poor environment [50], and the availability of amino acids and lipids as major carbon sources. This may reflect the invasion of microbial pathogens (e.g. *Prevotella intermedia* which is enriched in the diseased samples) into human cells (both epithelial cells and macrophages). The disease flora is rich in lipid degradation pathways, as well as other known virulence-related activities, such as LPS biosynthesis. In turn, the consistency of the intracellular environment across different patients may explain why the disease points tend to cluster together in the Principal Component Analysis (PCA) plots. The ensuing picture is that the disease state is an attractor in the space of metabolic functions, with enrichment in cytotoxic and parasitic functions.

De Novo Assembly of Oral Microbes

The analyses we presented above have focused either exclusively on organisms (16S rDNA diversity) or biological function (metabolic analysis), thus ignoring the important link between organisms and the functions they perform. This connection can only be made by reconstructing partial or entire organisms from the community through metagenomic assembly. Currently, no practical genome assemblers exist that are specifically designed for large-scale metagenomic assembly, thus we relied on a hybrid assembly approach that combined *de novo* assembly using SOAPdenovo [51] (assembler used in a recent metagenomic analysis of gut microbes [52]), and alignments against a collection of oral microbes (Methods). The results shown in Table 2 demonstrate the power of this hybrid approach, which leads to an average of 4.4 and 2.1 times larger (in terms of N50 contig size) assemblies than *de novo* assembly and comparative assembly, respectively. Despite the relatively low level of coverage in our data, we obtain fairly contiguous assemblies (average N50 contig size of 3.5 Kbp), and are able to assemble up to about 50% of the

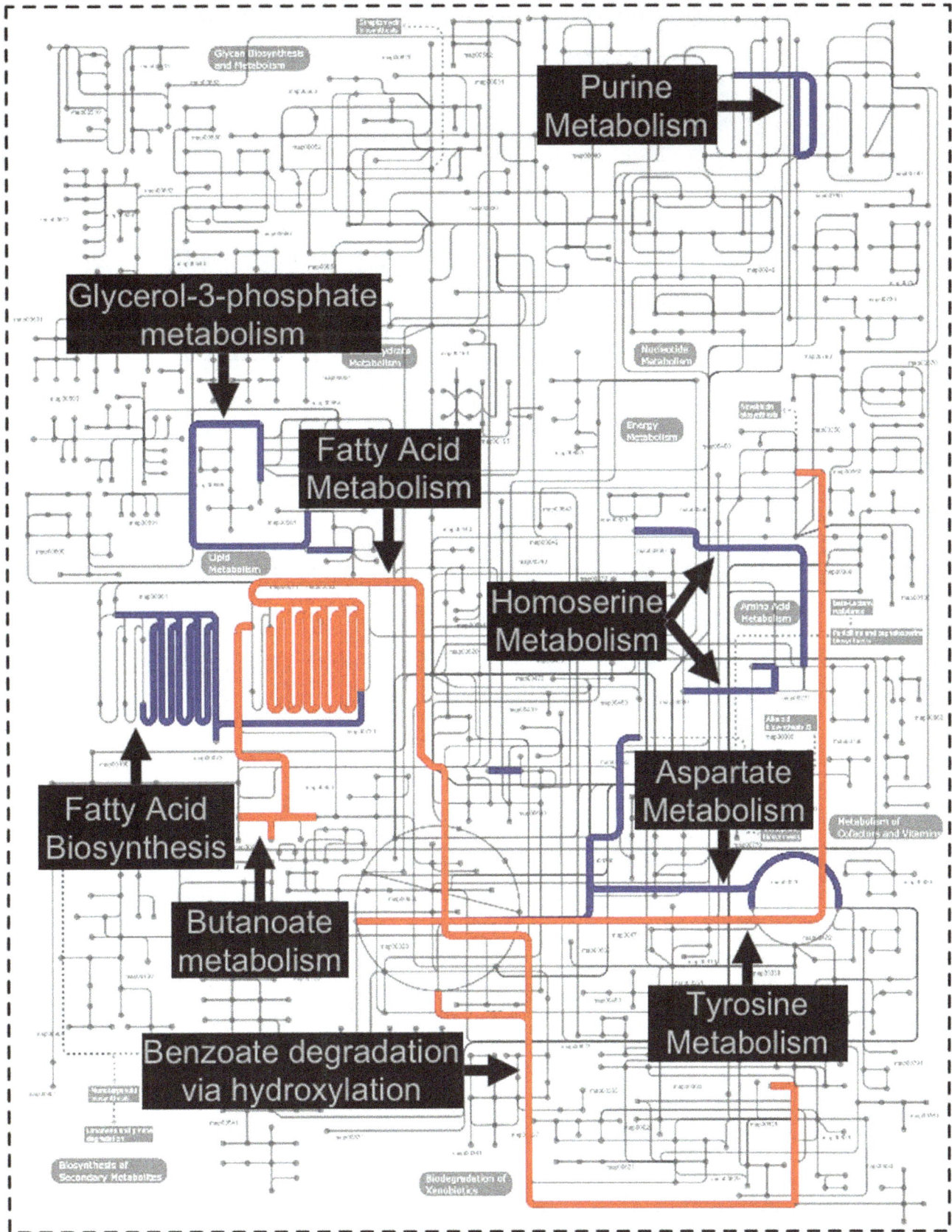

Figure 2. Metabolic pathways present in our samples. Dark blue – significantly enriched in healthy samples (p<0.05, MetaPath [84]); Dark red– significantly enriched in diseased samples (p<0.05, MetaPath). (Figure constructed with iPath [85]).

(A) Taxonomic Diversity

(B) Taxonomic Composition

(C) Enzyme Content

(D) K-mer Frequency

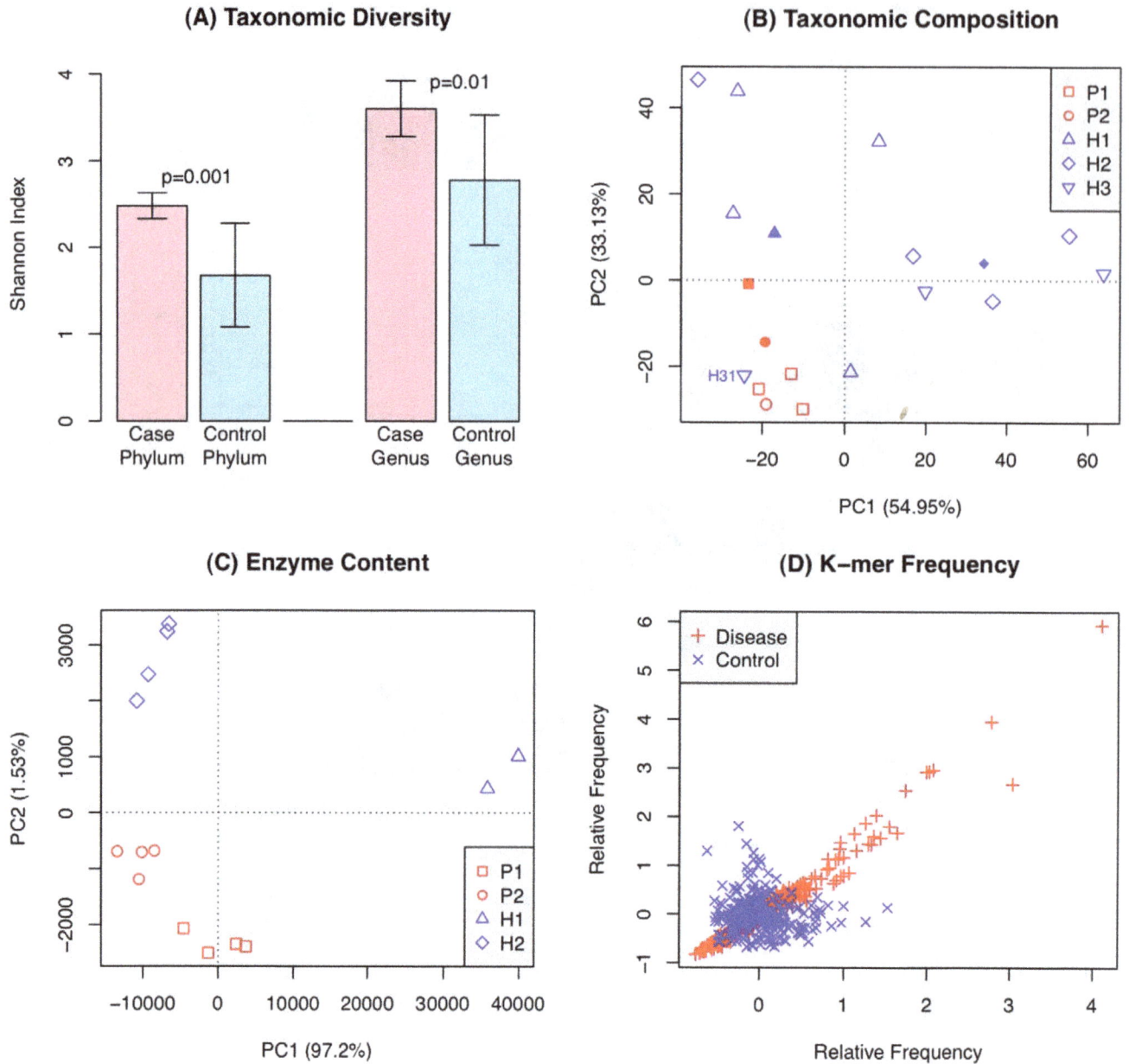

Figure 3. Systems-level analysis reveals the disease state to occupy a narrow region within the space of possible states for the microbiome. A – Shannon diversity calculated from 16S rDNA data is significantly higher in diseased samples (community is more diverse). B – Principal Component Analysis of the taxonomic compositions from 16S rDNA (empty symbols) and pooled WGS data (filled symbols). Disease samples cluster together in the bottom left corner. Sample H31 (tooth with incipient periodontal disease from an otherwise healthy patient) clusters together with the disease samples. C – Principal component analysis of the enzyme content of samples based on metagenomic sequencing. The PCA graph shows a tighter clustering of disease samples (red) relative to the healthy ones (blue). This suggests that the disease state may be linked to a specific metabolic configuration, and that the space of disease configurations is more constrained than the healthy one. Replicates (forward/reverse reads from one or two instrument lanes) are shown separately as identical symbols, and exhibit minimal metabolic variation within each sample. D – Comparison of relative frequencies of tetramers (4 bp motifs) in metagenomic reads across disease cases (in red, P1 vs. P2) and across control cases (in blue, H1 vs. H2). Based on the relative frequencies of tetramers, disease samples are more similar to each other (points lie along the diagonal) than controls are to each other.

total number of reads in our data-set. Furthermore, consistent with our previous observation that the periodontal disease samples are more diverse, the corresponding assemblies are also more fragmented (average N50 contig size is 1.2 Kbp in diseased samples versus 5.8 Kbp in healthy samples). In addition, a pooled assembly of all four samples results in dramatically increased contig sizes (max contig size is 16.9 Kbp in pooled assembly versus

7.6 Kbp in individual assemblies), indicating these samples contain closely related organisms.

Assembly of a TM7 Genome

As described above, we detected a higher presence of TM7 organisms in our samples than previously reported in literature. TM7 is a novel candidate bacterial phylum without cultivated

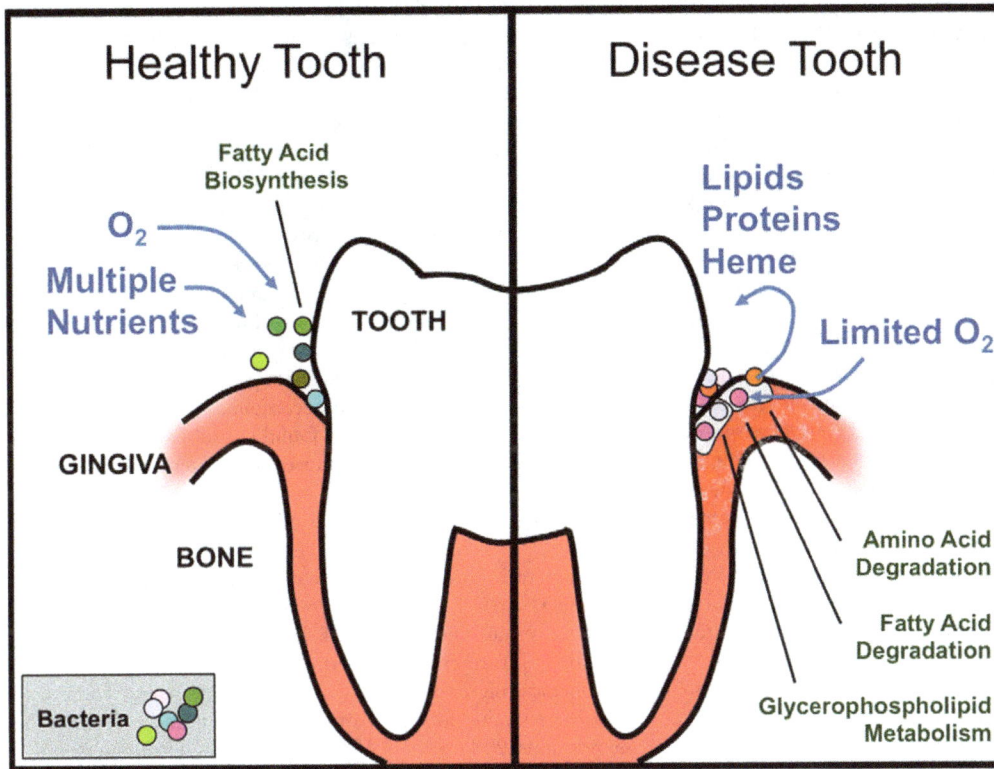

Figure 4. Schematic representation of the putative metabolic lifestyle shifts associated with the change in microbial flora around the tooth and gum tissue upon the transition from a healthy (A) to an advanced periodontal disease (B) state. The healthy state is dominated by the bacterial genera *Streptococcus, Fusobacterium, Actinomyces,* and *Corynebacterium,* whereas the disease state is primarily dominated by pathogenic genera such as *Prevotella, Leptotrichia, Treponema,* and *Fusobacterium.*

Table 2. Assembly statistics of metagenomic shotgun reads for contigs that are $>= 300$ bp using (1) SOAPdenovo, (2) comparative assembly and (3) a hybrid approach that uses MINIMUS to combine the contigs from the previous two methods.

Sample	Assembly approach	# Contigs	Length (Mbp)	Max (Kbp)	N50 (bp)	N90 (bp)	Reads assembled	
							# (M)	%
P1	SOAPdenovo	22,226	11.8	12.0	583	368	1.2	12.45
	Comparative	26,464	16.7	16.0	1113	598	1.3	13.21
	Hybrid	37,213	24.6	16.0	1829	1025	2.3	23.42
P2	SOAPdenovo	12,966	6.3	3.3	352	0	6.7	14.23
	Comparative	13,841	8.5	35.2	490	0	5.7	11.69
	Hybrid	21,835	12.5	37.6	647	396	10.5	21.39
H1	SOAPdenovo	45,658	3.1	22.6	3042	1648	5.0	40.20
	Comparative	46,036	3.3	18.6	2437	1559	3.5	28.21
	Hybrid	63,688	5.1	19.0	7567	3953	6.7	53.18
H2	SOAPdenovo	18,048	10.6	12.7	616	352	1.7	25.51
	Comparative	16,107	13.6	26.8	1543	689	2.2	32.33
	Hybrid	20,339	17.6	110.0	3934	1099	3.1	45.88
Pool	SOAPdenovo	98,051	54.9	15.7	2035	1342	8.1	24.12
	Comparative	63,506	60.1	44.6	8415	5474	8.4	24.89
	Hybrid	115,718	93.4	229.8	16896	9245	13.4	39.87

'Pool' represents the assembly of all four samples together. N50 or N90 is defined as the contig length such that equal or longer contigs produce 50% or 90% of 10 Mbp.

species, and previous studies have shown its high prevalence in human oral flora but with very low abundances [31,32]. The first sequence of a TM7 organism (TM7a) was generated through single-cell isolation in a microfluidic device, followed by whole genome amplification [53]. Due to the artifacts of the whole genome amplification approach, the resulting assembly is fairly fragmented (row 1 in Table 3). Here we relied on a hybrid assembly approach to reconstruct a more complete version of this genome, using the corresponding shotgun sequences generated in our project. Briefly, we started with the pooled assembly of all our samples and extracted all contigs that are mapped to the previously sequenced TM7a genome, and scaffolded these contigs using Bambus 2 [54]. Finally, we merged our TM7 assembly with the previously published assembly, derived from single-cell sequencing, in order to construct the most complete (to date) assembly of an organism from the TM7 group. The final assembly is still highly fragmented, comprising over 1,500 contigs (Table 3), however it contains almost 50% more sequence than the single-cell derived assembly (2.3 Mbp versus 1.7 Mbp), and the N50 contig size is two times larger (790 bp versus 389 bp). These results highlight the power of combining single-cell and metagenomic approaches when reconstructing the genomes of unculturable organisms from metagenomic samples (Figure S1 for the distribution of contig sizes).

In addition, this improved TM7 genome assembly allows us to identify 703 genes that were not present in the original assembly (Methods for details). In order to evaluate the additional information contained in these genes, we annotated them using the COMBREX [55] system (Table S4). The analysis revealed several potential virulence genes including an EmrB/QacA family drug resistance transporter gene (Gene ID: 681_1) and two phage proteins (Gene IDs: 386_2 and 1828_4). These genes are not necessarily omissions from the original assembly, rather they could represent *de novo* insertions into the TM7 genome present in our sample. The set of 'novel' TM7 genes does, however, included several housekeeping genes (e.g., 10 ribosomal protein genes not present in the original assembly) which should be conserved across TM7 genomes, thereby indicating that our assembly improves upon our current understanding of the structure of the TM7 genome in addition to revealing strain-specific genomic variants.

Genomic Variation in Actinomyces Naeslundii

Close analysis of one of the most abundant organisms in our samples (present at 24- and 6-fold coverage in samples H2 and H1, respectively, Table 4), a relative of *Actinomyces naeslundii* MG1 (sequence ID SEQF1063 in the Human Oral Microbiome

Database (HOMD) database), provides evidence for structural variations distinguishing this strain from the reference strain originally isolated from a patient with mild gingivitis [56]. The average similarity between the assembled metagenomic contigs from our project and the reference sequence is 96.2% and 95.2% for samples H1 and H2, respectively (second and sixth ring in Figure 5). A number of genomic deletions with respect to the reference strain are apparent in our samples, several of which contain potential virulence factors. These differences could be explained by the fact that the reference genome was isolated from a patient with gingivitis, while in our samples the *Actinomyces* strains are predominantly associated with healthy samples. Most striking is a deletion at 2120 kbp containing a putative mobile element encoding a mercury resistance locus (including a mercury resistance gene, a site-specific recombinase, and an integrase). Mercury resistance is commonly found in oral bacteria, frequently associated with antibiotic resistance [42]. Interestingly, gene set enrichment analysis of the entire metagenomic data-set reveals an enrichment of mercury resistance genes in the diseased samples (Table S2), possibly due to the association of these genes with virulence loci. Several other deletions also appear to encode virulence factors - a drug transporter (at position 580 kbp in the reference strain) and an alcohol dehydrogenase gene (at position 165 kbp) – further underscoring the difference between the pathogenic reference strain and the presumably commensal *Actinomyces* strains found in our samples. Another two deletions (at positions 20 kbp, and 1010 kbp) contain genes predicted to encode proteins involved in secretion and response regulation. These deletions occur at slightly different locations in the two samples we analyzed, suggesting they may be subject to rapid evolution.

Further evidence of the adaptation of *Actinomyces* to the oral environment is revealed by the analysis of single nucleotide polymorphism (SNP) densities. In Figure 5 (rings 6 and 8) we highlight the regions of the genome that have higher than expected SNP densities (>2 standard deviations from the mean). The most polymorphic regions (Table S3) correspond to genes predicted to be involved in the adaptation of an organism to its environment: transcriptional regulators, known to evolve rapidly in bacteria [57,58], and ABC transporters [59]. Another highly polymorphic region occurs within the glyceraldehyde-3-phosphate dehydrogenase (GAPDH) gene, a virulence-associated protein originally identified in Streptococci, which plays an important role in the colonization of periodontal pockets by interacting with plaque-forming bacteria [60]. GAPDH was also shown to mediate the interactions between Streptococci and

Table 3. Assembly statistics (calculated on contigs > = 300 bp) for HOMD TM7a reference sequences (row 1), hybrid assembly from metagenomic shotgun reads (row 2), Bambus scaffolding of hybrid assembly (row 3), assembly from combining hybrid assembly and the HOMD reference sequences (row 4), and Bambus scaffolding of 'combined reference' (row 5).

Assembly	# Contigs	Total Length	Max Contig	3Mbp	
				N25	N50
HOMD TM7a reference genome	1,780	1.7Mbp	17.5 Kbp	1.9 Kbp	0.4 Kbp
Hybrid assembly	1,340	1.5Mbp	13.9 Kbp	1.8 Kbp	NA
Scaffolds	874	1.6Mbp	20.9 Kbp	5.1K bp	0.5 Kbp
Combine reference	2,222	2.2Mbp	17.5 Kbp	2.9 Kbp	0.8 Kbp
Scaffolds	1,593	2.3Mbp	33.7 Kbp	7.2 Kbp	1.8 Kbp

The N25 and N50 are calculated assuming a 3 Mbp genome size.

Table 4. Assembly statistics (calculated on contigs >= 100 bp) for *Actinomyces naeslundii* MG1 in sample H1 and H2.

Reference genome	Length	Sample	# Contigs	Total length	Depth of coverage	Max Contig	N50	N90
Actinomyces naeslundii MG1	~3Mbp	H1	2850	~2.8Mbp	6.2	14.5 Kbp	1.7 Kbp	0.1 Kbp
		H2	1168	~2.9Mbp	24.3	28.6 Kbp	5.5 Kbp	0.9 Kbp

The N50 and N95 are calculated based on the MG1 genome size.

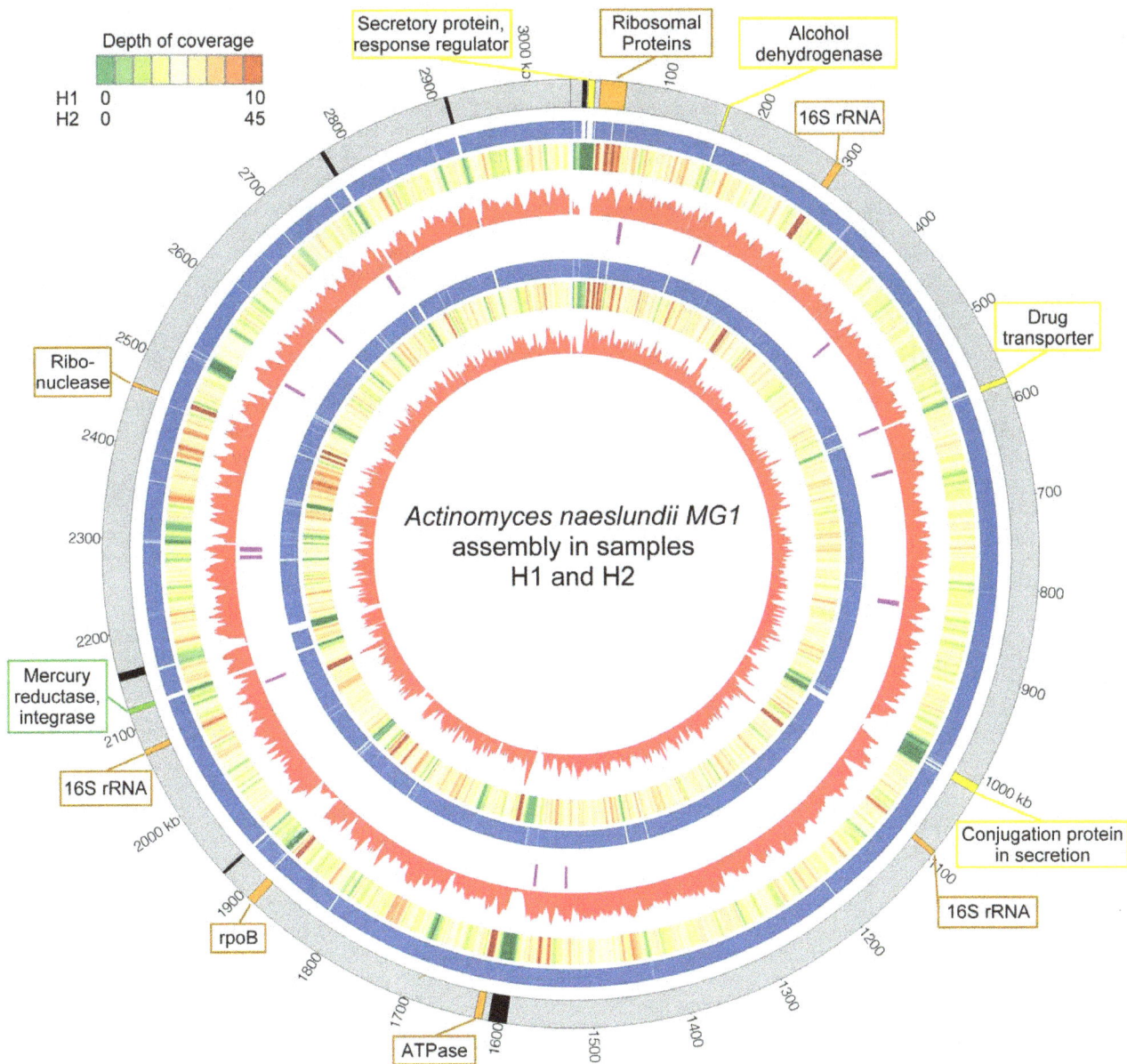

Figure 5. Comparative analysis of the *Actinomyces naeslundii* MG1 reference genome (HOMD SeqID SEQF1063), and assemblies from samples H1 and H2. Counting from outside, the first ring is the reference genome with genes annotated by colored bands: orange bands are conserved genes; green bands are genes involved in horizontal gene transfer; yellow bands are genes with known functions; black bands are genes with unknown functions. Only regions that are associated with genomic variations are colored and annotated. The second and sixth rings are the assembled contigs from sample H2 and H1. The heatmaps in the third and seventh rings represent the depth of coverage of the contigs with 5K bp window and 100 bp step for sample H2 and H1. The histograms in the fourth and eighth rings represent the scaled SNP rate with 5 Kbp window and 100 bp step for sample H2 (max = 0.08) and H1 (max = 0.03). The purple bands in the fifth ring represent regions with significantly higher theta values than average (p<=0.05). Image generated with Circos [86].

Porphyromonas gingivalis fimbriae [61,62], possibly contributing to the colonization of the subgingival pocket by *P. gingivalis*. These observations are consistent with previous findings of high-SNP densities within genomic regions surrounding recombination events [63].

Conclusions

Our study represents a novel step towards characterizing the genomic composition of the microbial communities associated with periodontal disease. We have demonstrated that the subgingival microbiome can be effectively interrogated through high-throughput sequencing, and that the resulting data provide valuable insights into the molecular underpinnings of periodontal disease.

Despite a relatively small amount of bacterial sequence data recovered from our samples (primarily due to the high level of human DNA contamination), a combination of comparative and *de novo* assembly approaches was able to reconstruct large genomic segments from several dominant organisms in our samples, thereby allowing a better reconstruction of an unculturable TM7 organism (in conjunction with data generated through single cell genomic approaches), and providing a glimpse at the genomic variation (and possible association with virulence) within *Actinomyces* genomes. Better assemblies were possible in samples that were sequenced more deeply (e.g., sample H1), indicating the need to sequence the oral environment more deeply than has been done in this study. Furthermore, assembly quality roughly correlated with disease status, partly confirming our observation (based on 16S rDNA data) that diseased samples had a higher microbial diversity. This observation also highlights a limitation of existing assembly tools in dealing with genomic diversity, further underscoring the need for the development of metagenomic-specific genome assemblers.

The analysis of the TM7 and *Actinomyces* genomes revealed signatures consistent with recombination events possibly associated with virulence factors. Lateral transfer of virulence determinants through phages and recombination is well documented in the bacterial world, leading to a partial separation between function and phylogeny, thus, suggesting the need for metagenomic and functional analyses as a complement to taxonomic surveys of host-associated microbiota.

Taxonomic analyses of the data we generated are consistent with a well-established community shift from a gram-positive dominated healthy microbiome to a gram-negative dominated diseased microbiome, which is also enriched in a number of oral pathogens. The molecular mechanisms that underlie and cause this transition are, however, unknown. Here we have shown that functional information derived from whole-metagenomic data provides a valuable complement to the taxonomic data and allows us to develop a novel theory of periodontal disease. The healthy state is highly regulated by the host immune system and interactions between community members to maintain a community dominated by few "good" microbes, usually gram-positive Actinobacteria or Streptococci. The transition to periodontal disease involves a disruption of the host-microbiome interactions that results in a more even community structure composed by a broad range of organisms that can thrive in the oral environment. The presence of pathogens within this community can lead to the clinical manifestations of periodontal disease, which in turn can lead to additional changes in the community due to the increased availability of nutrients released by the damaged tissue. As a result, the periodontal disease microbiome eventually settles into a state characterized by a diverse population of microbes adapted to a parasitic lifestyle made possible by the disrupted host homeostasis.

One of the samples from our study was characterized by a microbiota typical of a diseased state, yet the corresponding tooth was just starting to show some of the clinical symptoms of disease. This observation implies that dysbiosis precedes the clinical manifestation of disease, and that the oral microbiota could be a potential tool for the early diagnosis of periodontitis.

The large variability we observe between healthy samples, and even between different teeth of a same person, highlights the limitation of using data derived from cross-sectional studies to define what the core "normal microbiome" means. Furthermore, case-control studies are likely insufficient to determine the causal agents of periodontal disease – the organisms found to dominate the diseased microbiome (the "usual suspects" commonly described in the literature) may simply be a symptom of the disrupted subgingival environment rather than the primary cause of disease. The "usual suspects" approach considers presence and absence of specific bacteria to be the critical precondition for disease, however, our data support a more nuanced approach that considers quantitative and genomic differences as the critical factors when moving from health to a diseased state. Longitudinal studies are necessary to characterize the dynamic changes that occur in the oral microbiome in response to environmental changes (food intake, changes in the host, etc.) and to track the transition between the healthy and diseased states, and the return to health after treatment.

It is important to note that the analyses described above are a preliminary pilot project with limited sample size, and our observations must be confirmed in more extensive studies. Furthermore, we focus on whether the microbiome has the potential to perform certain biological functions, and on determining the relative fraction of the microbial population that can perform a particular function. These results (as well as those of similar metagenomic projects) must be complemented by experimental studies aimed at determining whether the biological processes statistically enriched in disease are actually active in the subgingival pocket.

As others have previously reported, and as observed in the data we have shown here, periodontal disease is the result of a disruption of the complex interactions occurring within the subgingival microbiome and between the microbiome and the host. A full understanding of the etiology of periodontal disease will only be possible through further in-depth systems-level analyses of the host-microbiome interaction.

Materials and Methods

Subject Population

The subject population consisted of 5 patients who were in good general health and were recruited between August and November 2009 at the Clinical Research Center, Boston University Goldman School of Dental Medicine. Written informed consent was obtained from all enrolled individuals. The study protocol was reviewed and approved by the Institutional Review Board at the Boston University Medical Center. All subjects had at least 12 natural teeth with >20 years of age (age range, 28–45 years). Subjects diagnosed with chronic periodontitis (n = 2) were selected among those who had at least six sites with probing depth ≥6 mm and attachment loss ≥5 mm. Subjects in the control (periodontally healthy) group had no pockets >3 mm and no attachment loss >2 mm at any site with no signs of periodontal inflammation characterized by bleeding on probing, redness, edema, and attachment loss, with the exception of subject 5 where one of the teeth (# 3, sample H31) exhibited mild bleeding at probing time consistent with initial periodontal disease. Sites with gingivitis were characterized by bleeding on probing, redness, edema, but no attachment loss (pocket depth ≤4 mm). Sites from chronic periodontitis subjects further characterized as mild, moderate or advanced periodontitis sites based on the pocket depth. Mild periodontitis was characterized with pockets >4 mm but not more than 5 mm; moderate periodontitis was characterized with pockets >5 but <7 mm while advanced periodontitis was characterized with pockets >7 mm. Healthy group consisted of subjects of Asian, Caucasian and African American origin, while periodontitis subjects were of Caucasian and African-American origin. Exclusion criteria included pregnancy, lactation, systemic conditions that could affect the progression or treatment of periodontal diseases. In addition, none of the subjects had received systemic antibiotics or periodontal therapy in the previous 6 months.

Subgingival Plaque Sampling and Isolation of Bacterial DNA

After the removal of supragingival plaque with sterile gauze, individual subgingival plaque samples were taken from the mesio-buccal aspect of four molar teeth in four quadrants (upper right, upper left, lower right and lower left) per subject using sterile periodontal curettes (Hu-Friedy, Chicago, IL). Each sample was placed in a separate sterile 1.5-ml tube containing 200 µl TE buffer (50 mM Tris-HCl, 1 mM EDTA; pH 7.6). Bacterial DNA extraction was performed using commercially available DNA purification kit (Epicentre MasterPure™, Madison, WI) according to manufacturer's guidelines. First, the debris was separated by centrifugation at 4°C and supernatant was transferred to another microcentrifuge tube and pellet was discarded. The collected supernatant was mixed with 500 µl of isopropanol and centrifuged at 4°C for DNA isolation. Isopropanol solution was carefully removed without dislodging the DNA pellet. The DNA pellet was rinsed with 75% ethanol and residual ethanol was removed. The sample was resuspended in 25 µl of TE buffer and stored at −80°C until analysis.

16S rDNA Sequencing Protocol

DNA samples were amplified using the primers: 5'-GCCTCCCTCGCGCCATCAGacacactgCATGCTGCCTCC-CGTAGGAGT and 5'-CCTATCCCCTGTGTGCCTTGG-CAGTCTCAGAGAGTTTGATCCTGGCTCAG to initiate the reaction. The underlined portions of the primers corresponded to 'universal' bacterial primers 338R and 27F primer, the small letters contained a barcode specific to each well and the 5' end of the primer was specific to the 454 specific protocols. Each reaction had 5 units of Choice DNA Taq polymerase (Denville Scientific), 100 uM of dNTPs, 1× reaction buffer and 2 mM MgCl$_2$ and occurred for 30 cycles of 94°C for 30 sec, 50°C for 30 sec, and 72°C for 30 sec. The presence of amplified products was confirmed by gel electrophoresis. Approximately equimolar amounts of product were pooled and gel purified. Sequencing was performed using the Lib-L kit following instructions from the manufacturer (Roche).

Data Collection, Sequencing and Preprocessing

16S rDNA sequences were processed and filtered based on quality with an in-house pipeline as follows. First, sequences containing at least one unrecognizable base-pair ('N'), and that were too short (<75 cycles of the 454 instrument) were excluded from further analysis. Then, barcode sequences were deconvoluted and removed.

Metagenomic sequencing was performed on pooled DNA from multiple teeth in order to obtain sufficient DNA concentrations for library construction. Metagenomic shotgun sequences were obtained from the Illumina instruments in fastq format and were trimmed for quality using the FastX Toolkit (Hannon Lab, CSHL) with the following parameters: (1) minimum length 25, and (2) q-value cutoff 20. Sequences containing at least one ambiguity character ('N') were also removed. The remaining sequences that passed the quality trimming outlined above were mapped to the human genome reference (NCBI build 37 v 1) downloaded from NCBI using Bowtie with parameters (−v 3; at most 3 mismatches) If one of the sequences from a paired end matched the human genome, then both sequences were removed from the data-set. The remaining reads were mapped against the human sequences in the NCBI *nr* database using Basic Local Alignment Search Tool (BLAST) in order to remove human sequences not present in the NCBI human genome reference. For this additional check we required at least 95% global identity (since BLAST is a local alignment algorithm, our calculation also takes into account the length of the unaligned segments flanking the 'hit' reported by BLAST).

Comparative Assembly

We mapped and assembled the samples against reference sequences for oral microbes extracted from the Human Oral Microbiome Database (HOMD, http://www.homd.org) [64] as follows:

1. We used MUMmer [65] (-maxmatch -l 20 -b) to map the individual reads against the HOMD reference database.
2. Reads that mapped with higher than 80% global identity were then assembled based on the mapped coordinates of the reads.
3. This process was repeated using a 90% similarity threshold, but mapping the reads against the assemblies generated at step 2, rather than against the HOMD database.
4. The resulting contigs were then combined with the results of a de novo assembly of the data, as described in more detail below.

All customized scripts used to run this analysis can be obtained by request from the authors and will soon be released as part of an open-source package for comparative assembly of metagenomic data [Liu et al. in preparation].

De Novo Assembly Using SOAPdenovo

We used SOAPdenovo V. 1.04 [66] with parameters −K 23 and −M 3, as previously used by the MetaHit project [52] to assemble gut microbiome data.

Combining Comparative and de Novo Assembly Data

Contig sequences longer than 100 bp, which were generated by our customized comparative assembly pipeline (workflow presented above) and by SOAPdenovo, were combined and assembled using MINIMUS [67] with the following parameters: (1) minimum overlap length 40 bp, and (2) overlap error rate is 0.1.

Assembly and Gene Prediction of TM7 Genome

The reference genome of TM7a was downloaded from HOMD (http://www.homd.org/). We pooled all available metagenomic sequences together, and performed comparative assemblies against the existing TM7a reference sequences as described above. The resulting contigs were combined together with the *de novo* assemblies of all metagenomic sequences using MINIMUS, resulting in a hybrid assembly for TM7a. The resulting assembly was then further combined with the HOMD TM7a reference genomic sequence. After assembly, scaffolds were created using BAMBUS 2 using the available mate-pair information.

We used MetaGene [68] to predict genes ($> = 300$ bp) in the TM7 reference genome (NCBI accession NZ_ABBV00000000) as well as in our combined assembly described above. We, then mapped (using BLASTN) the predicted genes from our assembly against the predicted genes from the TM7 reference genome. A match was defined as E-value$< = 0.00001$, % similarity $> = 90\%$, and more than 50% of the query sequence is aligned. Genes found in our assembly that did not match any gene in the reference strain were considered novel and subjected to functional annotation using COMBREX.

Estimation of SNP Rates and Genetic Diversity

After assembly, the shotgun reads were mapped back to the contigs using Bowtie [69] allowing at most 3 mismatches. To avoid sequencing and mapping errors we used a conservative approach as suggested in [70]: we only retained SNPs occurring in regions with a depth of coverage higher than 4, and with each individual haplotype represented in at least two different reads. The SNP rate was calculated using a 5 Kbp window and a 100 bp step size.

We adapted the approach used in [71,72] to infer the genetic diversity θ from metagenomic shotgun sequencing data using composite likelihood estimators while accounting for a constant sequencing error rate. First we classified the nucleotide positions of the assembled contigs into k groups, where k is the maximum depth of coverage of the contigs, and positions within the same group have the same depth of coverage. The number of nucleotide positions in each group is denoted by n_1, n_2, ..., n_k. Considering the large number of bacteria in the sampled community relative to the number of reads sequenced, the probability that each read derives from a different individual microorganism is close to one. Thus, we have a population size equal to the depth of coverage at every site in the assembled contigs [71]. Consequently, the estimator can be obtained by calculating the expected number of true SNPs and false SNPs due to sequencing errors [72]. Then for a particular nucleotide group with the same depth d, assuming an infinite sites model, the expected number of segregating sites is $\theta n_d \sum_{i=1}^{d-1} \frac{1}{i} = S_d - S_d^{error}$, where S_d is the observed number of segregating sites (SNPs) from data and S_d^{error} is the expected number of segregating sites induced by sequencing errors. For a nucleotide position with depth of coverage d, the probability of at least two mutations ($x > = 2$; considered as true SNPs) induced by sequencing error (e) is:

$$\sum_{x=2}^{d} B(d,e)$$

$$= \sum_{x=2}^{d} \binom{d}{x} e^x (1-e)^{d-x} = 1 - (1-e)^d - ne(1-e)^{d-1} = e_d$$

Since there are n_d such sites with depth of d, the expected number of segregating sites induced by error is $S_d^{error} = n_d e_d$. Hence the estimated $\hat{\theta}$ for regions with d depth of coverage is $\hat{\theta} = \dfrac{S_d - S_d^{error}}{n_d \sum_{i=1}^{d-1} \frac{1}{i}}$

Finally, summing over all groups we get the equation.

$$\hat{\theta} = \frac{S - \sum_{d=4}^{k} S_d^{error}}{\sum_{d=4}^{k} n_d \sum_{i=1}^{d-1} \frac{1}{i}} = \frac{S - \sum_{d=4}^{k} n_d \left[1 - (1-e)^d - ne(1-e)^{d-1} \right]}{\sum_{d=4}^{k} n_d \sum_{i=1}^{d-1} \frac{1}{i}}$$

In our calculation, we assume a constant sequencing error rate $e = 0.01$. The θ value is calculated using a 1 Kbp window moving average (which is roughly the average gene size in bacteria) with 100 bp step size.

Regions of the genome that had a value of θ more than 2 standard deviations higher than the average were flagged as potential polymorphism hotspots (Table S3).

Clustering and Annotation of 16S rDNA Sequences

The entire set of trimmed 16S rDNA sequences were clustered into Operational Taxonomic Units (OTUs) with the program DNACLUST [73], using a 1% radius ($-r$ 2). To obtain the taxonomic identities, the OTU centers were aligned using BLAST to the RDP database [74] augmented with oral clones from the HOMD database [64], and were annotated using the lowest common ancestor approach (similar to the approach in [75]). The assignment process is conservative: (1) only sequence with at least global 98% identity with the reference is classified; (2) if there are more than one equally good best hits, then the sequence is classified using the lowest common ancestor approach; (3) otherwise it is classified as unknown. Finally, the taxonomic label of the OTU center is transferred to the sequences from the same OTU cluster. The resulting data was organized in a collection of tables at different taxonomic levels containing each taxonomic group as a row and each sample as a column. These tables formed the substrate for the further statistical analyses.

Antibiotic Resistance Genes Annotation

Shotgun reads are annotated against the Antibiotic Resistance Genes Database (ARDB) reference genes [76] using BLASTX with the following thresholds: (1) at least 60 bp long high-scoring segment pairs, and (2) 90% or 95% similarity cutoff at the amino acid level.

Seed Functional Mapping

Sequences that were preprocessed for removal human contamination were uploaded to the MG-RAST online webtool (version 2.0 [77] metagenomics.anl.gov/v2). Results were downloaded and parsed into individual files, one per patient, using PERL. Only annotations with a confidence of 1E-5 or lower were kept for further processing resulting in 1,130,510 annotations (representing 75,742 distinct functional labels). In an attempt to correct for under-counting of low-abundance sequences, we used the Laplace correction and added one to all counts.

GSEA

To perform the gene set enrichment analysis (GSEA), we used the gene set enrichment analysis (GSEA) tool version 2.07 [78], downloaded from the Broad Institute website (www.broadinstitute. org/gsea/index.jsp). GSEA was used to identify functional categories that were enriched in disease or control patients. Functional sub-classes from SEED (Version 12) [79] were used as the gene sets (total of 669). We added two gene sets which were not represented in SEED, 'transposases', and 'transposon related', bringing the total to 671). These new gene sets were created by searching for the title term (i.e. 'transposases', or 'transposon related') in the functional descriptions of the full set of SEED functional categories. We used the default parameter settings of the GSEA software, with two exceptions. In our analysis, to rank the functional classes, we used a 'ratio of classes' rather than the 'signal to noise' metric, and for the significance testing we permuted the gene set instead of the phenotype. We selected and reported all gene sets that had a p-value less than 0.005, and with a false discovery rate q-value cut off of 0.01.

Calculating Tetramer Frequencies

K-mer frequencies, especially tetranucleotide frequencies in prokaryotic genomes, have been shown to carry a phylogenetic signal [80]. For each patient, we counted the occurrence of each sequence motif of length 4 for all the pre-processed sequence reads using a sliding window approach. The relative frequency of each motif was calculated as the number of occurrences of a specific motif (tetramer), divided by the total number of motifs of length 4. The number of expected motifs of length k based on the expectation from motifs of length k-1 was estimated using a Markov chain [81]. For example, the probability of observing a tetramer, such as "CTAG" is estimated from the transition probability of observing a "CTA" motif adjacent to a "TAG" motif at "TA" dinucleotides, or p(CTAG|CTA,TAG) = p(CTA) * p(TAG)/p(TA). The observed motif frequencies were normalized by subtracting the number of expected motifs from the number of observed motifs, and dividing the result by the number of expected motifs. Using these normalized values, we can visualize the tetramer frequency counts directly and compare them across samples. The tighter, linear grouping of the disease samples suggests that the corresponding communities are composed of organisms phylogenetically less diverse, compared to the larger, more diverse cluster of healthy samples.

Taxonomic Diversity Analysis

Relative abundance estimates obtained from the 16S rDNA sequencing data were used to compute the entropy (Shannon diversity) for each of the 15 samples for which 16S rDNA data were generated. Separate analyses were performed at the genus and phylum levels, and the results were aggregated across clinical status. The statistical significance of the observed differences was estimated using a standard t-test.

Taxonomy Based PCA

The taxonomic composition of the samples was estimated based on both 16S rDNA data (Methods above) and WGS data using MetaPhyler [82]. Each sample was represented as a vector of relative abundances of individual phyla, and the resulting vectors were subjected to Principal Component Analysis using the *princomp* function in R. Note that samples represented in both the 16S rDNA and the WGS data are represented twice in this analysis.

Enzyme Based PCA

After pre-processing, metagenomic sequences were annotated with specific Kyoto Encyclopedia of Genes and Genomes (KEGG) orthology (KO) codes using BLAST searches against the KEGG sequence repository [83]. The KO numbers for each protein were mapped to EC numbers, using a combination of custom Perl scripts and a conversion table. The table was generated from data available from the KEGG ftp server (ftp://ftp.genome.jp/pub/kegg/). An E-value cut-off of 1E-05 was applied to the resulting annotations to remove non-specific BLAST hits. For each sample, we constructed a count matrix containing the number of reads mapping to each enzyme. We carried out a principal component analysis on this matrix, using the 'princomp' function in Matlab implemented with the default parameters. We then displayed the sample position on the first and second principal components in Figure 3C to visualize each sample's relative distance.

Supporting Information

Figure S1 Histogram distribution of contig sizes. The upper plot shows the distribution of contig size from TM7 reference genome, which is assembled from single-cell sequencing. The lower plot shows the distribution of contig size from the assembly that combines the contigs from TM7 reference genome and metagenome. Contig sizes that are $>= 5000$ bp are plotted as 5000 bp.

Table S1 Differential abundance of genera between cases and controls. P-values were computed with Metastats [30].

Table S2 Summary of microbial functions enriched in diseased or control samples. CLINICAL – indicates whether enrichment occurs in disease or control samples; METHOD – method used to compute significance of enrichment; SIGNIFICANCE – Method-specific assessment of the significance of enrichment: for GSEA [87] we report both the p-value and the q-value obtained by correcting for the False Discovery Rate (FDR); for MetaPath [84] we report both the raw p-value for enrichment (p-abund) and p-value corrected for the structure of the metabolic network (p-struct).

Table S3 Genomic regions with nucleotide diversity θ values that are more than two standard deviations away from the mean.

Table S4 COMBREX [55] functional annotations of new genes predicted from TM7a metagenomic assembly.

Acknowledgments

We would like to thank Luke Tallon and Lisa Sadzewicz for assistance with Illumina and 454 sequencing.

Data Availability: The data described in this paper have been submitted to NCBI under project ID: PRJNA78025.

Author Contributions

Conceived and designed the experiments: SK DS MP SA. Performed the experiments: BL LF NK VM MG DDS TG TJT YCC SL OCS HH. Analyzed the data: SK DS MP SA. Contributed reagents/materials/analysis tools: BL LF NK VM MG DDS TG TJT YCC SL OCS HH SK DS MP SA. Wrote the paper: BL LF NK VM MG DDS TG TJT YCC SL OCS HH SK DS MP SA.

References

1. Turnbaugh P, Ley R, Hamady M, Fraser-Liggett C, Knight R, et al. (2007) The Human Microbiome Project. Nature 449: 804–810.

2. Ley RE, Peterson DA, Gordon JI (2006) Ecological and evolutionary forces shaping microbial diversity in the human intestine. Cell 124: 837–848.

3. Kuramitsu HK, He X, Lux R, Anderson MH, Shi W (2007) Interspecies interactions within oral microbial communities. Microbiology and molecular biology reviews : MMBR 71: 653–670.

4. Belda-Ferre P, Alcaraz LD, Cabrera-Rubio R, Romero H, Simón-Soro A, et al. (2011) The oral metagenome in health and disease. The ISME journal. pp 1–11.

5. Whitman WB, Coleman DC, Wiebe WJ (1998) Prokaryotes: the unseen majority. Proc Natl Acad Sci U S A 95: 6578–6583.

6. Zaura E, Keijser BJ, Huse SM, Crielaard W (2009) Defining the healthy "core microbiome" of oral microbial communities. BMC Microbiol 9: 259.

7. Conly J, Johnston B (2005) Where are all the new antibiotics? The new antibiotic paradox. The Canadian journal of infectious diseases & medical microbiology 16: 159–160.

8. Lipsitch M (2001) The rise and fall of antimicrobial resistance. Trends in microbiology 9: 438–444.

9. Jones KE, Patel NG, Levy MA, Storeygard A, Balk D, et al. (2008) Global trends in emerging infectious diseases. Nature 451: 990–993.

10. Bell T, Newman JA, Silverman BW, Turner SL, Lilley AK (2005) The contribution of species richness and composition to bacterial services. Nature 436: 1157–1160.

11. Ptacnik R, Solimini AG, Andersen T, Tamminen T, Brettum P, et al. (2008) Diversity predicts stability and resource use efficiency in natural phytoplankton communities. Proceedings of the National Academy of Sciences of the United States of America 105: 5134–5138.

12. Darveau RP (2010) Periodontitis: a polymicrobial disruption of host homeostasis. Nat Rev Microbiol 8: 481–490.

13. Koenig JE, Spor A, Scalfone N, Fricker AD, Stombaugh J, et al. (2011) Succession of microbial consortia in the developing infant gut microbiome. Proceedings of the National Academy of Sciences of the United States of America 108 Suppl 4578–4585.

14. Teles R, Wang CY (2011) Mechanisms involved in the association between peridontal diseases and cardiovascular disease. Oral diseases.

15. Ali J, Pramod K, Tahir MA, Ansari SH (2011) Autoimmune responses in periodontal diseases. Autoimmune reviews.

16. Bascones-Martinez A, Matesanz-Perez P, Escribano-Bermejo M, Gonzalez-Moles MA, Bascones-Ilundain J, et al. (2011) Periodontal disease and diabetes-Review of the Literature. Medicina oral, patologia oral y cirugia bucal.

17. Rodrigues RM, Goncalves C, Souto R, Feres-Filho EJ, Uzeda M, et al. (2004) Antibiotic resistance profile of the subgingival microbiota following systemic or local tetracycline therapy. Journal of clinical periodontology 31: 420–427.

18. van Winkelhoff AJ, Herrera D, Winkel EG, Dellemijn-Kippuw N, Vanden-broucke-Grauls CM, et al. (1999) [Antibiotic resistance in the subgingival microflora in patients with adult periodontitis. A comparative survey between Spain and the Netherlands]. Nederlands tijdschrift voor tandheelkunde 106: 290–294.

19. Edwards JS, Covert M, Palsson B (2002) Metabolic modelling of microbes: the flux-balance approach. Environmental Microbiology 4: 133–140.

20. Mazumdar V, Snitkin ES, Amar S, Segrè D (2009) Metabolic network model of a human oral pathogen. Journal of bacteriology 191: 74–90.

21. Wintermute EH, Silver PA (2010) Emergent cooperation in microbial metabolism. Molecular Systems Biology 6: 407.

22. Klitgord N, Segrè D (2010) Environments that induce synthetic microbial ecosystems. PLoS Computational Biology 6: e1001002.

23. Diaz-Torres ML, Villedieu A, Hunt N, McNab R, Spratt DA, et al. (2006) Determining the antibiotic resistance potential of the indigenous oral microbiota of humans using a metagenomic approach. FEMS microbiology letters 258: 257–262.

24. Voelkerding KV, Dames SA, Durtschi JD (2009) Next-generation sequencing: from basic research to diagnostics. Clin Chem 55: 641–658.

25. Keijser B, Zaura E, Huse S, van der Vossen J, Schuren F, et al. (2008) Pyrosequencing analysis of the Oral Microflora of healthy adults. Journal of Dental Research 87.

26. Paster BJ, Olsen I, Aas JA, Dewhirst FE (2006) The breadth of bacterial diversity in the human periodontal pocket and other oral sites. Periodontol 2000 42: 80–87.

27. Jenkinson HF (2011) Beyond the oral microbiome. Environmental Microbiology 13: 3077–3087.

28. Bik EM, Long CD, Armitage GC, Loomer P, Emerson J, et al. (2010) Bacterial diversity in the oral cavity of 10 healthy individuals. The ISME Journal 4: 962–974.

29. Ahn J, Yang L, Paster BJ, Ganly I, Morris L, et al. (2011) Oral Microbiome Profiles: 16S rRNA Pyrosequencing and Microarray Assay Comparison. PloS one 6: e22788.

30. White JR, Nagarajan N, Pop M (2009) Statistical methods for detecting differentially abundant features in clinical metagenomic samples. PLoS Comput Biol 5: e1000352.

31. Brinig MM, Lepp PW, Ouverney CC, Armitage GC, Relman DA (2003) Prevalence of bacteria of division TM7 in human subgingival plaque and their association with disease. Appl Environ Microbiol 69: 1687–1694.

32. Podar M, Abulencia CB, Walcher M, Hutchison D, Zengler K, et al. (2007) Targeted access to the genomes of low-abundance organisms in complex microbial communities. Appl Environ Microbiol 73: 3205–3214.

33. Faveri M, Mayer MP, Feres M, de Figueiredo LC, Dewhirst FE, et al. (2008) Microbiological diversity of generalized aggressive periodontitis by 16S rRNA clonal analysis. Oral Microbiol Immunol 23: 112–118.

34. Kumar PS, Griffen AL, Moeschberger ML, Leys EJ (2005) Identification of candidate periodontal pathogens and beneficial species by quantitative 16S clonal analysis. J Clin Microbiol 43: 3944–3955.

35. Darby I, Curtis M (2001) Microbiology of periodontal disease in children and young adults. Periodontol 2000 26: 33–53.

36. Mineoka T, Awano S, Rikimaru T, Kurata H, Yoshida A, et al. (2008) Site-specific development of periodontal disease is associated with increased levels of Porphyromonas gingivalis, Treponema denticola, and Tannerella forsythia in subgingival plaque. J Periodontol 79: 670–676.

37. Slots J (1979) Subgingival microflora and periodontal disease. J Clin Periodontol 6: 351–382.

38. Siqueira JF, Jr., Rocas IN (2006) Catonella morbi and Granulicatella adiacens: new species in endodontic infections. Oral Surg Oral Med Oral Pathol Oral Radiol Endod 102: 259–264.

39. Socransky S, Haffajee AD, Cugini MA, Smith C, Jr K, R L (1998) Microbial complexes in subgingival plaque. pp 134–144.

40. Cicek Y, Ozmen I, Canakci V, Dilsiz A, Sahin F (2005) Content and composition of fatty acids in normal and inflamed gingival tissues. Prostaglandins Leukot Essent Fatty Acids 72: 147–151.

41. Eisenreich W, Dandekar T, Heesemann J, Goebel W (2010) Carbon metabolism of intracellular bacterial pathogens and possible links to virulence. Nature reviews Microbiology 8: 401–412.

42. Pike R, Lucas V, Stapleton P, Gilthorpe MS, Roberts G, et al. (2002) Prevalence and antibiotic resistance profile of mercury-resistant oral bacteria from children with and without mercury amalgam fillings. J Antimicrob Chemother 49: 777–783.

43. Campan P, Planchand PO, Duran D (1997) Pilot study on n-3 polyunsaturated fatty acids in the treatment of human experimental gingivitis. J Clin Periodontol 24: 907–913.

44. Kesavalu L, Bakthavatchalu V, Rahman MM, Su J, Raghu B, et al. (2007) Omega-3 fatty acid regulates inflammatory cytokine/mediator messenger RNA expression in Porphyromonas gingivalis-induced experimental periodontal disease. Oral Microbiol Immunol 22: 232–239.

45. Rosenstein ED, Kushner LJ, Kramer N, Kazandjian G (2003) Pilot study of dietary fatty acid supplementation in the treatment of adult periodontitis. Prostaglandins Leukot Essent Fatty Acids 68: 213–218.

46. Barnes VM, Teles R, Trivedi HM, Devizio W, Xu T, et al. (2009) Acceleration of purine degradation by periodontal diseases. J Dent Res 88: 851–855.

47. Frias J, Olle E, Alsina M (2001) Periodontal pathogens produce quorum sensing signal molecules. Infect Immun 69: 3431–3434.

48. Jayaraman A, Wood TK (2008) Bacterial quorum sensing: signals, circuits, and implications for biofilms and disease. Annu Rev Biomed Eng 10: 145–167.

49. Cvitkovitch DG, Li YH, Ellen RP (2003) Quorum sensing and biofilm formation in Streptococcal infections. J Clin Invest 112: 1626–1632.

50. Stefanopoulos PK, Kolokotronis AE (2004) The clinical significance of anaerobic bacteria in acute orofacial odontogenic infections. Oral surgery, oral medicine, oral pathology, oral radiology, and endodontics 98: 398–408.

51. Li R, Zhu H, Ruan J, Qian W, Fang X, et al. (2010) De novo assembly of human genomes with massively parallel short read sequencing. Genome Res 20: 265–272.

52. Qin J, Li R, Raes J, Arumugam M, Burgdorf KS, et al. (2010) A human gut microbial gene catalogue established by metagenomic sequencing. Nature 464: 59–65.

53. Marcy Y, Ouverney C, Bik EM, Losekann T, Ivanova N, et al. (2007) Dissecting biological "dark matter" with single-cell genetic analysis of rare and uncultivated TM7 microbes from the human mouth. Proc Natl Acad Sci U S A 104: 11889–11894.

54. Koren S, Treangen TJ, Pop M (2011) Bambus 2: Scaffolding Metagenomes. Bioinformatics.

55. Roberts RJ, Chang YC, Hu Z, Rachlin JN, Anton BP, et al. COMBREX: a project to accelerate the functional annotation of prokaryotic genomes. Nucleic Acids Res 39: D11–14.

56. Delisle AL, Nauman RK, Minah GE (1978) Isolation of a bacteriophage for Actinomyces viscosus. Infect Immun 20: 303–306.

57. Lozada-Chavez I, Janga SC, Collado-Vides J (2006) Bacterial regulatory networks are extremely flexible in evolution. Nucleic Acids Research 34: 3434–3445.

58. Price MN, Dehal PS, Arkin AP (2007) Orthologous transcription factors in bacteria have different functions and regulate different genes. PLoS Computational Biology 3: 1739–1750.

59. Panina EM, Vitreschak AG, Mironov AA, Gelfand MS (2003) Regulation of biosynthesis and transport of aromatic amino acids in low-GC Gram-positive bacteria. FEMS microbiology letters 222: 211–220.

60. Madureira P, Baptista M, Vieira M, Magalhaes V, Camelo A, et al. (2007) *Streptococcus agalactiae* GAPDH is a virulence-associated immunomodulatory protein. Journal of immunology 178: 1379–1387.

61. Maeda K, Nagata H, Nonaka A, Kataoka K, Tanaka M, et al. (2004) Oral streptococcal glyceraldehyde-3-phosphate dehydrogenase mediates interaction with *Porphyromonas gingivalis* fimbriae. Microbes and infection/Institut Pasteur 6: 1163–1170.

62. Maeda K, Nagata H, Yamamoto Y, Tanaka M, Tanaka J, et al. (2004) Glyceraldehyde-3-phosphate dehydrogenase of *Streptococcus oralis* functions as a coadhesin for *Porphyromonas gingivalis* major fimbriae. Infection and Immunity 72: 1341–1348.

63. Chen Y, Stine OC, Badger JH, Gil AI, Nair GB, et al. (2011) Comparative genomic analysis of *Vibrio parahaemolyticus*: serotype conversion and virulence. BMC Genomics 12: 294.

64. Chen T, Yu WH, Izard J, Baranova OV, Lakshmanan A, et al. (2010) The Human Oral Microbiome Database: a web accessible resource for investigating oral microbe taxonomic and genomic information. Database: the journal of biological databases and curation 2010: baq013.

65. Kurtz S, Phillippy A, Delcher AL, Smoot M, Shumway M, et al. (2004) Versatile and open software for comparing large genomes. Genome Biol 5: R12.

66. Li Y, Hu Y, Bolund L, Wang J (2010) State of the art de novo assembly of human genomes from massively parallel sequencing data. Human genomics 4: 271–277.

67. Sommer DD, Delcher AL, Salzberg SL, Pop M (2007) Minimus: a fast, lightweight genome assembler. BMC Bioinformatics 8: 64.

68. Noguchi H, Park J, Takagi T (2006) MetaGene: prokaryotic gene finding from environmental genome shotgun sequences. Nucleic Acids Res 34: 5623–5630.

69. Langmead B, Trapnell C, Pop M, Salzberg SL (2009) Ultrafast and memory-efficient alignment of short DNA sequences to the human genome. Genome Biol 10: R25.

70. Kunin V, Copeland A, Lapidus A, Mavromatis K, Hugenholtz P (2008) A bioinformatician's guide to metagenomics. Microbiol Mol Biol Rev 72: 557–578, Table of Contents.

71. Johnson PL, Slatkin M (2006) Inference of population genetic parameters in metagenomics: a clean look at messy data. Genome Res 16: 1320–1327.

72. Hellmann I, Mang Y, Gu Z, Li P, de la Vega FM, et al. (2008) Population genetic analysis of shotgun assemblies of genomic sequences from multiple individuals. Genome Res 18: 1020–1029.

73. Ghodsi M, Liu B, Pop M (2011) DNACLUST: accurate and efficient clustering of phylogenetic marker genes. BMC Bioinformatics 12: 271.

74. Cole JR, Chai B, Farris RJ, Wang Q, Kulam SA, et al. (2005) The Ribosomal Database Project (RDP-II): sequences and tools for high-throughput rRNA analysis. Nucleic Acids Res 33: D294–296.

75. Huson DH, Auch AF, Qi J, Schuster SC (2007) MEGAN analysis of metagenomic data. Genome Res 17: 377–386.

76. Liu B, Pop M (2009) ARDB–Antibiotic Resistance Genes Database. Nucleic Acids Res 37: D443–447.

77. Glass EM, Wilkening J, Wilke A, Antonopoulos D, Meyer F (2010) Using the metagenomics RAST server (MG-RAST) for analyzing shotgun metagenomes. Cold Spring Harbor protocols 2010.

78. Subramanian A, Kuehn H, Gould J, Tamayo P, Mesirov JP (2007) GSEA-P: a desktop application for Gene Set Enrichment Analysis. Bioinformatics 23: 3251–3253.

79. Overbeek R, Begley T, Butler RM, Choudhuri JV, Chuang HY, et al. (2005) The subsystems approach to genome annotation and its use in the project to annotate 1000 genomes. Nucleic Acids Res 33: 5691–5702.

80. Pride DT, Meinersmann RJ, Wassenaar TM, Blaser MJ (2003) Evolutionary implications of microbial genome tetranucleotide frequency biases. Genome Research 13: 145–158.

81. Phillips GJ, Arnold J, Ivarie R (1987) The effect of codon usage on the oligonucleotide composition of the E. coli genome and identification of over- and underrepresented sequences by Markov chain analysis. Nucleic Acids Research 15: 2627–2638.

82. Liu B, Gibbons T, Ghodsi M, Treangen T, Pop M (2011) Accurate and fast estimation of taxonomic profiles from metagenomic shotgun sequences. BMC Genomics 12 Suppl 2: S4.

83. Kanehisa M, Goto S (2000) KEGG: kyoto encyclopedia of genes and genomes. Nucleic Acids Res 28: 27–30.

84. Liu B, Pop M (2011) MetaPath: identifying differentially abundant metabolic pathways in metagenomic datasets. BMC Proceedings 5 Suppl 2: S9.

85. Letunic I, Yamada T, Kanehisa M, Bork P (2008) iPath: interactive exploration of biochemical pathways and networks. Trends in biochemical sciences 33: 101–103.

86. Krzywinski M, Schein J, Birol I, Connors J, Gascoyne R, et al. (2009) Circos: an information aesthetic for comparative genomics. Genome Research 19: 1639–1645.

87. Subramanian A, Tamayo P, Mootha VK, Mukherjee S, Ebert BL, et al. (2005) Gene set enrichment analysis: a knowledge-based approach for interpreting genome-wide expression profiles. Proceedings of the National Academy of Sciences of the United States of America 102: 15545–15550.

11

Therapeutic Effect of TSG-6 Engineered iPSC-Derived MSCs on Experimental Periodontitis in Rats

Heng Yang[1], Raydolfo M. Aprecio[2], Xiaodong Zhou[2], Qi Wang[1], Wu Zhang[2], Yi Ding[3]*, Yiming Li[2]

1 State Key Laboratory of Oral Diseases, Sichuan University, Chengdu, Sichuan, China, 2 Center for Dental Research, Loma Linda University School of Dentistry, Loma Linda, California, United States of America, 3 Department of Periodontology, West China Hospital of Stomatology, Sichuan University, Chengdu, Sichuan, China

Abstract

Background: We derived mesenchymal stem cells (MSCs) from rat induced pluripotent stem cells (iPSCs) and transduced them with tumor necrosis factor alpha-stimulated gene-6 (TSG-6), to test whether TSG-6 overexpression would boost the therapeutic effects of iPSC-derived MSCs in experimental periodontitis.

Methods: A total of 30 female Sprague-Dawley (SD) rats were randomly divided into four groups: healthy control group (Group-N, n = 5), untreated periodontitis group (Group-P, n = 5), iPS-MSCs-treated and iPSC-MSCs/TSG-6-treated periodontitis groups (Group-P1 and P2, n = 10 per group). Experimental periodontitis was established by ligature and infection with *Porphyromonas gingivalis* around the maxillae first molar bilaterally. MSC-like cells were generated from rat iPSCs, and transducted with TSG-6. iPSC-MSCs or iPSC-MSCs/TSG-6 were administrated to rats in Group-P1 or P2 intravenously and topically, once a week for three weeks. Blood samples were obtained one week post-injection for the analysis of serum pro-inflammatory cytokines. All animals were killed 3 months post-treatment; maxillae were then dissected for histological analysis, tartrate-resistant acid phosphatase (TRAP) staining, and morphological analysis of alveolar bone loss.

Results: Administration of iPSC-MSC/TSG-6 significantly decreased serum levels of IL-1β and TNF-α in the Group-P2 rats (65.78 pg/ml and 0.56 pg/ml) compared with those in Group-P (168.31 pg/ml and 1.15 pg/ml respectively) ($p < 0.05$). Both alveolar bone loss and the number of TRAP-positive osteoclasts showed a significant decrease in rats that received iPSC-MSC/TSG-6 treatment compared to untreated rats in Group-P ($p < 0.05$),

Conclusions: We demonstrated that overexpression of TSG-6 in rat iPSC-derived MSCs were capable of decreasing inflammation in experimental periodontitis and inhibiting alveolar bone resorption. This may potentially serve as an alternative stem-cell-based approach in the treatment and regeneration of periodontal tissues.

Editor: Salomon Amar, Boston University, United States of America

Funding: This study was supported by Loma Linda University Grants for Research and School Partnerships (GRASP) number: 699310-2938. The funder had no role in study design, data collection and analysis, decision to publish, or preparation of the manuscript.

Competing Interests: The authors have declared that no competing interests exist.

* Email: jessie.yh@163.com

Introduction

Periodontitis is a chronic infectious disease, leading to periodontal tissue inflammation, attachment loss, alveolar bone resorption, and eventually tooth loss [1]. To date, several therapies, such as mechanical and chemical root conditioning, implantation of autografts, allografts and alloplastic materials, growth factors, guided tissue regeneration, and various combinations of these approaches, have been used in clinical practice with the aim of achieving true periodontal regeneration [2–5]. However, the clinical results vary widely and are often unpredictable. Currently, stem cell biology has become an important field for the understanding of regenerative medicine.

Multipotent mesenchymal stem cells (MSCs) are a population of postnatal stem cells that have been successfully isolated from various human tissues. MSCs have been shown to possess a self-renewing capacity and can differentiate several cell lineages, including osteocytes, chondrocytes, and adipocytes [6–9]. MSCs

are thus considered an attractive candidate for regenerative therapy. Recent reports indicate that MSCs are important guardian cells for modulating inflammation. Certain therapeutic effects of the cells seen in animal models are believed to be the result of MSCs being activated by signals from injured tissues to secrete anti-inflammatory factors [10,11]. Among these factors, the most interesting was tumor necrosis factor alpha-stimulated gene-6 (TSG-6) [12], which has been extensively studied in articular joint diseases [13–15]. The anti-inflammatory and chondroprotective effects of TSG-6 have been reported in numerous animal models [16–19]. However, the combined effect of MSCs and TSG-6 has not been investigated.

Although MSCs are recognized as having a great potential for regeneration, extended *in vitro* culture reduces the differentiation potential of MSCs, which limits their therapeutic efficacy [20]. Successful generation of induced pluripotent stem cells (iPSCs) by Yamanaka and co-workers [21], which can be expanded to large numbers before *in vitro* differentiation and transplantation, is an option to overcome such limitations seen with MSCs.

The objective of the present study was to derive MSCs from rat iPSCs and transduce them with TSG-6 to test our hypothesis that TSG-6 overexpression will boost the anti-inflammatory effects of iPSC-derived MSCs in experimental periodontitis.

Materials and Methods

iPSC-derived MSC (iPSC-MSC) generation

Based on our previous study, rat iPSCs were reprogrammed from female rat embryonic fibroblasts by transducing them with Oct4, Sox2, Myc, and Klf4-expressing lentiviral vectors [22]. iPSCs in passage 5 were cultured in a gelatin-coated six-well plate with Minimum Essential Medium (MEM; Gibco, Life Technologies, Grand Island, NY, USA) supplemented with 2% fetal bovine serum (FBS; Fisher Scientific, Pittsburgh, PA, USA), 1% Penicillin/Stremycin (Gibco), 5% knockout serum replacement (Gibco), 1% platelet-derived growth factor, 1% fibroblast growth factor-2, and 0.1% epidermal growth factor. Cytokines were purchased from ProSpec (East Brunswick, NJ, USA). Cells were cultured under hypoxic conditions [23] by placing culture plates in a Hypoxia Chamber (Stem cell Technologies, Vancouver, British Columbia, Canada) that was flushed with mixed air composed of 92% N_2, 3% O_2, and 5% CO_2. Media were replaced every another day. Cells were cultured and passaged until homogeneous fibroblastic morphology appeared.

Flow cytometry assay

The representative markers characteristic of rat MSCs were confirmed with flow cytometry following the previous protocol [22]. Briefly, cells were harvested by Accutase treatment (Innovative Cell Technologies, San Diego, CA, USA) and fixed for 30 minutes at room temperature in fixation buffer and permeabilization buffer (eBiosciences, San Diego, CA, USA). After washing, cells were stained at room temperature for 2 hours with antibodies followed by washing twice with permeabilization buffer. The following conjugated antibodies were used: fluorescein isothiocyanate (FITC)-conjugated against CD45, and PE-conjugated against CD29 and CD90 (BD Biosciences, San Jose, CA, USA). Flow cytometric analysis was performed using FACS Aria II (BD Biosciences) with a 488 nm laser. For each sample 30,000 events were collected.

Transfection and overexpression TSG-6 in iPSC-derived MSCs *in vitro*

The construction of the lentiviral vector was performed according to our previous study [24]. Subcultured iPSC-MSCs were transfected with TSG-6 lentiviral vector for 24 hours. Total RNA was isolated using RNeasy Mini Kit (QIAGEN, Valencia, CA, USA). First-strand complimentary DNA (cDNA) was synthesized using Super-Script III First-Strand Synthesis System and the OligodT primer (Invitrogen, Life Technologies, Grand Island, NY, USA). Real-time amplification was performed using Taqman Universal PCR master mix (Applied Biosystems, Grand Island, NY, USA) on RT-PCR System (ViiA 7 real-time PCR system, Applied Biosystems). An 18s ribosomal RNA (rRNA) probe (Taqman Gene Expression Assays ID, Hs03003631_g1) was used for normalization of gene expression. The PCR products were resolved by electrophoresis on 1.5% (w/v) agarose gels containing ethidium bromide (0.5 mg/mL) to visualize the PCR products.

Animal model of periodontitis and treatment

The experimental protocols were approved by Loma Linda University Institutional Animal Care and Use Committee (IACUC, permit number: 699310-2938). A total of 30, 7-week-old female Sprague-Dawley (SD) rats (SAS-SD rat; Charles River Laboratories International, Inc., Wilmington, MA, USA) were used. Animals were randomly assigned to four groups: healthy control (Group-N, n = 5), untreated periodontitis (Group-P, n = 5), iPSC-MSCs-treated periodontitis (Group-P1, n = 10), or iPSC-MSCs/TSG-6-treated periodontitis (Group-P2, n = 10).

Following anesthesia by intraperitoneal (i.p.) injection of ketamine/xylazine (Clipper Distributing Company, St. Joseph, MO, USA and Akorn, Inc., Decatur, IL, USA), orthodontic wire of 0.2 mm in diameter was bilaterally ligatured around the first molar of the rat maxilla in Group P, P1, and P2. Cultures of *Porphyromonas gingivalis* (*P. gingivalis* 381, ATCC, Manassas, VA, USA) at 10^{10} cfu/mL were inoculated into the oral cavity four times a week for 4 weeks to establish experimental periodontitis. The wires were then removed, and the treatment was applied as follows: rats in Groups P1 and P2 received iPSC-MSCs and iPSC-MSCs/TSG-6, respectively, through both systemic and topical injections. For systemic injections, rats received 5×10^6 cells in 200 μL of culture media via the tail vein; for topical injections, 10^6 cells in 20 μL of matrigel (BD Biosciences) were delivered around the maxilla first molar. Cells were injected once a week for 3 weeks. All animals were killed 3 months post-injection.

ELISA analysis

Rat tail blood samples were collected one week post-cell injections and centrifuged at 1,000 rpm for 15 minutes. The supernatant was collected and stored at −20°C. Samples were thawed at room temperature before analysis. Serum concentrations of interleukin-1β (IL-1β) and tumor necrosis factor-α (TNF-α) were analyzed using enzyme-linked immunosorbent assay (ELISA) (Rat quantikine ELISA kit, R&D, Minneapolis, MN, USA and BlueGene ELISA kit, Life Sciences Advanced Technologies Inc, Saint Petersburg, FL, USA).

TRAP staining

The rats were killed and the maxillae were dissected and fixed in 10% formalin for 48 hours. The left maxillae were decalcified in 15% EDTA solution for 2 weeks. Specimens were paraffin-embedded; and mesial-distal orientated 5 μm sections were prepared. Alternate slides were stained with hematoxylin and eosin (H&E) for descriptive histology. For enumeration of osteoclasts, tartrate-resistant acid phosphatase (TRAP) staining was carried out using a leukocyte acid phosphatase kit (Sigma, St. Louis, MO, USA). Active osteoclasts were defined as multinucleated (≥3) TRAP-positive cells in contact with the bone surface located between the first and second molars. Four continual sections were used for the enumeration of osteoclasts. Images were captured with an Aperio Scan Scope (Aperio Technologies, Vista, CA, USA), and cells were counted using Image J software (NIHImage).

Morphometric evaluation of alveolar bone loss

The 10% formalin-fixed right maxillae were dehydrated by passing through a graded series of ethanol solutions (from 30% to 100%). Specimens were incubated in a desiccator for 48 hours then coated with platinum and examined under a scanning electron microscope (VEGA II Tescan, Cranberry TWP., PA, USA) at an accelerating voltage of 10 kV. Alveolar bone loss was evaluated morphometrically by measuring the distance between the cemento-enamel junction (CEJ) and the palatal alveolar bone crest (ABC) at nine sites [25] from first to second molar for three times. For each animal, alveolar bone loss was defined as the mean of nine measurements. Images were analyzed using Image J software.

Statistical analysis

Data were expressed as mean±standard error of the mean (SEM). Comparison of parameters among the groups was performed using one-way analysis of variance (ANOVA) using SPSS software (SPSS 17.0, Chicago, IL, USA). A p-value of <0.05 was considered statistically significant.

Results

Derivation of MSCs from rat iPSCs

After five passages by culturing in MSC culture medium, rat iPSCs began to form MSC-like cells, which were similar to the morphology of rat BM-MSCs (Fig. 1). Subsequently, flow cytometry analysis showed that these cells expressed CD29 and CD90, but were negative for CD34 and CD45 (Fig. 2).

Overexpression of TSG-6 in iPSC-MSCs *in vitro*

After lentiviral transfection for 24 hours, iPSC-MSCs were harvested using Accutasefor total mRNA extraction and cDNA synthesis for RT-PCR. As a result, TSG-6 expression increased approximately 18-fold in transfected iPSC-MSCs, whereas TSG-6 expression in untransfected iPSC-MSCs was too low to be detected (Fig. 3).

Suppression of inflammation by systemic and topical injections of iPSC-MSCs/TSG-6

The systemic administration of iPSC-MSCs and iPSC-MSCs/TSG-6 significantly reduced periodontal inflammation. Histologically, the infiltration of inflammatory cells in the periodontal tissues was markedly decreased in the iPSC-MSCs/TSG-6-treated group (Fig. 4). The production of proinflammatory cytokines was also significantly decreased in serum samples that were measured by ELISA (Fig. 5). IL-1β and TNF-α were significantly decreased in the iPSC-MSCs/TSG-6-treated group compared to the untreated periodontitis group (p<0.001); but no significant difference was detected compared to the healthy control group.

Overexpression of TSG-6 inhibited osteoclast formation and alveolar bone loss

TRAP-positive osteoclasts (nuclei≥3) in the iPSC-MSCs/TSG-6-treated group significantly decreased compared to the untreated periodontitis group three months post-treatment (Fig. 6). Alveolar bone analysis showed that rats from the untreated periodontitis

group had significant bone loss compared to the healthy control group (p<0.001). Rats from the iPSC-MSCs/TSG-6 group had less bone loss than the untreated periodontitis group (p = 0.001) (Fig. 7).

Discussion

In 2006, iPS cells were first generated from mouse embryonic fibroblasts and adult mouse tail-tip fibroblasts by transfecting four transcription factors: Oct3/4, Sox2, Klf4, and c-Myc [21]. iPS cells have comparable properties to embryonic stem cells in terms of morphology, proliferation, and gene expression *in vitro* and teratoma formation *in vivo*, without many of the ethical concerns associated with embryonic stem cells. iPS cells can be used to regenerate different tissues and differentiate to different cell lineages, which promises great potential for cell therapy and regenerative medicine [26–28]. iPS cells, derived from somatic cells and reprogrammed to the pluripotent state by the induced expression of defined transcription factors, can be expanded to large numbers before *in vitro* differentiation and transplantation. Consequently, deriving MSCs from iPSCs represents an important alternative to overcome the limitations seen with MSCs. Recent studies have reported functional MSCs derived from human iPSCs, which expressed characteristic MSC makers and differentiated into osteoblasts, adipocytes and chondrocytes, promoted vascular and muscle regeneration [29], or formed bones in mice after transplantation *in vivo* [30].

In the present study, in order to use iPSC-derived MSCs for treating experimental periodontitis, we attempted to generate rat iPSCs first. We previously reported successful reprograming of human and mouse cells to iPSCs by transducing with Oct4, Sox2, Myc, and Klf4-expressing lentiviral vectors [24]; in the present study the same strategy was used to generate iPSCs from rat embryonic fibroblasts. After culturing rat iPSCs in MSC media for five passages, MSC-like cells were derived from rat iPSCs, as shown by the expression of typical rat MSC surface makers (Figs. 1 to 3) [31]. Subcultured cells of iPSC-derived MSCs were successfully differentiated into osteoblasts, adipocytes, and chondrocytes *in vitro*.

TSG-6 is a 35 kDa inflammation-induced protein that was first discovered by differential screening of a cDNA library prepared from TNF-stimulated human FS-4 fibroblasts. It is not constitutively expressed in normal tissues or cells, but up-regulated in response to pro-inflammatory mediators, such as TNF, IL-1, and IL-6 [13,14]. TSG-6 has been reported to have an anti-inflammatory effect in several animal models including arthritis, myocardial infarction, and chemical injury to cornea [15–17]; this finding has been attributed to its inhibitory effects on neutrophil migration and plasmin activity [32–34].

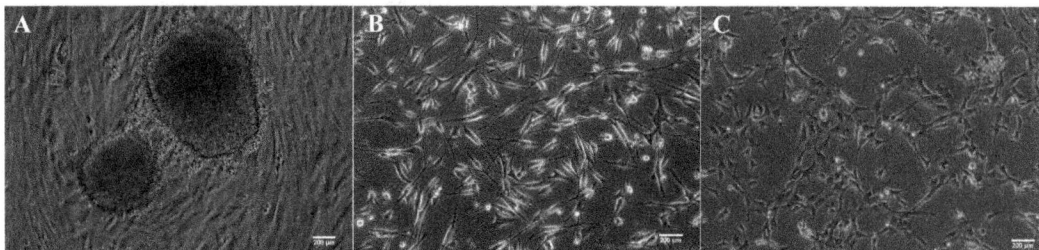

Figure 1. Cell culture: Morphology of cells under light microscopy. (A) Rat induced pluripotent stem cells (iPSCs). (B) Rat bone marrow mesenchymal stem cells (BM-MSCs), passage 3. (C) iPSC derived-MSCs, passage 3. Scale bar, 200 μm.

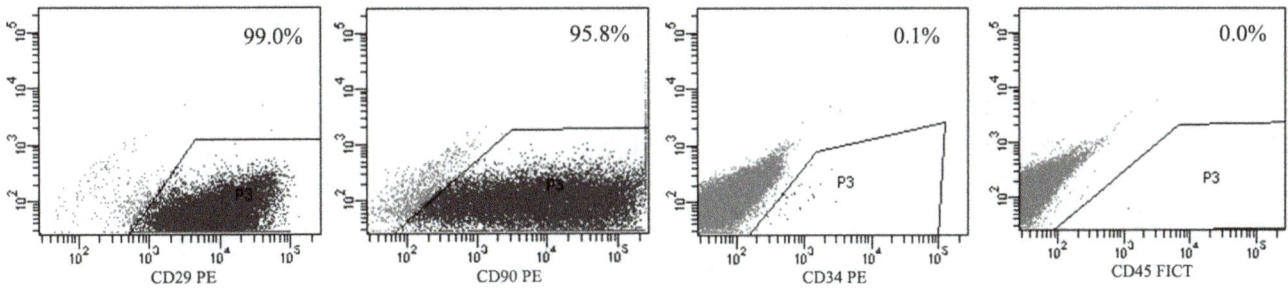

Figure 2. Flow cytometry assay. The characteristic cell surface makers of rat MSCs were detected by FACS. The iPSC derived MSCs at passage 5 revealed positivity for CD29 and CD90, negativity for CD34 and CD45.

In the present study, TSG-6 was transfected into iPS-MSCs to examine the hypothesis that overexpression of TSG-6 would boost the anti-inflammatory effects of iPS-MSCs. Our data demonstrate that systemic and topical administration of TSG-6 engineered iPSC-MSCs significantly decreased the serum concentrations of proinflammatory cytokines, which indicates an anti-inflammatory effect in experimental periodontitis. In addition, histologic results showed less inflammatory infiltration in periodontal tissues after treatment. iPSC-MSCs without TSG-6 also had an anti-inflammatory effect on the experimental periodontitis which, however, was significantly weaker compared to the TSG-6-modified iPSC-MSC-treated group, indicating that TSG-6 enhanced the anti-inflammatory function of iPS-MSCs. The mechanism of the anti-inflammatory action of MSCs through secretion of TSG-6 has been indicated in Choi's study: MSCs introduced a negative feedback loop into the inflammatory response in which the MSCs and TSG-6 suppressed the initial production of pro-inflammatory cytokines (TNF-α and IL-1) from zymosan-activated macrophages [35]. Morphological analysis of alveolar bone loss (Fig. 7) also showed anti-bone resorption of TSG-6-modified iPS-MSCs by suppressing osteoclast formation and inhibiting alveolar bone resorption in this investigation. Previous study has shown that TSG-6 could regulate bone remodeling though the inhibition of osteoclast activity and the synergistic formation with osteoprotegerin [18,19]. They indicated an autocrine mechanism of TSG-6 inhibiting osteoclasts activation; that is, osteoclast precursors and mature osteoclasts produced TSG-6 in response to pro-inflamma-

tory cytokines (i.e. TNF-α, IL-1, and IL-6) and thereby limit their own ability to anchor to and resorb bone.

Previous work showed that the four factor-derived (Oct3/4, Sox2, Klf4, and c-Myc) iPSCs can cause tumor formation on reactivation of c-Myc [36]. My et al. [37] showed that rat iPSCs derived without c-Myc did not develop tumors, strongly suggesting that the presence of the *c-Myc* gene is a serious problem for their biomedical and clinical application. Thus c-Myc-free or non-viral reprogrammed iPSCs may be important for the future application in our further study. Although MSCs or TSG-6 have an anti-inflammatory effect, the combination of TSG-6 and iPSC-MSCs could enhance the therapeutic effect of MSCs, at the same time, iPSC-derived MSCs will maintain their multipotentiality to reconstruct periodontium destruction. Base on our pilot investigation, further studies on regulating periodontal regeneration using tissue-engineering approaches on bone defection models are in progress.

In summary, we demonstrated that overexpression of TSG-6 in rat iPSC-derived MSCs are capable of decreasing inflammation in

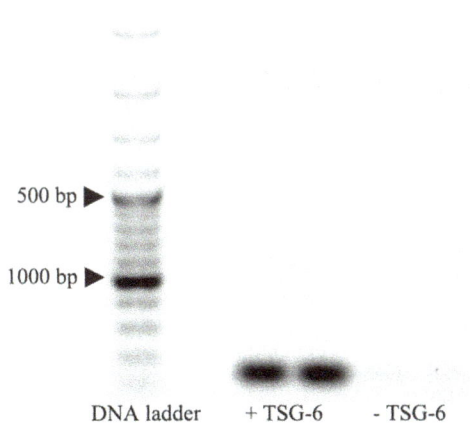

Figure 3. Overexpression TSG-6 in iPSC-derive MSCs in vitro. Overexpression TSG-6 in iPSC-MSCs in vitro. After 24 hrs transfection, TSG-6 was overexpressed in iPSC-MSCs in vitro, detected by PCR.

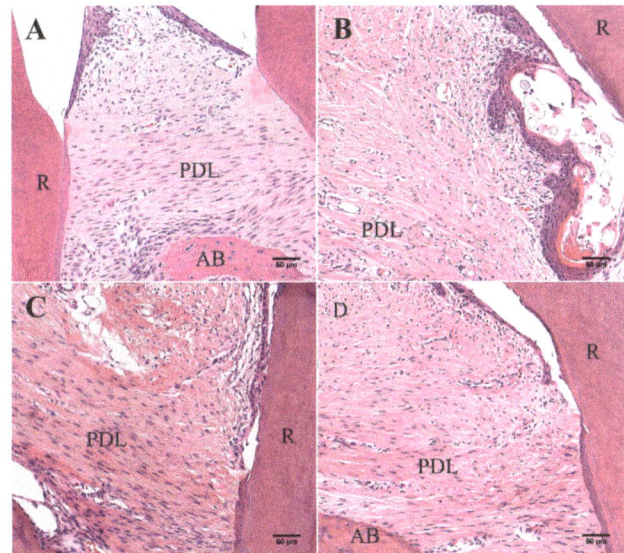

Figure 4. Histological analysis. Histological analysis showed severe inflammation in untreated periodontitis rats (B), while no inflammation was observed in healthy control animals (A); inflammatory infiltration in periodontal tissue decreased in rats received iPSC-MSCs (C) or iPSC-MSCs/TSG-6 (D) (H&E staining, scale bar, 50 μm; AB = alveolar bone, PDL = periodontal ligament, R = tooth root).

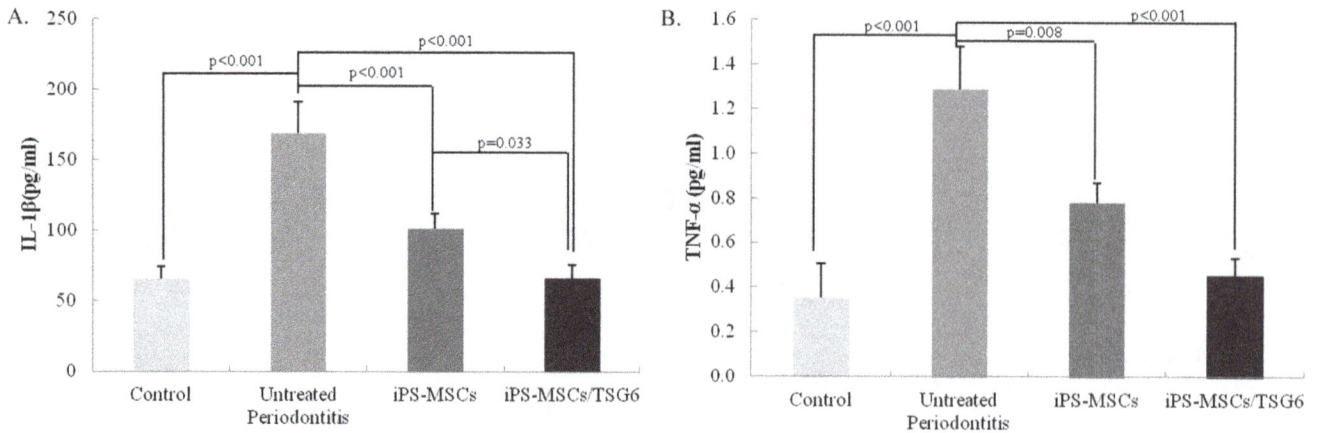

Figure 5. Pro-inflammation cytokine. Pro-inflammatory cytokine IL-1β and TNF-α in serum was detected by ELISA. The serum concentration of IL-1β and TNF-α showed a significant decrease after iPS-MSCs/TSG-6 treated when compared to untreated periodontitis group; and no significant differences compared to healthy control group.

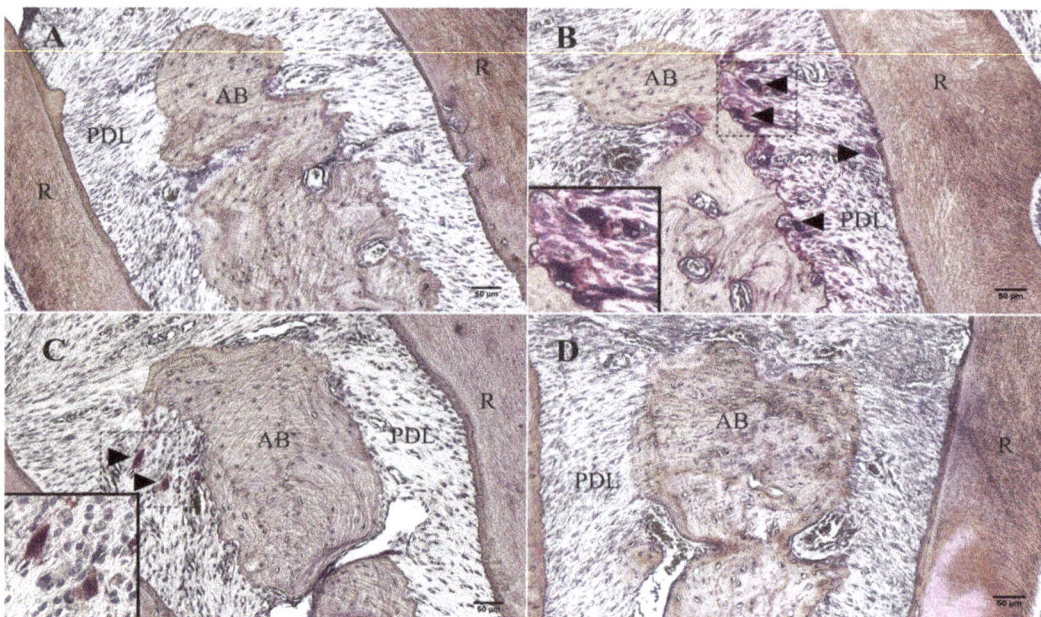

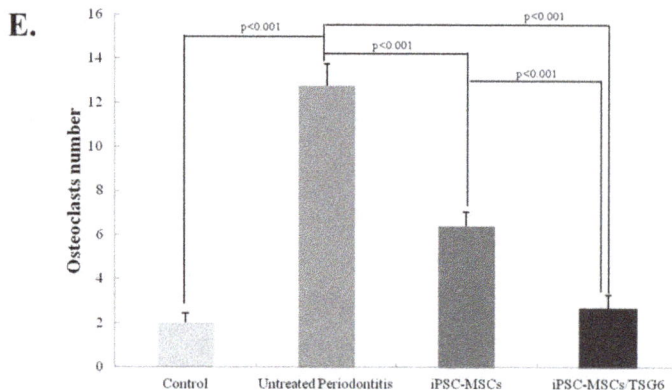

Figure 6. TRAP staining: Osteoclasts formation in different groups. (A) Healthy control group. (B) Untreated periodontitis group. (C) iPSC-MSCs treated periodontitis group. (D) iPSC-MSCs/TSG-6 treated periodontitis group. TRAP-positive osteoclasts in rat maxillae showed a significant decrease in iPSC-MSCs/TSG-6 treated group. (AB = alveolar bone, PDL = periodontal ligament, R = tooth root, black arrow = TRAP-positive osteoclasts) (TRAP staining, scale bar, 50 μm). (E) Quantitative analysis of TRAP-positive osteoclasts (nuclei≥3) showed a significantly decreased number of osteoclasts in iPSC-MSCs and iPSC-MSCs/TSG-6 treated group, compared to untreated periodontitis group; the decrease number of osteoclasts showed a significant differences between iPSC-MSCs/TSG-6 and iPSC-MSCs treated group.

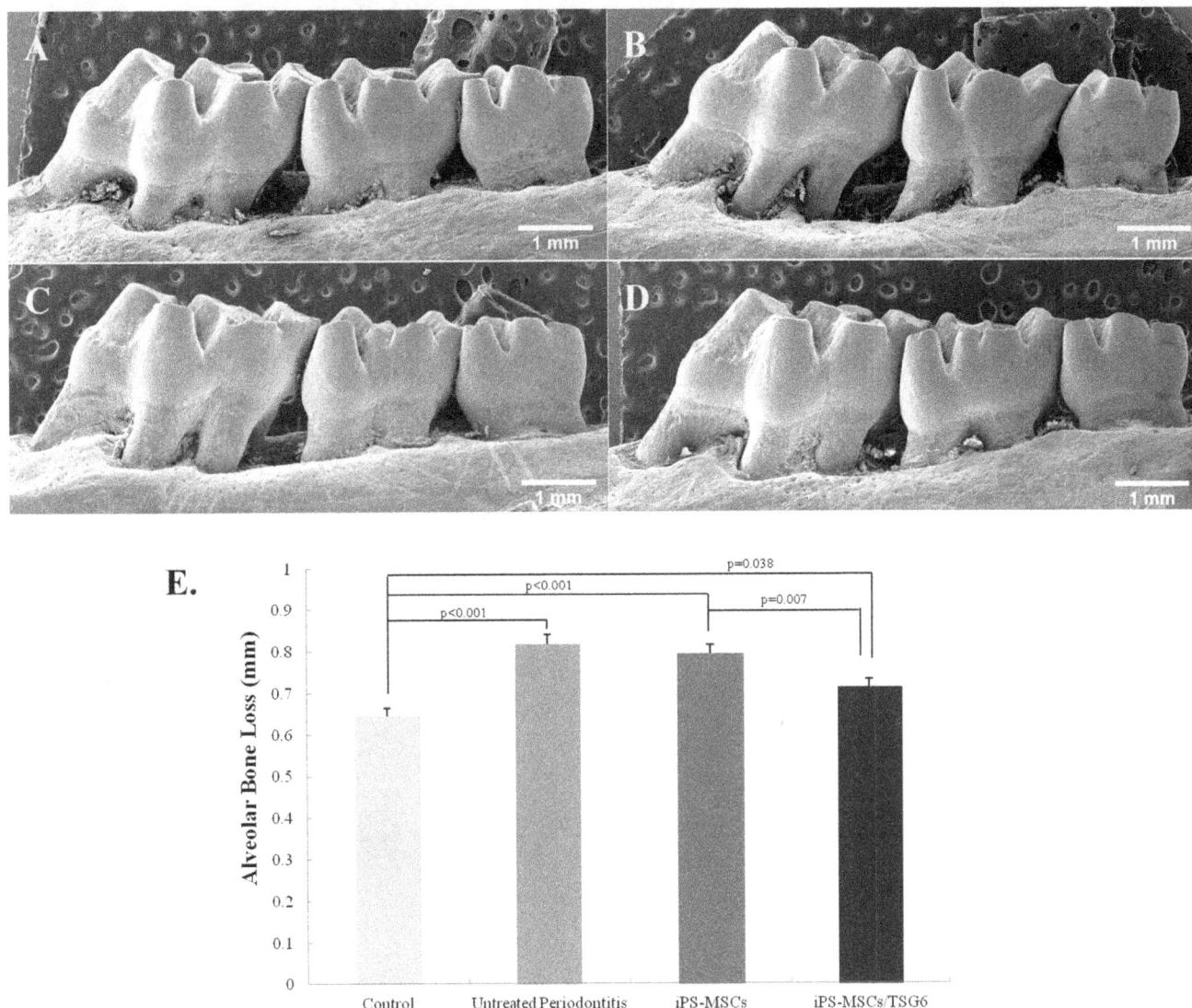

Figure 7. Alveolar bone loss: Alveolar bone loss analysis. (A) Healthy control group. (B) Untreated periodontitis group. (C) iPSC-MSCs treated periodontitis group. (D) iPSC-MSCs/TSG-6 treated periodontitis group. Scale bar, 1 mm. (E) Alveolar bone loss (ABL) was analyzed by measuring the distance between the cementum-enamel junction (CEJ) and the palatal alveolar bone crest (ABC) at 9 sites from first to second molar. The ABL in iPSC-MSCs/TSG-6 treated group showed a significant difference compared to the other groups.

experimental periodontitis, and inhibiting alveolar bone resorption, and may potentially serve as an alternative stem-cell-based approach in the treatment and regeneration of periodontal tissues.

Author Contributions

Conceived and designed the experiments: HY RA XZ QW WZ YL YD. Performed the experiments: HY RA XZ WZ. Analyzed the data: HY XZ. Contributed reagents/materials/analysis tools: HY RA XZ WZ. Wrote the paper: HY.

References

1. Pihlstrom BL, Michalowicz BS, Johnson NW (2005) Periodontal disease. Lancet 366:1809–1820.
2. Yilmaz S, Cakar G, Yildirim B, Sculean A (2010) Healing of two and three wall intrabony periodontal defects following treatment with an enamel matrix derivative combined with autogenous bone. J Clin Periodontol 37:544–550.
3. Emerton KB, Drapeau SJ, Prasad H, Rohrer M, Roffe P, et al. (2011) Regeneration of periodontal tissues in non-human primates with rhGDF-5 and beta-tricalcium phosphate. J Dent Res 90:1416–1421.
4. Stavropoulos A, Chiantella G, Costa D, Steigmann M, Windisch P, et al. (2011) Clinical and histologic evaluation of a granular bovine bone biomaterial used as an adjunct to GTR with a bioresorbable bovine pericardium collagen membrane in the treatment of intrabony defects. J Periodontol 82:462–470.

5. Tu YK, Needleman I, Chambrone L, Lu HK, Faggion CM Jr (2012) A Bayesian network meta-analysis on comparisons of enamel matrix derivatives, guided tissue regeneration and their combination therapies. J Clin Periodontol 39:303–314.
6. Pittenger MF, Mackay AM, Beck SC, Jaiswal RK, Douglas R, et al Multilineage potential of adult human mesenchymal stem cells. (1999) Science 284:143–147.
7. Prockop DJ (1997) Marrow stromal cells as stem cells for nonhematopoietic tissues. Science 276:71–74.
8. Chen J, Zhang ZG, Li Y, Wang L, Xu YX, et al. (2003) Intravenous administration of human bone marrow stromal cells induces angiogenesis in the ischemic boundary zone after stroke in rats. Circ Res 92:692–699.
9. Horwitz EM, Prockop DJ, Fitzpatripnck LA, Koo WWK, Gordon PL, et al. (1999) Transplantability and therapeutic effects of bone marrow-derived

mesenchymal cells in children with osteogenesis imperfecta. Nat Med 5:309–313.

10. Bianco P, Sacchetti B, Riminucci M (2011) Osteoprogenitors and the hematopoietic microenvironment. Best Pract Res Clin Haematol 24:37–47.

11. Méndez-Ferrer S, Michurina TV, Ferraro F, Mazloom AR, MacArthur BD, et al. (2010) Mesenchymal and haematopoietic stem cells form a unique bone marrow niche. Nature 466: 829–834.

12. Prockopl DJ, Oh JY (2012) Mesenchymal Stem/Stromal Cells (MSCs): Role as Guardians of Inflammation. Mol Ther. 20:14–20.

13. Milner CM, Day AJ (2003) TSG-6: a multifunctional protein associated with inflammation. J Cell Sci 116:1863–1873.

14. Wisniewski HG, Maier R, Lotz M, Lee S, Klampfer L, et al. (1993) TSG-6: a TNF-, IL-1-, and LPS-inducible secreted glycoprotein associated with arthritis. J Immunol 151:6593–6601.

15. Bardos T, Kamath RV, Mikecz K, Glant TT (2001) Anti-inflammatory and chondroprotective effect of TSG-6 (tumor necrosis factor stimulated gene-6) in murine models of experimental arthritis. Am J Pathol 159:1711–1721.

16. Lee RH, Pulin AA, Seo MJ, Kota DJ, Ylostalo J, et al. (2009) Intravenous hMSCs improve myocardial infarction in mice because cells embolized in lung are activated to secrete the anti-inflammatory protein TSG-6. Cell Stem Cell 5:54–63.

17. Roddy GW, Oh JY, Lee RH, Bartosh TJ, Ylostalo J, et al. (2011) Action at a distance: systemically administered adult stem/progenitor cells (MSCs) reduce inflammatory damage to the cornea without engraftment and primarily by secretion of TNF-α stimulated gene/protein 6. Stem Cells 29:1572–1579.

18. Mahoney DJ, Mikecz K, Ali T, Mabilleau G, Benayahu D, et al. (2008) TSG-6 regulates bone remodeling through inhibition of osteoblastogenesis and osteoclast activation. J Biol Chem 283:25952–25962.

19. Mahoney DJ, Swales C, Athanasou NA, Bombardieri M, Pitzalis C, et al. (2011) TSG-6 inhibits osteoclast activity via an autocrine mechanism and is functionally synergistic with ostioprotegerin. Arthritis Rheum 63:1034–1043.

20. Katsara O, Mahaira LG, Iliopoulou EG, Moustaki A, Antsaklis A, et al. (2011) Effects of donor age, gender, and in vitro cellular aging on the phenotypic, functional, and molecular characteristics of mouse bone marrow-derived mesenchymal stem cells. Stem Cells Dev 20:1549–1561.

21. Takahashi K, Yamanaka S (2006) Induction of pluripotent stem cells from mouse embryonic and adult fibroblast cultures by defined factors. Cell 126:663–676.

22. Meng X, Neises A, Su RJ, Payne KJ, Ritter L, et al. (2012) Efficient Reprogramming of Human Cord Blood CD34+ Cells Into Induced Pluripotent Stem Cells With OCT4 and SOX2 Alone. Mol Ther 20:408–416.

23. Yoshida Y, Takahashi K, Okita K, Ichisaka T, Yamanaka S (2009) Hypoxia enhances the generation of induced pluripotent stem cells. Cell Stem Cell 5:237–241.

24. Meng X, Baylink DJ, Sheng M, Wang H, Gridley DS, et al. (2012) Erythroid promoter confines FGF2 expression to the marrow after hematopoietic stem cell gene therapy and leads to enhanced endosteal bone formation. PLoS One 7: e37569.

25. Pontes Andersen CC, Buschard K, Flyvbjerg A, Stoltze K, Holmstrup P (2006) Periodontitis deteriorates metabolic control in type 2 diabetic Goto-Kakizaki rats. J Periodontol 77:350–356.

26. Dimos JT, Rodolfa KT, Niakan KK, Weisenthal LM, Mitsumoto H, et al. (2008) Induced pluripotent stem cells generated from patients with ALS can be differentiated into motor neurons. Science 321:1218–1221.

27. Mauritz C, Schwanke K, Reppel M, Neef S, Katsirntaki K, et al. (2008) Generation of functional murine cardiac myocytes from induced pluripotent stem cells. Circulation 118:507–17.

28. Furth ME, Atala A (2009) Stem cell sources to treat diabetes. J Cell Biochem 106:507–511.

29. Lian Q, Zhang Y, Zhang J, Zhang HK, Wu X, et al. (2010) Functional mesenchymal stem cells derived from human induced pluripotent stem cells attenuate limb ischemia in mice. Circulation 121:1113–1123.

30. Villa-Diaz LG, Brown SE, Liu Y, Ross AM, Lahann J, et al. (2012) Derivation of mesenchymal stem cells from human induced pluripotent stem cells cultured on synthetic substrates. Stem Cells 30:1174–1181.

31. de Hemptinne I, Vermeiren C, Maloteaux JM, Hermans E (2004) Induction of glial glutamate transporters in adult mesenchymal stem cells. J Neurochem 91:155–166.

32. Wisniewski HG, Hua JC, Poppers DM, Naime D, Vilcek J, et al. (1996) TNF/IL-1-inducible protein TSG-6 potentiates plasmin inhibition by inter-alpha-inhibitor and exerts a strong anti-inflammatory effect in vivo. J Immunol 156:1609–15.

33. Getting SJ, Mahoney DJ, Cao T, Rugg MS, Fries E, et al. (2002) The link module from human TSG-6 inhibits neutrophil migration in a hyaluronan- and inter-alpha-inhibitor-independent manner. J Biol Chem 277:51068–76.

34. Cao TV, La M, Getting SJ, Day AJ, Perretti M (2004) Inhibitory effects of TSG-6 Link module on leukocyte-endothelial cell interactions in vitro and in vivo. Microcirculation 11:615–24.

35. Choi H, Lee RH, Bazhanov N, Oh JY, Prockop DJ (2011) Anti-inflammatory protein TSG-6 secreted by activated MSCs attenuates zymosan-induced mouse peritonitis by decreasing TLR2/NF-κB signaling in resident macrophages. Blood 118:330–338.

36. Okita K, Ichisaka T, Yamanaka S (2007) Generation of germline-competent induced pluripotent stem cells. Nature 448:313–317.

37. Chang M-Y, Kim D, Kim C-H, Kang H-C, Yang E, et al. (2010) Direct reprogramming of rat neural precursor cells and fibroblasts into pluripotent stem cells. PLoS One 5:e9838.

12

The Personal Human Oral Microbiome Obscures the Effects of Treatment on Periodontal Disease

Karen Schwarzberg[1], Rosalin Le[1], Balambal Bharti[2], Suzanne Lindsay[2], Giorgio Casaburi[3,4], Francesco Salvatore[3,4], Mohamed H. Saber[5], Faisal Alonaizan[5], Jørgen Slots[6], Roberta A. Gottlieb[7], J. Gregory Caporaso[8,9], Scott T. Kelley[1]*

1 Department of Biology, San Diego State University, San Diego, California, United States of America, 2 Graduate School of Public Health, San Diego State University, San Diego, California, United States of America, 3 CEINGE-Biotecnologie Avanzate, Napoli, Italy, 4 Dipartimento di Medicina Molecolare e Biotecnologie Mediche, Università di Napoli Federico II, Napoli, Italy, 5 Section of Endodontics, Herman Ostrow School of Dentistry of USC, Los Angeles, California, United States of America, 6 Professor of Dentistry and Microbiology, Herman Ostrow School of Dentistry of USC, Los Angeles, California, United States of America, 7 BioScience Center, San Diego State University, San Diego, California, United States of America, 8 Department of Biological Sciences, Northern Arizona University, Flagstaff, Arizona, United States of America, 9 Institute for Genomics and Systems Biology, Argonne National Laboratory, Argonne, Illinois, United States of America

Abstract

Periodontitis is a progressive disease of the periodontium with a complex, polymicrobial etiology. Recent Next-Generation Sequencing (NGS) studies of the microbial diversity associated with periodontitis have revealed strong, community-level differences in bacterial assemblages associated with healthy or diseased periodontal sites. In this study, we used NGS approaches to characterize changes in periodontal pocket bacterial diversity after standard periodontal treatment. Despite consistent changes in the abundance of certain taxa in individuals whose condition improved with treatment, post-treatment samples retained the highest similarity to pre-treatment samples from the same individual. Deeper phylogenetic analysis of periodontal pathogen-containing genera *Prevotella* and *Fusobacterium* found both unexpected diversity and differential treatment response among species. Our results highlight how understanding interpersonal variability among microbiomes is necessary for determining how polymicrobial diseases respond to treatment and disturbance.

Editor: Stefan Bereswill, Charité-University Medicine Berlin, Germany

Funding: This work received financial support from the following sources: NIH Grant U26IHS300292 (PI: Calac; Project Leader: Gottlieb); "Native American Research Centers for Health (NARCH5): Periodontal Disease, Atherosclerosis, and the Oral Microbiome". The funders had no role in study design, data collection and analysis, decision to publish, or preparation of the manuscript.

Competing Interests: The authors have declared that no competing interests exist.

* E-mail: skelley@mail.sdsu.edu

Introduction

Periodontitis is a complex, polymicrobial infection of the periodontium. The disease is caused by dental plaque microorganisms that migrate into the periodontal pocket and give rise to inflammation of the gingiva [1]. Left untreated, the inflammatory process may lead to loss of tooth-supporting connective tissue and bone, and eventually to edentulism [2]. While oral microbes are the principal cause of periodontitis, factors such as tobacco use, osteoporosis, obesity, and diabetes exacerbate the disease [3]. Periodontitis has also been associated with systemic diseases, including atherosclerosis, preterm birth, and diabetes [4].

Conventional diagnostic techniques in periodontics are based on clinical examination and occasionally on laboratory tests. Clinical examination assesses gingival health status, periodontal pocket depth, clinical attachment loss, radiographic alveolar bone level, oral hygiene performance, and other clinical variables [5]. Laboratory testing may include microbiological analysis for periodontal pathogens, blood tests for systemic health status, and histological evaluation of tissue changes. The obtained information allows a classification of periodontal disease into gingivitis and mild, moderate and severe periodontitis. However, the current diagnostic tests are not particularly sensitive and specific for periodontal disease activity and have limited prognosticative value. Rapid molecular techniques capable of identifying periodontal bacteria and viruses with great accuracy may eventually provide a better classification and diagnosis of various types of periodontal disease and aid significantly in clinical decision-making [5].

Thus far, most of what we know about bacteria in periodontal disease has been learned through anaerobic culturing, but the immense bacterial diversity in periodontal pockets will require molecular methods able to simultaneously investigate all members of periodontal pocket communities, including those that we cannot currently grow in culture [6,7,8]. Recent studies by Griffen et al. (2012) and Abusleme et al. (2013) using Next-Generation Sequencing (NGS) of bacterial small-subunit ribosomal RNA (16S rRNA) genes showed the promise of these methods for investigating periodontal disease. [9,10]. These studies analyzed patterns of microbial diversity in healthy and diseased periodontal pockets and showed clear community level differences among, and even within, individuals.

Here, we used NGS methods to determine how standard periodontal disease treatment, namely scaling and root planing and oral hygiene instruction, altered polymicrobial diversity in periodontal pockets. The study design and analytical methods allowed us to investigate differences in microbial community

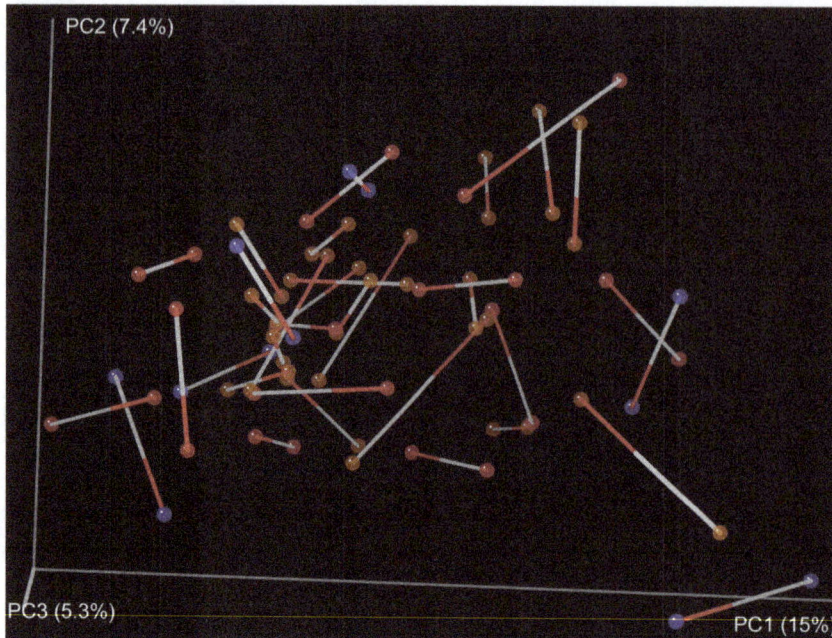

Figure 1. Procrustes analysis of samples before and after periodontal treatment, Procrustes M^2 value = 0.420 (dissimilarity of the two datasets), *P*-value = 0.00 based on 1000 Monte Carlo iterations. This analysis is a visualization of a principal coordinates analysis (PCoA) of the Unifrac distances between samples, showing the best superimposition of one Unifrac plot on the other. Samples collected from the same patient before and after treatment are connected by a line, the white end indicating the before-treatment sample red end indicating the after-treatment sample. Patients were classified as improved (red circles), worsened (brown circles) or no change (blue circles). Determination of patient improvement or decline was based on changes in observed pocket depth, a standard approach used in periodontal research [12,13].

diversity among periodontal health and disease states, and whether there were consistent associations of particular bacteria with health or disease.

Materials and Methods

Ethics Statement

The supporting TREND checklist for this study is available in the supplemental materials (Figure S1). The San Diego State Institutional Review Board obtained full ethical approval on August 11, 2008. Written informed consent was obtained from each participant. The study was registered as "Assess the Effect of Treating Periodontal Disease on Cardiovascular Function in Young Adults" on ClinicalTrials.gov under the identifier NCT01376791.

Study Population, Clinical Assessment and Treatment

Thirty-six subjects aged 21–40 with gingivitis, mild-to-moderate periodontitis, or severe periodontitis, along with 4 healthy controls were recruited from an American Indian/Alaska Native (AIAN) population in Southern California. The AIAN population is known to have a higher incidence of periodontal disease than the general population, making it an important subject of study for this community [11]. Degree of periodontal disease was assessed by measuring probing pocket depths (PD), clinical attachment loss (CAL), plaque scores, and bleeding on probing (BOP). Twenty-three patients aged 21–40 with gingivitis (CAL≤3 mm, PD≤ 4 mm, BOP>10%), twelve patients with mild-moderate periodontitis (CAL≥4 mm, PD≥5 mm, BOP≥30%), one patient with severe periodontitis (CAL≥6 mm, pocket depths ≥7 mm, BOP≥30%), along with 4 healthy controls (CAL≤3 mm, PD≤ 3 mm, BOP≤10%) all aged 21–40 were enrolled in the study.

Following completion of periodontal treatment (at least 6 weeks later), patients returned for a follow-up visit.

Patients received a baseline dental examination which included a full dental screening and measurement of periodontal pocket depths of all teeth. Following the clinical examination, microbial samples were collected from the two deepest periodontal pockets of the dentition using a periodontal scaler. The sample material was wiped onto sterile Whatman filters and submerged into 10 mL of sterile Sodium-Magnesium buffer (SM buffer) and kept at 4°C. DNA was extracted with the NucleoSpin Tissue Nucleic Acid and Protein Purification Kit (Macherey-Nagel GmbH & Co, Germany) from the supernatant after vigorous vortexing. The same procedure was repeated at least six weeks following completion of standard periodontal disease treatment. Patients were classified as improved if their average pocket depth decreased (twelve patients), worsened if their average pocket depth increased (eighteen patients), and no change if their average pocket depth remained the same (6 patients) [12,13].

Next-Generation Sequencing and Bioinformatics

The 27F and 338R primers targeting the V1–V2 hypervariable regions of 16S rRNA genes were used in the PCR reactions [14]. The primers were barcoded following Fierer *et al.* (2008), using the same PCR thermocycling parameters. PCR products were submitted to the core sequencing facility at the University of Pennsylvania for purification, equimolar dilution and pyrosequencing on a Roche 454 GS FLX instrument. The dataset sequences were deposited into the publicly accessible QIIME Database at http://www.microbio.me/qiime. The study name in QIIME is: Schwarzberg_periodontal_disease. The study ID is: 2083. The sequences were also deposited into figshare at http://

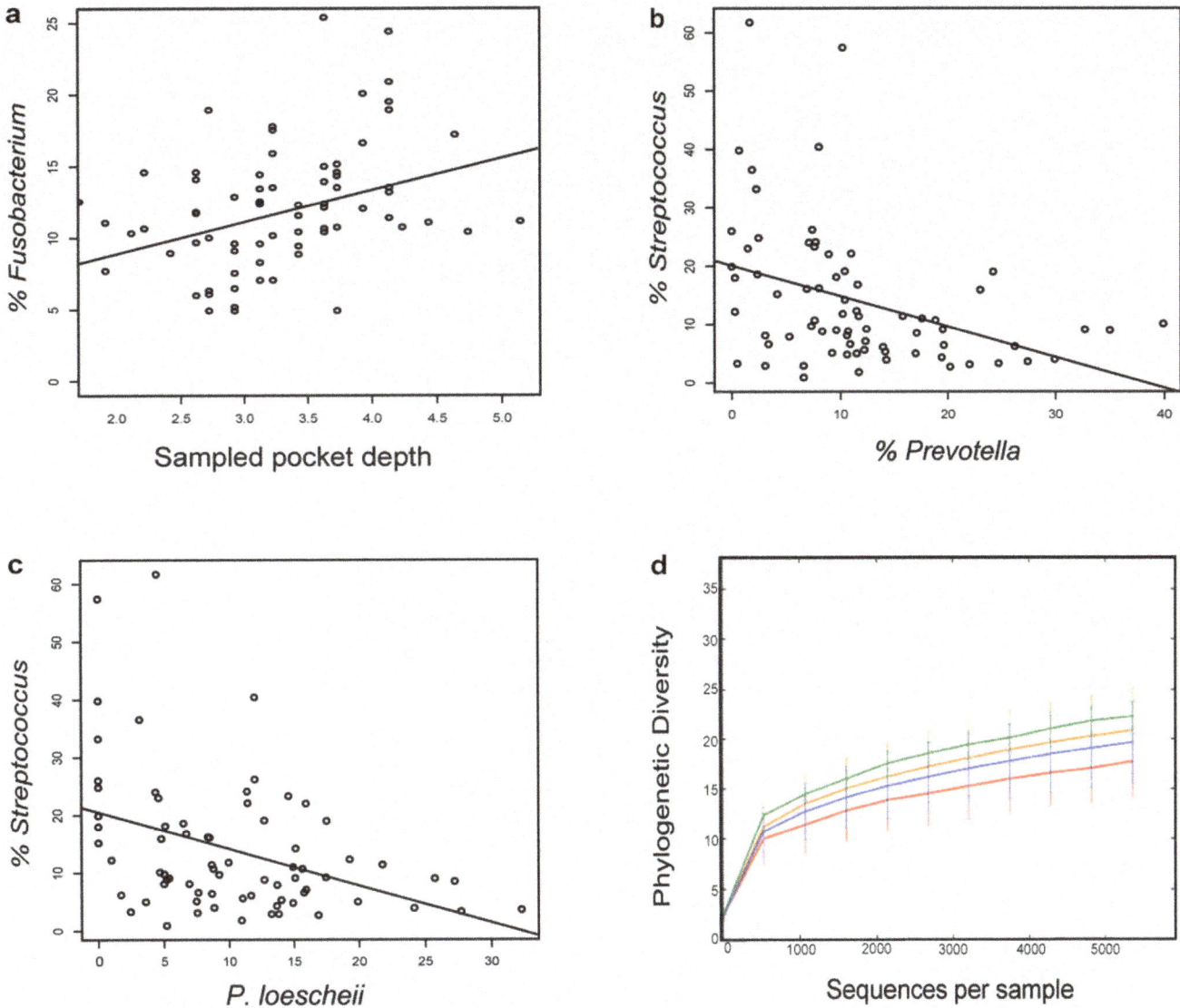

Figure 2. Statistical trends and alpha diversity of samples. a Percent of *Fusobacterium* relative to pocket depth of sampled teeth (r = 0.2413, *P* = 0.0411). **b** Percent of *Streptococcus* relative to *Prevotella* (r = −0.3846, *P* = 0.0008). **c** Percent of *Streptococcus* relative to single *Prevotella* species, *P. loescheii* (r = −0.3055, *P* = 0.0090). **d** Rarefaction trends: distribution of number of sequences per sample. Samples were classified as Healthy Controls (red line), gingivitis (blue line), mild/moderate periodontitis (orange line) and severe periodontitis (green line).

dx.doi.org/10.6084/m9.figshare.855613 along with the mapping file at http://dx.doi.org/10.6084/m9.figshare.855612.

Sequencing data were analyzed using QIIME 1.6.0-dev [15]. Briefly, sequences were clustered into 97% using a uclust-based [16] open-reference OTU picking protocol using the Greengenes 12_10 reference sequences [17]. Taxonomy was assigned to sequences using the RDP Classifier [18], retrained on Greengenes 12_10, via QIIME. Representative sequences, which were selected as the centroid sequence of each OTU, were aligned with PyNAST [19], and trees were constructed using FastTree [20] for phylogenetic diversity calculations. Procrustes analysis [21] was performed using QIIME with 1000 Monte Carlo iterations. OTU counts for specific taxonomic groups (e.g., *Streptococcus*) were exported from QIIME for statistical analyses in R version 2.15.1 [22]. Representative *Fusobacterium* and *Prevotella* sequences were exported for multiple sequence alignment and phylogenetic analyses (Figures S3 and S4).

Results and Discussion

A total of 76 periodontal pocket microbial community samples were analyzed via 454 pyrosequencing of bacterial 16S rRNA amplicons (Figure S2). Pyrosequencing yielded a combined total of 759,717 sequences across all samples with a median sequence count of 9,676. From these data, we identified 87 bacterial genera belonging to 12 different divisions, the majority of which were common members of periodontal pocket microbiota. Community-level analyses (Unifrac-based PCoA) did not uncover clear differences between samples collected prior to treatment with those collected post-treatment, even after accounting for the treatment effectiveness. On the contrary, post-treatment samples remained most similar to pre-treatment samples from the same individual (Figure 1).

Deeper analyses of the distributions of specific bacterial taxa associated with either health (*Streptococcus*, *Veillonella*) or disease (*Fusobacterium*, *Prevotella* and *Leptotrichia*) [6,9,10] found only

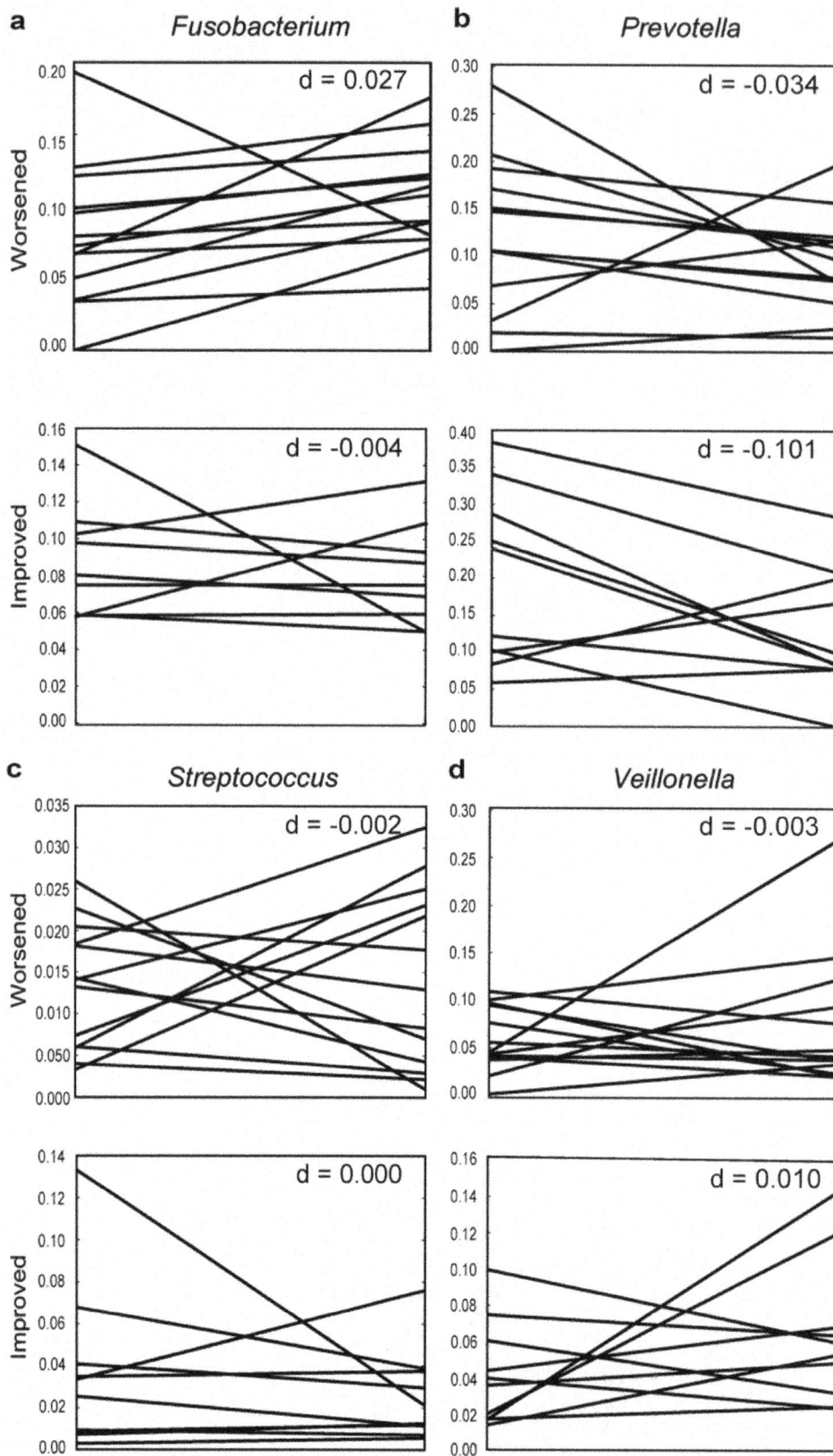

Figure 3. Trends of bacterial genera associated with health or disease, separated by whether individuals improved or worsened after treatment. An analysis of average periodontal pocket depth before and after treatment showed that less than half (N = 12) the treated individuals improved post-treatment, while the rest stayed the same (N = 6) or worsened (N = 18). Lines indicate the proportion for a particular individual. The d-scores indicate the median line slope. **a** *Fusobacterium*, **b** *Prevotella*, **c** *Streptococcus*, **d** *Veillonella*. Note that the scale of the y-axis differs to highlight difference in individual responses to treatment.

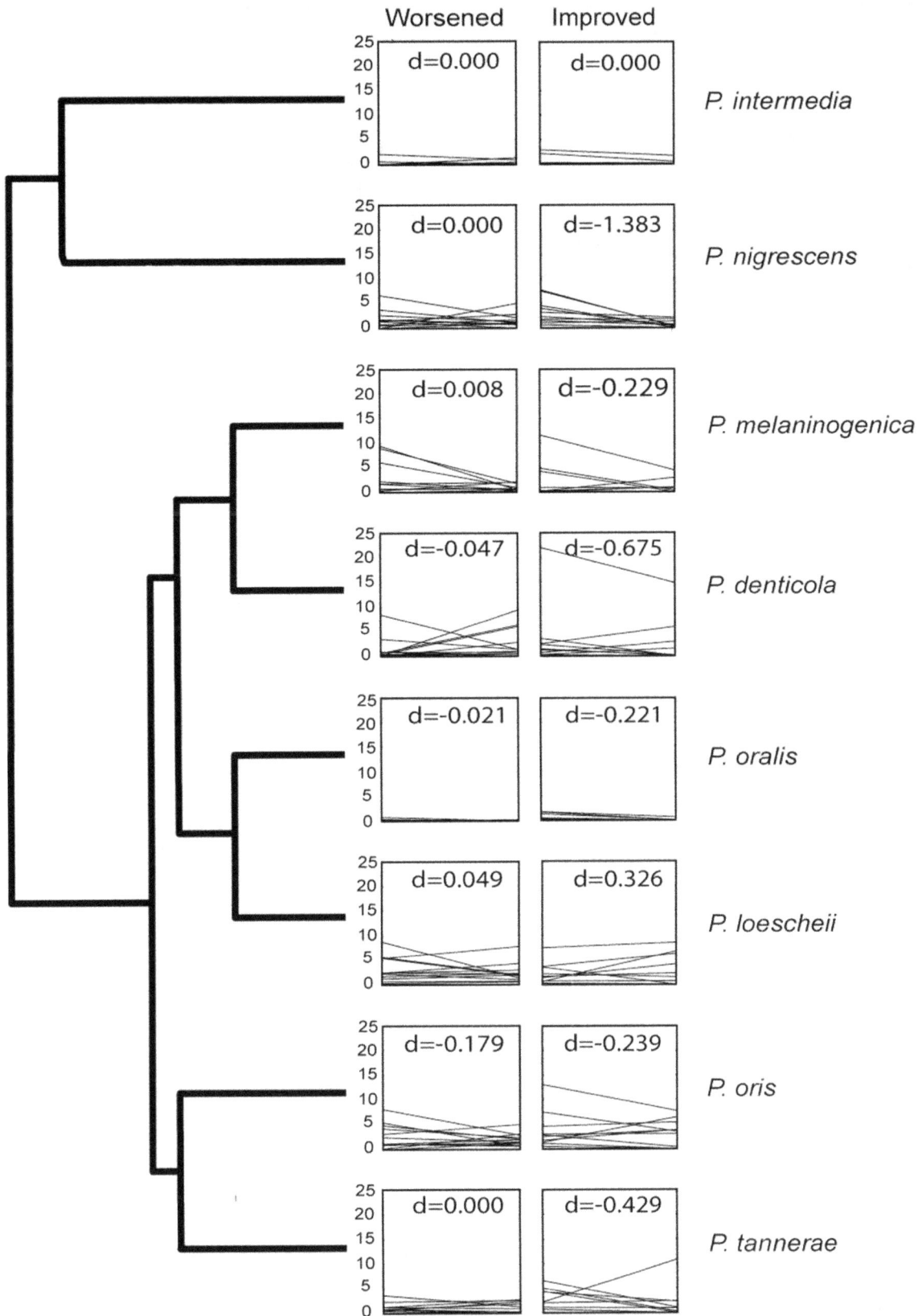

Figure 4. Representative cladogram of *Prevotella* species determined in this study (based on phylogenetic analysis shown in Figure S2) with plots of relative abundance of specific species divided into patients that improved and patients that worsened. The d-scores indicate the median line slope. In many cases, changes in relative proportions before and after treatment appeared to be species dependent.

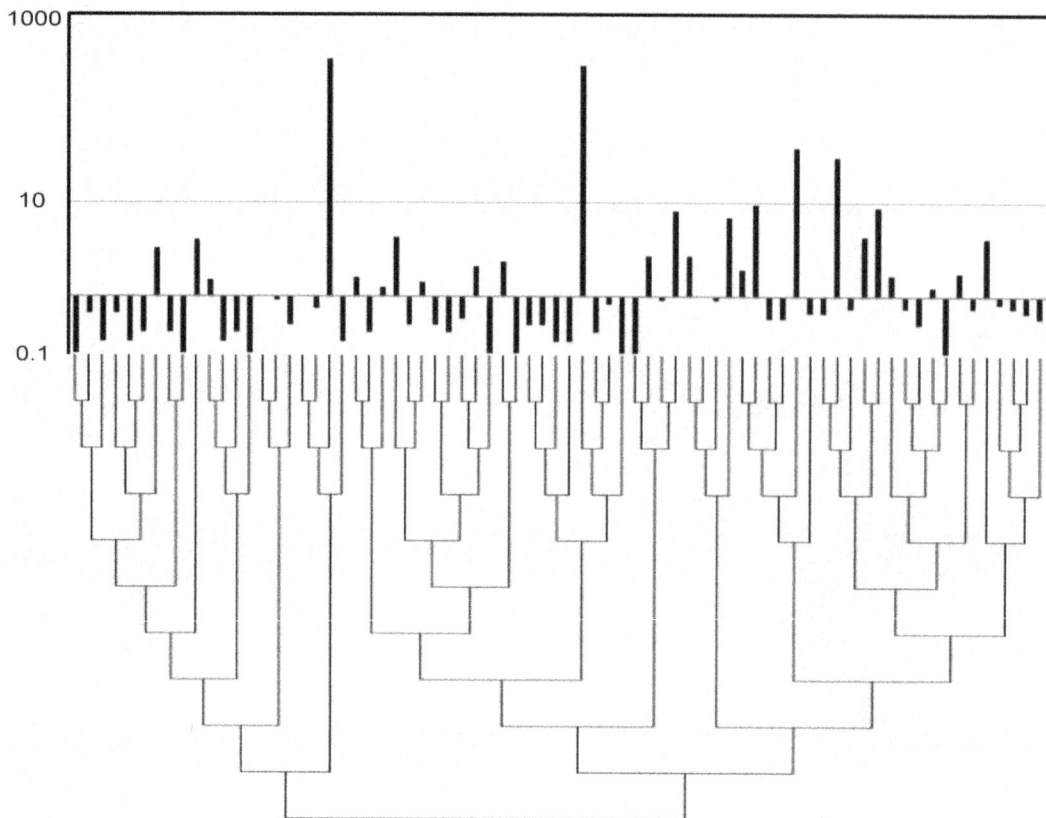

Figure 5. Cladogram of 73 different *Fusobacterium*-species (OTUs clustered at 97%) sequences along with a histogram showing the log OTU-count abundance of these same species. Most OTUs were sparse and the overall diversity within and among pockets was considerable.

Fusobacterium to be significantly correlated with pocket depth over all samples (Figure 2a). As expected, we found an inverse correlation between the abundance of *Fusobacterium* and *Streptococcus* (data not shown) and between *Streptococcus* and *Prevotella* (Figure 2b), with the association primarily driven by the negative correlation between *Streptococcus* and *P. loescheii* (Figure 2c). *Fusobacterium*, especially *F. nucleatum*, plays a key role in periodontal biofilm development by bridging early and late colonizers, according to the successional integration theory [23]. *Streptococcus* species establish the biofilm and *P. loescheii* attaches directly to *Streptococcus*, unlike the other *Prevotella* species. The roles played by these bacterial genera may make them particularly responsive to biofilm disturbance, and perhaps make them useful indicators of periodontal treatment efficacy.

In interpreting patient response to treatment, accounting for the personal microbiome of individual patients proved critical. This interpersonal variability also explains why we do not observe pre- and post-treatment clustering in PCoA space (Figure 1). While there are consistent changes associated with recovery from periodontal disease (e.g., a decrease in *Prevotella* abundance), the "healthy" amount of *Prevotella* differs on an individual basis. Moreover, the flora of some individuals changed contrary to the prevailing trends, notably in the *Fusobacterium* and *Prevotella*. *Streptococcus* remained steady or slightly increased in patients that improved, except two individuals who experienced dramatic declines post-treatment (Figure 3c). We also did not observe an expected increase in *Veillonella* in improving individuals post-treatment (Figure 3d).

Understanding the behavior of the biofilm response also appeared, at least in the case of *Prevotella*, to require more species-specific knowledge. Having successfully differentiated a number of oral *Prevotella* species (Figure S3), we found the abundance of *P. melaninogenica* and *P. loescheii* changed in opposite directions, while other *Prevotella* showed highly variable response post-treatment (Figure 4). A closer examination of *Fusobacterium* diversity also provided intriguing insight into periodontal biofilms. OTU clustering and phylogenetic analysis determined as many as 73 different species (Figure 5; Figure S4). Only four of these were abundant across all samples, and only two were found in every sample (Figure 5), supporting recent findings that the core human microbiome in unrelated individuals tends to be minimal at lower taxonomic levels [24]. These rarer species may increase the overall immune response and metabolic activity, but our data also suggest the presence of biofilm "cheaters" who contribute little to actual biofilm stability.

In the past, it was common to focus on the presence or absence of the bacteria that comprise the "red complex" (*Porphyromonas gingivalis*, *Tannerella forsythia* and *Treponema denticola*), which were implicated in disease [26]. However, it is clear from recent studies that culturing and emphasis on specific bacteria will not capture all the variability in the diseased periodontium [6,9,10]. This leads us to question the use of antibiotics in treatment of periodontal disease due to the variability of bacteria found in different diseased patients and the varied susceptibility of bacteria to different kinds of antibiotics.

Systemic antibiotic therapy is often used in periodontics to reduce or eradicate periodontopathic bacteria that are invading gingiva or are otherwise not reachable by topical antimicrobial treatment [25]. The selection of antibiotics is challenging because deep periodontal pockets can harbor several pathogens which exhibit diverse susceptibility to common antibiotics. Reference laboratories are available to identify periodontal pathogens and their antibiotic susceptibility, but most dentists institute antibiotic therapy empirically based on the best estimate of the most probable pathogen(s) and their usual antibiotic susceptibility pattern. Combination antibiotic therapy is frequently employed to cover a broader spectrum of pathogens. However, even though properly prescribed antibiotics can help provide resolution of severe periodontitis, the widespread use of antibiotics carries risks of inducing antibiotic resistance in important medical pathogens. It is expected that increased insights into the composition of the periodontal microbiome will lead to a better definition of patients who may, or may not, benefit from adjunctive antibiotic therapy.

Altogether, our results highlight the importance of understanding each patient's personal oral microbiome, a goal achievable by collecting and analyzing pre- and post-treatment samples. Furthermore, they lead us to believe that there is not a single composition that represents a healthy periodontal state and that recovery from periodontal disease appears to reflect a shift from a personalized disease state to a personalized healthy state. While there is consensus that particular communities should shift with response to disease, there may not be a "healthy amount" of these bacteria that is consistent across individuals. Further research with a larger patient sample size and more sampling over a longer time period will be necessary to confirm this hypothesis.

Supporting Information

Figure S1 TREND checklist for non-randomized trials.

Figure S2 Table describing the distribution of patients by disease classification.

Figure S3 Maximum likelihood tree of *Prevotella*-related small-subunit ribosomal RNA gene sequences. The sequences highlighted in red were obtained in this study, while the rest include both cultured and uncultured sequences obtained from GenBank. To be included in the phylogenetic analysis, sequences identical to the representative OTU had to be found in at least three independent periodontal pocket samples. Sequences from cultured and uncultured organisms were also included in the alignments. Alignments were trimmed to ~300 nucleotides and checked for accuracy and edited manually. Maximum-likelihood trees were created using RAxML HPC-BlackBox on CIPRES ([27]; http://www.phylo.org/). Black circles indicate bootstrap values of >70% while white circles indicate bootstrap values between 50 and 70%.

Figure S4 Maximum likelihood tree of *Fusobacterium*-related small-subunit ribosomal RNA gene sequences. The sequences highlighted in red were obtained in this study. The orange highlighted sequences were obtained from a study of bacteria in periradicular lesions by Saber *et al.* (2012) [27]. See Figure S3 for details on the phylogenetic methods.

Acknowledgments

We would like to thank the staff at the American Indian/Alaska Native (AIAN) population clinic, specifically to the medical, dental and administrative staff for all of their hard work and dedication. We thank Mike Furlan for his consultation on this project. We also thank the many willing participants in this study.

Author Contributions

Conceived and designed the experiments: KS RL BB SL RAG JGC STK. Performed the experiments: KS RL. Analyzed the data: KS GC FS JGC STK. Contributed reagents/materials/analysis tools: MHS FA JS. Wrote the paper: KS SL JS RAG JGC STK.

References

1. Dentino A, Lee S, Mailhot J, Hefti AF (2013) Principles of periodontology. Periodontology 2000 61: 16–53.
2. Teles R, Teles F, Frias-Lopez J, Paster B, Haffajee A (2013) Lessons learned and unlearned in periodontal microbiology. Periodontology 2000 62: 95–162.
3. Genco RJ, Borgnakke WS (2013) Risk factors for periodontal disease. Periodontology 2000 62: 59–94.
4. Cullinan MP, Seymour GJ (2013) Periodontal disease and systemic illness: will the evidence ever be enough? Periodontology 2000 62: 271–286.
5. Slots J (2013) Periodontology: past, present, perspectives. Periodontology 2000 62: 7–19.
6. Liu B, Faller LL, Klitgord N, Mazumdar V, Ghodsi M, et al. (2012) Deep sequencing of the oral microbiome reveals signatures of periodontal disease. Plos One 7.
7. Paster BJ, Olsen I, Aas JA, Dewhirst FE (2006) The breadth of bacterial diversity in the human periodontal pocket and other oral sites. Periodontology 2000 42: 80–87.
8. Keijser BJF, Zaura E, Huse SM, van der Vossen JMBM, Schuren FHJ, et al. (2008) Pyrosequencing analysis of the oral microflora of healthy adults. Journal of Dental Research 87: 1016–1020.
9. Abusleme L, Dupuy AK, Dutzan N, Silva N, Burleson JA, et al. (2013) The subgingival microbiome in health and periodontitis and its relationship with community biomass and inflammation. ISME J 2013 Jan 10 doi: 101038/ismej2012174: T - aheadofprint.
10. Griffen AL, Beall CJ, Campbell JH, Firestone ND, Kumar PS, et al. (2012) Distinct and complex bacterial profiles in human periodontitis and health revealed by 16S pyrosequencing. Isme Journal 6: 1176–1185.
11. Skrepcinski FB, Niendorff WJ (2000) Periodontal Disease in American Indians and Alaska Natives. Journal of Public Health Dentistry 60: 261–266.
12. Badersten A, Nilveus R, Egelberg J (1981) Effect of nonsurgical periodontal therapy. I. Moderately advanced periodontitis. Journal of Clinical Periodontology 8: 57–72.
13. Cobb CM (2002) Clinical significance of non-surgical periodontal therapy: an evidence-based perspective of scaling and root planing. Journal of Clinical Periodontology 29: 22–32.
14. Fierer N, Hamady M, Lauber CL, Knight R (2008) The influence of sex, handedness, and washing on the diversity of hand surface bacteria. Proceedings of the National Academy of Sciences 105: 17994–17999.
15. Caporaso JG, Kuczynski J, Stombaugh J, Bittinger K, Bushman FD, et al. (2010) QIIME allows analysis of high-throughput community sequencing data. Nature Methods 7: 335–336.
16. Edgar RC (2010) Search and clustering orders of magnitude faster than BLAST. Bioinformatics 26: 2460–2461.
17. McDonald D, Price MN, Goodrich J, Nawrocki EP, DeSantis TZ, et al. (2012) An improved Greengenes taxonomy with explicit ranks for ecological and evolutionary analyses of bacteria and archaea. ISME J 6: 610–618.
18. Wang Q, Garrity GM, Tiedje JM, Cole JR (2007) Naive Bayesian classifier for rapid assignment of rRNA sequences into the new bacterial taxonomy. Appl Environ Microbiol 73: 5261–5267.
19. Caporaso JG, Bittinger K, Bushman FD, DeSantis TZ, Andersen GL, et al. (2010) PyNAST: a flexible tool for aligning sequences to a template alignment. Bioinformatics 26: 266–267.
20. Price MN, Dehal PS, Arkin AP (2010) FastTree 2–approximately maximum-likelihood trees for large alignments. Plos One 5: e9490.
21. Gower JC (1975) Generalized procrustes analysis. Psychometrika 40: 33–51.
22. Team RC (2008) R: A language and environment for statistical computing. R Foundation Statistical Computing, Vienna, Austria.
23. Kolenbrander PE, Palmer RJ, Jr., Rickard AH, Jakubovics NS, Chalmers NI, et al. (2006) Bacterial interactions and successions during plaque development. Periodontology 2000 42: 47–79.
24. Faith JJ, Guruge JL, Charbonneau M, Subramanian S, Seedorf H, et al. (2013) The Long-Term Stability of the Human Gut Microbiota. Science 341.
25. Slots J (2012) Low-cost periodontal therapy. Periodontology 2000 60: 110–137.

13

Effects of Aging on Endotoxin Tolerance Induced by Lipopolysaccharides Derived from *Porphyromonas gingivalis* and *Escherichia coli*

Ying Sun[1,2], Hui Li[1,2], Mi-Fang Yang[1], Wei Shu[2], Meng-Jun Sun[1,2], Yan Xu[1,2]*

1 Institute of Stomatology, Nanjing Medical University, Nanjing, China, **2** Department of Periodontology, Stomatology Hospital affiliated to Nanjing Medical University, Nanjing, China

Abstract

Background: Periodontitis is a bacterially induced chronic inflammatory disease. Exposure of the host to periodontal pathogens and their virulence factors induces a state of hyporesponsiveness to subsequent stimulations, termed endotoxin tolerance. Aging has a profound effect on immune response to bacteria challenge. The aim of this study was to explore the effects of aging on endotoxin tolerance induced by *Porphyromonas gingivalis* (*P. gingivalis*) lipopolysaccharide (LPS) and *Escherichia coli* (*E. coli*) LPS in murine peritoneal macrophages.

Methodology/Principal Findings: We studied the cytokine production (TNF-α and IL-10) and Toll-like receptor 2, 4 (TLR2, 4) gene and protein expressions in peritoneal macrophages from young (2-month-old) and middle-aged (12-month-old) ICR mice following single or repeated *P. gingivalis* LPS or *E. coli* LPS stimulation. Pretreatment of peritoneal macrophages with *P. gingivalis* LPS or *E. coli* LPS resulted in a reduction in TNF-α production and an increase in IL-10 production upon secondary stimulation (p<0.05), and the markedly lower levels of TNF-α and higher levels of IL-10 were observed in macrophages from young mice compared with those from middle-aged mice (p<0.05). In addition, LPS restimulations also led to the significantly lower expression levels of TLR2, 4 mRNA and protein in macrophages from young mice (p<0.05).

Conclusions/Significance: Repeated LPS stimulations triggered endotoxin tolerance in peritoneal macrophages and the ability to develop tolerance in young mice was more excellent. The impaired ability to develop endotoxin tolerance resulted from aging might be related to TLR2, 4 and might lead to the incontrollable periodontal inflammation in older adults.

Editor: Markus M. Heimesaat, Charité, Campus Benjamin Franklin, Germany

Funding: This work was supported by the National Natural Science Foundation of China through Project 81000444 (https://isis.nsfc.gov.cn), the Natural Science Foundation of Jiangsu Province through Project BK2008363 (http://www.jskjjh.gov.cn/) and the Priority Academic Program Development of Jiangsu Higher Education Institutions (http://jsycw.ec.js.edu.cn/). The funders had no role in study design, data collection and analysis, decision to publish, or preparation of the manuscript.

Competing Interests: The authors have declared that no competing interests exist.

* E-mail: yanxu@njmu.edu.cn

Introduction

Periodontitis is one of the most common oral diseases in humans, which is characterized by the loss of tooth-supporting structures. It is a bacterially induced chronic destructive inflammatory disease and is difficult to treat [1]. Gram-negative bacteria, including *Porphyromonas gingivalis* (*P. gingivalis*), *Prevotella intermedia* (*P. intermedia*), *Fusobacterium nucleatum* (*F. nucleatum*) and *Aggregatibacter actinomycetemcomitans* (*A. actinomycetemcomitans*), have been considered to be the important periodontopathic bacteria. Among them, *P. gingivalis* can be frequently isolated from periodontal pockets in patients with chronic periodontitis, which is the most common form of periodontiis [2,3]. The cell-wall components of periodontal pathogens, especially lipopolysaccharide (LPS), can trigger a wide range of host responses, including the production of pro-inflammatory cytokines, anti-inflammatory cytokines, and chemokines. Excessive and prolonged immune responses can lead to the destruction of periodontal tissues and may be very important in the progression of periodontitis [4,5].

Endotoxin tolerance is a phenomenon whereby previous exposure of cells or organisms to microbial products induces a hyporesponsiveness to subsequent challenge and is characterized by diminished release of proinflammatory cytokines, such as TNF-α and IL-1ß [6]. The hyporesponsiveness to a secondary challenge with a different LPS (heterotolerance) is usually weaker than that with the same LPS (homotolerance) [7]. Endotoxin tolerance represents a selective reprogramming aimed at limiting inflammatory damage resulted from activation of the immune system by bacteria or their virulence factors [8]. Therefore, tolerance induced by persistent periodontopathic bacteria stimulations might be essential to maintain homeostasis in periodontal tissues. Accumulating evidence suggested the possible involvement of Toll-like receptors (TLRs) pathways in endotoxin tolerance [9,10]. However, the exact mechanism, especially for endotoxin tolerance in periodontitis, still remains obscure.

TLRs are type I transmembrane proteins found on the surface of mammalian cells and are implicated in the recognition of conserved bacterial cell-wall components [11]. To date, at least 11 human TLRs and 13 murine TLRs have been described. Among them, TLR2 and 4 function as the principal innate sensors for cell-wall components of gram-negative bacteria in mammals [12–14], and might be very important in endotoxin tolerance induced by periodontal pathogens [9,10].

Aging is associated with poor periodontal health and some studies have disclosed the potential relationship between advanced age and the increased prevalence and severity of periodontitis [15,16]. In old individuals, alterations of both innate and adaptive immunity lead to increased susceptibility to infections, including periodontal inflammation [17,18]. Age-related changes in the adaptive immune system are well-documented, such as altered cytokine patterns and a decline in Ag-presenting cell function [19]. Researches have also indicated the decreased functions of macrophages, NK cells and lymphocytes with aging, including chemotaxis, phagocytic and scavenger receptor activity, production of reactive oxygen species, the inflammatory wound healing response, and induction of certain cytokine responses [20–22]. Macrophages, which play an important role in the innate host response in periodontitis as well as other chronic infections [23], are known to develop endotoxin tolerance [24,25]. Little is known about the influence of aging on endotoxin tolerance in macrophages. In addition, it is still not fully understood the relationship between age-related alterations in innate immunity and the prognosis of periodontitis.

It is hypothesized that 1) aging might have an effect on endotoxin tolerance, which might be related with the development of periodontitis in aged individuals; and 2) age-related alteration in TLR2, 4 might be associated with the impact of aging on endotoxin tolerance. To better understand the effects of aging on endotoxin tolerance and their underlying mechanisms, endotoxin tolerance was induced by LPS derived from *P. gingivalis* and *E. coli* in peritoneal macrophages from young and middle-aged mice. Then, we explored the production of pro-inflammatory cytokine TNF-α and anti-inflammatory cytokine IL-10 in these cells by enzyme-linked immunosorbent assays (ELISA), and examined the changes of TLR2, 4 expressions by real-time PCR and flow cytometry. Our results revealed the impaired ability to develop endotoxin tolerance resulted from aging, which might have an influence on the development of periodontitis in old individuals. In addition, this impaired ability might be related to the aged-associated changes in TLR2, 4.

Results

Cytokine Production in Peritoneal Macrophages upon a Primary or Secondary Exposure to LPS

To explore the secretions of pro-inflammatory cytokine TNF-α and anti-inflammatory cytokine IL-10 by murine peritoneal macrophages, the levels of these cytokines in the culture supernatants were measured by ELISA. Our results revealed that without stimulation, there were no significant differences in the production of all cytokines between peritoneal macrophages from young and middle-aged mice (p>0.05). Stimulations with *P. gingivalis* LPS or *E. coli* LPS for 24 h resulted in marked increases in the levels of TNF-α and IL-10 (p<0.05), and the production of all cytokines secreted by peritoneal macrophages from young mice were significantly higher than those from middle-aged mice (p<0.05). In addition, the secretions of all cytokines induced by *E. coli* LPS were significantly higher than those induced by *P. gingivalis* LPS (p<0.05) (Figure 1).

Next, to investigate the effects of aging on the ability of peritoneal macrophages to develop endotoxin tolerance, cells were pretreated with *P. gingivalis* LPS or *E. coli* LPS for 24 h, then restimulated after washing for an additional 24 h and assayed for cytokine production. When macrophages from both young and middle-aged mice were restimulated with *P. gingivalis* LPS or *E. coli* LPS, significant reductions were observed in the levels of TNF-α compared with those seen following single stimulation (p<0.05), except TNF-α production in the cells from middle-aged mice pretreated with *E. coli* LPS and treated with *P. gingivalis* LPS (p>0.05). Importantly, upon repeated LPS stimulations, the secretions of TNF-α by macrophages from young mice were significantly lower than those from middle-aged mice (p<0.05), which indicated that the ability to develop tolerance to endotoxin in young mice was more excellent. In addition, our study demonstrated that in macrophages from both young and middle-aged mice, homotolerance was much stronger than hetero-tolerance at the levels of TNF-α (p<0.05) (Figure 1A).

However, the changes of anti-inflammatory cytokine IL-10 levels was not as same as the those of TNF-α. *P. gingivalis* LPS and *E. coli* LPS homotolerance resulted in a significant increase in IL-10 secretions in peritoneal macrophages from both young and middle-aged mice (p<0.05), and the levels of IL-10 secreted by the cells from young mice were significantly higher than those from middle-aged mice (p<0.05). Moreover, in macrophages from young mice, but not middle-aged mice, precondition with *P. gingivalis* LPS and subsequent stimulation with *E. coli* LPS also led to a markedly increased IL-10 production (p<0.05) (Figure 1B).

Expression of TLR2, 4 in Peritoneal Macrophages after a Primary or Secondary LPS Exposure

We next examined whether the impaired ability of middle-aged mice to develop endotoxin tolerance was associated with the age-related changes in TLR2, 4. Quantitative real-time PCR analysis of total RNA and flow cytometry detection of TLR2, 4 surface expressions demonstrated that without stimulation, there were no significant differences in the mRNA and protein expressions of TLR2, 4 between peritoneal macrophages from young and middle-aged mice (p>0.05). *P. gingivalis* LPS stimulation led to the significant increases in the mRNA and protein expressions of TLR2 in macrophages from both young and middle-aged mice (p<0.05), and the expression levels in the cells from young mice were much higher than those from middle-aged mice (p<0.05). Similar to the expressions of TLR2, in macrophages from young and middle-age mice upon *E. coli* LPS stimulation, marked increases in the expressions of TLR4 mRNA and protein could also be observed (p<0.05), and the expression levels of TLR4 in the cells from young mice were significantly higher than those from middle-aged mice too (p<0.05) (Figure 2, 3). The representative result of five independent flow cytometry detections was shown in Figure 4.

Furthermore, the reduced mRNA and protein expressions of TLR2 or 4 were observed in macrophages from both young and middle-aged mice after *P. gingivalis* LPS or *E. coli* LPS restimulation respectively (homotolerance) (p<0.05), and the expression levels of TLR2, 4 in the cells from young mice were significantly lower than those from middle-aged mice (p<0.05) (Figure 2, 3, 4).

Our results also revealed the down-regulation of TLR2, 4 protein in macrophages from both young and middle-aged mice after different LPS restimulation (heterotolerance) (p<0.05). However, in heterotolerance groups, there were no significant differences in TLR2, 4 protein expressions between macrophages from young and middle-aged mice (p>0.05). In addition, in macrophages from young mice, but not middle-aged mice, the protein expressions of TLR2, 4 after repeated stimulation with the same LPS (homotolerance) were much

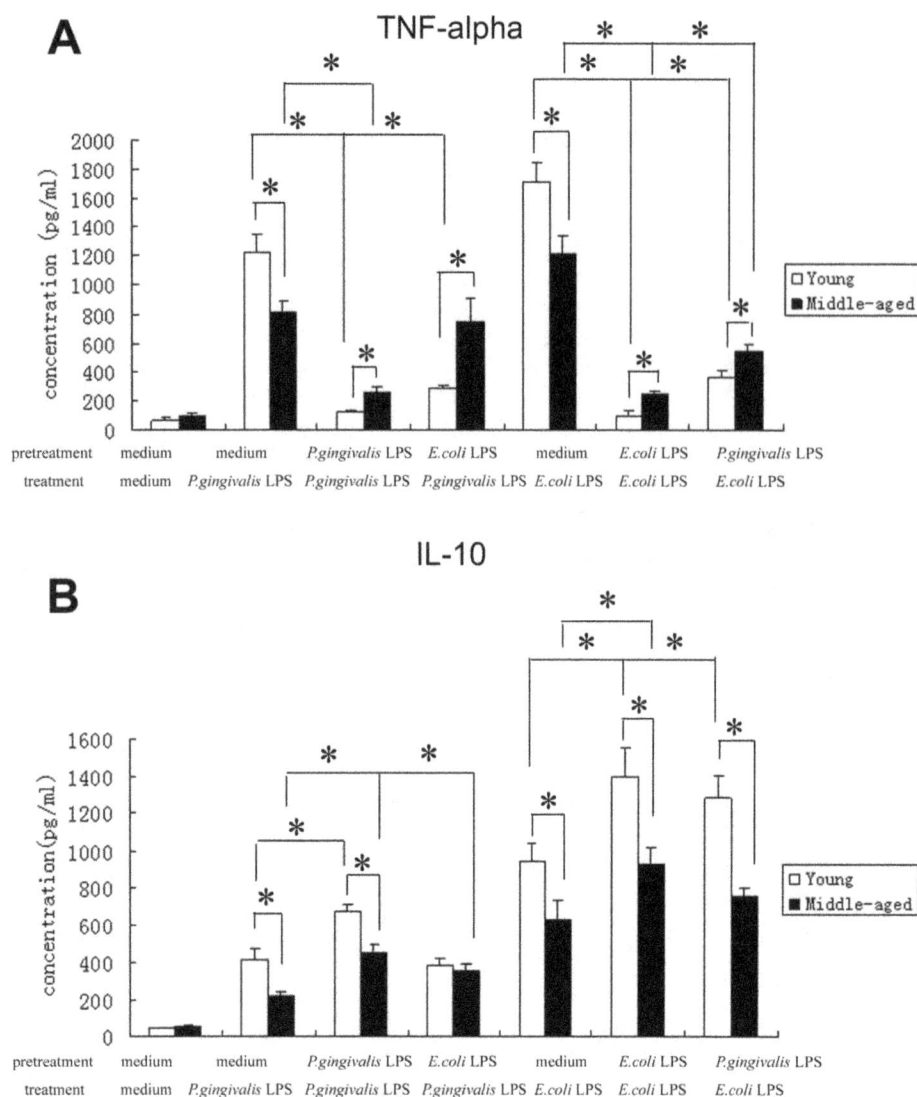

Figure 1. Cytokine production in peritoneal macrophages from young and middle-aged mice stimulated with LPS. Peritoneal macrophages from both young and middle-aged mice were pretreated with medium, 1 μg/ml *P.gingivalis* LPS or 1 μg/ml *E.coli* LPS for 24 h, washed, and then incubated with medium, 1 μg/ml *P.gingivalis* LPS or 1 μg/ml *E.coli* LPS for another 24 h. The levels of TNF-α (1A) and IL-10 (1B) in the culture supernatants were measured by ELISA. Data are expressed as mean±SD (n = 5 per group). *$P<0.05$.

lower than those after different LPS restimulation (heterotolerance) ($p<0.05$) (Figure 3, 4).

Discussion

The primary etiologic factor of periodontitis is bacterial biofilm. Accumulating evidence indicates that specific microorganisms in subgingival plaque, including *P. gingivalis, P. intermedia,F. nucleatum* and *A. actinomycetemcomitans*, initiate the disease [26]. LPS is one of the most important virulence factors of gram-negative bacteria, and plays an essential role in triggering periodontal inflammation [27,28]. Endotoxin tolerance induced by repeated LPS stimulations could lead to the reprogramming of the immune system, such as the downregulation of TNF-α and IL-1β, and the preservation of IL-10. It could play a protective role against inflammatory tissue destruction [29] and might have an effect on the development of periodontitis. Aging, which is characterized by the gradual decline in immune function, might also be associated with the prevalence

and severity of periodontitis, at least in part [30,31]. However, the influences of aging on endotoxin tolerance induced by periodontal pathogens and their underlying mechanisms still remain poorly characterized.

This is the first report on the effects of aging on endotoxin tolerance induced by LPS derived from periodontal bacteria. Our results provided evidence that the ability to develop tolerance in response to the repeated stimulation with LPS from both periodontal bacteria and non-periodontal bacteria was impaired in peritoneal macrophages from middle-aged mice. In addition, the different sensitivity to repeated LPS exposure in the cells from young and middle-aged mice might be partly associated with the different expressions levels of TLR2, 4.

In this present study, endotoxin tolerance was induced by *P. gingivalis* LPS and *E.coli* LPS. Although there are many common grounds on the biochemical and immunobiological properties of LPS from different gram-negative bacteria, differences in biological potency and pathogenicities still exist. It is not surprising

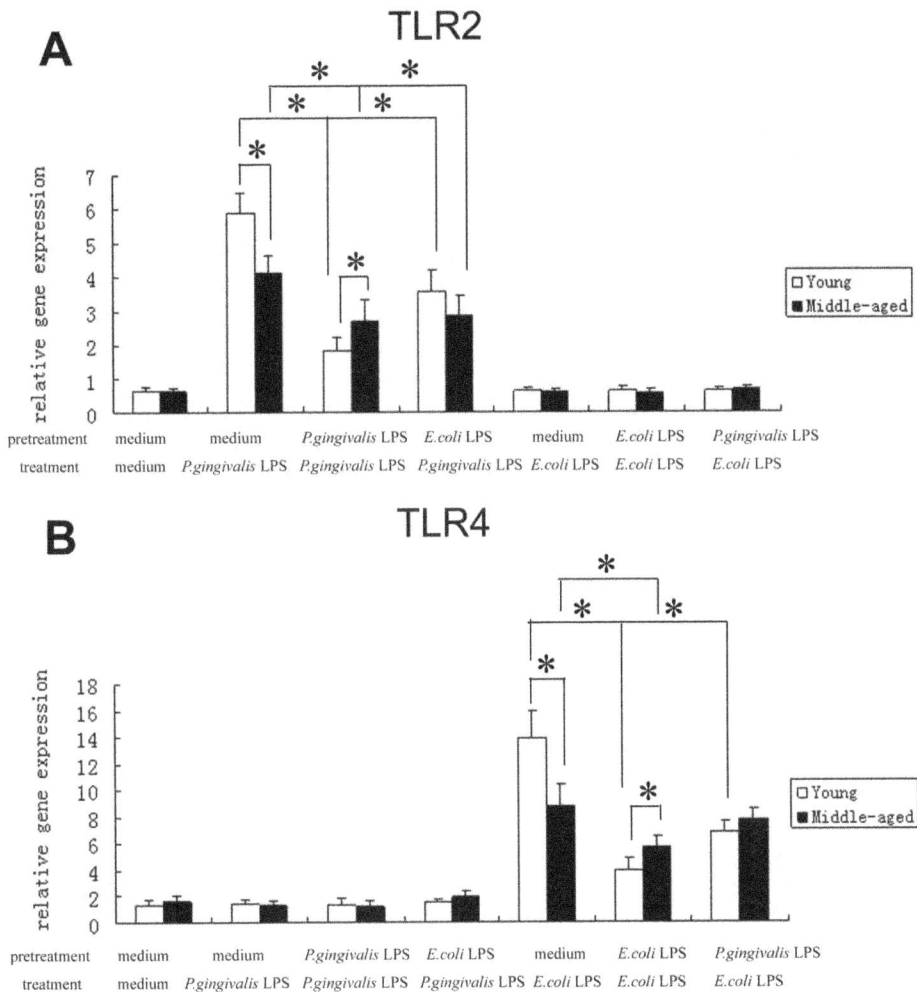

Figure 2. Gene expression changes of TLR2, 4 in peritoneal macrophages from young and middle-aged mice stimulated with LPS. Peritoneal macrophages from both young and middle-aged mice were pretreated with medium, 1 μg/ml *P.gingivalis* LPS or 1 μg/ml *E.coli* LPS for 24 h, washed, and then restimulated with medium, 1 μg/ml *P.gingivalis* LPS or 1 μg/ml *E.coli* LPS for 6 h. Real-time PCR was used to quantify TLR2 (2A) and TLR4 (2B) mRNA expression levels. The absolute mRNA levels of all the genes were normalized to ß-actin levels of individual samples. Data are expressed as mean±SD (n = 5 per group). *P<0.05.

that there are quantitative and/or qualitative differences in triggering TLRs and developing endotoxin tolerance between *E.coli* LPS and *P. gingivalis* LPS. *E.coli* LPS represents the classic LPS derived from gram-negative bacteria and is the optimal TLR4 agonist. LPS from many periodontopathic bacteria, such as *F. nucleatum* and *A. actinomycetemcomitans*, can also activate TLR4, and there are some similarities in triggering inflammation between *E. coli* LPS and these periodontopathic bacteria LPS [32,33]. *P. gingivalis* LPS is an unusual pattern recognition receptor ligand for the innate defense system and expresses a low level of endotoxic activity relative to *E. coli* LPS. The protein structure of *P. gingivalis* LPS lacks heptose and 2-keto-3-deoxyoctonate, which are unique to enterobacterial LPS. Moreover, its lipid A exhibits a phosphorylation and acylation pattern, and contains branched and relatively longer fatty acids (15–17 carbon atoms). It is a TLR2 agonist, and its biochemical and immunobiological properties are quite different from *E. coli* LPS [34,35]. Therefore, we chose two different LPS, *P. gingivalis* LPS and *E. coli* LPS, as the stimulators in this study to explore the reprogramming of the immune system resulted from endotoxin tolerance, which might take place in the development of periodontal inflammation.

Secretion of pro-inflammatory cytokines, including TNF-α, IL-1β and IL-6, and chemokine, such as IL-8, is one of the most important strategies utilized by the host to resist periodontal microorganisms. However, an orchestrated balance of pro-inflammatory cytokine, chemokine and anti-inflammatory cytokine release is critical for an innate immune response sufficient to resist periodontopathic bacteria without excessive damage to periodontal tissues. Endotoxin tolerance is an important protective mechanism, which could lead to the reprogramming of cytokine network to limit immune damage and maintain periodontal homeostasis. Therefore, it might be closely related to the progression of periodontitis. The impaired ability to develop endotoxin tolerance in old persons might be associated with the incontrollable periodontal inflammation.

Our findings demonstrated the diversity in different cytokine production after repeated LPS stimulations. Therefore, endotoxin tolerance is a case of reprogramming and immunomodulation rather than a global downregulation of cytokine expression and function. It is often linked with up-regulated expression of anti-inflammatory cytokines, such as IL-10 and TGF-ß, which contribute to the deactivation of monocytes/macrophages and

A

B

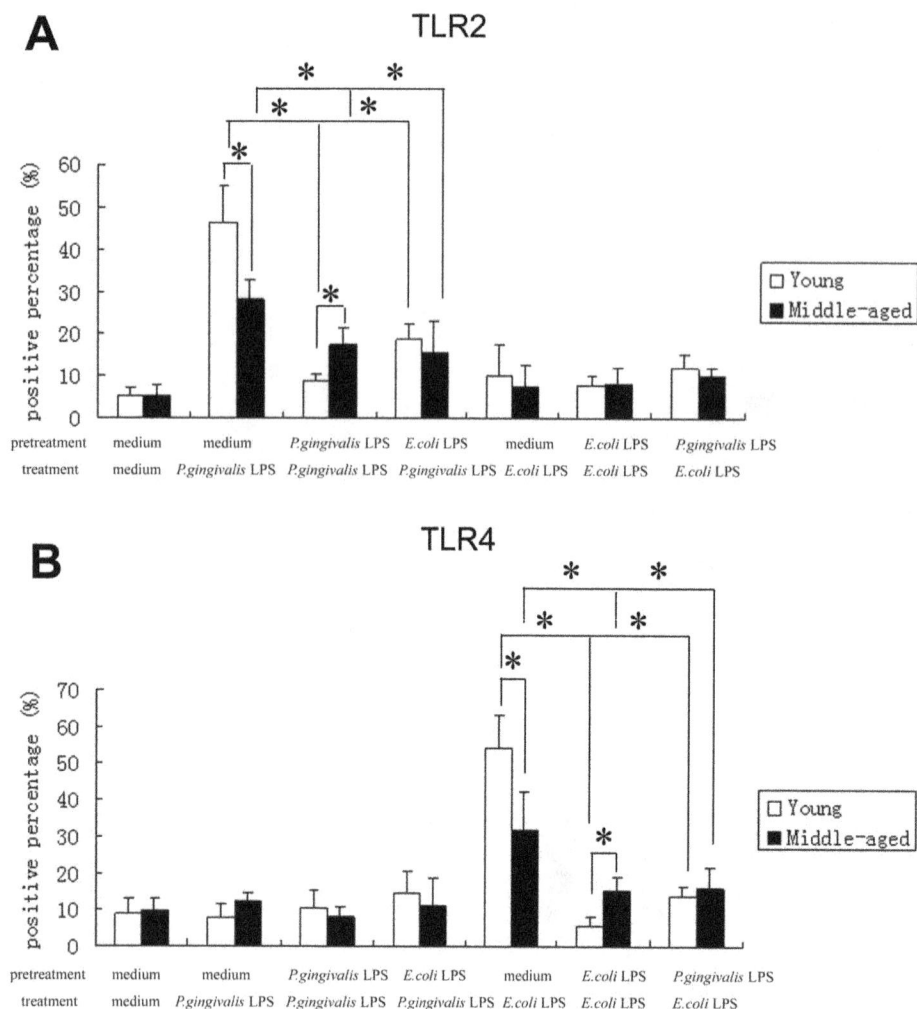

Figure 3. Protein expression changes of TLR2, 4 in peritoneal macrophages from young and middle-aged mice stimulated with LPS.
Peritoneal macrophages from both young and middle-aged mice were stimulated with medium or LPS as described in the legends to Figure 1. Flow cytometry was used to quantify TLR2 (4A) and TLR4 (4B) protein expression levels. Data are expressed as mean±SD (n=5 per group). *$P<0.05$.

the suppression of pro-inflammatory cytokine production in these cells [36,37]. Our research indicated the higher expression levels of IL-10 in peritoneal macrophages from young mice after second LPS challenges compared with those in middle-aged mice, which might be responsible for the more excellent ability to develop endotoxin tolerance in the younger.

Periodontitis is an inflammatory disease resulted from poly-infection and there are many other virulence factors in period-onpathic bacteria than LPS. Therefore, heterotolerance might be more universal than homotolerance in the developmemt of periodontitis. Our results indicated that the heterotolerance was much weaker than homotolerance at the levels of TNF-α, which was consistent with previous research partially [7], but the interesting finding was that there were no significant differences between homotolerance and heterotolerance at the levels of IL-10, which disclosed the complexity of reprogramming in endotoxin tolerance.

Another finding of our study was that there were no effects of aging on the expression levels of TLR2, 4 in murine peritoneal macrophages without any stimulation. Our results are consistent with some previous studies. In Murciano's researches, no significant differences between aged and young donors were

observed on cell surface TLR2, 4 and 6 expression on lymphocytes, monocytes and granulocytes [38]. Similar finding was also reported in paper concerning TLR4 expression on macrophages from older and younger mice [39]. In addition, the decreased secretions of TNF-α and IL-10 by peritoneal macro-phages from middle-aged mice stimulated with *E.coli* LPS or *P.gingivalis* LPS indicated the impaired functions of TLR2, 4 in these cells, which might be associated with the age-related changes in TLR2, 4 signaling transduction.

TLR2, 4 signaling pathway involves a cascade of intermediates, including myeloid differentiation factor-88 (MyD88), IL-1 re-ceptor-associated kinase (IRAK) and TNF receptor-associated factor-6 (TRAF-6). Signaling transduction triggered by TLR2, 4 ligands leads to the activation of two distinct signaling pathways. One pathway leads to the activation of activator protein-1 through mitogen-activated protein kinase (MAPK), and the other enhances the activity of inhibitor of nuclear factor-κB kinase complex, which induces the release of nuclear factor-κB (NF-κB) and the expression of cytokines and chemokines [40].

TLR2, 4 signaling transductions are so complicated that any signaling molecule in these pathways might have influences on the production of cytokines and chemokines. Therefore, it is

A pretreatment isotype / treatment medium
B medium / medium
C medium / P.gingivalis LPS
D P.gingivalis LPS / P.gingivalis LPS
E pretreatment E.coli LPS / treatment P.gingivalis LPS
F medium / E.coli LPS
G E.coli LPS / E.coli LPS
H P.gingivalis LPS / E.coli LPS
I pretreatment isotype / treatment
J medium / medium
K medium / P.gingivalis LPS
L P.gingivalis LPS / P.gingivalis LPS
M pretreatment E.coli LPS / treatment P.gingivalis LPS
N medium / E.coli LPS
O E.coli LPS / E.coli LPS
P P.gingivalis LPS / E.coli LPS

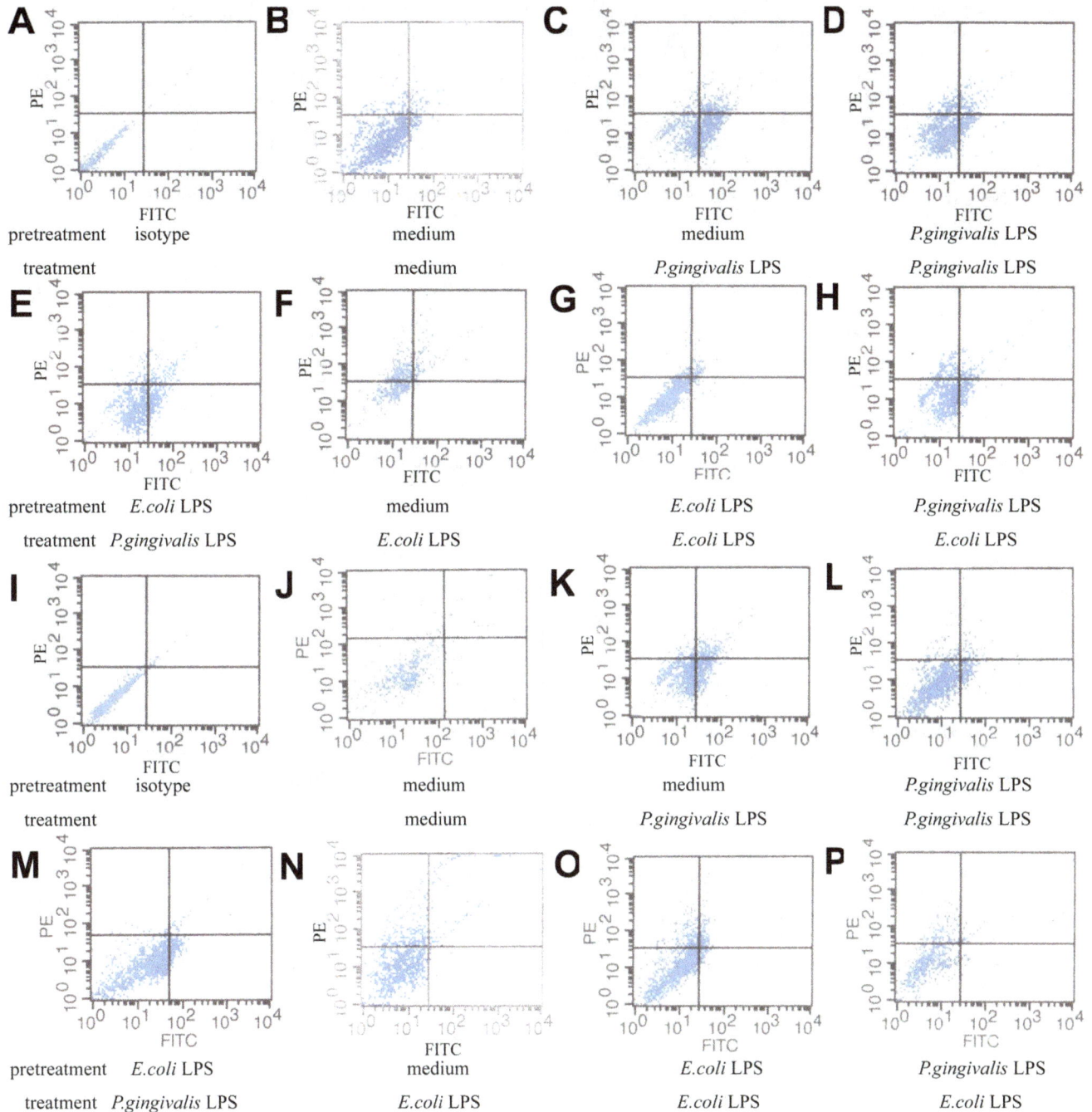

Figure 4. Protein expression of TLR2, 4 in peritoneal macrophages from young and middle-aged mice stimulated with LPS detected by flow cytometry. Peritoneal macrophages from both young (3A-3H) and middle-aged mice (3I-3P) were stimulated with medium or LPS as described in the legends to Figure 1. Protein expression levels of TLR2 (FITC-conjugated) and TLR4 (PE-conjugated) were detected by flow cytometry. One representative result of five independent experiments is shown.

hypothesized that there might be age-dependent changes in intermediates in TLR2, 4 signaling pathways, which might be associated with the differences in the function of TLR2, 4 between peritoneal macrophages from young and middle-aged mice. In an early research, Boehmer disclosed that levels of activated MAPKs did not differ by age in unstimulated macrophages, but LPS-stimulated macrophages from aged mice had <70% activated p38 and JNK than those of young controls, which might be related to the decreased production of proinflammatory cytokines, such as

TNF-α and IL-6, in old mice [39]. Several years later, a gene expression microarray study from Chelvarajan indicated that aging influenced several downstream signaling molecules. It was found in his study that in macrophages from old mice, MyD88 and TRAF6 gene expressions were decreased and the levels of NF-κB components, p50, p52 and p65, were also reduced. However, the gene expression levels of negative regulatory molecules, Toll-interleukin-1 receptor–associated-protein (TIRAP) and IRAK-M, were enhanced. These findings contributed to disclosing the molecular basis of cytokine dysregulation in aged mice [41]. Therefore, age-associated alterations in signaling pathways might be responsible for the age-related deterioration of TLR2, 4. In contrast to these studies, there were some other researchers who believed that aging critically impaired intrinsic adaptive T-cell function, but preserved TLR-mediated immune responses [42].

Based on these understandings, we attempted to further explore the involvement of TLR2, 4 in endotoxin tolerance. Our study disclosed the less decreased expressions of TLR2, 4 and proinflammatory cytokine and the less enhanced production of anti-inflammatory cytokine in peritoneal macrophages from middle-aged mice treated with the second LPS stimulation, which implied that TLR2, 4 might interfere with the ability of the host to develop endotoxin tolerance. Our results were consistent with some early researches. Wang and Kim indicated that pretreatment of monocytes/macrophages with LPS or the other virulence factors strongly inhibited TLR2 or 4 activation in response to subsequent stimulation, then they drew the conclusion that tolerance could develop through down-regulation of TLR2 or 4 expression [9,10].

Signaling through TLR2 and (or) 4 is one of the principal molecular mechanisms for the detection of gram-negative bacteria and their virulence factors by host cells. As discussed above, the effects of aging on TLR2, 4 signaling are so complicated that TLR2 and 4 are not the unique regulatory components that can modulate the development of endotoxin tolerance. Downstream signaling pathways and native cytokine profiles are also involved in the regulation of endotoxin tolerance. Recent in vitro studies have identified that impairment of IRAK activity and defects in the activation of MAPKs and NF-$_k$B were associated with endotoxin tolerance in mouse macrophages and human monocytes [43–45]. New insights into the regulation of inflammation also disclosed the molecular mechanism of endotoxin tolerance, which involved some novel signaling molecules, such as protein kinase R (PKR) and phosphatidylinositol-3′-kinase (PI3K) [46–48]. In addition, our study revealed that even if the heterotolerance was much weaker than homotolerance at the levels of TNF-α, the surface expressions of TLR2, 4 in heterotolerance were not always much higher than those in homotolerance in both age groups. Therefore, we presumed that the age-dependent changes in some other signaling molecules in TLR2, 4 signaling pathways might be associated with the impaired ability of the host to develop endotoxin tolerance and heterotolerance might develop through the regulation of the downstream signaling pathways other than down-regulation of TLR2, 4 expression.

Periodontal infections are polymicrobial in nature, and numerous virulence factors are involved in it. The effects and mechanisms of heterotolerance in periodontal tissues might be more complex than those in vitro. Up to now, most of the studies about endotoxin tolerance are in vitro. Even though there were some in vivo researches concerning homotolerance [49,50], reports on in vivo heterotolerance are very scarce and it is still not clear the effects of aging on endotoxin tolerance in vivo. Astiz's early research demonstrated the reduced concentrations of IL-6, IL-8 and TNF-α in normal human volunteers pretreated with lipid A and treated with E. coli LPS [51]. Several years later, Lehner developed a mice model challenged with LPS and restimulated with serovar Typhimurium. In his research, an attenuation of cytokine production (TNF-α, IFN-γ and IL-6) and an increased capacity to recruit neutrophilic granulocytes in tolerant mice were revealed [52]. However, the mechanisms of heterotolerance in vivo still need to be explored.

In summary, the present study showed that peritoneal macrophages from middle-aged mice were more sensitive to repeated LPS stimulations, and the impaired ability to develop endotoxin tolerance might be related to the less decreased expressions of TLR2, 4. The effects of aging on tolerance in vivo might be much complicated. Therefore, further investigations of different sensitivity between young and aged subjects to repeated bacteria exposure are necessary for a better understanding of immune mechanisms of periodontitis in older adults.

Materials and Methods

Ethics Statement

This study was approved by the Ethical Committee of Nanjing Medical University (Permit Number: 2010-018) and all experiments were performed in agreement with national regulations on animal welfare and animal experiments. All efforts were made to minimize suffering.

Animals

Young (2-month-old) and middle-aged (12-month-old) ICR mice were purchased from Vital River (Beijing, China) and maintained in an environmentally controlled facility at 21°C under a 12 h light : 12 h dark cycle.

Reagents

P. gingivalis ATCC 33277 LPS and E. coli O127:B8 LPS were purchased from Invivogen (CA, USA) and Sigma Aldrich (Missouri, USA) separately. ELISA kit was obtained from Biosource (CO, USA). SYBR Premix Ex Taq was purchased from Takara (Dalian, China), and FITC-conjugated anti-TLR2 antibodies, PE-conjugated anti-TLR4 antibodies, FITC-conjugated IgG2b isotype control and PE-conjugated IgG1 isotype control were obtained from eBioscience (CA, USA).

Cell Culture and LPS Stimulation

1.5 ml 4% thioglycollate broth (Sigma, USA) was injected intraperitoneally in ICR mice. Three days later, the mice were sacrificed. Peritoneal macrophages were isolated by lavage of the peritoneal cavity with cold phosphate-buffered saline (PBS) and collected by centrifugation. Cells were then cultured in RPMI 1640 (GIBCO, USA) supplemented with 10% fetal calf serum (Hyclone, USA) at a concentration of 2×10^6 cells/ml in 6-well plates. 2 h later, non-adherent cells were discarded. The remaining adherent cells were maintained in culture for 24 h until they were used for experiments [53].

Peritoneal macrophages from both young and middle-aged mice were divided into seven groups separately (n = 5 per group). Group 1 was cultured in medium alone. Groups 2 and 5 were treated with medium for 24 h, washed three times with fresh medium and stimulated with 1 µg/ml P. gingivalis LPS or 1 µg/ml E. coli LPS respectively for 6 h to determine TLR2, 4 mRNA or 24 h for analysis of TLR2, 4 proteins and cytokines. Group 3, 4, 6 and 7 were incubated for 24 h with an initial LPS challenge (1 µg/ml P. gingivalis LPS？or 1 µg/ml E. coli LPS), washed, and then restimulated with either 1 µg/ml P. gingivalis LPS or 1 µg/ml E. coli LPS for the subsequent detections as described in group 2 and 5. All cells were washed three times with cold PBS and collected for real-time PCR and flow cytometry analysis. Cell-free supernatants were harvested and stored at −20°C for cytokine assays.

Cytokine Detection

Cytokine levels (TNF-α and IL-10) in the culture supernatants were measured by ELISA according to the manufacturer's instruction. The plates were read in an ELISA-reader (Bio-Hit, Helsinki, Finland) at 490 nm.

Real-time PCR

Total RNA was prepared from peritoneal macrophages, which were stimulated with LPS or medium. cDNA was synthesized using a reverse transcription kit (Takara, China). Levels of ß-actin mRNA served as internal controls. The primer sequences were as follows (F/R): TLR2 (GAGTCAGACGTAGTGAGCA/AGTGTTCCTGCTGATGTCAAG); TLR4 (GCAGCAGGTG-GAATTGTATC/TGTTCTCCTCTGCTGTTTG); and ß-actin (GCTACAGCTTCACCACCACAG/GGTCTTTACG-GATGTCAACGTC).

Real-time PCR analysis was performed in duplicates in an ABI PRISM 7300 Real-Time PCR System (Applied Biosystems, USA). The reaction product was quantified by the standard curve method [54]. A standard curve with predetermined concentrations and serial diluted respective PCR amplification products from 1×10^{-1} to 1×10^{-10} was constructed for each transcript analyzed.

Flow Cytometry

Peritoneal macrophages were scraped off from 6-well plates and washed in washing buffer (PBS containing 1% fetal calf serum). To analyze TLR2, 4 surface expressions, cells were incubated with FITC-conjugated anti-TLR2 antibodies and PE-conjugated anti-TLR4 antibodies for 30 min at 4°C in the dark. Corresponding isotypes to the above antibodies, conjugated to the appropriate fluorochromes, were used as controls for nonspecific binding of antibodies. After this incubation, cells were washed twice in washing buffer and then fixed in 1% formalin in PBS [55]. Expressions of TLR2, 4 on 10,000 viable cells were then gated and analyzed by a FACSCalibur (BD Biosciences,USA).

Statistical Analysis

Statistical analysis of ELISA data was performed using ANOVA and Dunnett's T3 test was used to compare differences between groups. The data of real-time PCR and flow cytometry were analyzed using the Kruskal–Wallis test, and subsequently the Mann–Whitney test was performed as a post-hoc test. All data are presented as means±SD. The level of significance was set at $p < 0.05$.

Acknowledgments

The authors thank Mrs Ling Wang, Zi-Lu Wang and Yang-Yu Zheng for their excellent technical assistance.

Author Contributions

Conceived and designed the experiments: YS YX. Performed the experiments: YS HL MFY MJS. Analyzed the data: YS HL WS YX. Contributed reagents/materials/analysis tools: YS HL MFY MJS. Wrote the paper: YS YX.

References

1. Oliver RC, Brown LJ, Loe H (1998) Periodontal diseases in the United States population. J Periodontol 69: 9–13.
2. Braga RR, Carvalho MA, Bruña-Romero O, Teixeira RE, Costa JE, et al. (2010) Quantification of five putative periodontal pathogens in female patients with and without chronic periodontitis by real-time polymerase chain reaction. Anaerobe 16: 234–239.
3. Komiya Ito A, Ishihara K, Tomita S, Kato T, Yamada S (2010) Investigation of subgingival profile of periodontopathic bacteria using polymerase chain reaction. Bull Tokyo Dent Coll 51: 139–144.
4. Cardoso CR, Garlet GP, Moreira AP, Júnior WM, Rossi MA, et al. (2008) Characterization of CD4+CD25+ natural regulatory T cells in the inflammatory infiltrate of human chronic periodontitis. J Leukoc Biol 84: 311–318.
5. Garlet GP (2010) Destructive and protective roles of cytokines in periodontitis: a re-appraisal from host defense and tissue destruction viewpoints. J Dent Res 89: 1349–1363.
6. Parker LC, Jones EC, Prince LR, Dower SK, Whyte MK, et al. (2005) Endotoxin tolerance induces selective alterations in neutrophil function. Leukoc Biol 78: 1301–1305.
7. Dobrovolskaia MA, Medvedev AE, Thomas KE, Cuesta N, Toshchakov V, et al. (2003) Induction of in vitro reprogramming by Toll-like receptor (TLR)2 and TLR4 agonists in murine macrophages: effects of TLR "homotolerance" versus "heterotolerance" on NF-kappa B signaling pathway components. J Immunol 170: 508–519.
8. Melo ES, Barbeiro DF, Gorjão R, Rios EC, Vasconcelos D, et al. (2010) Gene expression reprogramming protects macrophage from septic-induced cell death. Mol Immunol 47: 2587–2593.
9. Wang JH, Doyle M, Manning BJ, Di Wu Q, Blankson S, et al. (2002) Induction of bacterial lipoprotein tolerance is associated with suppression of toll-like receptor 2 expression. J Biol Chem 277: 36068–36075.
10. Kim HG, Kim NR, Gim MG, Lee JM, Lee SY, et al. (2008) Lipoteichoic acid isolated from Lactobacillus plantarum inhibits lipopolysaccharide-induced TNF-alpha production in THP-1 cells and endotoxin shock in mice. J Immunol 180: 2553–2561.
11. Medzhitov R, Preston-Hurlburt P, Janeway CA Jr (1997) A human homologue of the Drosophila Toll protein signals activation of adaptive immunity. Nature 388: 394–397.
12. Suzuki T, Kobayashi M, Isatsu K, Nishihara T, Aiuchi T, et al. (2007) Mechanisms involved in apoptosis of human macrophages induced by lipopolysaccharide from Actinobacillus actinomycetemcomitans in the presence of cycloheximide. Infect Immun 72: 1856–1865.
13. Gaddis DE, Michalek SM, Katz J (2009) Requirement of TLR4 and CD14 in dendritic cell activation by Hemagglutinin B from Porphyromonas gingivalis. Mol Immunol 46: 2493–2504.
14. Gelani V, Fernandes AP, Gasparoto TH, Garlet TP, Cestari TM, et al. (2009) The role of toll-like receptor 2 in the recognition of Aggregatibacter actinomyce-temcomitans. J Periodontol 80: 2010–2019.
15. Beck JD, Lainson PA, Field HM, Hawkins BF (1984) Risk factors for various levels of periodontal disease and treatment needs in Iowa. Community Dent Oral Epidemiol 12: 17–22.
16. Krustrup U, Erik Petersen P (2006) Periodontal conditions in 35–44 and 65–74-year-old adults in Denmark. Acta Odontol Scand 64: 65–73.
17. Miller RA (1996) The aging immune system: primer and prospectus. Science 273: 70–74.
18. Goldstein DR (2010) Aging, imbalanced inflammation and viral infection. Virulence 1: 295–298.
19. Grubeck-Loebenstein B, Wick G (2002) The aging of the immune system. Adv Immunol 80: 243–284.
20. Plackett TP, Boehmer ED, Faunce DE, Kovacs EJ (2004) Aging and innate immune cells. J Leukoc Biol 76: 291–299.
21. Desai A, Grolleau-Julius A, Yung R (2010) Leukocyte function in the aging immune system. J Leukoc Biol 87: 1001–1009.
22. Mahbub S, Brubaker AL, Kovacs EJ (2011) Aging of the Innate Immune System: An Update. Curr Immunol Rev 7: 104–115.
23. Teng YT (2006) Protective and Destructive Immunity in the Periodontium: Part 1–Innate and Humoral Immunity and the Periodontium. J Dent Res 85: 198–208.
24. Nussbaum G, Ben-Adi S, Genzler T, Sela M, Rosen G (2009) Involvement of Toll-like receptors 2 and 4 in the innate immune response to Treponema denticola and its outer sheath components. Infect Immun 77: 3939–3947.
25. Sato S, Takeuchi O, Fujita T, Tomizawa H, Takeda K, et al. (2002) A variety of microbial components induce tolerance to lipopolysaccharide by differentially affecting MyD88-dependent and -independent pathways. Int Immunol 14: 783–791.
26. Haffajee AD, Socransky SS (1994) Microbial etiological agents of destructive periodontal diseases. Periodontol 2000 5: 78–111.
27. Roberts HC, Moseley R, Sloan AJ, Youde SJ, Waddington RJ (2008) Lipopolysaccharide alters decorin and biglycan synthesis in rat alveolar bone osteoblasts: consequences for bone repair during periodontal disease. Eur J Oral Sci 116: 207–216.
28. Sun Y, Shu R, Li CL, Zhang MZ (2010) Gram-negative Periodontal Bacteria Induce the Activation of Toll-like Receptor 2, 4 and Cytokine Production in Human Periodontal Ligament Cells. J Periodontol 81: 1488–1496.
29. Broad A, Jones DE, Kirby JA (2006) Toll-like receptor (TLR) response tolerance: a key physiological "damage limitation" effect and an important potential opportunity for therapy. Curr Med Chem. 13: 2487–2502.
30. Beck JD, Lainson PA, Field HM, Hawkins BF (1984) Risk factors for various levels of periodontal disease and treatment needs in Iowa. Community Dent Oral Epidemiol 12: 17–22.
31. Krustrup U, Erik Petersen P (2006) Periodontal conditions in 35–44 and 65–74-year-old adults in Denmark. Acta Odontol Scand 64: 65–73.
32. Yoshimura A, Hara Y, Kaneko T, Kato I (1997) Secretion of IL-1 beta, TNF-alpha, IL-8 and IL-1ra by human polymorphonuclear leukocytes in response to

lipopolysaccharides from periodontopathic bacteria. J Periodontal Res 32: 279–286.

33. Gutiérrez-Venegas G, Kawasaki-Cárdenas P, Cruz-Arroyo SR, Pérez-Garzón M, Maldonado-Frías S (2006) *Actinobacillus actinomycetemcomitans* lipopolysaccharide stimulates the phosphorylation of p44 and p42 MAP kinases through CD14 and TLR-4 receptor activation in human gingival fibroblasts. Life Sci 78: 2577–2583.

34. Netea MG, van Deuren M, Kullberg BJ, Cavaillon JM, Van der Meer JW (2002) Does the shape of lipid A determine the interaction of LPS with Toll-like receptors? Tends Immunol 23: 135–139.

35. Barksby HE, Nile CJ, Jaedicke KM, Taylor JJ, Preshaw PM (2009) Differential expression of immunoregulatory genes in monocytes in response to *Porphyromonas gingivalis* and *Escherichia coli* lipopolysaccharide. Clin Exp Immunol 156: 479–487.

36. Schröder M, Meisel C, Buhl K, Profanter N, Sievert N, et al. (2003) Different modes of IL-10 and TGF-beta to inhibit cytokine-dependent IFN-gamma production: consequences for reversal of lipopolysaccharide desensitization. J Immunol 170: 5260–5267.

37. Chang J, Kunkel SL, Chang CH (2009) Negative regulation of MyD88-dependent signaling by IL-10 in dendritic cells. Proc Natl Acad Sci U S A 106: 18327–18332.

38. Murciano C, Villamón E, Yáñez A, Murciano J, Mir A, et al. (2007) In vitro response to *Candida albicans* in cultures of whole human blood from young and aged donors. FEMS Immunol Med Microbiol 51: 327–335.

39. Boehmer ED, Goral J, Faunce DE, Kovacs EJ (2004) Age-dependent decrease in Toll-like receptor 4-mediated proinflammatory cytokine production and mitogen-activated protein kinase expression. J Leukoc Biol 75: 342–349.

40. Mahanonda R, Pichyangkul S (2007) Toll-like receptors and their role in periodontal health and disease. Periodontol 2000 43: 41–55.

41. Chelvarajan RL, Liu Y, Popa D, Getchell ML, Getchell TV, et al. (2006) Molecular basis of age-associated cytokine dysregulation in LPS-stimulated macrophages. J Leukoc Biol 79: 1314–1327.

42. Tesar BM, Walker WE, Unternaehrer J, Joshi NS, Chandele A, et al. (2006) Murine [corrected] myeloid dendritic cell-dependent toll-like receptor immunity is preserved with aging. Aging Cell 5: 473–486.

43. Biswas SK, Tergaonkar V (2007) Myeloid differentiation factor 88-independent Toll-like receptor pathway: Sustaining inflammation or promoting tolerance? Int J Biochem Cell Biol 39: 1582–1592.

44. Ben-Othman R, Dellagi K, Guizani-Tabbane L (2009) Leishmania major parasites induced macrophage tolerance: implication of MAPK and NF-kappaB pathways. Mol Immunol 46: 3438–3444.

45. De Nardo D, Nguyen T, Hamilton JA, Scholz GM (2009) Down-regulation of IRAK-4 is a component of LPS- and CpG DNA-induced tolerance in macrophages. Cell Signal 21: 246–252.

46. Perkins DJ, Qureshi N, Vogel SN (2010) A Toll-like receptor-responsive kinase, protein kinase R, is inactivated in endotoxin tolerance through differential K63/K48 ubiquitination. MBio 1: pii: e00239-10.

47. Pan H, Ding E, Hu M, Lagoo AS, Datto MB, et al. (2010) SMAD4 is required for development of maximal endotoxin tolerance. J Immunol 184: 5502–5509.

48. Yang Q, Calvano SE, Lowry SF, Androulakis IP (2011) A dual negative regulation model of Toll-like receptor 4 signaling for endotoxin preconditioning in human endotoxemia. Math Biosci 232: 151–163.

49. Qu J, Zhang J, Pan J, He L, Ou Z, et al. (2003) Endotoxin tolerance inhibits lipopolysaccharide-initiated acute pulmonary inflammation and lung injury in rats by the mechanism of nuclear factor-kappaB. Scand J Immunol 58: 613–619.

50. Zhang J, Qu JM, He LX (2009) IL-12 suppression, enhanced endocytosis and up-regulation of MHC-II and CD80 in dendritic cells during experimental endotoxin tolerance. Acta Pharmacol Sin 30: 582–588.

51. Astiz ME, Rackow EC, Still JG, Howell ST, Cato A, et al. (1995) Pretreatment of normal humans with monophosphoryl lipid A induces tolerance to endotoxin: a prospective, double-blind, randomized, controlled trial. Crit Care Med 23: 9–17.

52. Lehner MD, Ittner J, Bundschuh DS, van Rooijen N, Wendel A, et al. (2001) Improved innate immunity of endotoxin-tolerant mice increases resistance to Salmonella enterica serovar typhimurium infection despite attenuated cytokine response. Infect Immun 69: 463–471.

53. da Silva PT, Pappen FG, Souza EM, Dias JE, Bonetti Filho I, et al. (2008) Cytotoxicity evaluation of four endodontic sealers. Braz Dent J 19: 228–231.

54. Sun Y, Guo QM, Liu DL, Zhang MZ, Shu R (2010) In vivo expression of Toll-like receptor 2, Toll-like receptor 4, CSF2 and LY64 in Chinese chronic periodontitis patients. Oral Dis 16: 343–350.

55. Liu QY, Yao YM, Zhang SW, Yan YH, Wu X (2011) Naturally existing CD11c(low)CD45RB(high) dendritic cells protect mice from acute severe inflammatory response induced by thermal injury. Immunobiology 216: 47–53.

14

Phosphorylated Dihydroceramides from Common Human Bacteria Are Recovered in Human Tissues

Frank C. Nichols[1]*, Xudong Yao[2], Bekim Bajrami[2], Julia Downes[3], Sydney M. Finegold[3], Erica Knee[1], James J. Gallagher[4,5], William J. Housley[6], Robert B. Clark[6]

1 Department of Oral Health and Diagnostic Sciences, University of Connecticut School of Dental Medicine, Farmington, Connecticut, United States of America, **2** Department of Chemistry, University of Connecticut, Storrs, Connecticut, United States of America, **3** Division of Infectious Diseases, VA Greater Los Angeles Healthcare System, Los Angeles, California, United States of America, **4** Department of Surgery, University of Connecticut School of Medicine, Farmington, Connecticut, United States of America, **5** Connecticut Vascular Institute, Hartford, Connecticut, United States of America, **6** Departments of Immunology and Medicine, School of Medicine, University of Connecticut, Farmington, Connecticut, United States of America

Abstract

Novel phosphorylated dihydroceramide (PDHC) lipids produced by the periodontal pathogen *Porphyromonas gingivalis* include phosphoethanolamine (PE DHC) and phosphoglycerol dihydroceramides (PG DHC) lipids. These PDHC lipids mediate cellular effects through Toll-like receptor 2 (TLR2) including promotion of IL-6 secretion from dendritic cells and inhibition of osteoblast differentiation and function *in vitro* and *in vivo*. The PE DHC lipids also enhance (TLR2)-dependent murine experimental autoimmune encephalomyelitis (EAE), a model for multiple sclerosis. The unique non-mammalian structures of these lipids allows for their specific quantification in bacteria and human tissues using multiple reaction monitoring (MRM)-mass spectrometry (MS). Synthesis of these lipids by other common human bacteria and the presence of these lipids in human tissues have not yet been determined. We now report that synthesis of these lipids can be attributed to a small number of intestinal and oral organisms within the *Bacteroides*, *Parabacteroides*, *Prevotella*, *Tannerella* and *Porphyromonas* genera. Additionally, the PDHCs are not only present in gingival tissues, but are also present in human blood, vasculature tissues and brain. Finally, the distribution of these TLR2-activating lipids in human tissues varies with both the tissue site and disease status of the tissue suggesting a role for PDHCs in human disease.

Editor: Olivier Neyrolles, Institut de Pharmacologie et de Biologie Structurale, France

Funding: This work was supported by a grant from the National Multiple Sclerosis Society (RG4070-A-6). The funders had no role in study design, data collection and analysis, decision to publish, or preparation of the manuscript.

Competing Interests: The authors have declared that no competing interests exist.

* E-mail: nichols@nso.uchc

Introduction

Porphyromonas gingivalis is a periodontal pathogen strongly associated with development of destructive periodontal disease in adults. We have recently characterized the structures of novel phosphorylated dihydroceramide (PDHC) lipids produced by this organism [1]. PDHCs include both low mass (LM) and high mass (HM) forms of phosphoglycerol dihydroceramide (PG DHC) and phosphoethanolamine dihydroceramide (PE DHC) lipids. These lipids have unique non-mammalian structures [1] which allow for their specific quantification in bacteria and human tissues using multiple reaction monitoring (MRM)-mass spectrometry (MS). These PDHC lipids are important because of their capacity to engage Toll-like receptor 2 (TLR2) resulting in dendritic cell secretion of IL-6 [2] and inhibition of osteoblast differentiation and function [3]. In addition, we have shown that the PG DHC lipids markedly stimulate proinflammatory secretory responses in human gingival fibroblasts [1] and the PE DHC lipids enhance murine experimental autoimmune encephalomyelitis (EAE), a model for multiple sclerosis [2]. Others have shown that these lipids promote apoptosis in HUVEC cells in culture through activation of caspases 3, 6 and 9 [4]. In these previously reported studies, the PDHC lipid classes were isolated only from *P. gingivalis*. Little is known regarding the capacity of other common human

bacteria to produce these lipids and most importantly, whether these lipids can be identified in human tissues distant from sites normally colonized by these bacteria. Therefore, the purpose of this investigation was to evaluate intestinal bacterial species as well as other periodontal organisms for their capacity to produce PDHCs and to examine blood and human tissue samples for the presence of these novel TLR2-activating bacterial lipids.

Results

We analyzed lipid extracts derived from greater than 240 individual human isolates representing over 90 intestinal bacterial species. Of the intestinal bacterial species evaluated, only approximately 5% produced PDHCs. Furthermore, only intestinal organisms of the *Bacteroides*, *Parabacteroides* or *Prevotella* genera produced PDHCs and of these, most produced predominantly PE DHC lipids (see Table S1 for the data set). Furthermore, the predominant PE DHC lipids produced by these intestinal organisms were usually the LM PE DHC form (see Figure 1 for lipid structures and Figure 2A for recovery of these lipids in intestinal and oral bacteria). Of the intestinal bacteria examined, only *Parabacteroides distasonis* and *Parabacteroides merdea* produced the PG DHC lipids, with *P. distasonis* producing primarily LM PG DHCs and *P. merdea* producing primarily HM PG DHCs

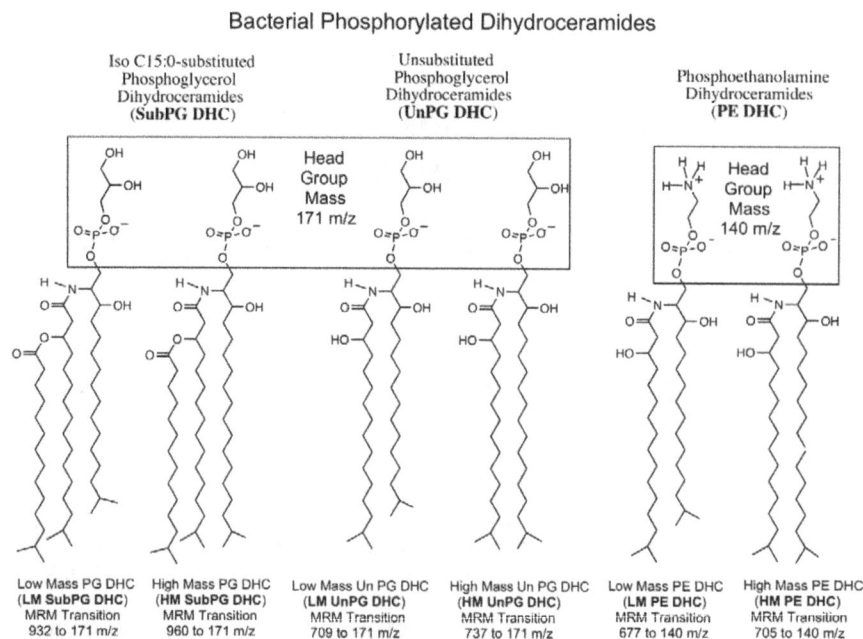

Figure 1. Structures of bacterial phosphorylated dihydroceramides (PDHC) lipids. Each lipid species was quantified using multiple reaction monitoring (MRM) mass spectrometry, via monitoring an MRM transition from the precursor lipid ion to the phosphorylated head group fragment ion generated upon collision-induced dissociation. The structures of low and high mass PDHC lipids are based on previously published reports [1,5]. Though PG DHC and PE DHC lipids normally exist in high, medium and low masses, we elected to quantify only the high and low mass products because these vary most strongly between different bacterial species.

(Figure 2A). We also examined lipid extracts from three bacterial species known to be associated with inflammatory periodontal disease in humans including *Porphyromonas gingivalis*, *Tannerella forsythia* and *Prevotella intermedia*. Figure 2A shows that these species vary in their capacity to produce either PE DHC or PG DHC lipids and also vary in their production of the HM versus the LM forms of these PDHCs. For example, the PDHC lipid constituents produced by *P. gingivalis* are predominantly HM PE DHC lipids whereas *T. forsythia* produces primarily LM PG DHC forms. Though individual intestinal and oral organisms vary in their capacity to produce specific PDHC lipids, combinations of these organisms also have the potential to deposit unique mixtures of PDHCs in human tissues and blood.

We next quantified bacterial PDHCs in human blood and tissue samples (see Table S2 for the data set). We examined blood plasma samples from periodontally healthy subjects, blood plasma samples from subjects with generalized severe destructive periodontal disease (chronic periodontitis), subgingival microbial plaque samples, and normal human brain samples. For carotid endarterectomy samples, we excised the patent segment of the common carotid artery (control samples) from the grossly apparent atheroma of the carotid body and quantified PDHCs within the lipid extracts of these paired carotid samples. The patent carotid artery samples showed no apparent gross atheroma formation though these artery segments usually were variably but significantly calcified within the artery wall.

We observed deposition of PDHCs in all of the human tissues examined, but the distribution of PDHCs in these tissues showed distinctive patterns. While the PDHCs derived directly from bacterial samples tended to contain primarily either HM or LM PDHCs, PDHC lipids in human tissue samples showed a mixture of HM and LM forms suggesting a heterogenous bacterial source (see Figure 2B). Nevertheless, tissue-associated patterns described below suggest that it may be possible to attribute a relatively specific distribution of bacterial PDHCs to various human tissues in health and in disease.

PG DHC lipids (both the HM and LM forms) can exist with three aliphatic chains (the substituted or "Sub" form) or can be de-esterified to a lipid class with 2 aliphatic chains (the unsubstituted or "Un" form) [1,5]. We next compared the de-esterification status of the PG DHCs derived from bacteria with the PG DHCs derived from human tissue samples. Of the intestinal and periodontal organisms observed to produce PG DHCs, only *P. merdea* produced a small amount of the UnPG DHC lipids (<10% of total PDHC), whereas the remaining intestinal and oral bacteria produced negligible amounts of UnPG DHC lipids (Figure 2A).

In contrast, human tissue samples revealed significant percentages of both LM or HM UnPG DHC lipids (Figure 2B and Figure 3). We next examined blood plasma samples from periodontally healthy subjects and subjects with chronic periodontitis, and found that both revealed substantial percentages of both LM and HM UnPG DHC lipids (Figure 2B and Figure 3). In evaluating PG DHC de-esterification in atherosclerosis, we found that the lipid extracts from atheroma artery segments revealed significantly higher percentages of HM or LM UnPG DHC when compared with the control artery extracts. This suggests that atheroma formation is associated with greater de-esterification of deposited SubPG DHC lipids.

Of note, the average total ion abundances of PDHC lipids per microgram of total lipid extract were at least 33 times higher in the control artery segments than the atheroma segments (see Table S3 for the data set). In fact, the highest levels of PDHC lipids in lipid extracts from human tissue samples were observed in control artery segments, not gingival tissue samples from periodontal disease sites. The average levels of HM PE DHC and LM PE DHC lipids were at least 44 times higher in the control artery segments than the atheroma segments. This observation suggests that the vascular system proximal to (or upstream from) the site of atheroma formation is heavily contaminated with PDHC lipids. Since the control artery segments demonstrated variable degrees of

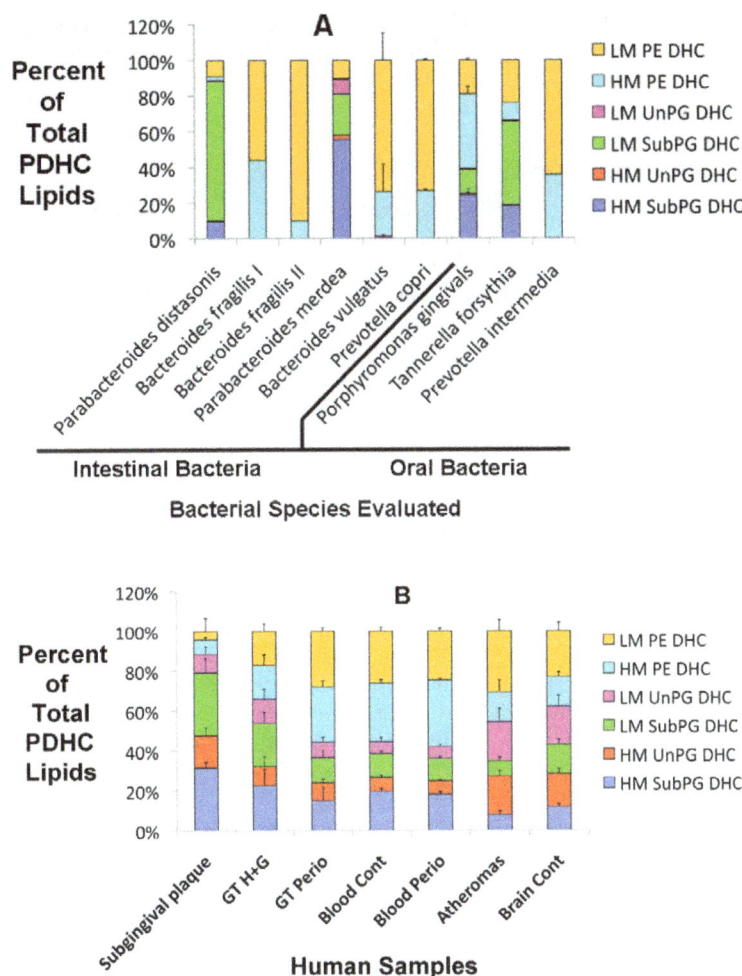

Figure 2. Recovery of bacterial phosphorylated dihydroceramides in intestinal and oral bacteria, subgingival plaque samples, blood plasma, atheroma and brain samples. Individual bacterial, blood and tissue samples were processed as described in the Methods section. The ion abundances of high and low mass PDHC lipid classes were summed and the recovery of each lipid class is depicted as the percent of the total ion abundance of the quantified PDHC lipids. Standard deviation bars are shown for lipid extracts from *Bacteroides vulgatus* (n = 13), *Prevotella copri* (n = 2), *Porphyromonas gingivalis* (n = 6), subgingival plaque (n = 2), healthy/mildly inflamed gingival tissue (GT H+G, n = 7), periodontitis gingival tissue samples (GT Perio, n = 6), control blood plasma (Blood Cont, n = 8), blood plasma from patients with generalized severe periodontitis (Blood Perio, n = 6), carotid atheroma (Atheroma, n = 11) and brain samples from deceased, neurologically-normal subjects (Brain Control, n = 14). Recovery of each lipid class is depicted as percent of the total PDHC ion recovery. Two-factor ANOVA indicated significant differences between categories of human samples. Comparison of PDHC lipid distributions in healthy/mildly inflamed versus periodontitis gingival tissue samples revealed significant differences for the percentage of HM SubPG DHC lipids, LM UnPG DHC lipids, LM PE DHC lipids.

mineralization based on the resistance to sectioning with a scalpel, the possibility exists that the elevated bacterial lipid accumulation is related to the process of mineralization in arterial walls without grossly evident atheroma development. The reduced levels of bacterial lipids in the atheroma lipid extracts compared to control carotid lipid extracts is probably accounted for by the overwhelming accumulation of cholesterol and cholesterol esters that are known to accompany atheroma formation. It is also possible that substantial cholesterol accumulation during atheroma formation could either prevent bacterial lipid accumulation in arterial walls or cause release of bacterial lipids from artery walls. These possibilities will be the subject of future research.

Lipid extracts of brain samples showed a mean percentage of UnPG DHC lipids comparable to or higher than those observed in carotid atheromas. In contrast, subgingival microbial plaque samples taken from gingival crevices at periodontitis sites showed only minimal levels of UnPG DHC. Subgingival plaque samples

are known to contain microbial organisms as well as desquamated epithelial cells and inflammatory cells, and this combination apparently possesses the capability to partially de-esterify PG DHC lipids. These results suggest that metabolic conversion of the SubPG DHC lipids to the UnPG DHC lipids, while not occurring in the relevant bacteria, occurs both in blood and in some but not all human tissues. The percentage of UnPG DHC lipids in blood plasma samples compared with that in patent arterial samples and paired atheroma samples further suggests that the UnPG DHC lipids are not simply transported from blood to all tissues but may undergo specific metabolic conversion within certain tissues. Importantly, the biological properties of the SubPG DHC versus the UnPG DHC lipids remain to be evaluated.

We next compared the distribution of PDHC lipids in gingival tissue samples excised either from healthy/mildly inflamed or destructive periodontal disease (periodontitis) sites. We also evaluated blood plasma samples taken from periodontally healthy

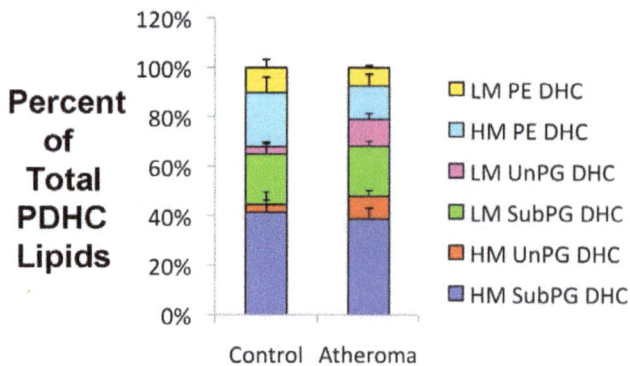

Figure 3. Recovery of bacterial phosphorylated dihydrocer-amides in paired patent artery and atheroma samples. For each carotid endarterectomy sample, the patent artery segment of the proximal common carotid artery was excised from the grossly evident atheroma located within the carotid sinus. The paired tissue samples were separately extracted for lipids as described in the Methods. A defined amount (approximately 3 µg of total lipids in 5 µl of HPLC solvent) of each lipid extract was analyzed by MRM-MS and the recovery of each lipid class is depicted as the percent of the total ion abundance of the quantified PDHC lipids. The percentages of PDHC lipids are depicted (means and standard errors) for five paired control and atheroma lipid extracts. Significant differences between control versus atheroma lipid extracts were shown only for the percentages of HM UnPG DHC and LM UnPG DHC lipids ($p = 0.0144$ and $p = 0.0258$, respectively, by paired t test). Though not shown, the mean abundances of PDHC ions per µg of total lipid extract were at least 33 times higher for the control artery samples compared with the atheroma samples.

subjects or subjects with destructive periodontal disease. Two-factor ANOVA revealed significantly lower percentages of HM and LM SubPG DHC lipids and significantly higher percentages of HM and LM PE DHC lipids in periodontitis gingival tissue samples versus healthy samples (Figure 2B). Similarly, blood plasma samples demonstrated a significant increase in the percentage of HM PE DHC lipids in periodontitis plasma versus healthy plasma samples (though SubPG DHC percentages were not lower in plasma samples from periodontitis patients).

For quantification of absolute PDHC lipid levels in control and periodontitis gingival tissue samples, each tissue lipid extract was supplemented with 1.5 µg of synthetic phospholipid internal standard before analysis by MRM/MS. This analysis revealed that lipid extracts of periodontitis tissue samples contained significantly higher mean levels of HM PE DHC and LM PE DHC lipids than that recovered in healthy gingival tissue samples ($p = 0.0062$ and $p = 0.0056$, respectively, by one factor ANOVA, see Table S2). However, all other PDHC lipids were not significantly altered between periodontitis and healthy gingival tissue samples. Therefore, we now show that shifts in the deposition of specific bacterial lipids (PE DHCs) in gingival tissues is directly correlated with expression of destructive periodontal disease and that this specific increase in PE DHC is also reflected in blood plasma levels. Given that we have demonstrated that PE DHC can enhance murine autoimmunity [2], these results further suggest both a pro-inflammatory and tissue destructive role for PE DHC lipids and show that the absolute amount of PE DHC lipids in gingival tissues could be an important bacterial marker for expression of destructive periodontal disease in humans.

Overall, our findings indicate that human periodontal bacteria and a small percentage of human intestinal bacterial produce PDHC lipids, that these bacteria differ in the specific forms of PDHCs they produce, that PDHCs accumulate in numerous human tissues, and that the pattern of deposition varies not only among the tissue sites involved but also with the state of inflammation in those sites.

Discussion

We have recently demonstrated that unique bacterially-derived lipids, termed PDHC lipids, promote cell activation through TLR2 [2,3]. We now report that these bacterial lipids are recovered in human tissue samples and blood, making it plausible that PDHCs play a role in disease via acute and chronic activation of the immune system. The varying percentages of PDHC lipid species observed in either periodontal or intestinal bacterial species suggests that a mixture of bacterial species normally account for the overall blood and tissue deposition of these novel lipid classes. The fact that bacterial lipids are prevalent in patent artery segments suggests significant systemic exposure to these lipids. This may occur through release of PDHCs upon bacterial death, phagocytic engulfment of the PDHC-producing bacteria at their sites of origin, and/or through intermittent bacteremias. Recent studies have demonstrated that soluble bacterial peptidoglycan originating from the intestinal microflora can be recovered in the circulation and can subsequently prime neutrophils in bone marrow [6,7]. Furthermore, ^{13}C-labeled bacterial dihydrocera-mides ingested by experimental animals were shown to be distributed in skin, liver, skeletal muscle and brain, and a portion of the bacterial dihydroceramides were metabolized in liver to ceramides [8]. Therefore, our results demonstrating bacterial PDHC lipids in human tissues and de-esterification of SubPG DHC lipids in blood and tissues are consistent with these previous reports. That bacterial PDHC lipids are known to engage TLR2 in promoting cell activation of dendritic cells, macrophages or osteoblasts [2,3] and are prevalent even in patent artery segments, raises the possibility that bacterial lipid deposition predisposes major arteries to the development of atherosclerosis. Furthermore, the relative predominance of PDHC lipids in control vessels suggests that bacterial lipid accumulation in the vasculature occurs before the majority of cholesterol and other mammalian lipids accumulate within atheromas. Whether blood and tissue PDHCs demonstrate transient variation in levels or fractional compositions and whether such variations correlate with inflammatory or other human diseases remains to be clarified.

We have demonstrated that PDHCs can promote autoimmune disease in mice and that this process is dependent on expression of TLR2 [2]. The role of the intestinal flora in both gastrointestinal and systemic immune activation has received considerable attention [9,10,11,12,13,14]. We postulate that the intestinal and perhaps periodontal microbial production of PDHC lipids may also play a role in both the systemic immune homeostasis of the host and in disease mechanisms. For example, the relationship between severity of periodontal disease and rheumatoid arthritis [15,16,17,18,19] may relate to immune cell exposure to these lipids either systemically or through the direct deposition of these bacterial lipids in synovial sites.

Overall, our present findings provide a compelling rationale for future studies investigating the relationship between bacterial colonization of oral and intestinal sites, tissue deposition of PDHC lipids and the capacity of these uniquely structured, TLR2-activating lipids to promote human disease.

Materials and Methods

For research involving human participants, written informed consent was obtained. The University of Connecticut Health

Center Institutional Review Board specifically approved the human subject components of this study. Human atheroma, blood and plaque samples were stored frozen ($-20°C$) until the time of lipid extraction. Human brain specimens were obtained as postmortem samples from the Colorado Brain Bank, Denver, CO.

Intestinal bacterial samples that were previously stored frozen were grown on blood agar plates after demonstrating purity of bacterial isolates. The plates were scraped to recover the bacterial colonies and were extracted using the phospholipid extraction procedure of Bligh and Dyer [20] as modified by Garbus et al. [21]. *Porphyromonas gingivalis* (type strain, ATCC#33277), *Tannerella forsythia* (generously provided by Dr. Sigmund Socransky) and *Prevotella intermedia* (VPI 8944, generous gift of L.V. Moore) were grown in broth culture and after pelleting bacteria by centrifugation, the bacterial pellets were stored frozen until processing. At the time of lipid extraction, samples of bacterial pellets were removed and extracted using the same phospholipid extraction procedure.

All tissue and blood samples were stored frozen until processing. Gingival tissue, atheroma and brain samples were thawed and at least 20 mg of tissue was minced and extracted for several days in organic solvent according the method of Bligh and Dyer [20]. After drying organic solvent extracts under nitrogen, the lipid extracts were reconstituted in hexane:isopropanol:water (HPLC solvent, 6:8:0.75, v/v/v), vortexed and centrifuged. The resultant supernatants were recovered, a sample of defined volume (5μl) was dried and weighed, and a defined amount of each sample was transferred to a clean glass vial either for further processing or for MRM-MS analysis. For brain samples, 10 mg of each lipid extract was fractionated by normal phase HPLC as previously described [1] and the fractions expected to contain the PDHC lipids were pooled and dried. Each brain lipid isolate was then reconstituted in 300 μl of HPLC solvent and 5 μl was analyzed by MRM-MS for the bacterial lipids of interest. For each subgingival plaque sample, 50 μg of lipid extract was dissolved in 200 μl of HPLC solvent and 5 μl of each sample was analyzed by MRM-MS. For gingival tissue samples, each gingival lipid sample (1 mg) was supplemented with 50 μg of 1,2-di-(3,7,11,15-tetramethylhexadecanoyl)-sn-glycero-3-phosphoserine and the characteristic 847 to 311 m/z ion transition of this internal standard was used to correct for bacterial lipid levels between gingival tissue lipid samples. Each gingival lipid extract was then dissolved in 300 μl of HPLC solvent and 5 μl of each sample was analyzed by MRM-MS. Citrated blood samples, obtained by venipuncture from dental patients, were diluted 2:1 in saline and subjected to Ficoll-Hypaque centrifugation. The recovered plasma samples were stored frozen until lipid extraction. For lipid extraction, the plasma samples were thawed and 0.5 ml of each sample was extracted for lipids as described above. The dried lipid samples were reconstituted in 300 μl of HPLC solvent and analyzed by MRM-MS.

Individual lipid samples were analyzed using a QTrap 4000 mass spectrometer (ABSciex). A standard volume of each lipid sample (5 μl) was analyzed by flow injection and HPLC solvent was run at a rate of 80 μl/min. Using previously purified lipid preparations of each phosphorylated dihydroceramide class, the instrument parameters were optimized for detection of each lipid component based on gas phase transitions depicted in Figure 1. The instrument parameters are listed in Table S4. Standard curves were generated using serially diluted lipid standards of known quantity and linearity of lipid quantification was observed

(regression coefficients >0.98). In addition, carryover of individual lipid ion transitions into other monitored transitions was not observed. Using the optimized instrument parameters, each lipid extract from tissue, blood and bacterial samples was individually analyzed.

Each lipid ion transition peak was electronically integrated and the percentage abundance of each lipid class was calculated from the integrated lipid ion transition peaks. For each category of tissue or blood samples, all samples within a particular tissue or blood category were analyzed during a single analysis session. One or two-factor ANOVA, or the paired student t test was used to test for significance differences between sample categories.

Supporting Information

Table S1 Ion abundances of bacterial phosphorylated dihydroceramides recovered from each intestinal and oral bacterial isolate. The individual bacterial samples were processed as described in the Materials and Methods and individual lipid extracts were evaluated by MRM-MS. Electronically integrated peaks depicted here for each bacterial isolate were used to generate the summary results shown in Figure 2A. Bacterial lipids that were not detected are listed as ND.

Table S2 Ion abundances of bacterial phosphorylated dihydroceramides recovered from individual lipid extracts of subgingival plaque samples, and human gingival tissue, blood, atheroma and brain samples. The individual tissue and blood specimens were processed as described in the Materials and Methods and individual lipid extracts were evaluated by MRM-MS. Electronically integrated peaks depicted here were used to generate the summary results shown in Figure 2B.

Table S3 Ion abundances of bacterial phosphorylated dihydroceramides in lipid extracts of paired common carotid (control) and carotid atheroma samples derived from human endarterectomy samples. The individual tissue specimens were processed as described in the Materials and Methods and individual lipid extracts were evaluated by MRM-MS. Electronically integrated peaks depicted here were used to generate the summary results shown in Figure 3.

Table S4 Mass spectrometric calibration parameters used to quantify bacterial lipids in bacterial or human specimens. The instrument parameters for the MRM-MS analysis are listed for the 4000QTrap Instrument (ABSciex). These parameters were defined using highly purified preparations of each PDHC lipid class.

Author Contributions

Conceived and designed the experiments: FN XY BB JD SF EK JG WH RC. Performed the experiments: FN XY BB JD SF EK JG WH RC. Analyzed the data: FN XY BB JD SF EK RC. Contributed reagents/materials/analysis tools: FN XY BB JD SF JG RC. Wrote the paper: FN XY BB JD SF EK WH RC.

References

1. Nichols FC, Riep B, Mun J, Morton MD, Bojarski MT, et al. (2004) Structures and biological activity of phosphorylated dihydroceramides of *Porphyromonas gingivalis*. J Lipid Res 45: 2317–2330.

2. Nichols FC, Housley WJ, O'Conor CA, Manning T, Wu S, et al. (2009) Unique lipids from a common human bacterium represent a new class of Toll-like receptor 2 ligands capable of enhancing autoimmunity. Am J Pathol 175: 2430–2438.

3. Wang YH, Jiang J, Zhu Q, Alanezi AZ, Clark RB, et al. (2010) *Porphyromonas gingivalis* lipids inhibit osteoblastic differentiation and function. Infect Immun 78: 3726–3735.

4. Zahlten J, Riep B, Nichols FC, Walter C, Schmeck B, et al. (2007) *Porphyromonas gingivalis* dihydroceramides induce apoptosis in endothelial cells. J Dent Res 86: 635–640.

5. Nichols FC, Rojanasomsith K (2006) *Porphyromonas gingivalis* lipids and diseased dental tissues. Oral Microbiol Immunol 21: 84–92.

6. Clarke TB, Davis KM, Lysenko ES, Zhou AY, Yu Y, et al. (2010) Recognition of peptidoglycan from the microbiota by Nod1 enhances systemic innate immunity. Nat Med 16: 228–231.

7. Philpott DJ, Girardin SE (2010) Gut microbes extend reach to systemic innate immunity. Nat Med 16: 160–161.

8. Fukami H, Tachimoto H, Kishi M, Kaga T, Waki H, et al. (2010) Preparation of ^{13}C-labeled ceramide by acetic acid bacteria and its incorporation in mice. J Lipid Res.

9. Aumeunier A, Grela F, Ramadan A, Pham Van L, Bardel E, et al. (2010) Systemic Toll-like receptor stimulation suppresses experimental allergic asthma and autoimmune diabetes in NOD mice. PLoS One 5: e11484.

10. Mazmanian SK, Kasper DL (2006) The love-hate relationship between bacterial polysaccharides and the host immune system. Nat Rev Immunol 6: 849–858.

11. Mazmanian SK, Liu CH, Tzianabos AO, Kasper DL (2005) An immunomodulatory molecule of symbiotic bacteria directs maturation of the host immune system. Cell 122: 107–118.

12. Round JL, Mazmanian SK (2009) The gut microbiota shapes intestinal immune responses during health and disease. Nat Rev Immunol 9: 313–323.

13. Round JL, O'Connell RM, Mazmanian SK (2010) Coordination of tolerogenic immune responses by the commensal microbiota. J Autoimmun 34: J220–225.

14. Wen L, Ley RE, Volchkov PY, Stranges PB, Avanesyan L, et al. (2008) Innate immunity and intestinal microbiota in the development of Type 1 diabetes. Nature 455: 1109–1113.

15. Arkema EV, Karlson EW, Costenbader KH (2010) A Prospective Study of Periodontal Disease and Risk of Rheumatoid Arthritis. J Rheumatol.

16. de Pablo P, Chapple IL, Buckley CD, Dietrich T (2009) Periodontitis in systemic rheumatic diseases. Nat Rev Rheumatol 5: 218–224.

17. de Pablo P, Dietrich T, McAlindon TE (2008) Association of periodontal disease and tooth loss with rheumatoid arthritis in the US population. J Rheumatol 35: 70–76.

18. Mikuls TR, Payne JB, Reinhardt RA, Thiele GM, Maziarz E, et al. (2008) Antibody responses to *Porphyromonas gingivalis* (*P. gingivalis*) in subjects with rheumatoid arthritis and periodontitis. Int Immunopharmacol.

19. Pischon N, Pischon T, Kroger J, Gulmez E, Kleber BM, et al. (2008) Association among rheumatoid arthritis, oral hygiene, and periodontitis. J Periodontol 79: 979–986.

20. Bligh EG, Dyer WJ (1959) A rapid method of total lipid extraction and purification. Can J Biochem Physiol 37: 911–917.

21. Garbus J, DeLuca HF, Loomas ME, Strong FM (1968) Rapid incorporation of phosphate into mitochondrial lipids. J Biol Chem 238: 59–63.

15

Activity of 25-Hydroxylase in Human Gingival Fibroblasts and Periodontal Ligament Cells

Kaining Liu, Huanxin Meng*, Jianxia Hou

Department of Periodontology, Peking University School and Hospital of Stomatology, Beijing, China

Abstract

Background: We previously demonstrated that 25-hydroxyvitamin D_3 concentrations in gingival crevicular fluid are 300 times higher than those in the plasma of patients with aggressive periodontitis. Here we explored whether 25-hydroxyvitamin D_3 can be synthesized by periodontal soft tissue cells. We also investigated which of the two main kinds of hydroxylases, CYP27A1 and CYP2R1, is the key 25-hydroxylase in periodontal soft tissue cells.

Methodology/Principal Findings: Primary cultures of human gingival fibroblasts and periodontal ligament cells from 5 individual donors were established. CYP27A1 mRNA, CYP2R1 mRNA and CYP27A1 protein were detected in human gingival fibroblasts and periodontal ligament cells, whereas CYP2R1 protein was not. After incubation with the 25-hydroxylase substrate vitamin D_3, human gingival fibroblasts and periodontal ligament cells generated detectable 25-hydroxyvitamin D_3 that resulted in the production of $1\alpha,25$-dihydroxyvitamin D_3. Specific knockdown of CYP27A1 in human gingival fibroblasts and periodontal ligament cells using siRNA resulted in a significant reduction in both 25-hydroxyvitamin D_3 and $1\alpha,25$-dihydroxyvitamin D_3 production. Knockdown of CYP2R1 did not significantly influence 25-hydroxyvitamin D_3 synthesis. Sodium butyrate did not influence significantly CYP27A1 mRNA expression; however, interleukin-1β and *Porphyromonas gingivalis* lipopolysaccharide strongly induced CYP27A1 mRNA expression in human gingival fibroblasts and periodontal ligament cells.

Conclusions: The activity of 25-hydroxylase was verified in human gingival fibroblasts and periodontal ligament cells, and CYP27A1 was identified as the key 25-hydroxylase in these cells.

Editor: Andrzej T. Slominski, University of Tennessee, United States of America

Funding: This research was funded by National Natural Science Foundations of China (http://www.nsfc.gov.cn/Portal0/default152.htm) (30772420, 81100749) and Beijing Natural Science Foundation (http://www.bjkw.gov.cn/n1143/n1240/n1465/n2276/index.html) (7102164). The funders had no role in study design, data collection and analysis, decision to publish, or preparation of the manuscript.

Competing Interests: The authors have declared that no competing interests exist.

* E-mail: kqhxmeng@bjmu.edu.cn

Introduction

Vitamin D plays an important role in the regulation of bone metabolism and immunological reactions [1,2]. In humans, vitamin D, in the form of vitamin D_3, is derived from dietary sources or made from 7-dehydrocholesterol in the skin by exposure to ultraviolet rays [3,4,5,6,7]. Then, vitamin D_3 is metabolized by two-step hydroxylations: first 25-hydroxylation in the liver to form 25-hydroxyvitamin D_3 ($25OHD_3$), the major circulating metabolite of vitamin D_3, followed by $1,\alpha$-hydroxylation in the kidney to form $1\alpha,25$-dihydroxyvitamin D_3 ($1,25OH_2D_3$), the biologically active metabolite of vitamin D_3 [6,7].

In the early years of biochemical research, a mitochondrial cytochrome P450 (CYP27A1), an important enzyme in the bile acid synthesis pathway [8,9], was demonstrated to be 25-hydroxylase. Afterwards, Cheng et al. identified a microsomal cytochrome P450 (CYP2R1) with vitamin D 25-hydroxylase activity [10,11]. In addition, other cytochrome P450 enzymes, such as CYP2C11, CYP2D25, CYP3A4 and CYP2J2, were all identified as vitamin D 25-hydroxylases [12,13,14], and the two most active 25-hydroxylases were found to be CYP27A1 and

CYP2R1 [10]. It was reported that CYP27A1 was the more abundant 25-hydroxylase in the liver [10,15]. However, mutations in human and mouse genes encoding CYP27A1 protein influenced bile acid synthesis, but had no consequence on vitamin D metabolism [15,16,17,18]. Thus, the question as to which of these proteins is the key 25-hydroxylase in the liver remains controversial. In addition, it was reported that, besides the liver, there are extra-hepatic sites of $25OHD_3$ synthesis, including the skin [7,19,20,21], prostate [22,23], macrophages [24,25,26], and endothelial cells [24].

Human gingival fibroblasts (hGF) and human periodontal ligament cells (hPDLC) are two kinds of periodontal fibroblasts and are important components of periodontal soft tissues. Our previous study demonstrated that local $25OHD_3$ levels in gingival crevicular fluid were about 300 times higher than that in the plasma of patients with aggressive periodontitis [27,28]. Since there is abundant $25OHD_3$ around periodontal soft tissues, it was hypothesized that hGF and hPDLC have 25-hydroxylase activity, and can synthesize $25OHD_3$. The objective of this study was to test this hypothesis.

Results

CYP27A1 and CYP2R1 mRNA were detected in all the cells of the five donors, and no significant difference was found between the mRNA levels in hGF and hPDLC (Fig. 1). CYP27A1 protein was also detected in all cells of the five donors, whereas CYP2R1 was not detected, with the premise that anti-CYP2R1 antibody was able to recognize the protein in PC-3 cells, which were used as a positive control (Fig. 2). This indicated that CYP27A1 might be the key 25-hydroxylase in hGF and hPDLC.

After confirming the expression of 25-hydroxylase in hGF and hPDLC, the function of 25-hydroxylase was investigated. Whereas 1000 nM vitamin D_3 did not have a significant cytotoxic effect on any of the cells within 48 h, hGF and hPDLC generated $25OHD_3$ in response to vitamin D_3 (Figs. 3A, B). The fact that extra- and intracellular $25OHD_3$ was generated in the presence of vitamin D_3 provides direct and convincing evidence of the existence of 25-hydroxylase in hGF and hPDLC. At all time points, there was no significant difference in the levels of intracellular and extracellular $25OHD_3$ between the two cell types.

Additionally, exposure to vitamin D_3 also resulted in the synthesis of $1,25OH_2D_3$ in hGF and hPDLC (Fig. 4). The observation that hGF and hPDLC could synthesize $1,25OH_2D_3$ when exposed to $25OHD_3$ [29] is further evidence of 25-hydroxylase activity in hGF and hPDLC.

Based on the above direct evidence for 25-hydroxylase activity in hGF and hPDLC, we examined the effect of 25-hydroxylase knockdown. The efficiency of RNA interference against both CYP27A1 and CYP2R1 was both over 70% (Fig. 5). The generation of $25OHD_3$ increased with increasing vitamin D_3 concentrations, but dropped significantly when CYP27A1 was knocked down using specific siRNA (Figs. 6A–D). However, knockdown of CYP2R1 did not significantly influence $25OHD_3$ generation by hGF (Figs. 6A, C), and only slightly influenced $25OHD_3$ generation by hPDLC (Figs. 6B, D). These results suggest that CYP27A1 might be the key 25-hydroxylase in hGF and hPDLC. In addition, knockdown of CYP27A1 resulted in a

significant reduction of $1,25OH_2D_3$ generation (Figs. 7A–B). This is additional evidence for the activity of CYP27A1 as the 25-hydroxylase in hGF and hPDLC.

After the comprehensive confirmation of 25-hydroxylase activity in hGF and hPDLC, and the verification of CYP27A1 as the key 25-hydroxylase, the regulation of CYP27A1 in hGF and hPDLC was investigated. Interleukin-1β (IL-1β) and *Porphyromonas gingivalis* lipopolysaccharide (*Pg*-LPS) strongly induced CYP27A1 expression (Fig. 8). Additionally, dose-dependent increases in expression of CYP27A1 mRNA in hGF and hPDLC following incubation with IL-1β or *Pg*-LPS were demonstrated (Fig. 8). By contrast, sodium butyrate did not influence significantly CYP27A1 mRNA expression in hGF and hPDLC (Fig. 8). In addition, no significant differences between hGF and hPDLC were observed in the regulation of CYP27A1.

Discussion

In the present study, our hypothesis that hGF and hPDLC have 25-hydroxylase activity, and that they can synthesize $25OHD_3$ was verified. Therefore, the origin of high $25OHD_3$ concentrations in gingival crevicular fluid [27,28] might be hGF and hPDLC. Having demonstrated 1α-hydroxylase activity in hGF and hPDLC [29], we could consider that the conversion of vitamin D_3 to $1,25OH_2D_3$ in hGF and hPDLC consisted of two steps: ① from vitamin D_3 to $25OHD_3$, under the action of 25-hydroxylase CYP27A1; ② from $25OHD_3$ to $1,25OH_2D_3$, under the action of 1α-hydroxylase CYP27B1. This two-step conversion is similar to that observed in human keratinocytes [7,19,30,31,32]. In addition, Slominski et al. reported an alternate pathway of vitamin D_3 metabolism by cytochrome P450scc (CYP11A1) [33,34,35,36]. P450scc activity in hGF and hPDLC is worth further investigation in our future study.

We can then calculate and compare the amount of $1,25OH_2D_3$ synthesized from 1000 nM vitamin D_3 and from 1000 nM $25OHD_3$. According to the present study, the amount of $1,25OH_2D_3$ generated would be: ① In hGF exposed to 1000 nM vitamin D_3 for 48 h, 9 fmol/10000 cells in supernatants +14 fmol/10000 cells in cell lysates = 23 fmol/10000 cells (Fig. 4). ② In hPDLC exposed to 1000 nM vitamin D_3 for 48 h, 13 fmol/10000 cells in supernatants +16 fmol/10000 cells in cell lysates = 29 fmol/10000 cells (Fig. 4). According to our previous study [29], the amount of $1,25OH_2D_3$ generated would be the following: ③ In hGF exposed to 1000 nM $25OHD_3$ for 48 h, 5 fmol/10000 cells in supernatants +13 fmol/10000 cells in cell lysates = 18 fmol/10000 cells. ④ In hPDLC exposed to 1000 nM $25OHD_3$ for 48 h, 13 fmol/10000 cells in supernatants +14 fmol/10000 cells in cell lysates = 27 fmol/10000 cells. It is interesting that 1000 nM vitamin D_3 could induce hGF and hPDLC to generate even more $1,25OH_2D_3$ than 1000 nM $25OHD_3$. Particular attention should be paid to the observation that after 1000 nM vitamin D_3 treatment for 48 h, the $25OHD_3$ concentration in the cell supernatants of hGF and hPDLC were only about 45 nM–64 nM and 30 nM–50 nM respectively, much lower than the added 1000 nM vitamin D_3. So, why was less $25OHD_3$ converted to more $1,25OH_2D_3$? One reason might be that after vitamin D_3 treatment, $25OHD_3$ is found not only in the supernatant, but also in the cell lysates, allowing intracellular $25OHD_3$ to act directly as substrate of 1α-hydroxylase. On the other hand, exogenous $25OHD_3$ should enter the cells before eliciting a response. Thus, the direct availability at the site of action might be of great importance.

After comprehensive verification of 25-hydroxylase activity and the demonstration of CYP27A1 as the key 25-hydroxylase in hGF

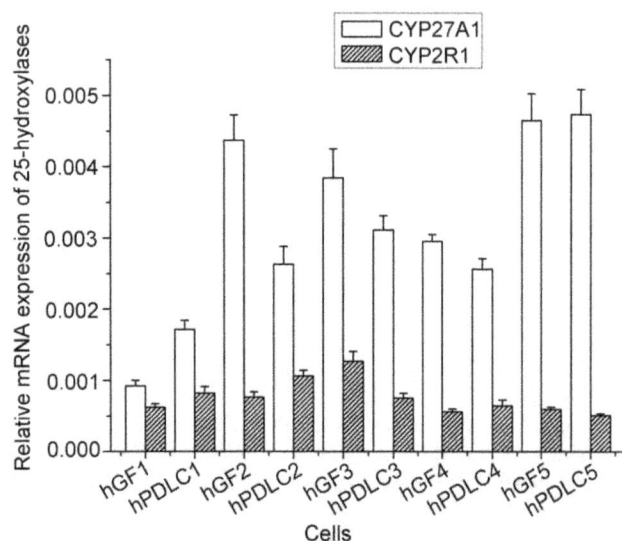

Figure 1. Expression of CYP27A1 and CYP2R1 mRNA in hGF and hPDLC. Expression of CYP27B1 mRNA was detected by real-time PCR in hGF and hPDLC from all five donors (donors are numbered 1–5). The expression levels of CYP27A1 and CYP2R1 mRNA were not significantly different in the two kinds of cells. The data are presented as the mean ± SD.

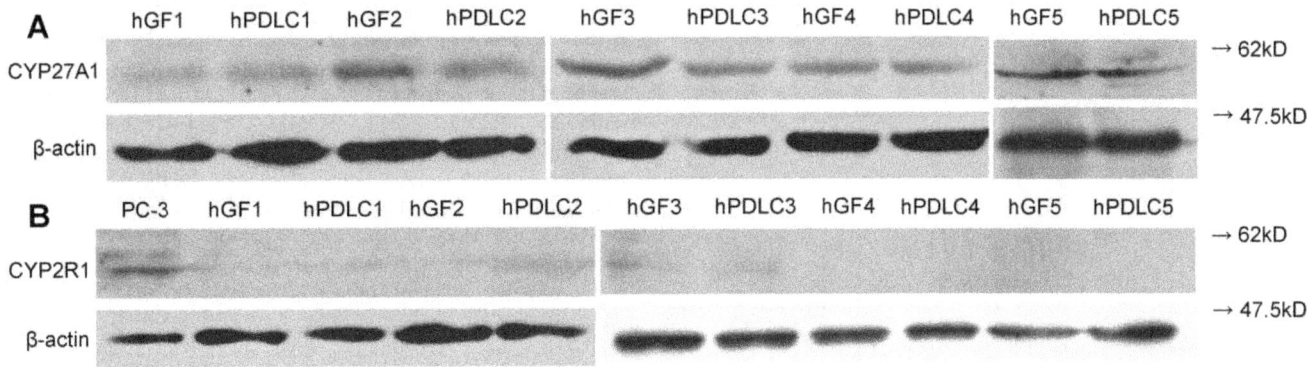

Figure 2. Protein expression of CYP27A1 and CYP2R1 in hGF and hPDLC. Protein expression of CYP27A1 was detected by Western blot in hGF and hPDLC from all five donors (donors are numbered 1–5). Protein expression of CYP2R1 was detected by Western blot in PC-3 cells, which were used as a positive control, but was not detected in hGF and hPDLC. β-actin was used as an internal control.

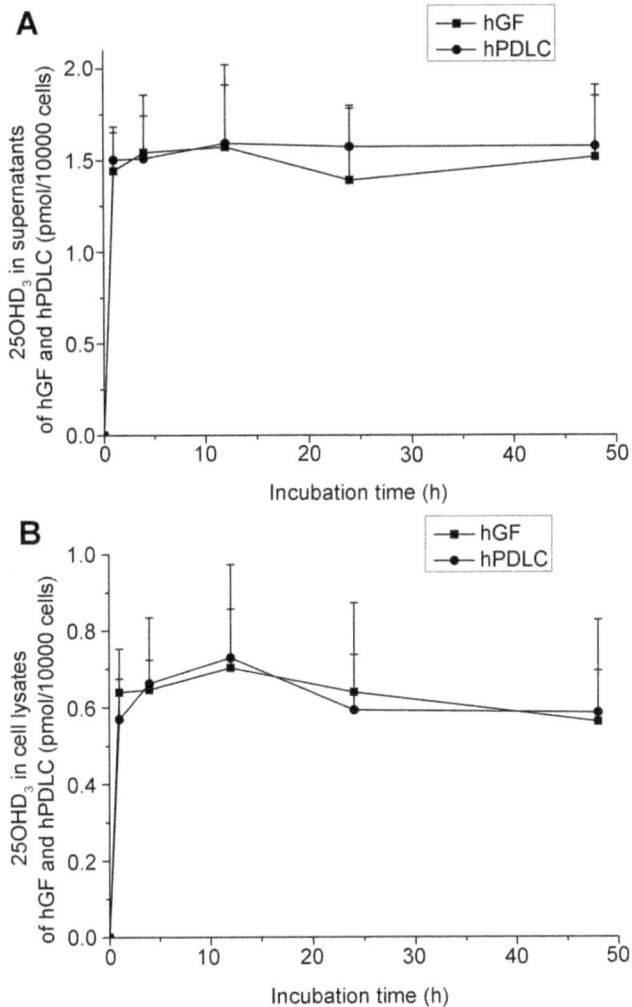

Figure 3. Activity of 25-hydroxylases in hGF and hPDLC. hGF and hPDLC from donors 2, 4 and 5 were incubated with 1000 nM vitamin D_3 for the times indicated, and the production of $25OHD_3$ was determined in supernatants(A) and cell lysates (B). After incubation, the production of $25OHD_3$ was detected. The amount of $25OHD_3$ generated was not significantly different between hGF and hPDLC. The data are presented as the mean ± SE.

and hPDLC, the regulation of CYP27A1 in these cells was preliminarily investigated. IL-1β in gingival crevicular fluids of patients with periodontitis decreases significantly after initial periodontal therapy, indicating that IL-1β is associated with periodontitis [28]. *Porphyromonas gingivalis* is an important pathogen of periodontitis and butyrate is one of its metabolites [37]. It was demonstrated that the butyrate concentrations in gingival crevicular fluids of patients with periodontitis are significantly higher than those of healthy controls, and that butyrate concentrations in gingival crevicular fluids are significantly correlated with periodontal inflammation [38,39]. To investigate the regulation of CYP27A1 in hGF and hPDLC, IL-1β, *Pg*-LPS and sodium butyrate were chosen for the present study. It should be considered, however, that although stimuli with periodontal characteristics were used to simulate a periodontitis-like condition, this does not properly model the chronic disease situation *in vivo*, and can only help to investigate the regulation of CYP27A1 in hGF and hPDLC. The NF-κB activator, IL-1β, was demonstrated to be a potent up-regulator of CYP27A1 mRNA in hGF and hPDLC (Fig. 8). *Pg*-LPS could also up-regulate significantly the

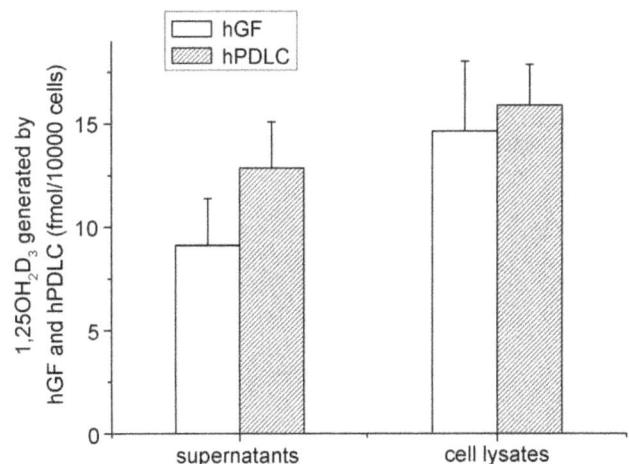

Figure 4. 1,25OH₂D₃ generation by hGF and hPDLC. hGF and hPDLC from donors 2, 4 and 5 were incubated with 1000 nM vitamin D_3 for 48 h, and the production of $1,25OH_2D_3$ was determined in supernatants and cell lysates. The amount of $1,25OH_2D_3$ generated was not significantly different between hGF and hPDLC. The data are presented as the mean ± SE.

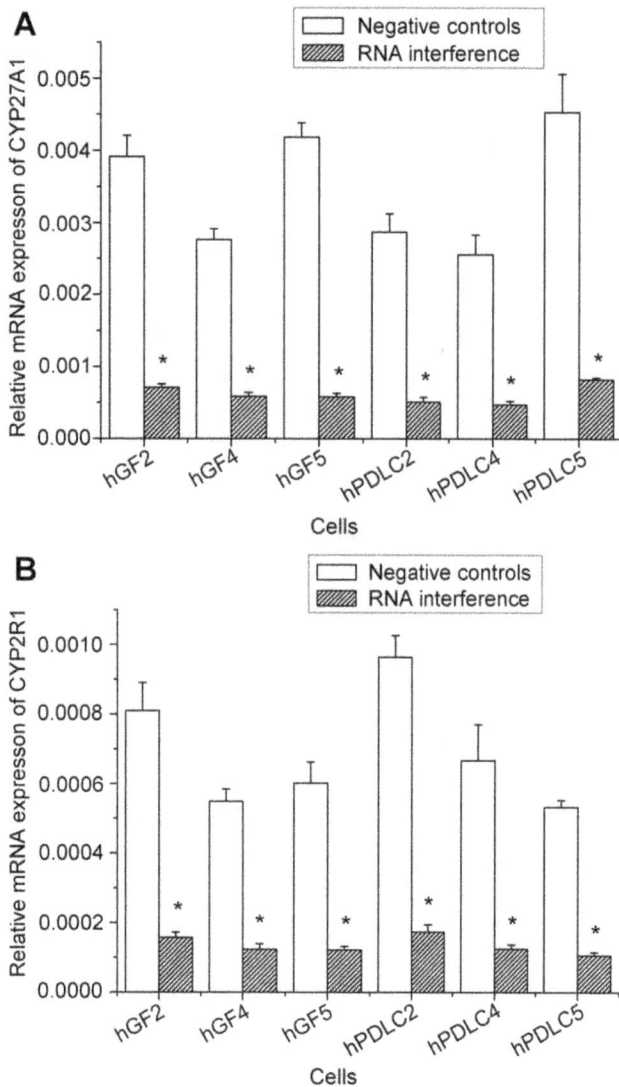

Figure 5. The efficiency of RNA interference against CYP27A1 and CYP2R1. hGF and hPDLC from donors 2, 4 and 5 were transfected with a siRNA oligonucleotide for CYP27B1, a siRNA oligonucleotide for CYP2R1, or a non-silencing control. Using real-time PCR as a measure, the efficiency of RNA interference against CYP27A1 and CYP2R1 was over 70% in hGF and hPDLC. The data are presented as the mean ± SD. * denotes difference from negative controls ($p < 0.05$).

expression of CYP27A1 mRNA, whereas sodium butyrate could not. It was reported that Pg-LPS is the ligand of Toll-like receptor 2 (TLR2) and TLR4 [40,41] and that both hGF and hPDLC expressed TLR2 and TLR4 [42]. Upon ligand binding, TLR2 or TLR4-mediated signaling could activate signal transduction, leading to NF-κB activation [43,44]. Thus, NF-κB might be involved in the regulation of CYP27A1 expression, an observation that warrants further investigation.

Each donor supplied both hGF and hPDLC in the present study. Although hGF and hPDLC are two different kinds of cells, they shared many features in 25-hydroxylase expression, activity and regulation, and only subtle differences were detected. As shown in Fig. 6, when CYP2R1 was knocked down, 25OHD$_3$ generation by hGF was not changed significantly, whereas 25OHD$_3$ generation by hPDLC was affected slightly. However,

the difference did not affect our conclusion that CYP27A1 might be the key 25-hydroxylase in hGF and hPDLC.

Since 1,25OH$_2$D$_3$ may enhance the antibacterial defense of human gingival epithelial cells [45] and hGF and hPDLC could synthesize 1,25OH$_2$D$_3$ with 25OHD$_3$ [29], the confirmation of 25-hydroxylase activity in hGF and hPDLC implies that these cells could generate 25OHD$_3$ as a substrate for 1,25OH$_2$D$_3$. From this perspective, 25-hydroxylase activity in hGF and hPDLC may be involved in the innate immune defense of the oral cavity. Recently, it was reported that oral calcium and vitamin D supplementation have a positive effect on periodontal health [46,47]. However, topical application of vitamin D has not been reported. Since hGF and hPDLC have the ability to synthesize 25OHD$_3$ and then to synthesize 1,25OH$_2$D$_3$, the topical application of vitamin D$_3$ might fulfill the function of 1,25OH$_2$D$_3$. Thus, our data suggest a potential benefit of topical application of vitamin D$_3$ in periodontal therapy.

In conclusion, hGF and hPDLC were identified as new extra-hepatic sites of 25OHD$_3$ synthesis for the first time, and CYP27A1 might be the key 25-hydroxylase in these cells.

Materials and Methods

Ethics Statement

The study protocol was approved by the institutional review board of Peking University School and Hospital of Stomatology (PKUSSIRB-2011007) and written informed consent was obtained from each participant in accordance with the Declaration of Helsinki.

Cell Culture

Primary culture of hGF and hPDLC was carried out according to our previous methods [29]. In brief, hPDLC were obtained from extracted third molars of 5 young healthy volunteers, and hGF was isolated from the gingiva of the same 5 donors. The periodontal ligament tissues attached to the middle third of the roots were curetted gently by a surgical scalpel, minced and placed in 24-well plates. Gingivae were also minced and transferred into 24-well plates. Tissue explants were cultured in Dulbecco's Modified Eagle's Medium (DMEM; Gibco, Grand Island, NY, USA) supplemented with 10% (v/v) fetal bovine serum (FBS; PAA, Coelbe, Germany), 100 U/mL penicillin G and 100 μg/mL streptomycin. Cultures were maintained in a humidified atmosphere of 5% (v/v) CO$_2$ at 37°C. After reaching 80% confluence, hGF and hPDLC were digested with a mixture of 0.25% (w/v) trypsin and 0.02% (w/v) EDTA, and subcultured at a 1:3 ratio. DMEM without phenol red (Sigma, St. Louis, MO, USA), 10% (v/v) dextran-coated, charcoal-stripped FBS (DCC-FBS; TBD, Tianjin, China) and hGF and hPDLC of passage 4 were used in all the following experiments. All experiments were conducted in triplicate.

The prostate cancer cell line, PC-3 (American Type Culture Collection, Rockville, MD, USA), was cultured in RPMI 1640 (Gibco, Gaithersburg, MD, USA) supplemented with 10% (v/v) FBS (FBS; PAA, Coelbe, Germany) in a humidified atmosphere of 5% CO$_2$ at 37°C and was used when the cells were in the logarithmic phase and reached 80% confluence.

Cytotoxicity Test of Vitamin D$_3$

hGF and hPDLC of three donors were used in the cytotoxicity test. hGF and hPDLC in their logarithmic growth phase were plated into 96-well plates at a density of 3000 cells/well in DMEM with 10% DCC-FBS, and the medium was replaced by DMEM without DCC-FBS after 24 h. After another 24 h, the medium

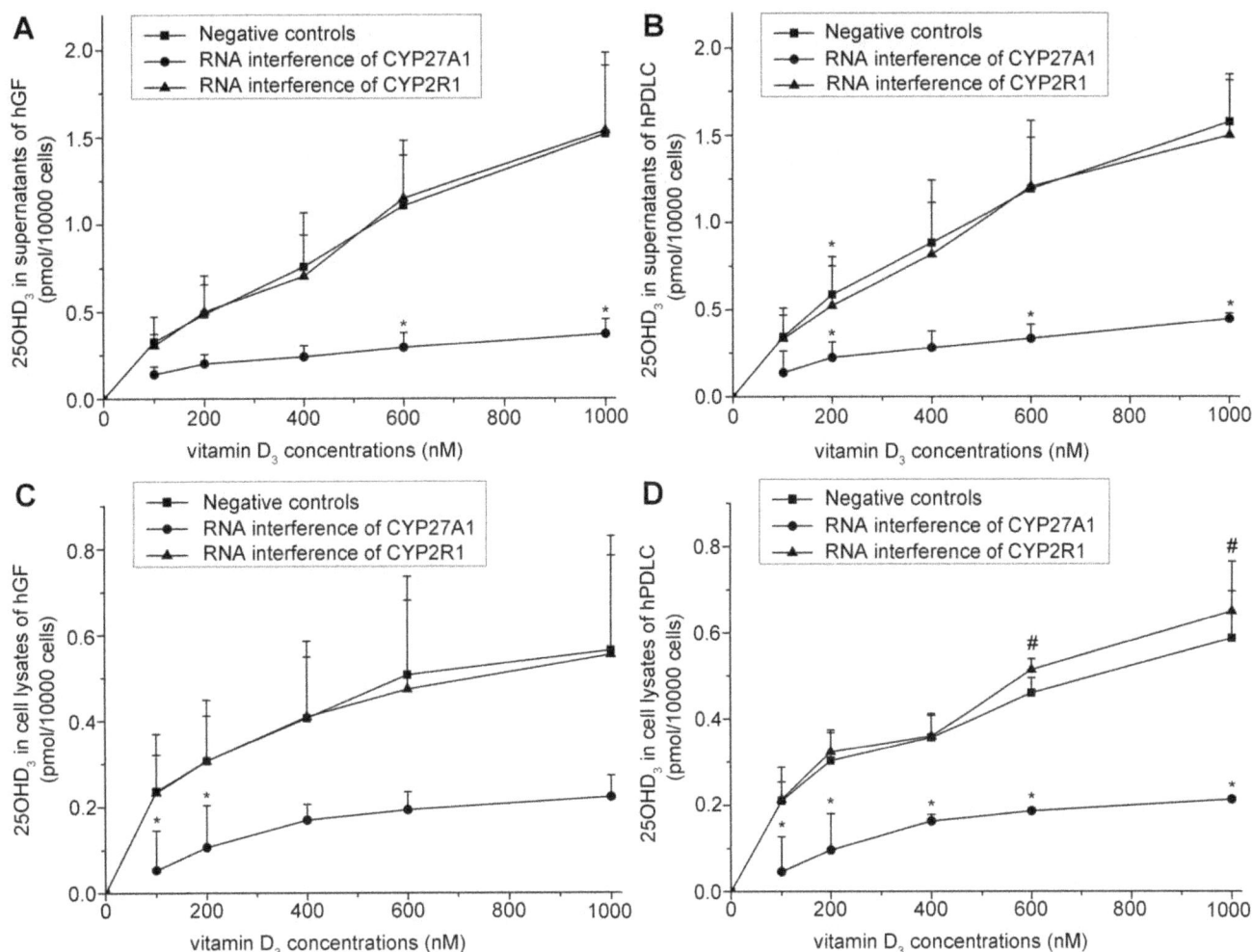

Figure 6. Effect of knockdown of 25-hydroxylases on 25OHD₃ generation. hGF and hPDLC from donors 2, 4 and 5 were treated with vitamin D₃ at various concentrations indicated in the figure for 12 h after transfection with a siRNA oligonucleotide for CYP27A1, a siRNA oligonucleotide for CYP2R1, or a non-silencing control. 25OHD₃ production was measured in supernatants of hGF (A), supernatants of hPDLC (B), cell lysates of hGF (C), and cell lysates of hPDLC (D). When CYP27A1 or CYP2R1 was not knocked down, the production of 25OHD₃ increased with an increasing concentration of 25OHD₃. When CYP27A1 was knocked down in hGF and hPDLC, the generation of 25OHD₃ decreased significantly compared to when CYP27A1 was not knocked down. When CYP2R1 was knocked down in hGF (A, C), the generation of 25OHD₃ was not significantly different from that when CYP2R1 was not knocked down. When CYP2R1 was knocked down in hPDLC (B, D), the generation of 25OHD₃ was only slightly different at some time points from that when CYP2R1 was not knocked down. The data are presented as the mean ± SE. * hGF or hPDLC generated significantly less 25OHD₃ with the same amount of added vitamin D₃ when CYP27A1 or CYP2R1 was knocked down ($p<0.05$). # hGF or hPDLC generated significantly more 25OHD₃ with the same amount of added vitamin D₃ when CYP27A1 or CYP2R1 was knocked down ($p<0.05$).

was changed to DMEM with 10% DCC-FBS, and supplemented with 1000 nM vitamin D₃ or vehicle, respectively. The cytotoxicity test was carried out according to the Cell Counting Kit-8 protocol (CCK-8; Dojindo, Kumamoto, Japan). At hours 0, 24 and 48, cells were incubated with CCK-8 for the last 3 h of the culture period, after which the optical density values (OD values) were detected at 490 nm with a microplate reader (Bio-Rad Model 550, Hercules, CA, USA).

Detection of 25-hydroxylase Expression

hGF and hPDLC from all five donors were seeded into six-well plates at a density of 5000 cm^{-2} in DMEM supplemented with 10% DCC-FBS. Four days later, a portion of the cells were harvested using Trizol agent (Dongsheng Biotech, Guangzhou, China). RNA was extracted using Trizol according to the manufacturer's instructions, and was reverse transcribed to cDNA

using a reverse transcription kit (Bio-Rad, Hercules, CA, USA). Real-time PCR reactions were accomplished using SYBR® Premix Ex Taq™ II (TaKaRa Biotechnology, Dalian, China) in an ABI 7500 real-time Thermocycler (Applied Biosystems, Foster City, CA, USA). The data were analyzed using the SDS software, according to the manufacturer's instructions.

Glyceraldehyde-3-phosphate-dehydrogenase (GAPDH) was used as an internal control. Data were presented as relative mRNA levels calculated by the equation $2^{-\Delta Ct}$ ($\Delta Ct = Ct$ of target gene minus Ct of GAPDH) [48]. The primers used are listed in Table 1.

PC-3 cells and the remaining hGF and hPDLC were harvested using lysis buffer [20 mM Tris (pH 7.4), 150 mM NaCl, 1 mM EDTA, 1 mM EGTA, 1% (v/v) Triton X-100, 2.5 mM sodium pyrophosphate, 1 mM β-glycerol phosphate and 2 mM Na₃VO₄ supplemented with a protease inhibitor cocktail (Roche, Mannheim, Germany)] [29] for Western blotting. The protein

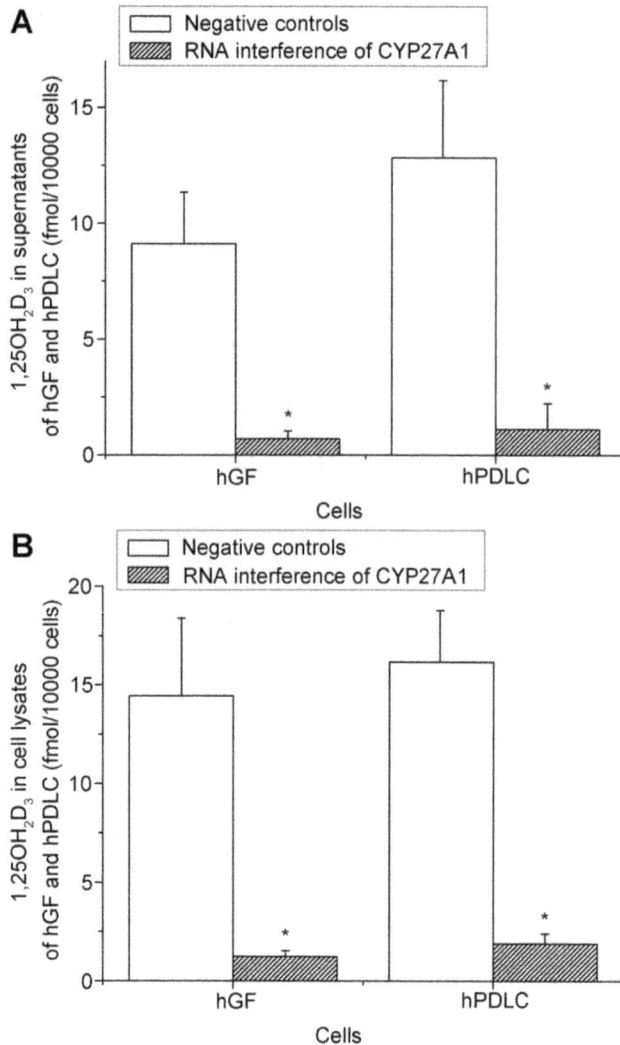

Figure 7. The effect of 25-hydroxylase knockdown on 1,25OH$_2$D$_3$ generation. hGF and hPDLC from donors 2, 4 and 5 were treated with 1000 nM vitamin D$_3$ for 48 h after transfection with a siRNA oligonucleotide for CYP27A1 or a non-silencing control, and 1,25OH$_2$D$_3$ production was measured in supernatants(A) and cell lysates (B). When CYP27A1 was knocked down, the generation of 1,25OH$_2$D$_3$ decreased significantly compared to when CYP27A1 was not knocked down. The data are presented as the mean ± SE. * hGF or hPDLC generated significantly less 1,25OH$_2$D$_3$ with 1000 nM vitamin D$_3$ when CYP27A1 was knocked down ($p < 0.05$).

Figure 8. Preliminary investigation of CYP27A1 regulation by inflammatory stimuli in hGF and hPDLC. hGF and hPDLC from donors 2, 3, 4 and 5 were stimulated with different treatments indicated in the figure for 24 h, and CYP27A1 mRNA expression was determined by real-time PCR. IL-1β and Pg-LPS significantly up-regulated CYP27A1 mRNA expression and the higher dose of IL-1β or Pg-LPS raised higher CYP27A1 mRNA up-regulation in both hGF and hPDLC. Sodium butyrate did not significantly influence CYP27A1 mRNA expression. Additionally, the characteristics of CYP27A1 regulation in hGF and hPDLC were not significantly different. The data are presented as the mean ± SE. * CYP27A1 mRNA expression was significantly different from that of the vehicle group ($p < 0.05$). # CYP27A1 mRNA expression was significantly different from that of the 1 ng/mL IL-1β group ($p < 0.05$). ^ CYP27A1 mRNA expression was significantly different from that of the 1 μg/mL Pg-LPS group ($p < 0.05$). IL-1ß : interleukin-1β. Pg-LPS: *Porphyromonas gingivalis* lipopolysaccharide.

concentration was determined using the Bicinchoninic Acid Protein Assay Kit (Applygen, Beijing, China). Twenty micrograms of total protein from each sample were loaded onto a gel comprising a 5% (w/v) stacking gel and a 10% (w/v) running gel. At the end of the electrophoresis, samples were transferred onto nitrocellulose blotting membranes (Hybond^{TM}; Amersham Pharmacia, Little Chalfont, UK). Blots were probed with a goat polyclonal antibody to CYP27A1 (diluted 1:200; Santa Cruz Biotechnology, Santa Cruz, CA, USA), a mouse polyclonal antibody to CYP2R1 (diluted 1:500; ABCAM, Cambridge, UK) or a mouse monoclonal antibody to β-actin (diluted 1:1000; Santa Cruz Biotechnology, Santa Cruz, CA, USA). After washing, blots were incubated with horseradish peroxidase-linked secondary antibody. The secondary antibodies against sheep (Kirkegaard & Perry Laboratories, Inc., Maryland, USA) and mouse (Beijing

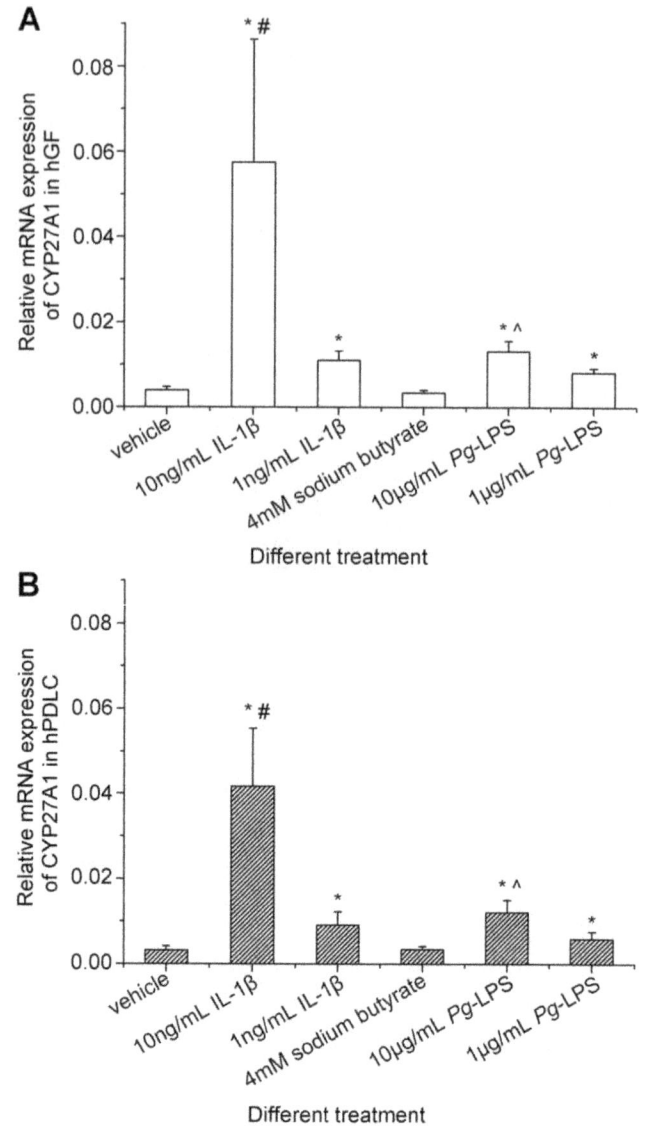

Zhongshan Golden Bridge Biotechnology, Beijing, China) IgG were both diluted 1:2500. Antigen-antibody complexes were detected using the Enhanced Chemiluminescence reagent (Applygen, Beijing, China).

Table 1. Primer sequences used for PCR or real-time PCR.

Target genes	Forward primer (5′ →3′)	Reverse primer (5′ →3′)	Products (bp)
CYP27A1	GCTCTTGGAGCAAGTGATG	AGCATCCGTATAGAGCGC	196
CYP2R1	TTGGAGGCATATCAACTGTGGT	CTCGGCCATATCTGGAATTGAG	153
GAPDH	GAAGGTGAAGGTCGGAGTC	GAAGATGGTGATGGGATTTC	226

Detection of 25OHD$_3$ Production

Cells from 3 donors were treated with 1000 nM vitamin D$_3$ (Sigma, St. Louis, MO, USA) for 1, 4, 12, 24 or 48 h, after which supernatants were collected, and the cells were scraped in PBS containing 0.2% Triton X-100 and stored at -80°C. Prior to use, cell lysates were sonicated on ice in a sonifier cell disrupter for 2×15 s. The levels of 25OHD$_3$ in cell supernatants and cell lysates were detected using a 25OHD$_3$ radioimmunoassay kit (DiaSorin, Stillwater, MN, USA) with a sensitivity of 1.5 ng/mL.

Detection of 1,25OH$_2$D$_3$ Production

Cells from 3 donors were treated with 1000 nM vitamin D$_3$ (Sigma, St. Louis, MO, USA) for 48 h and then supernatants were collected and cells were scraped in PBS containing 0.2% Triton X-100 and stored at -80°C. Prior to use, cell lysates were sonicated on ice in a sonifier cell disrupter for 2×15 s. The levels of 1,25OH$_2$D$_3$ in cell supernatants and cell lysates were determined using a 1,25OH$_2$D$_3$ radioimmunoassay kit (DiaSorin, Stillwater, MN, USA). The sensitivity of the assay was 2.0 pg/mL.

RNA Interference of 25-hydroxylase

To confirm the dependence of vitamin D$_3$ conversion to 25OHD$_3$ on 25-hydroxylase, the highly specific technique of RNA interference was utilized. Cells were seeded at a density of 15000 cm^{-2} in six-well plates. Eight hours later, the cells were transfected with either CYP27A1 siRNA (10 nM) or CYP2R1 siRNA (10 nM), or a non-silencing control siRNA using Hiperfect^{TM} transfection reagent (Qiagen, Duesseldorf, Germany), according to the manufacturer's instructions. The target sequence of CYP27A1 siRNA was 5′- CACGCTGACATGGGCCCTGTA -3′, the target sequence of CYP2R1 siRNA was 5′-TGGGTTGATCACAGACGATTA -3′, and the non-silencing control was a non-homologous, scrambled sequence equivalent.

Sixty hours after transfection, cells were harvested, RNA and cDNA were obtained, and real-time PCR was performed as described earlier to test the effect of RNAi.

After confirming the effect of RNAi, 25OHD$_3$ production after RNAi was determined. Cells were first transfected with CYP27A1 siRNA (10 nM) or CYP2R1 siRNA (10 nM), or non-silencing control siRNA. Twelve hours after transfection, these cells were treated with 100 nM, 200 nM, 400 nM, 600 nM or 1000 nM

vitamin D$_3$ (Sigma, St. Louis, MO, USA) for another 12 h. Then, the 25OHD$_3$ concentrations in the cell supernatants and cell lysates were determined as described earlier.

Some other cells were first transfected with CYP27A1 siRNA (10 nM), or non-silencing control siRNA, and 12 h after transfection, these cells were treated with 1000 nM vitamin D$_3$ (Sigma, St. Louis, MO, USA) for another 48 h. Then, the 1,25OH$_2$D$_3$ concentrations in the cell supernatants and cell lysates were detected as described earlier.

Regulation of CYP27A1 in hGF and hPDLC

Cells from four donors were seeded into six-well plates at a density of 5000 cm^{-2} in DMEM supplemented with 10% DCC-FBS. Four days later, cells were incubated with IL-1β (PeproTech, London, UK; 1 ng/mL and 10 ng/mL), Pg-LPS (Invivogen, San Diego, CA, USA; 1 μg/mL and 10 μg/mL) or sodium butyrate (SCRC, Shanghai, China; 4 mM) for 24 h. Then mRNA expression was detected by real-time PCR as described previously.

Statistical Methods

The Shapiro-Wilk test was used to determinate the distribution of the variants. The paired samples t-test was used to compare differences of the mRNA expression levels of CYP27A1 and CYP2R1 between hGF and hPDLC, differences of 25OHD$_3$ generation by hGF and hPDLC, and the effect of RNA interference. Comparison of 25OHD$_3$ generation with and without knockdown of 25-hydroxylase, and 1,25OH$_2$D$_3$ generation with and without knockdown of CYP27A1 were also performed using a paired samples t-test. The impact of stimulation on CYP27A1 mRNA expression was analyzed using a paired-samples t-test, and the difference between CYP27A1 regulation in hGF and hPDLC was analyzed using a Wilcoxon test.

Statistical analyses were accomplished using the SPSS 11.5 software package (SPSS Inc., Chicago, IL, USA). A p value <0.05 was considered statistically significant.

Author Contributions

Conceived and designed the experiments: KNL HXM JXH. Performed the experiments: KNL. Analyzed the data: KNL HXM. Contributed reagents/materials/analysis tools: KNL JXH. Wrote the paper: KNL HXM JXH.

References

1. Christakos S, Dhawan P, Liu Y, Peng X, Porta A (2003) New insights into the mechanisms of vitamin D action. J Cell Biochem 88: 695–705.
2. von EM, Kongsbak M, Schjerling P, Olgaard K, Odum N, et al. (2010) Vitamin D controls T cell antigen receptor signaling and activation of human T cells. Nat Immunol 11: 344–349.
3. Holick MF, Clark MB (1978) The photobiogenesis and metabolism of vitamin D. Fed Proc 37: 2567–2574.
4. Holick MF, MacLaughlin JA, Clark MB, Holick SA, Potts JJ, et al. (1980) Photosynthesis of previtamin D3 in human skin and the physiologic consequences. Science 210: 203–205.
5. Holick MF (1981) The cutaneous photosynthesis of previtamin D3: a unique photoendocrine system. J Invest Dermatol 77: 51–58.
6. Jones G, Strugnell SA, DeLuca HF (1998) Current understanding of the molecular actions of vitamin D. Physiol Rev 78: 1193–1231.
7. Bikle DD (2011) Vitamin D metabolism and function in the skin. Mol Cell Endocrinol 347: 80–89.
8. Cali JJ, Russell DW (1991) Characterization of human sterol 27-hydroxylase. A mitochondrial cytochrome P-450 that catalyzes multiple oxidation reaction in bile acid biosynthesis. J Biol Chem 266: 7774–7778.
9. Okuda K, Usui E, Ohyama Y (1995) Recent progress in enzymology and molecular biology of enzymes involved in vitamin D metabolism. J Lipid Res 36: 1641–1652.

10. Cheng JB, Motola DL, Mangelsdorf DJ, Russell DW (2003) De-orphanization of cytochrome P450 2R1: a microsomal vitamin D 25-hydroxilase. J Biol Chem 278: 38084–38093.

11. Cheng JB, Levine MA, Bell NH, Mangelsdorf DJ, Russell DW (2004) Genetic evidence that the human CYP2R1 enzyme is a key vitamin D 25-hydroxylase. Proc Natl Acad Sci U S A 101: 7711–7715.

12. Yamasaki T, Izumi S, Ide H, Ohyama Y (2004) Identification of a novel rat microsomal vitamin D3 25-hydroxylase. J Biol Chem 279: 22848–22856.

13. Gupta RP, Hollis BW, Patel SB, Patrick KS, Bell NH (2004) CYP3A4 is a human microsomal vitamin D 25-hydroxylase. J Bone Miner Res 19: 680–688.

14. Aiba I, Yamasaki T, Shinki T, Izumi S, Yamamoto K, et al. (2006) Characterization of rat and human CYP2J enzymes as Vitamin D 25-hydroxylases. Steroids 71: 849–856.

15. Bjorkhem I, Holmberg I (1978) Assay and properties of a mitochondrial 25-hydroxylase active on vitamine D3. J Biol Chem 253: 842–849.

16. Skrede S, Bjorkhem I, Kvittingen EA, Buchmann MS, Lie SO, et al. (1986) Demonstration of 26-hydroxylation of C27-steroids in human skin fibroblasts, and a deficiency of this activity in cerebrotendinous xanthomatosis. J Clin Invest 78: 729–735.

17. Cali JJ, Hsieh CL, Francke U, Russell DW (1991) Mutations in the bile acid biosynthetic enzyme sterol 27-hydroxylase underlie cerebrotendinous xanthomatosis. J Biol Chem 266: 7779–7783.

18. Rosen H, Reshef A, Maeda N, Lippoldt A, Shpizen S, et al. (1998) Markedly reduced bile acid synthesis but maintained levels of cholesterol and vitamin D metabolites in mice with disrupted sterol 27-hydroxylase gene. J Biol Chem 273: 14805–14812.

19. Lehmann B, Pietzsch J, Kampf A, Meurer M (1998) Human keratinocyte line HaCaT metabolizes 1alpha-hydroxyvitamin D3 and vitamin D3 to 1alpha,25-dihydroxyvitamin D3 (calcitriol). J Dermatol Sci 18: 118–127.

20. Schuessler M, Astecker N, Herzig G, Vorisek G, Schuster I (2001) Skin is an autonomous organ in synthesis, two-step activation and degradation of vitamin D(3): CYP27 in epidermis completes the set of essential vitamin D(3)-hydroxylases. Steroids 66: 399–408.

21. Holick MF (2007) Vitamin D deficiency. N Engl J Med 357: 266–281.

22. Flanagan JN, Young MV, Persons KS, Wang L, Mathieu JS, et al. (2006) Vitamin D metabolism in human prostate cells: implications for prostate cancer chemoprevention by vitamin D. Anticancer Res 26: 2567–2572.

23. Tang W, Norlin M, Wikvall K (2007) Regulation of human CYP27A1 by estrogens and androgens in HepG2 and prostate cells. Arch Biochem Biophys 462: 13–20.

24. Bjorkhem I, Andersson O, Diczfalusy U, Sevastik B, Xiu RJ, et al. (1994) Atherosclerosis and sterol 27-hydroxylase: evidence for a role of this enzyme in elimination of cholesterol from human macrophages. Proc Natl Acad Sci U S A 91: 8592–8596.

25. Quinn CM, Jessup W, Wong J, Kritharides L, Brown AJ (2005) Expression and regulation of sterol 27-hydroxylase (CYP27A1) in human macrophages: a role for RXR and PPARgamma ligands. Biochem J 385: 823–830.

26. Hansson M, Wikvall K, Babiker A (2005) Regulation of sterol 27-hydroxylase in human monocyte-derived macrophages: up-regulation by transforming growth factor beta1. Biochim Biophys Acta 1687: 44–51.

27. Liu K, Meng H, Tang X, Xu L, Zhang L, et al. (2009) Elevated plasma calcifediol is associated with aggressive periodontitis. J Periodontol 80: 1114–1120.

28. Liu K, Meng H, Lu R, Xu L, Zhang L, et al. (2010) Initial periodontal therapy reduced systemic and local 25-hydroxy vitamin D(3) and interleukin-1beta in patients with aggressive periodontitis. J Periodontol 81: 260–266.

29. Liu K, Meng H, Hou J (2012) Characterization of the autocrine/paracrine function of vitamin d in human gingival fibroblasts and periodontal ligament cells. PLoS One 7: e39878. doi:10.1371/journal.pone.0039878.

30. Bikle DD, Nemanic MK, Gee E, Elias P (1986) 1,25-Dihydroxyvitamin D3 production by human keratinocytes. Kinetics and regulation. J Clin Invest 78: 557–566.

31. Bikle DD, Nemanic MK, Whitney JO, Elias PW (1986) Neonatal human foreskin keratinocytes produce 1,25-dihydroxyvitamin D3. Biochemistry 25: 1545–1548.

32. Lehmann B, Rudolph T, Pietzsch J, Meurer M (2000) Conversion of vitamin D3 to 1alpha,25-dihydroxyvitamin D3 in human skin equivalents. Exp Dermatol 9: 97–103.

33. Slominski A, Zjawiony J, Wortsman J, Semak I, Stewart J, et al. (2004) A novel pathway for sequential transformation of 7-dehydrocholesterol and expression of the P450scc system in mammalian skin. Eur J Biochem 271: 4178–4188.

34. Slominski A, Semak I, Zjawiony J, Wortsman J, Li W, et al. (2005) The cytochrome P450scc system opens an alternate pathway of vitamin D3 metabolism. FEBS J 272: 4080–4090.

35. Tuckey RC, Li W, Zjawiony JK, Zmijewski MA, Nguyen MN, et al. (2008) Pathways and products for the metabolism of vitamin D3 by cytochrome P450scc. FEBS J 275: 2585–2596.

36. Slominski AT, Janjetovic Z, Fuller BE, Zmijewski MA, Tuckey RC, et al. (2010) Products of vitamin D3 or 7-dehydrocholesterol metabolism by cytochrome P450scc show anti-leukemia effects, having low or absent calcemic activity. PLoS One 5: e9907. doi:10.1371/journal.pone.0009907.

37. Kurita-Ochiai T, Ochiai K, Suzuki N, Otsuka K, Fukushima K (2002) Human gingival fibroblasts rescue butyric acid-induced T-cell apoptosis. Infect Immun 70: 2361–2367.

38. Li QQ, Meng HX, Gao XJ, Wang ZH (2005) Analysis of volatile fatty acids in gingival crevicular fluid of patients with chronic periodontitis. Zhonghua Kou Qiang Yi Xue Za Zhi 40: 208–210.

39. Lu RF, Meng HX, Gao XJ, Feng L, Xu L (2008) Analysis of short chain fatty acids in gingival crevicular fluid of patients with aggressive periodontitis. Zhonghua Kou Qiang Yi Xue Za Zhi 43: 664–667.

40. Darveau RP, Pham TT, Lemley K, Reife RA, Bainbridge BW, et al. (2004) Porphyromonas gingivalis lipopolysaccharide contains multiple lipid A species that functionally interact with both toll-like receptors 2 and 4. Infect Immun 72: 5041–5051.

41. Kocgozlu L, Elkaim R, Tenenbaum H, Werner S (2009) Variable cell responses to P. gingivalis lipopolysaccharide. J Dent Res 88: 741–745.

42. Hatakeyama J, Tamai R, Sugiyama A, Akashi S, Sugawara S, et al. (2003) Contrasting responses of human gingival and periodontal ligament fibroblasts to bacterial cell-surface components through the CD14/Toll-like receptor system. Oral Microbiol Immunol 18: 14–23.

43. Akira S, Takeda K, Kaisho T (2001) Toll-like receptors: critical proteins linking innate and acquired immunity. Nat Immunol 2: 675–680.

44. Mahanonda R, Pichyangkul S (2007) Toll-like receptors and their role in periodontal health and disease. Periodontol 2000 43: 41–55.

45. McMahon L, Schwartz K, Yilmaz O, Brown E, Ryan LK, et al. (2011) Vitamin D-mediated induction of innate immunity in gingival epithelial cells. Infect Immun 79: 2250–2256.

46. Garcia MN, Hildebolt CF, Miley DD, Dixon DA, Couture RA, et al. (2011) One-year effects of vitamin D and calcium supplementation on chronic periodontitis. J Periodontol 82: 25–32.

47. Bashutski JD, Eber RM, Kinney JS, Benavides E, Maitra S, et al. (2011) The impact of vitamin D status on periodontal surgery outcomes. J Dent Res 90: 1007–1012.

48. Livak KJ, Schmittgen TD (2001) Analysis of relative gene expression data using real-time quantitative PCR and the 2(-Delta Delta C(T)) Method. Methods 25: 402–408.

16

Impaired Phagocytosis in Localized Aggressive Periodontitis: Rescue by Resolvin E1

Gabrielle Fredman[1,2], **Sungwhan F. Oh**[2], **Srinivas Ayilavarapu**[1¤], **Hatice Hasturk**[1], **Charles N. Serhan**[2], **Thomas E. Van Dyke**[1]*

1 Department of Periodontology, The Forsyth Institute, Cambridge, Massachusetts, United States of America, 2 Department of Anesthesiology, Perioperative, and Pain Medicine, Center for Experimental Therapeutics and Reperfusion Injury, Brigham and Women's Hospital Harvard Medical School, Boston, Massachusetts, United States of America

Abstract

Resolution of inflammation is an active temporally orchestrated process demonstrated by the biosynthesis of novel proresolving mediators. Dysregulation of resolution pathways may underlie prevalent human inflammatory diseases such as cardiovascular diseases and periodontitis. Localized Aggressive Periodontitis (LAP) is an early onset, rapidly progressing form of inflammatory periodontal disease. Here, we report increased surface P-selectin on circulating LAP platelets, and elevated integrin (CD18) surface expression on neutrophils and monocytes compared to healthy, asymptomatic controls. Significantly more platelet-neutrophil and platelet-monocyte aggregates were identified in circulating whole blood of LAP patients compared with asymptomatic controls. LAP whole blood generates increased pro-inflammatory LTB4 with addition of divalent cation ionophore A23187 (5 µM) and significantly less, 15-HETE, 12-HETE, 14-HDHA, and lipoxin A$_4$. Macrophages from LAP subjects exhibit reduced phagocytosis. The pro-resolving lipid mediator, Resolvin E1 (0.1–100 nM), rescues the impaired phagocytic activity in LAP macrophages. These abnormalities suggest compromised resolution pathways, which may contribute to persistent inflammation resulting in establishment of a chronic inflammatory lesion and periodontal disease progression.

Editor: Dominik Hartl, Ludwig-Maximilians-Universität München, Germany

Funding: This study was supported in part by National Institutes of Health Grants DE-019938 (C.N. Serhan and T.E. Van Dyke), DE-015566 (T.E. Van Dyke) and GM38765 (C.N. Serhan). No additional external funding was received for this study. The funders had no role in study design, data collection and analysis, decision to publish, or preparation of the manuscript.

Competing Interests: The authors have read the journal's policy and have the following conflicts: C.N.S. is an inventor on patents assigned to Brigham and Women's Hospital on the resolvins, related compounds, and their analogs and uses (C.N.S. and T.E.V.D.) that are licensed for clinical development. There are several patents, details of which can be provided on request. C.N.S. and T.E.V.D. retain founder stock in Resolvyx Pharmaceuticals. There are no products in development or marketed products to declare. This does not alter the authors' adherence to all the PLoS ONE policies on sharing data and materials, as detailed online in the guide for authors.

* E-mail: tvandyke@forsyth.org

¤ Current address: Department of General Dentistry, Boston University Henry M. Goldman School of Dental Medicine, Boston, Massachusetts, United States of America

Introduction

Periodontitis and other periodontal diseases (PD) comprise a unique and complex group of inflammatory conditions that result in the destruction of the supporting structures of the dentition [1]. PD is a chronic inflammatory disease initiated by bacterial biofilms that naturally form on the teeth that is associated with, and is thought to exacerbate, the symptoms of several inflammatory disorders such as arthritis, Type II diabetes, preeclampsia, conditions associated with preterm low birth weight, and cardiovascular diseases (CVD) [2,3,4,5,6]. PD is a major public health concern given that it is among the most prevalent human diseases [7]. Since the pathogenesis of PD has strikingly similar aspects to many other inflammatory diseases, it has become a recognized model for examining effector cell mediated inflammation [8].

The etiology of PD is bacterial plaque and specific Gram-negative micro-organisms, such as *Porphyromonas gingivalis* and *Tannerella forsythensis* in the case of chronic periodontitis, and *Aggregatobacter actinomycetemcomitans* in the case of Localized

Aggressive Periodontitis, are associated with the subgingival biofilm in disease. [1,9]. The bacteria are necessary, but not always sufficient to produce disease [10] expression of disease is associated with modifiable risk factors such as smoking and genetic risk factors such as the inflammatory response. PD progresses in periodic, relatively short episodes of rapid tissue destruction followed by some repair, and prolonged intervening periods of disease remission [11]. Despite the apparent stochastic distribution of episodes of disease activity, the resulting tissue breakdown results in alveolar bone loss and pocket formation, which is common to several forms of PD. While LAP is clinically distinct from other types of periodontitis, it seems to represent the extreme with regard to inflammatory abnormalities. Chronic periodontitis is also associated with impaired phagocytosis [12] as well as other hyper-inflammatory traits. LAP is characterized by functional abnormalities of host cells, particularly neutrophils [13,14] that possess a hyper-activated or primed phenotype [1,15]. The functional consequences of neutrophil priming include dysregulated chemotaxis, phagocytic abnormalities, and heightened pro-inflammatory activity including increased oxidative stress and secretion of inflammatory mediators [16,17,18]. Hence, LAP PMN hyperfunction yields its inability to clear bacteria resulting in tissue damage and chronic lesions [1]. Of note, the cells used in several of these reports are circulating PMN, not just of those within the inflammatory milieu. Hyperactive circulating PMN indicates an underlying systemic component to this disease, suggesting persistent inflammation that does not resolve.

Resolution of inflammation is crucial for tissue homeostasis and necessary for ongoing health [19]. Resolution programs require the local biosynthesis of endogenous specialized pro-resolving lipid mediators (SPMs). These SPM include the lipoxins, resolvins, protectins and maresins [19], which are enzymatically synthesized via sequential steps involving lipoxygenases (LOX), and cyclooxygenases (COX). Arachidonic acid (AA) derived Lipoxin A_4 (LXA$_4$), as an example, is generated through two distinct transcellular pathways; a 15-LOX and 5-LOX biosynthetic pathway or a 5-LOX and 12-LOX pathway [20,21]. Cell: cell interactions determine the source of the LOX isoforms. The lipoxygenases are critical enzymes for the formation of LXA$_4$ as well as the omega-3 EPA and DHA derived resolvins, protectins are maresins [19]. SPM are dual functioning because they limit neutrophil accumulation and stimulate non-phlogistic activation of macrophages *in vivo* [19,22]. SPM have actions on selective cellular targets and act via specific G-protein coupled receptors [19]. It is noteworthy that EPA-derived Resolvin E1 (RvE1) is protective in several inflammatory disease models, including experimental periodontitis [8].

Recent evidence suggests that a failure in mounting endogenous resolution programs may be a key feature in various inflammatory disorders such as atherosclerosis [23,24]. The mechanisms underlying failed resolution are not known, but increasing evidence suggests an imbalance between pro- inflammatory and pro-resolving mediators to be a factor [25]. Here, we present an example of a human disease that exhibits a pro-inflammatory cellular phenotype and a malfunction in the capacity to generate LXA$_4$ and SPM precursors. LAP has activated circulating platelets and leukocytes and increased platelet-leukocyte aggregates compared to healthy, asymptomatic controls. There is also an imbalance in the release pro-inflammatory and anti-inflammatory LOX-derived lipid mediators from stimulated whole blood of LAP. Additionally, phagocytosis of opsonized zymosan particles by LAP macrophages was markedly reduced compared to healthy controls and RvE1 rescued the impairment. Hence, these results with LAP suggest an inability to effectively mount resolution pathways contributing to persistent, non-resolving, chronic lesion and periodontal disease progression.

Results

LAP has increased platelet–leukocyte aggregates in whole blood

Platelets, like neutrophils, are key cellular mediators of innate immune responses [26]. It is known that neutrophils from LAP patients are primed [27], thus it was of interest to assess whether platelets in LAP blood are hyperactive as well. Whole blood from healthy control volunteers or patients diagnosed with LAP was characterized based on cellular morphology and select antibody staining (Figure 1A–C). In unstimulated whole blood, platelet P-selectin was significantly increased (~50%) on the surface of LAP platelets as compared to healthy control (Figure 1D).

Aberrant formation of platelet-neutrophil and platelet-monocyte aggregates is associated with inflammatory diseases, such as cardiovascular diseases [28] and chronic periodontitis [29]. Since P-selectin is increased on LAP platelets, it was of interest to

monitor whether whole blood from LAP donors exhibited increased platelet-leukocyte aggregates as compared to healthy control. LAP exhibited significant increases in platelet-PMN and platelet-monocyte (~50% and ~30% respectively) aggregates (Figure 1B, E, and C, F respectively) compared to healthy control. Representative dot plots demonstrate platelet-leukocyte aggregates where platelets (CD41$^+$) are represented as green spots from healthy control (Figure 1B) or LAP (Figure 1C).

Leukocyte recruitment to inflamed areas requires a precise sequence of events that initially involves the interaction of platelets, leukocytes and activated endothelial cells via selectins and integrins [26]. Therefore, here we assessed integrin surface expression on leukocytes as a marker for activated of leukocytes. LAP exhibited higher surface expression of CD18 on PMN (Figure 2A, C) and monocytes (Figure 2B, D) as compared to healthy control. Representative histograms demonstrate that LAP (black) has a higher surface expression of CD18 on PMN (Figure 2C) and monocytes (Figure 2D) as compared to healthy controls (light gray). Together, these results indicate that LAP resting cells within whole blood are circulating in a hyperactive or primed state.

Imbalance in LOX biosynthetic markers in LAP

LTB$_4$ and other pro-inflammatory mediators were detected in the gingival crevicular fluid (GCF) of chronic periodontitis [30] and LAP patients [31]. We next questioned the pro-inflammatory and pro-resolving mediator formation within whole blood. To investigate the capacity of whole blood cells to generate and release lipid mediators, whole blood was stimulated with A23187 (5 µM) or vehicle, plasma was collected, subjected to solid-phase extraction followed by LC-MS/MS analysis (Table 1). Representative donor pairs demonstrated increased LTB$_4$ and 5-HETE (Figure 3A), and decreased 15-HETE (Figure 3B), 12-HETE (Figure 3C) and 14-HDHA (Figure 3D) levels plasma obtained from whole blood of LAP patients with the addition of A23187 (*ex vivo*) as compared to healthy controls (Table 1). A representative chromatogram is shown in Figure 3E. LAP, compared to its age, gender and race matched asymptomatic controls, has increased 5-LOX products including LTB$_4$ (47.7%±9.8) and 5-HETE (34.6%±7.2) indicating a hyperactive phenotype (Figure 3F). Of note, 12-LOX and 15-LOX products including 12HETE, 14HDHA and 15-HETE (48.5%±17.9, 79.8%±5.6, and 43.5%±8.5, respectively) were all significantly lower in stimulated LAP plasma compared to healthy controls (Figure 3F).

Since there is aberrant production of 5-,12-,and 15-LOX products, it was of interest to investigate the pro-resolving transcellular biosynthesis product, LXA$_4$. There was significantly less LXA$_4$ generation (375 pg/mL in healthy controls, 242 pg/mL in LAP) in A23187-stimulated whole blood of LAP donors (Figure 3G). These results suggest an imbalance between pro-inflammatory and pro-resolving mediator generation.

RvE1 Rescues Impaired Phagocytosis in LAP macrophages

Host defense mechanisms are abnormal in LAP [32]. Macrophages are essential for host defense because of their capacity to clear cellular debris and pathogens for the eventual return to homeostasis. LAP macrophage phagocyte function has not been investigated; therefore, it was of interest to determine whether LAP has normal phagocytic activity as compared to healthy control. There were no differences in viability of LAP and healthy control macrophages after isolation and Wright-Giemsa staining revealed no apparent difference in morphology between LAP and healthy control macrophages. Figure 4A demonstrates that LAP macrophages are impaired at phagocytizing serum

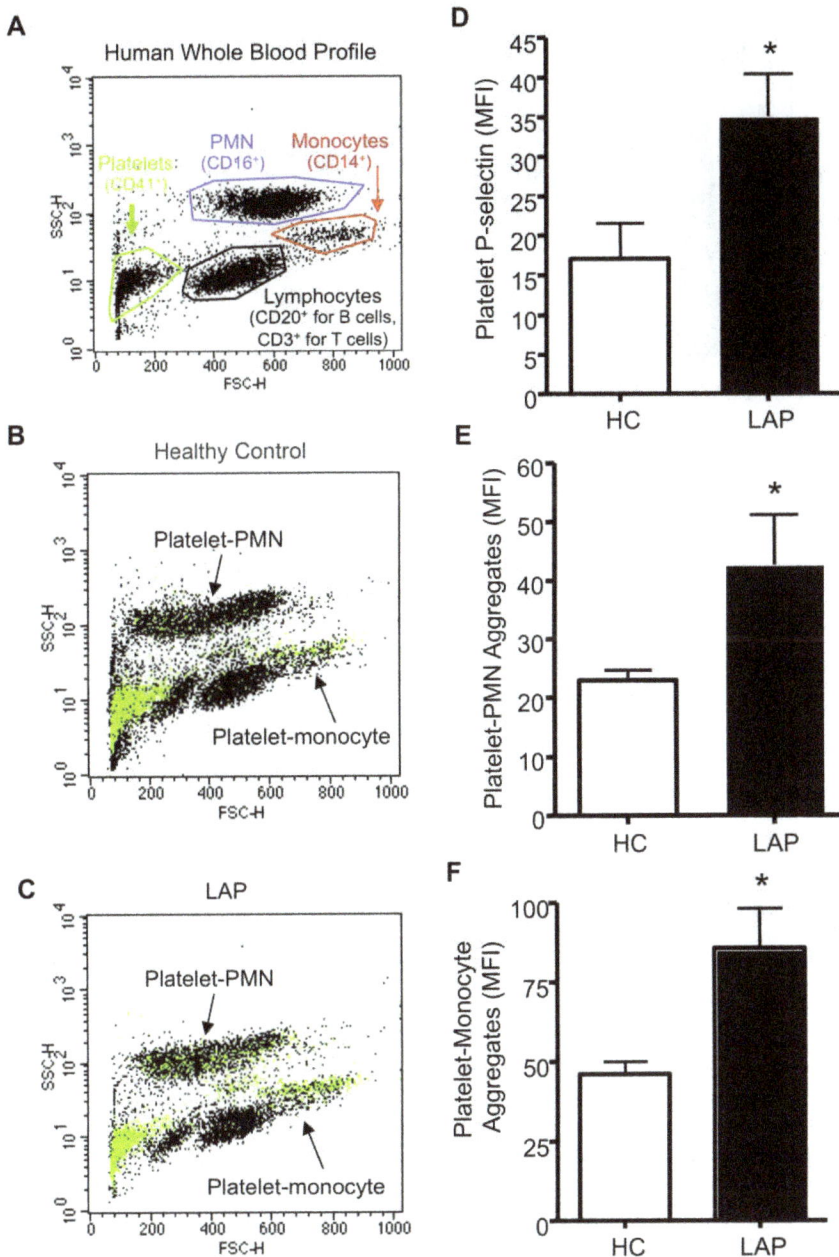

Figure 1. LAP platelets and leukocytes in whole blood. Venous whole blood was collected from LAP or healthy control donors. (A) Platelets, PMN or monocytes were characterized based on positive staining of cell specific antibodies (CD41, CD16, CD14, respectively) and characteristic cell morphology (representative dot plot). (B,C) Representative dot plots of platelet-leukocyte aggregates. Green spots indicate $CD41^+$ platelets. (D) $CD41^+CD62P^+$ were assessed and quantified via flow cytometry and Cell Quest software (LAP platelets, black bar; healthy control, white bar). (E) PMN or (F) monocyte populations with $CD41^+$ staining. Results are mean ± SEM, n = 4, *p<0.05.

treated FITC-zymosan (SZ). Since RvE1 is known to stimulate macrophages to enhance phagocytosis [22,33], it was of interest to investigate whether RvE1 would rescue the phagocytic defect observed in LAP. When incubated 15 minutes prior to SZ addition, RvE1 enhanced phagocytosis in healthy control (Figure 4B) and LAP macrophages (Figure 4C). Of note, RvE1 as low as 1 nM restored phagocytic activity of LAP macrophages to levels comparable to healthy controls (Figure 4C). ChemR23, an RvE1 receptor, has lower surface expression on circulating monocytes in whole blood (Figure 4 D). These results indicate that although LAP has impaired phagocytosis, RvE1, when added exogenously, can rescue the phagocytic defect.

Discussion

Periodontal diseases, such as LAP, result in the inflammatory destruction of the supporting tissues of the dentition. While the etiology of periodontitis is bacterial, it is becoming clear that the pathogenesis of disease is mediated by the host response [34]. Given the essential role of the innate immune system in regulating immunity, it is conceivable that dysfunction of the components of resolution can contribute to disease [35]. Hence, it was of interest to investigate whether distinct cellular and molecular pathways of resolution from LAP subjects were aberrantly regulated. Here, we report that (i) LAP platelets, neutrophils and monocytes in whole

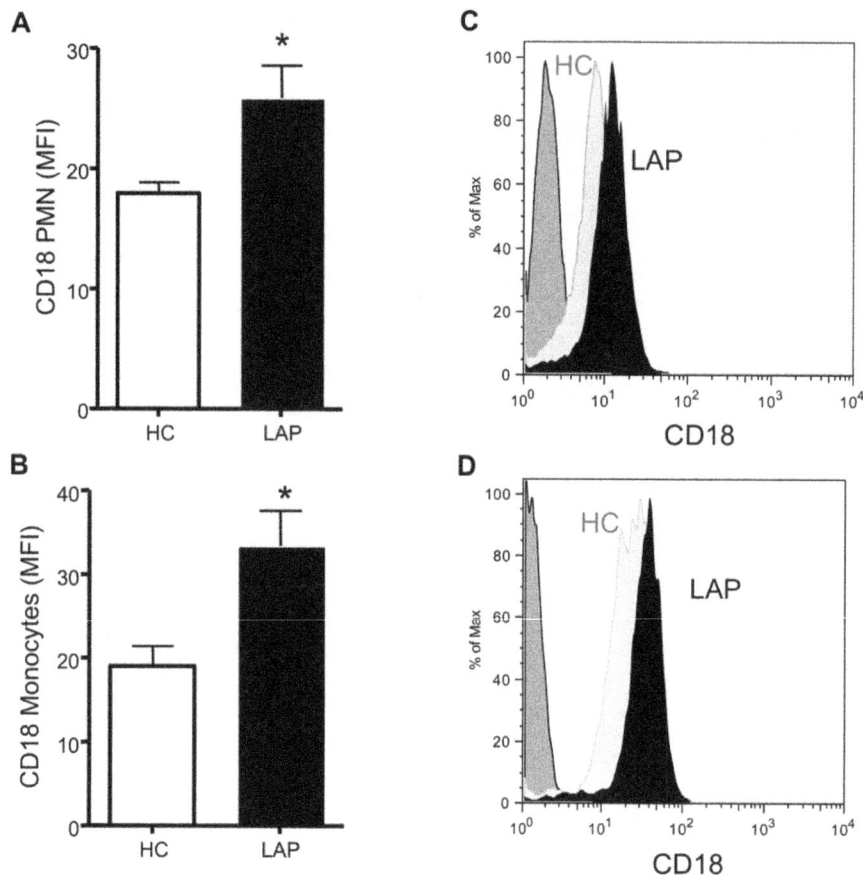

Figure 2. LAP patients display activated leukocytes in whole blood as compared to healthy control. CD18 was monitored on (A) PMN or (B) monocytes in whole blood without the addition of exogenous stimuli from healthy control (white) versus LAP (black). Results are mean ± SEM, n = 4, *p<0.05. Representative histograms of CD18 surface expression on (C) PMN and (D) monocytes. HC, healthy control, light grey; LAP, solid black; IgG dark grey.

blood display increased integrin and selectin surface expression compared to healthy control, as well as increased platelet-neutrophil and platelet-monocyte aggregates, (ii) the generation of LXA$_4$ and maresin precursor, 14-HDHA was compromised in LAP whole blood and (iii) macrophages from LAP patients exhibit impaired phagocytosis as compared to healthy control.

Inflammation, a common feature of periodontal and cardiovascular diseases [36,37], can be assessed at the cellular level by investigating the interactions between platelets and leukocytes. Figure 1 displays significantly elevated levels of P-selectin on platelets as well as increased platelet-leukocyte aggregates in LAP subject blood compared to healthy control blood. Since P-selectin is mobilized to the platelet surface upon activation, our results suggest that LAP platelets are circulating in a hyperactive state. In addition, platelets and leukocytes generally aggregate during inflammation or in a pathological milieu, such as those associated with CVD. In fact, circulating monocyte-platelet aggregates have been reported to be an early marker of myocardial infarction [28]. Therefore, the hyperactive state of LAP platelets as well as their increased association with leukocytes provides a further mechanistic link between periodontal and cardiovascular diseases [37].

To corroborate our finding that leukocytes are circulating in an activated state, we also profiled pro-inflammatory chemical mediators. LAP blood produced increased 5-LO products such as 5-HETE and LTB$_4$ (Figure 3), which is consistent with earlier reports that demonstrate LTB$_4$ within inflammatory periodontal

exudates. In addition to periodontal disease, elevated LTB$_4$ levels have also been associated with other non-communicable chronic inflammatory disease such as atherosclerosis [38]. Patients with atherosclerosis were found to possess a 5-LO gene variant leading to increased LTB$_4$ especially when on an omega-6 rich diet [39]. Of note, when these patients were placed on an omega-3 diet, there was significantly less LTB$_4$ generation [39].

12- and 15-LOX released products were decreased in LAP stimulated blood as compared to healthy controls (Figure 3). Of relevance, in a rabbit model of experimental periodontitis, overexpression of 15-LOX was protective against *P. gingivalis* induced bone loss [40]. Importantly, these rabbits were also resistant to CVD. The protective role of these lipoxygenase-derived products extends beyond that of periodontal disease models. In a pre-clinical disease model of atherosclerosis, 12/15 LOX knockout mice displayed increased atherosclerosis as compared to wild type [23]. 12- and 15- LOX are also critical enzymes for the biosynthesis of lipoxins. LXA$_4$ is generated via transcellular biosynthesis between PMN (5-LOX) and platelet (12-LOX) [20,41] or 15-lipoxygenase (15-LOX) and PMN (5-LOX) [20] interactions. LXA$_4$ levels were decreased in LAP compared to healthy control (Figure 3E) most likely due a result of aberrant activation of 12- or 15-LOX. Decreased generation of LXA$_4$ was also seen in cystic fibrosis (CF), where CF patients displayed increased platelet-leukocyte aggregates, yet compromised LXA$_4$ generation compared to healthy controls [25]. Hence, it is possible

Table 1. LAP whole blood LOX capacity versus healthy donors.

Donor Pairs	LTB$_4$	20-OH LTB$_4$	5-HETE	15-HETE	12-HETE	14-HDHA
Healthy control	1205.0	393.5	1335.0	365.5	3280.0	2273.6
LAP	2432.9	363.6	1878.3	246.4	2851.5	326.6
Healthy control	2120.4	682.9	4367.4	1057.4	33430.6	6903.4
LAP	5760.6	1191.8	8584.2	660.4	12699.0	107.1
Healthy control	1761.5	369.3	2407.4	839.6	17615.2	1361.1
LAP	2498.8	489.9	3253.3	332.1	5193.6	427.7

*Whole blood (1 mL) was incubated with A23187 (5 μM) for 20 mins, 37°C. Incubations were stopped on ice and plasma was collected for C-18 solid phase extraction and subjected to LC-MS/MS based lipidomics. Values are represented as pg/sample.

that compromised lipoxygenase pathways and the generation of lipoxin or other pro-resolving mediators may be an underlying component of several inflammatory diseases.

Since LAP is an inflammatory disease exacerbated by microbes, functional phagocytes to clear pathogens is of utmost importance for the return to homeostasis. Here, we report that LAP macrophages do not phagocytize opsonized zymosan A as readily as healthy control (Figure 4). The impairment in phagocytosis of opsonized zymosan may be attributed to the known polymorphisms of Fcγ receptors on leukocytes of periodontal disease patients [42]. Omega-3 EPA-derived RvE1 that rescued the phagocytic activity of LAP macrophages (Figure 4) was also shown to enhance efferocytosis *in vitro and in vivo* [22]. RvE1 was also reported to be protective on LAP PMN by dampen ingfMLP-stimulated O$_2^-$ release from LAP PMN [8]. RvE1 is protective for *P. gingivalis* -induced bone loss in experimental periodontitis [8,43]. Of note, RvE1 is also protective in asthma [44] and acute lung injury [45] models underscoring its role as regulator of several inflammatory diseases. Recent work demonstrated that RvE1 initiates direct activation of the ChemR23 receptor on human macrophages and signals receptor dependent phosphorylation during phagocytosis of opsonized zymosan [46].

Several investigations suggest that bone loss in PD is linked to an imbalance between omega-6 and omega-3 fatty acids [47]. Increased levels of omega-6 AA-derived products, including prostaglandin E$_2$ (PGE$_2$), thromboxane, prostacyclin and leukotriene B$_4$ (LTB$_4$) were found in inflamed gingival tissues and gingival crevicular fluid (GCF) [48,49]. Clinical studies investigating serum polyunsaturated fatty acid (PUFA) levels in periodontal disease patients demonstrated that omega-6 fatty acids were higher in patients with bone loss than in the control group; reduced bone loss was seen in patients with increased serum omega-3 levels [47]. Additionally, daily supplementation of omega-3 fatty acids showed a reduction in periodontal disease gingival pocket formation with an increase of attachment in periodontal disease patients indicating that omega-3 fatty acids are protective against inflammatory bone loss [50].

In addition to environmental factors, there is compelling evidence for genetic components associated with disease progression in LAP [51] (reviewed in [52]). As mentioned earlier LAP PMN exhibit a number of functional abnormalities including impaired chemotaxis, phagocytic abnormalities, and increased ROS generation to name a few [16,17,18]. As an example, LAP PMN that display decreased chemotaxis to n-formylated peptides like fMLP can at least in part be explained by a genetic variants associated with FPR receptors [53,54]. The phenotypic abnormalities presented in this report imply that our patient population may also have a genetic abnormality pertaining to a deficiency in

the biosynthesis of lipoxygenase pathways involved in the production of pro-resolving mediators.

Together, these findings demonstrate that cells from LAP patients present a heightened pro-inflammatory phenotype with a compromised capacity to generate SPM. LAP has hyperactive platelets, PMN and monocytes and increased platelet-leukocyte aggregates in the circulation compared to healthy controls. In addition, essential host defense mechanisms, such as removal of pathogens via macrophage phagocytosis are compromised in LAP. A resolution agonist, RvE1 rescues this critical impairment. In view of these findings, pro-resolving lipid mediators, such as RvE1 may be of interest for future clinical application in the treatment of inflammatory diseases like periodontitis.

Materials and Methods

Antibodies and Reagents

Antibodies. Phycoerythrin (PE)-conjugated mouse anti-human CD62P was obtained from Pharmingen (San Jose, CA) and mouse anti-human FITC-CD41 from BD Biosciences (Rockville, MD). (PE)-conjugated mouse anti-human CD18, FITC-conjugated mouse anti-human CD14, mouse anti-human CD16, Cy5-conjugated mouse anti-human CD3, and mouse anti-human CD20 were all purchased from Pharmingen (San Jose, CA). GM-CSF was obtained from R&D Systems (Minneapolis, MN), and FITC–zymosan from *Saccharomyces cerevisiae* was obtained from Molecular Probes (Carlsbad, CA). Lipoxin A$_4$ ELISA was purchased from Neogen Corporation (Lexington, KY). RBC Lysis buffer was purchased from eBioscience (San Diego, CA). Histopaque 1077 and Zymosan A were purchased from Sigma-Aldrich (St. Louis, MO).

Whole blood analysis

Human samples were obtained following informed consent under a Boston University (Boston, MA, USA) Institutional Review Board. The Boston University IRB approved our study in writing (protocol number H-23425). Venous blood (1:10 sodium citrate anticoagulant) was collected from healthy volunteers (n = 10) or patients with a diagnosis of aggressive periodontitis (LAP), n = 10 with no other known disease. All blood donors were non-smokers, between the age of 19–48 years of age who had denied taking any non steroidal anti-inflammatory drugs (NSAIDs) for at least two weeks prior to the experiment. The LAP subjects were all of African descent and were characterized by periodontal infection with multiple organisms including *Porphyromonas gingivalis* and *Aggregatibacter actinomycetemcomitans*, and a hyper-responsive neutrophil phenotype (elevated fMLP induced superoxide generation) [8]. Clinically, subjects presented with

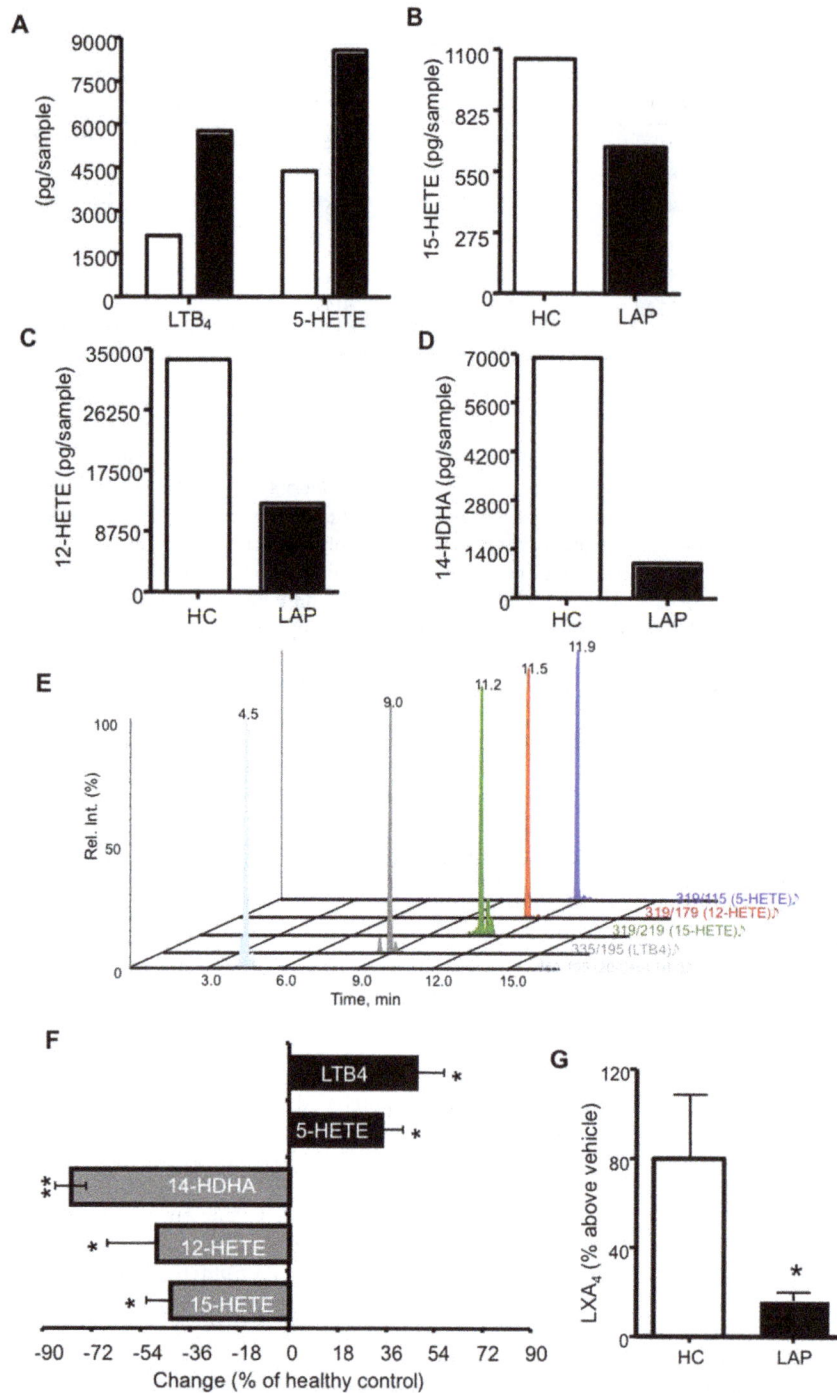

Figure 3. LAP whole blood displays increased capacity for 5-HETE and LTB₄ levels, and decreased for 12-HETE, 14-HDHA, 15-HETE and LXA₄. Whole blood was stimulated A23187 (5 μM) for 20 minutes, 37°C. Incubations were stopped on ice and plasma was collected for LC-MS/MS or ELISA analysis. (A–D) Representative LC-MS/MS quantitation of A23187-stimulated whole blood from healthy control (HC, white bars) and LAP (black bars) pairs. (E) Representative chromatogram. (F) Percent change of indicated lipid mediators. Results are meant ± SEM n=3, *p<0.05, **p<0.01. (G) Percent increase compared to vehicle of LXA₄ was analyzed by ELISA. Results are mean ± SEM, n=10, *p≤0.05, healthy control versus LAP.

severe, early-onset bone loss around first molars and incisor teeth only [13]. The patients were diagnosed by a licensed periodontist in the Clinical Research Center of Boston University School of Dental Medicine. Healthy control donors showed no signs of periodontal disease and were matched to LAP donor based on age, sex and race.

Red blood cells were lysed using 1×RBC Lysis buffer diluted 25:1 with blood for 10 minutes on ice [55]. Direct immunofluorescence labeling was performed using anti-human CD41 and CD62P, CD16, CD14, CD20, CD3 in combination with the corresponding isotype controls to detect platelets, neutrophils, monocytes, B cells and T cells, respectively. Cells were analyzed via flow cytometry (Becton, Dickinson

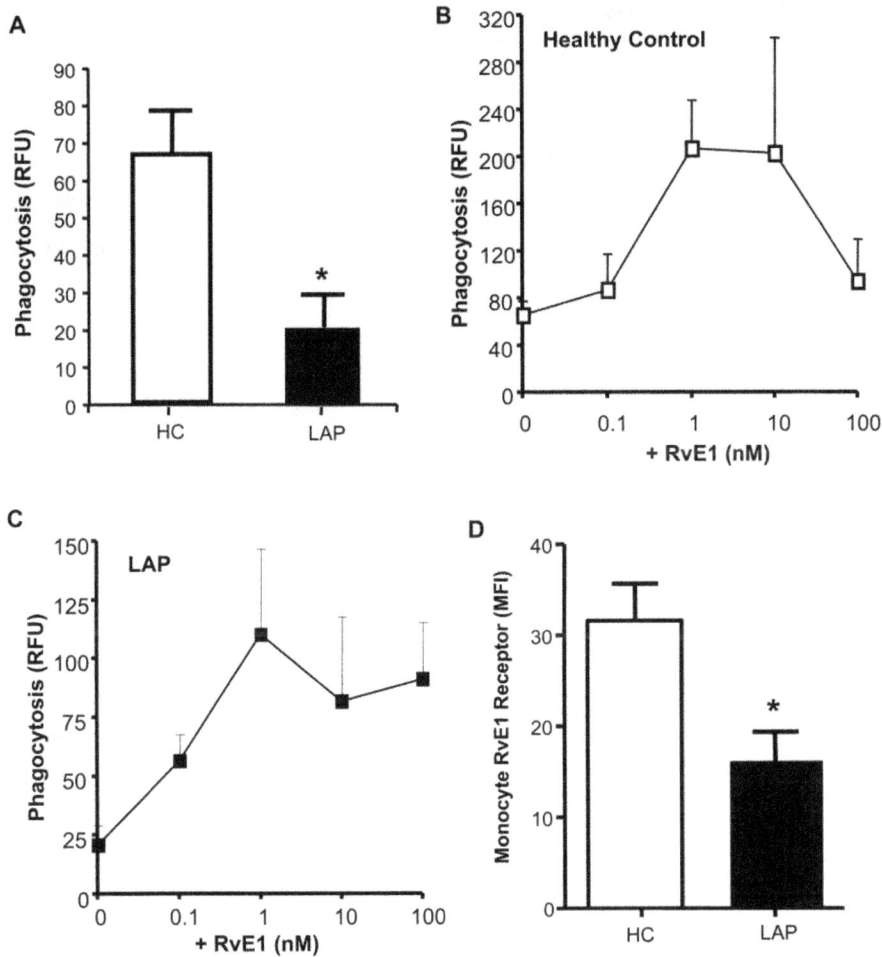

Figure 4. LAP Macrophages display impaired phagocytosis of opsonized zymosan particles. Monocytes were collected from venous whole blood and differentiated into macrophages in the presence of GMCSF (10 ng/mL) for 7 days. After differentiation macrophages were incubated with vehicle or RvE1 (0.1–100 nM) for 15 minutes. Phagocytosis was carried out for 30 minutes, 37°C and analyzed by a Victor3 fluorescent plate reader. (A) Healthy control (white bar) and LAP (black bar) baseline phagocytosis. RvE1 (0.1–100 nM) dose response, (B) HC (C) LAP. (D) Monocytes in whole blood were stained with anti-human ChemR23 and analyzed by flow cytometry. Results are mean ± SEM, n = 4, *p<0.05.

and Company, Franklin Lakes, NJ) and CellQuest software. Platelet-leukocyte aggregates were determined based on double positive staining for CD41 and corresponding leukocyte marker.

Human whole blood incubations

Freshly prepared blood (1 mL, anticoagulated with Heparin) was collected and incubated with A23187 (5 µM) for 20 minutes, 37°C. Incubations were stopped on ice and plasma was immediately collected by centrifugation (350×g, 5 minutes, 4°C). Two volumes of cold methanol and deuterated internal standards (PGE$_2$-d4 and 5(S)-HETE-d8) were then added. Samples were taken to C-18 solid phase extraction. Methyl formate fractions were collected, dried under nitrogen and subjected to LC-MS/MS [56].

LC-MS/MS-based lipid mediator lipidomics

LC-MS/MS was performed with a Shimadzu LC-20AD HPLC (Shimadzu Scientific Instruments, Columbia, MD) equipped with an Agilent Eclipse Plus C18 column (4.6 mm×50 mm×1.8 µm) paired with an ABI Sciex Instruments 3200 Qtrap linear ion trap triple quadrupole mass spectrometer (Applied Biosystems, Foster City, CA). Instrument control and data acquisition were performed using AnalystTM 1.5 software (Applied Biosystems). The mobile phase

consisted of methanol/water/acetic acid (60/40/0.01; v/v/v) and was ramped to 80/20/0.01 (v/v/v) after 10 min, 100/0/0.01 (v/v/v) after 12 min, and 90:10 (v/v/v) after 1.5 minutes to wash and equilibrate the column. Ion pairs from reported multiple reaction monitoring (MRM) methods [56] were used for profiling and quantification of various lipid mediators, including LTB$_4$, 20-OH-LTB$_4$, 5-HETE, 12-HETE, 15-HETE, and internal standards. The MRM transitions were LTB$_4$ (335/195), 20-OH-LTB4 (351/195), 5-HETE (319/115), 12-HETE (319/179), 15-HETE (319/219), 14-HDHA (343/205), PGE$_2$ (351/189), d8-5-HETE (327/116), and d4-PGE$_2$ (355/193). The criteria used for positive identification of compounds of interest were matching retention time and matching of 6 diagnostic ions to synthetic standards. Quantification was performed using standard calibration curves for each compound, and recovery was calculated using deuterated internal standards (PGE$_2$-d4 and 5(S)-HETE-d8) [56]. LXA$_4$ was confirmed by LC-MS/MS and quantified by ELISA using a ThermoMax microplate reader (Molecular Devices, Sunnyvale, CA).

Macrophage Phagocytosis of opsonized FITC-zymosan

Macrophage phagocytosis experiments were carried out as in [57]. Briefly, monocytes were isolated from human whole blood and cultured in RPMI with 10 ng/mL human GM–CSF at 37°C for 7 days. Macrophages were enumerated in a hemocytometer and viability was determined by Trypan blue exclusion. For phagocytosis of serum-opsonized zymosan A (SZ) experiments, macrophages $(0.1 \times 10^6$ cells/well in a 24-well plate) were incubated with RvE1 or vehicle for 15 min at 37°C. FITC–SZ from *Saccharomyces cerevisiae* was then added to cells $(0.5 \times 10^6$ particles/well) and incubated (30 min at 37°C) in the dark. Supernatants were aspirated, and Trypan blue (0.03% in PBS+/+ for ~60 s) was added to quench extracellular FITC–STZ. Fluorescence was measured using a Victor plate reader (Perki-nElmer).

References

1. Van Dyke TE, Serhan CN (2003) Resolution of inflammation: a new paradigm for the pathogenesis of periodontal diseases. J Dent Res 82: 82–90.
2. The J, Ebersole JL (1991) Rheumatoid factor (RF) distribution in periodontal disease. Journal of Clinical Immunology 11: 132–142.
3. Boggess KA, Lieff S, Murtha AP, Moss K, Beck J, et al. (2003) Maternal periodontal disease is associated with an increased risk for preeclampsia. Obstetrics and Gynecology 101: 227–231.
4. Offenbacher S, Boggess KA, Murtha AP, Jared HL, Lieff S, et al. (2006) Progressive periodontal disease and risk of very preterm delivery. Obstetrics and Gynecology 107: 29–36.
5. Taylor GW, Burt BA, Becker MP, Genco RJ, Shlossman M, et al. (1996) Severe periodontitis and risk for poor glycemic control in patients with non-insulin-dependent diabetes mellitus. Journal of Periodontology 67: 1085–1093.
6. Friedewald VE, Kornman KS, Beck JD, Genco R, Goldfine A, et al. (2009) The American Journal of Cardiology and Journal of Periodontology editors' consensus: periodontitis and atherosclerotic cardiovascular disease. Journal of Periodontology 80: 1021–1032.
7. Page RC, Eke PI (2007) Case definitions for use in population-based surveillance of periodontitis. Journal of Periodontology 78: 1387–1399.
8. Hasturk H, Kantarci A, Ohira T, Arita M, Ebrahimi N, et al. (2006) RvE1 protects from local inflammation and osteoclast- mediated bone destruction in periodontitis. FASEB J 20: 401–403.
9. Offenbacher S (1996) Periodontal diseases: pathogenesis. Ann Periodontol 1: 821–878.
10. Page RC, Kornman KS (1997) The pathogenesis of human periodontitis: an introduction. Periodontol 2000 14: 9–11.
11. Goodson JM, Tanner AC, Haffajee AD, Sornberger GC, Socransky SS (1982) Patterns of progression and regression of advanced destructive periodontal disease. Journal of Clinical Periodontology 9: 472–481.
12. Van Dyke TE, Warbington M, Gardner M, Offenbacher S (1990) Neutrophil surface protein markers as indicators of defective chemotaxis in LJP. J Periodontol 61: 180–184.
13. (2000) Parameter on aggressive periodontitis. American Academy of Periodontology. J Periodontol 71: 867–869.
14. Meng H, Xu L, Li Q, Han J, Zhao Y (2007) Determinants of host susceptibility in aggressive periodontitis. Periodontol 2000 43: 133–159.
15. Kantarci A, Oyaizu K, Van Dyke TE (2003) Neutrophil-mediated tissue injury in periodontal disease pathogenesis: findings from localized aggressive periodontitis. J Periodontol 74: 66–75.
16. Van Dyke TE, Zinney W, Winkel K, Taufiq A, Offenbacher S, et al. (1986) Neutrophil function in localized juvenile periodontitis. Phagocytosis, superoxide production and specific granule release. J Periodontol 57: 703–708.
17. Shapira L, Gordon B, Warbington M, Van Dyke TE (1994) Priming effect of Porphyromonas gingivalis lipopolysaccharide on superoxide production by neutrophils from healthy and rapidly progressive periodontitis subjects. J Periodontol 65: 129–133.
18. Shapira L, Warbington M, Van Dyke TE (1994) TNF alpha and IL-1 beta in serum of LJP patients with normal and defective neutrophil chemotaxis. J Periodontal Res 29: 371–373.
19. Serhan CN (2007) Resolution phase of inflammation: novel endogenous anti-inflammatory and proresolving lipid mediators and pathways. Annu Rev Immunol 25: 101–137.
20. Serhan CN, Hamberg M, Samuelsson B (1984) Lipoxins: novel series of biologically active compounds formed from arachidonic acid in human leukocytes. Proc Natl Acad Sci U S A 81: 5335–5339.
21. Serhan CN (2005) Lipoxins and aspirin-triggered 15-epi-lipoxins are the first lipid mediators of endogenous anti-inflammation and resolution. Prostaglandins Leukot Essent Fatty Acids 73: 141–162.
22. Schwab JM, Chiang N, Arita M, Serhan CN (2007) Resolvin E1 and protectin D1 activate inflammation-resolution programmes. Nature 447: 869–874.
23. Merched AJ, Ko K, Gotlinger KH, Serhan CN, Chan L (2008) Atherosclerosis: evidence for impairment of resolution of vascular inflammation governed by specific lipid mediators. FASEB Journal 22: 3595–3606.
24. Tabas I (2010) Macrophage death and defective inflammation resolution in atherosclerosis. Nature Reviews Immunology 10: 36–46.
25. Mattoscio D, Evangelista V, De Cristofaro R, Recchiuti A, Pandolfi A, et al. (2010) Cystic fibrosis transmembrane conductance regulator (CFTR) expression in human platelets: impact on mediators and mechanisms of the inflammatory response. FASEB Journal 24: 3970–3980.
26. Majno G, Joris I (2004) Cells, tissues, and disease : principles of general pathology. New York: Oxford University Press, xxviii, 1005 p.
27. Gronert K, Kantarci A, Levy BD, Clish CB, Odparlik S, et al. (2004) A molecular defect in intracellular lipid signaling in human neutrophils in localized aggressive periodontal tissue damage. J Immunol 172: 1856–1861.
28. Furman MI, Barnard MR, Krueger LA, Fox ML, Shilale EA, et al. (2001) Circulating monocyte-platelet aggregates are an early marker of acute myocardial infarction. J Am Coll Cardiol 38: 1002–1006.
29. Nicu EA, Van der Velden U, Nieuwland R, Everts V, Loos BG (2009) Elevated platelet and leukocyte response to oral bacteria in periodontitis. J Thromb Haemost 7: 162–170.
30. Heasman PA, Collins JG, Offenbacher S (1993) Changes in crevicular fluid levels of interleukin-1 beta, leukotriene B4, prostaglandin E2, thromboxane B2 and tumour necrosis factor alpha in experimental gingivitis in humans. Journal of Periodontal Research 28: 241–247.
31. Pouliot M, Clish CB, Petasis NA, Van Dyke TE, Serhan CN (2000) Lipoxin A(4) analogues inhibit leukocyte recruitment to Porphyromonas gingivalis: a role for cyclooxygenase-2 and lipoxins in periodontal disease. Biochemistry 39: 4761–4768.
32. Dennison DK, Van Dyke TE (1997) The acute inflammatory response and the role of phagocytic cells in periodontal health and disease. Periodontology 2000 14: 54–78.
33. Oh SF, Pillai PS, Recchiuti A, Yang R, Serhan CN (2011) Pro-resolving actions and stereoselective biosynthesis of 18S E-series resolvins in human leukocytes and murine inflammation. Journal of Clinical Investigation 121: 569–581.
34. Kantarci A, Hasturk H, Van Dyke TE (2006) Host-mediated resolution of inflammation in periodontal diseases. Periodontol 2000 40: 144–163.
35. Medzhitov R, Janeway C, Jr. (2000) Innate immunity. N Engl J Med 343: 338–344.
36. Dave S, Batista EL, Jr., Van Dyke TE (2004) Cardiovascular disease and periodontal diseases: commonality and causation. Compend Contin Educ Dent 25: 26–37.
37. Friedewald VE, Kornman KS, Beck JD, Genco R, Goldfine A, et al. (2009) The American Journal of Cardiology and Journal of Periodontology Editors' Consensus: periodontitis and atherosclerotic cardiovascular disease. American Journal of Cardiology 104: 59–68.
38. Spanbroek R, Grabner R, Lotzer K, Hildner M, Urbach A, et al. (2003) Expanding expression of the 5-lipoxygenase pathway within the arterial wall during human atherogenesis. Proc Natl Acad Sci U S A 100: 1238–1243.
39. Dwyer JH, Allayee H, Dwyer KM, Fan J, Wu H, et al. (2004) Arachidonate 5-lipoxygenase promoter genotype, dietary arachidonic acid, and atherosclerosis. N Engl J Med 350: 29–37.
40. Serhan CN, Jain A, Marleau S, Clish C, Kantarci A, et al. (2003) Reduced inflammation and tissue damage in transgenic rabbits overexpressing 15-lipoxygenase and endogenous anti-inflammatory lipid mediators. J Immunol 171: 6856–6865.
41. Serhan CN, Sheppard KA (1990) Lipoxin formation during human neutrophil-platelet interactions. Evidence for the transformation of leukotriene A4 by platelet 12-lipoxygenase in vitro. J Clin Invest 85: 772–780.
42. Yamamoto K, Kobayashi T, Grossi S, Ho AW, Genco RJ, et al. (2004) Association of Fcgamma receptor IIa genotype with chronic periodontitis in Caucasians. Journal of Periodontology 75: 517–522.
43. Hasturk H, Kantarci A, Goguet-Surmenian E, Blackwood A, Andry C, et al. (2007) Resolvin E1 regulates inflammation at the cellular and tissue level and restores tissue homeostasis in vivo. J Immunol 179: 7021–7029.
44. Haworth O, Cernadas M, Yang R, Serhan CN, Levy BD (2008) Resolvin E1 regulates interleukin 23, interferon-gamma and lipoxin A4 to promote the resolution of allergic airway inflammation. Nat Immunol 9: 873–879.
45. Seki H, Fukunaga K, Arita M, Arai H, Nakanishi H, et al. (2010) The anti-inflammatory and proresolving mediator resolvin E1 protects mice from bacterial pneumonia and acute lung injury. J Immunol 184: 836–843.

Data analysis

The significance of difference between groups was evaluated using the 2-tailed Student's *t*-test. P values of less than 0.05 were considered to be statistically significant.

Author Contributions

Conceived and designed the experiments: GF TEVD. Performed the experiments: GF SFO SA. Analyzed the data: GF SFO SA HH CNS TEVD. Contributed reagents/materials/analysis tools: GF SFO SA HH CNS TEVD. Wrote the paper: GF TEVD.

46. Ohira T, Arita M, Omori K, Recchiuti A, Van Dyke TE, et al. (2009) Resolvin E1 receptor activation signals phosphorylation and phagocytosis. Journal of Biological Chemistry.

47. Requirand P, Gibert P, Tramini P, Cristol JP, Descomps B (2000) Serum fatty acid imbalance in bone loss: example with periodontal disease. Clin Nutr 19: 271–276.

48. Dewhirst FE, Moss DE, Offenbacher S, Goodson JM (1983) Levels of prostaglandin E2, thromboxane, and prostacyclin in periodontal tissues. J Periodontal Res 18: 156–163.

49. Offenbacher S, Odle BM, Gray RC, Van Dyke TE (1984) Crevicular fluid prostaglandin E levels as a measure of the periodontal disease status of adult and juvenile periodontitis patients. J Periodontal Res 19: 1–13.

50. El-Sharkawy H, Aboelsaad N, Eliwa M, Darweesh M, Alshahat M, et al. (2010) Adjunctive treatment of chronic periodontitis with daily dietary supplementation with omega-3 Fatty acids and low-dose aspirin. J Periodontol 81: 1635–1643.

51. Hart TC, Marazita ML, McCanna KM, Schenkein HA, Diehl SR (1993) Reevaluation of the chromosome 4q candidate region for early onset periodontitis. Human Genetics 91: 416–422.

52. Kinane DF, Hart TC (2003) Genes and gene polymorphisms associated with periodontal disease. Critical Reviews in Oral Biology and Medicine 14: 430–449.

53. Zhang Y, Syed R, Uygar C, Pallos D, Gorry MC, et al. (2003) Evaluation of human leukocyte N-formylpeptide receptor (FPR1) SNPs in aggressive periodontitis patients. Genes Immun 4: 22–29.

54. Maney P, Emecen P, Mills JS, Walters JD (2009) Neutrophil formylpeptide receptor single nucleotide polymorphism 348T>C in aggressive periodontitis. Journal of Periodontology 80: 492–498.

55. Dona M, Fredman G, Schwab JM, Chiang N, Arita M, et al. (2008) Resolvin E1, an EPA-derived mediator in whole blood, selectively counterregulates leukocytes and platelets. Blood 112: 848–855.

56. Yang R CN, Oh SF, Serhan CN (2011) Metabolomics-lipidomics of eicosanoids and docosanoids generated by phagocytes. Curr Protoc Immunol.

57. Krishnamoorthy S, Recchiuti A, Chiang N, Yacoubian S, Lee CH, et al. (2010) Resolvin D1 binds human phagocytes with evidence for proresolving receptors. Proceedings of the National Academy of Sciences of the United States of America.

17

Both 25-Hydroxyvitamin-D$_3$ and 1,25-Dihydroxyvitamin-D$_3$ Reduces Inflammatory Response in Human Periodontal Ligament Cells

Oleh Andrukhov[1]*, Olena Andrukhova[2], Ulamnemekh Hulan[1,3], Yan Tang[1,4], Hans-Peter Bantleon[5], Xiaohui Rausch-Fan[1,5]*

1 Division of Oral Biology, Bernhard Gottlieb School of Dentistry, Medical University of Vienna, Vienna, Austria, 2 Department of Biomedical Science, University of Veterinary Medicine, Vienna, Austria, 3 Department of Restorative Science, School of Dentistry, Health Science University of Mongolia, Ulan Bator, Mongolia, 4 Department of Stomatology, Xuanwu Hospital, Capital Medical University, Beijing, China, 5 Division of Orthodontics, Bernhard Gottlieb School of Dentistry, Medical University of Vienna, Vienna, Austria

Abstract

Periodontitis is an inflammatory disease leading to the destruction of periodontal tissue. Vitamin D$_3$ is an important hormone involved in the preservation of serum calcium and phosphate levels, regulation of bone metabolism and inflammatory response. Recent studies suggest that vitamin D$_3$ metabolism might play a role in the progression of periodontitis. The aim of the present study was to examine the effects of 25(OH)D$_3$, which is stable form of vitamin D$_3$ in blood, and biologically active form 1,25(OH)$_2$D$_3$ on the production of interleukin-6 (IL-6), interleukin-8 (IL-8), and monocyte chemotactic protein-1 (MCP-1) by cells of periodontal ligament. Commercially available human periodontal ligament fibroblasts (hPdLF) and primary human periodontal ligament cells (hPdLC) were used. Cells were stimulated with either *Porphyromonas gingivalis* lipopolysaccharide (LPS) or heat-killed *P. ginigvalis* in the presence or in the absence of 25(OH)D$_3$ or 1,25(OH)$_2$D$_3$ at concentrations of 10–100 nM. Stimulation of cells with either *P. gingivalis* LPS or heat-killed *P. gingivalis* resulted in a significant increase of the expression levels of IL-6, IL-8, and MCP-1 in gene as well as in protein levels, measured by qPCR and ELISA, respectively. The production of these pro-inflammatory mediators in hPdLF was significantly inhibited by both 25(OH)D$_3$ and 1,25(OH)$_2$D$_3$ in a dose-dependent manner. In primary hPdLCs, both 25(OH)D$_3$ and 1,25(OH)$_2$D$_3$ inhibited the production of IL-8 and MCP-1 but have no significant effect on the IL-6 production. The effect of both 25(OH)D$_3$ and 1,25(OH)$_2$D$_3$ was abolished by specific knockdown of vitamin D$_3$ receptor by siRNA. Our data suggest that vitamin D$_3$ might play an important role in the modulation of periodontal inflammation via regulation of cytokine production by cells of periodontal ligament. Further studies are required for better understanding of the extents of this anti-inflammatory effect and its involvement in the progression of periodontal disease.

Editor: Makoto Makishima, Nihon University School of Medicine, Japan

Funding: The study was supported by authors' institution (Bernhard Gottlieb School of Dentistry, Medical University of Vienna) and by International Team of Implantology Foundation (Project No. 781_2011). The funders had no role in study design, data collection and analysis, decision to publish or preparation of the manuscript.

Competing Interests: The authors have declared that no competing interests exist.

* E-mail: oleh.andrukhov@meduniwien.ac.at (OA); xiaohui.rausch-fan@meduniwien.ac.at (XR-F)

Introduction

Vitamin D$_3$ is known to play an important role in the bone metabolism and mineral homeostasis [1]. The major sources of vitamin D$_3$ in organism are production by skin on the sun exposure and dietary supplements. To become metabolically active, vitamin D$_3$ is first converted by liver to 25(OH)D$_3$ (calcifediol), which has a half life time of about 15 day [2]. Calcifideol could be further converted into the active form of vitamin D$_3$ calcitriol (1,25(OH)$_2$D$_3$) by specific enzyme 25(OH)D-1α-hydroxylase. The half life time of 1,25(OH)$_2$D$_3$ is about 15 h [2] and its biological effects are mediated by activation of the vitamin D$_3$ receptor (VDR), a member of the nuclear receptor superfamily [3]. For a long time it was thought that the expression of 1α-hydroxylase is limited to kidney, but now this enzyme is also found to be expressed in numerous extrarenal tissues [4]. There

are accumulating evidences that vitamin D$_3$ is also involved in the regulation of immune response [5].

Periodontitis is a chronic bacterial infectious disease that affects tooth supporting tissues of periodontium [6,7]. Periodontitis is caused by overgrow of some anaerobic Gram-negative bacteria, which trigger host responses causing most of the tissue damages, and might lead to substantial loss of alveolar bone and eventually the loss of teeth [8]. Especially "red complex bacteria" that include the periodontal pathogens *Porphyromonas gingivalis*, *Treponema denticola*, and *Tannerella forsythia* have been strongly associated with clinical measurements of periodontitis [9]. The association between vitamin D$_3$ and periodontitis is currently under investigation and its role in the progression of periodontitis is not entirely understood [10]. Some studies report decreased serum levels of vitamin D$_3$ in periodontitis as well as a negative correlation between serum vitamin D$_3$ levels and severity of periodontal inflammation [11,12]. In contrast, other studies show the

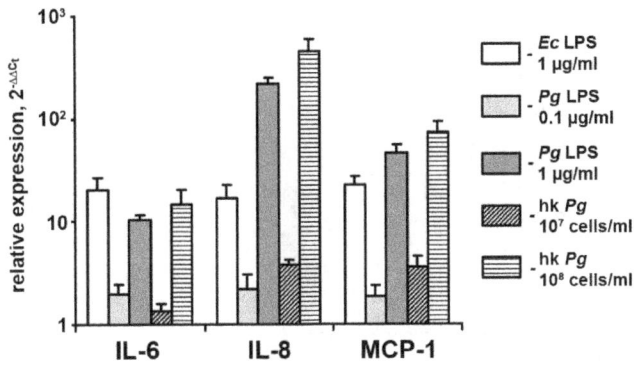

Figure 1. Gene expression levels of pro-inflammatory mediators in hPdLF in response to stimulation with *E. coli* LPS, *P. gingivalis* LPS, and heat-killed *P. gingivalis*. Cells were stimulated with *E. coli* LPS (1 µg/ml), *P. gingivalis* LPS (0.1–1 µg/ml), or heat-killed *P. gingivalis* (10^7–10^8 cells/ml) for 24 h. Gene expression levels of IL-6 (A), IL-8 (B), and MCP-1 (C) were measured using q-PCR. Y-axes represent the n-fold expression levels of target gene in relation to non-stimulated cells (control).

increased serum levels of vitamin D_3 in patients with aggressive periodontitis and positive association between serum vitamin D_3 concentration and periodontal disease severity [13,14]. Thus, the role of vitamin D_3 in periodontal disease needs to be further investigated.

Periodontal ligament is a structure connecting teeth to the alveolar bone and seems to actively participate in alveolar bone remodelling [15]. Periodontal ligament cells (PDLs) are fibroblast-like cells characterized by collagen production but also possessing some osteoblastic features (for review, see [16]). In addition, periodontal ligament cells produce several pro-inflammatory mediators when stimulated with *Porphyromonas gingivalis* and/or its components [16,17,18]. Periodontal ligament cells isolated from *P. gingivalis*-positive periodontitis patients exhibit increased cytokine production in response to *P. gingivalis* [19]. Due to the proximity of periodontal ligament to alveolar bone, the cytokine production by periodontal ligament cells might influence the processes of bone resorption in periodontal disease. Vitamin D_3 might have an important role in the function of periodontal ligament in periodontal disease, because periodontal ligament cells express 1α-hydroxylase and convert 25(OH)D_3 into 1,25(OH)$_2$D$_3$ [20,21]. A recent study shows that 1,25(OH)$_2$D$_3$ inhibits production of

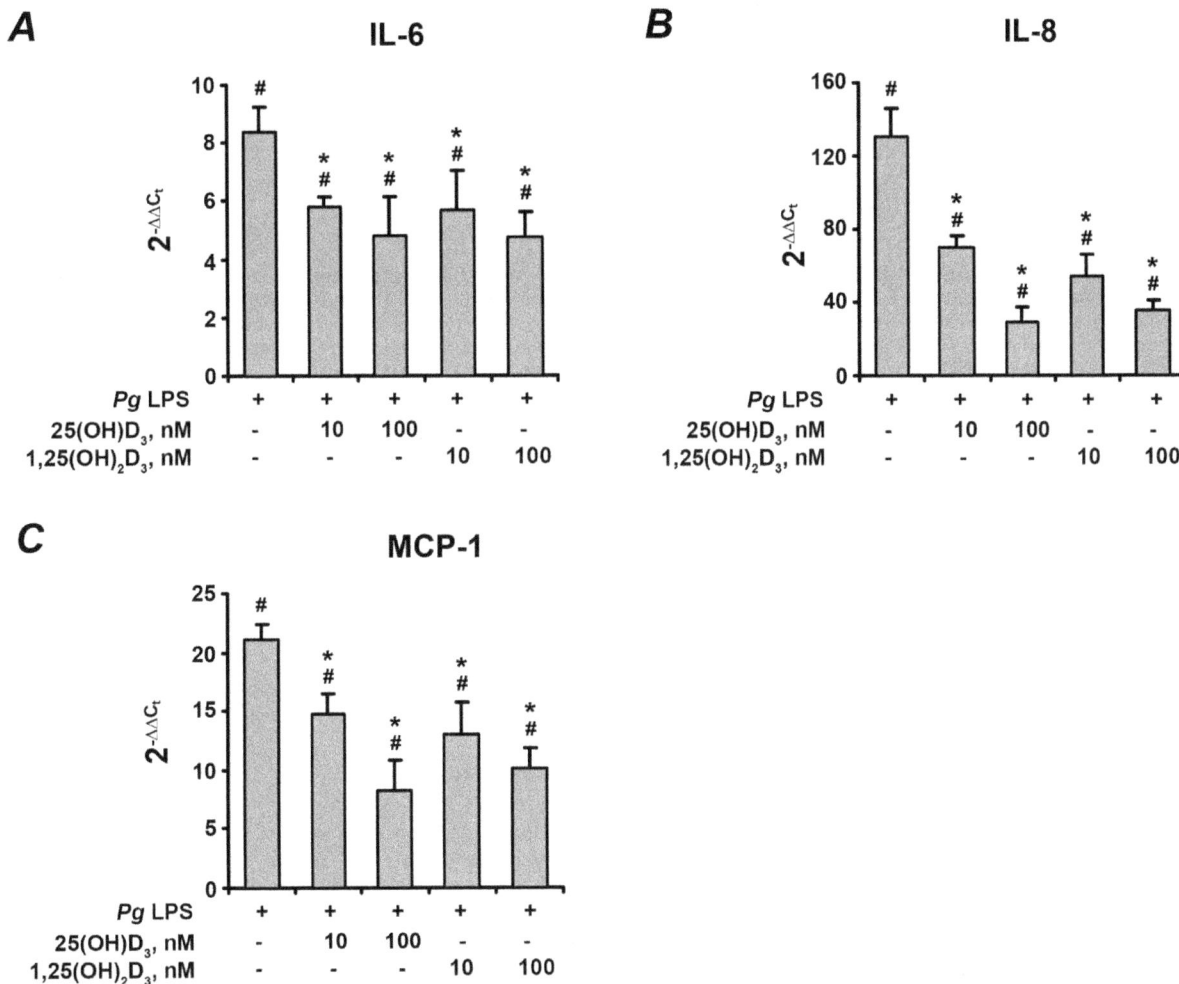

Figure 2. Effect of 25(OH)D$_3$ and 1,25(OH)$_2$D$_3$ on the gene-expression levels of pro-inflammatory mediators in hPdLF in response to stimulation with *P. gingivalis* LPS. Cells were stimulated with *P. gingivalis* LPS (*Pg* LPS, 1 µg/ml) for 24 h in the presence or in the absence of different concentrations of 25(OH)D$_3$ or 1,25(OH)$_2$D$_3$. Gene expression levels of IL-6 (A), IL-8 (B), and MCP-1 (C) were measured using q-PCR. Y-axes represent the n-fold expression levels of target gene in relation to non-stimulated cells (control). $^{#}$ means significantly different from control group ($2^{-\triangle\triangle Ct} = 1$). * means significantly different from cells stimulated with *P. gingivalis* LPS only.

A IL-6

B IL-8

C MCP-1

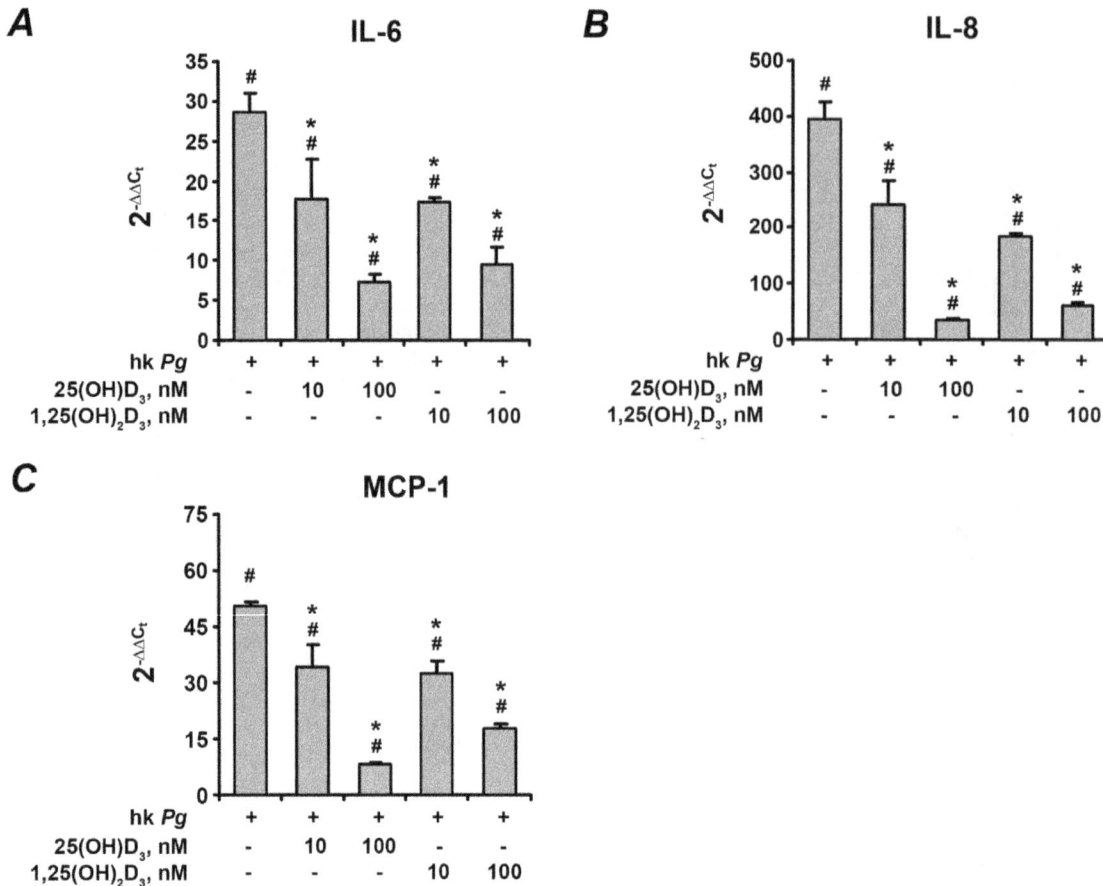

Figure 3. Effect of 25(OH)D$_3$ and 1,25(OH)$_2$D$_3$ on the gene-expression levels of pro-inflammatory mediators in hPdLF in response to stimulation with heat-killed *P. gingivalis*. Cells were stimulated with heat-killed *P. gingivalis* (hk *Pg*, 10^8 cells/ml) for 24 h in the presence or in the absence of different concentrations of 25(OH)D$_3$ or 1,25(OH)$_2$D$_3$. Gene expression levels of IL-6 (A), IL-8 (B), and MCP-1 (C) were measured using q-PCR. Y-axes represent the n-fold expression levels of target gene in relation to non-stimulated cells (control). $^\#$ means significantly different from control group (2$^{-\delta\delta Ct}$ = 1). * means significantly different from cells stimulated with heat-killed *P. gingivalis* only.

interleukin-8 by primary human periodontal ligament cells but has no effect on production of IL-6 [22]. Yet, it is not known if 25(OH)D$_3$, which is a biological precursor of 1,25(OH)$_2$D$_3$ and main form of vitamin D$_3$ in blood, could also influence the inflammatory response in cells of human periodontal ligament.

The main aim of the present study was to investigate if 25(OH)D$_3$ as well as 1,25(OH)$_2$D$_3$ influence the production of pro-inflammatory mediators in cells of human periodontal ligament in response to stimulation with periodontal pathogens. To answer this question we investigated the effect of 25(OH)D$_3$ and 1,25(OH)$_2$D$_3$ on the production of interleukin-6 (IL-6), interleukin-8 (IL-8), and monocyte chemoattractant protein 1 (MCP-1) by cells of human periodontal ligament in response to stimulation with *P. gingivalis* LPS or heat-killed *P. gingivalis*. The contribution of VDR on the effect of both vitamin D$_3$ forms was investigated in the experiments with deletion of this protein using small interfering RNA (siRNA).

In the present study, we use commercially available primary human periodontal ligament fibroblasts (hPdLF), which represent standardized model of periodontal ligament cells. In addition, the effect of both vitamin D$_3$ forms was investigated on the primary human periodontal ligament cells (hPdLC) isolated from six different donors. Our results revealed that both 25(OH)D$_3$ and

1,25(OH)$_2$D$_3$ might modulate periodontal inflammation via regulation of cytokine production by cells of periodontal ligament.

Materials And Methods

Ethic Statement

Protocol for primary human periodontal ligament cells isolation was approved by the Ethics Committee of the Medical University of Vienna. Patients were informed in details before the surgical procedures and gave their written agreement.

Cell Culture and reagents

Primary commercially available Clonetics human periodontal ligament fibroblasts (hPdLF) isolated from 16-year old male (Lonza, Switzerland) were used in the present study. These cells were shown to produce pro-inflammatory mediators and express osteogenesis-related genes, which is characteristic for periodontal ligament cells [23,24,25]. In addition, primary human periodontal ligament cells (hPdLC) were isolated from periodontally healthy donors undergoing routine extraction of their third molar teeth by outgrow method [26]. hPdLC were isolated by scraping the ligament tissue from the teeth root surface and cultured in Dulbecco's modified Eagle's medium (DMEM), supplemented with 10% fetal bovine serum (FBS), streptomycin (50 μg/ml) and

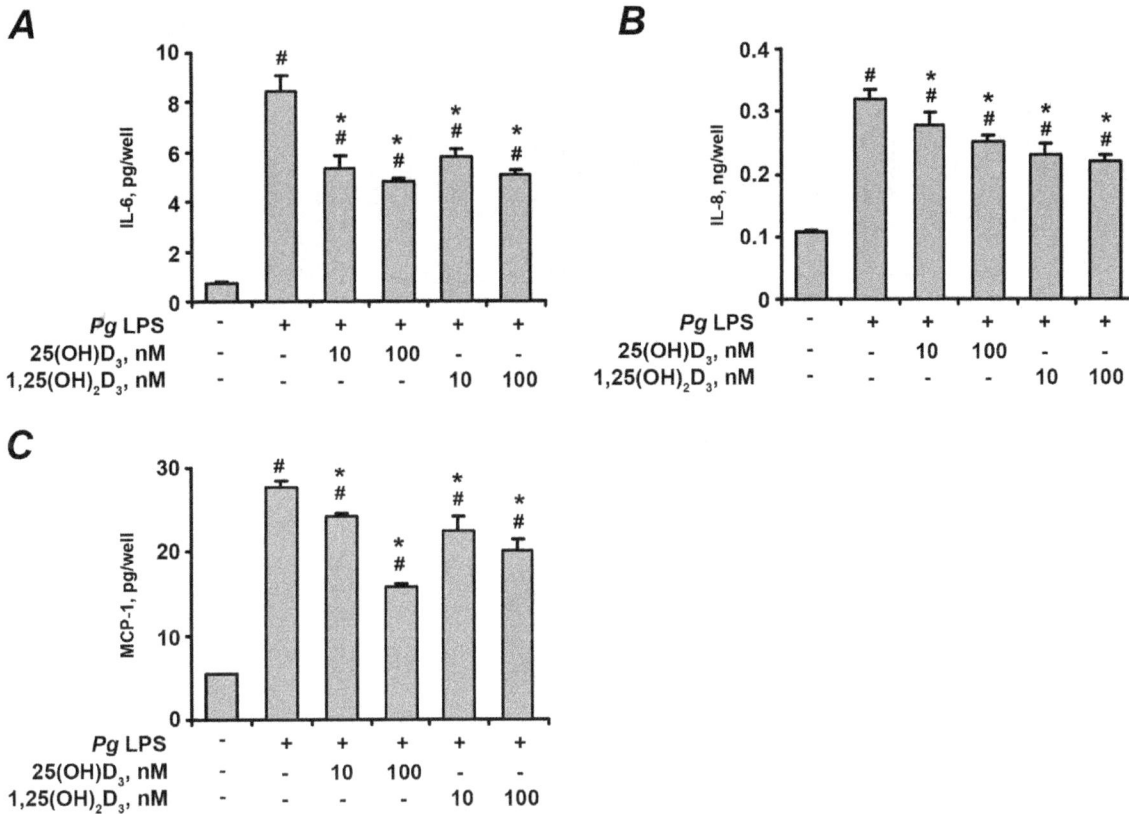

Figure 4. Effect of 25(OH)D₃ and 1,25(OH)₂D₃ on the production of pro-inflammatory mediators by hPdLF in response to stimulation with *P. gingivalis* LPS. Cells were stimulated with *P. gingivalis* LPS (*Pg* LPS, 1 µg/ml) for 24 h in the presence or in the absence of different concentrations of 25(OH)D₃ or 1,25(OH)₂D₃. The levels of IL-6 (A), IL-8 (B), and MCP-1 (C) were measured in cell supernatants using ELISA. # means significantly different from control group (non stimulated cells). * means significantly different from group stimulated with *P.gingivalis* LPS only

penicillin (100 U/ml) under humidified air atmosphere of 5% CO_2 at 37°C. Cells were cultured in Dulbecco's modified Eagle's medium (DMEM; Invitrogen), supplemented with 10% of FBS, 100 U/mL penicillin, and 100 µg/mL streptomycin at 37°C in a humidified atmosphere containing 5% CO_2. Cells from passage levels 3–6 were used in this study.

Commercially available ultrapure *P. gingivalis* LPS, heat-killed *P. gingivalis*, and ultrapure *E. coli* LPS (all from Invivogen, San Diego, USA) were used in the present study. As reported by other study [27], LPS preparations are free from contaminating lipoproteins.

Cells stimulation

Cells were seeded in a 24-well plate at a density of 5×10^4 cells per well containing 0.5 mL of DMEM medium supplemented with 10% FBS. After 24 h, cells were stimulated with either *P. gingivalis* LPS (1 µg/ml) or heat-killed *P. gingivalis* (10^8 cells/ml) in DMEM supplemented with 2% FBS. Stimulation was performed either in the presence or in the absence of 25(OH)D₃ (10–100 nM, Cayman Chemicals, Ann Arbor, USA) or 1,25(OH)₂D₃ (10–100 nM, Sigma, San Diego, USA). Each experimental group included three wells. After stimulation for 24 h, the cellular mRNA expression levels of IL-6, IL-8 and MCP-1 in cells as well as the content of corresponding proteins in the conditioned media were determined.

Quantitative PCR

The mRNA expression levels of IL-6, IL-8, and MCP-1 were determined by qPCR as described previously [28,29], taking the β-actin encoding gene as internal reference. Isolation of mRNA and transcription into cDNA was performed using the TaqMan Gene Expression Cells-to-CT kit (Ambion/Applied Biosystems, Foster City, CA, USA) according to the manufacturer's instructions. This kit provides good accuracy and superior sensitivity of gene-expression analysis [30]. qPCR was performed on an ABI StepOnePlus device (Applied Biosystems) in paired reactions using the Taqman gene expression assays with following ID numbers (all from Applied Biosystems): IL-6, Hs00985639_m1; IL-8, Hs00174103_m1; MCP-1, Hs00234140_m1; β-actin, Hs9999 9903_m1. qPCR reactions were performed in triplicate in 96-well plates using the following thermocycling conditions: 95°C for 10 min; 40 cycles, each for 15 s at 95°C and at 60°C for 1 min. The point at which the PCR product was first detected above a fixed threshold (cycle threshold, C_t), was determined for each sample. Changes in the expression of target genes were calculated using the $2^{-\triangle\triangle Ct}$ method, where $\triangle\triangle C_t = (C_t^{target} - C_t^{\beta-actin})_{sample} - (C_t^{target} - C_t^{\beta-actin})_{control}$, taking an untreated sample as a control.

Measurements of cytokines in supernatants

Commercially available ELISA kits (Hoelzel Diagnostika, Cologne, Germany) were used for measurements of IL-6, IL-8, and MCP-1 levels in the conditioned media. For measurement of IL-6 and MCP-1 samples were not diluted, whereas for measurements of IL-8 samples were diluted 1:10.

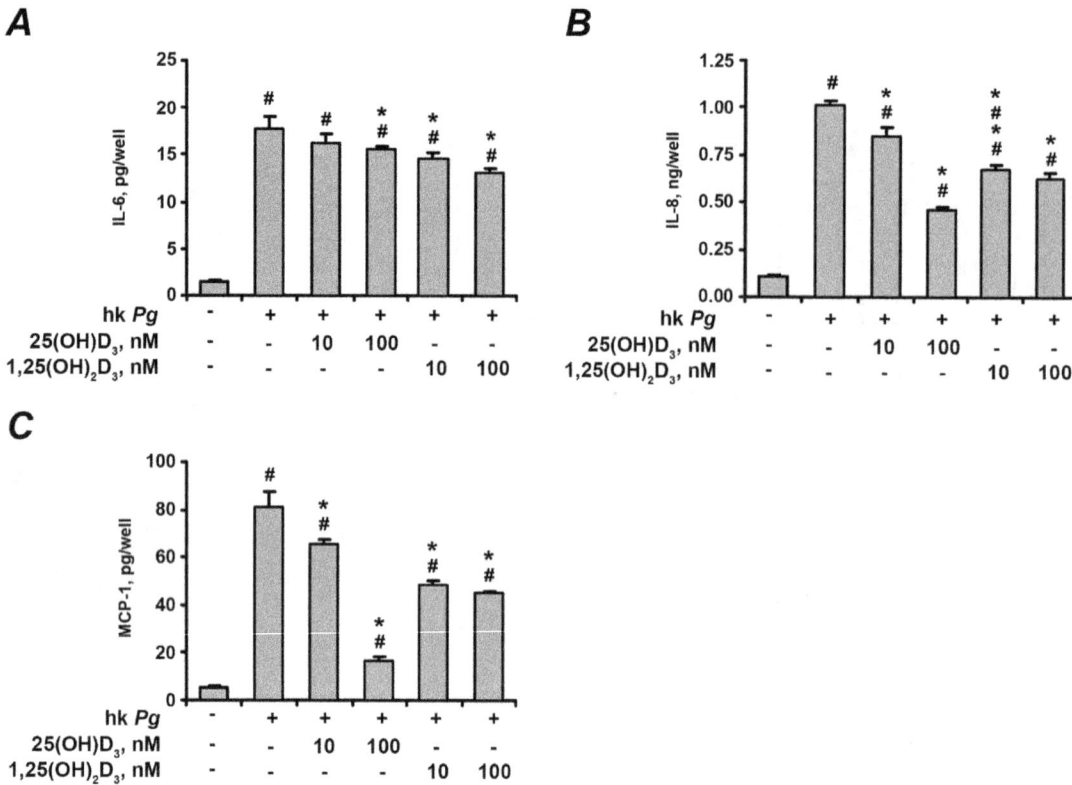

Figure 5. Effect of 25(OH)D$_3$ and 1,25(OH)$_2$D$_3$ on the production of pro-inflammatory mediators by hPdLF in response to stimulation with heat-killed *P. gingivalis*. Cells were stimulated with heat-killed *P. gingivalis* (hk *Pg*, 10^8 cells/ml) for 24 h in the presence or in the absence of different concentrations of 25(OH)D$_3$ or 1,25(OH)$_2$D$_3$. The levels of IL-6 (A), IL-8 (B), and MCP-1 (C) were measured in cell supernatants using ELISA. [#] means significantly different from control group (non-stimulated cells). [*] means significantly different from group stimulated with heat-killed *P.gingivalis* only

RNA Interference of VDR

The highly specific technique of small interfering RNA (siRNA) was used to knockdown the expression of VDR in hPdLF. Cells were seeded at a density of 3×10^4 cells per well containing 0.5 mL of DMEM medium supplemented with 10% FBS without antibiotics. 24 h later, the cells were transfected with either VDR siRNA (Cat. Nr. Sc-106692, Santa Cruz Biotechnology, Heidelberg, Germany) or a non-silencing control siRNA (Cat. Nr. Sc-37007, Santa Cruz Biotechnology) using siRNA Reagent System (Cat. Nr. Sc-45064, Santa Cruz Biotechnology) according to the manufacturers protocol. 48 h after transfection, cells were stimulated by *P. gingivalis* LPS or heat-killed *P. gingivalis* in the presence or in the absence of 25(OH)D$_3$ (100 nM) or 1,25(OH)$_2$D$_3$ (100 nM). Stimulation was performed in DMEM containing 2% of FBS, 100 U/mL penicillin, and 100 µg/mL streptomycin. After 24 h, the gene expression levels of pro-inflammatory mediators IL-6, IL-8, and MCP-1 as well as the content of corresponding proteins in conditioned media were investigated. The effectivity of siRNA transfection was controlled by western blot. Protein samples were collected from cells, fractionated on SDS-PAGE and transferred to a nitrocellulose membrane. Immunoblots were incubated for 3 hours at room temperature with primary antibodies anti-VDR (Abcam) or anti-β-actin (Sigma). Then, membranes were incubated with anti-rabbit horseradish peroxidase-conjugated secondary antibodies (Amersham Life Sciences). Specific signal was visualized by ECL kit (Amersham Life Sciences). The protein bands (~48 kDa for VDR and ~42 kDa for β-actin, respectively) were quantified by Image Quant 5.0 software (Molecular Dynamics). Equal sample loading was

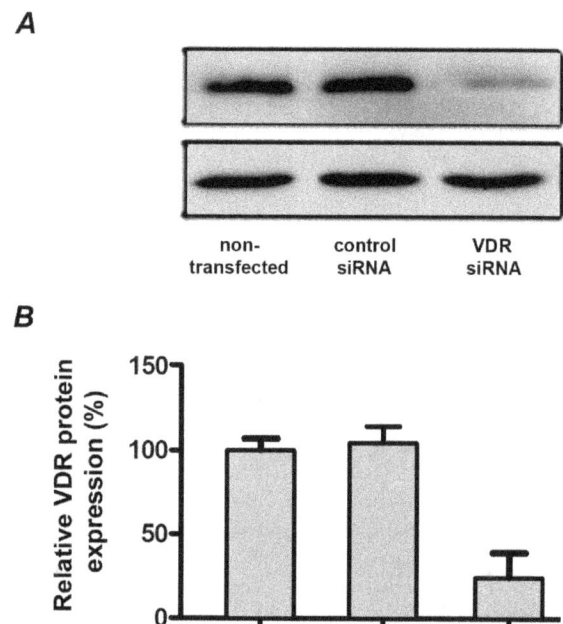

Figure 6. Western blot of VDR in hPdLF after transfection with VDR siRNA. (A) Original western-blots of hPdLF. Protein samples were collected from cells, and the expression of VDR and β-actin was detected using specific antibodies. (B) Quantification of western blot analysis. The protein bands of VDR and β-actin were quantified by Image Quant 5.0 software (Molecular Dynamics). The expression levels were normalized to β-actin.

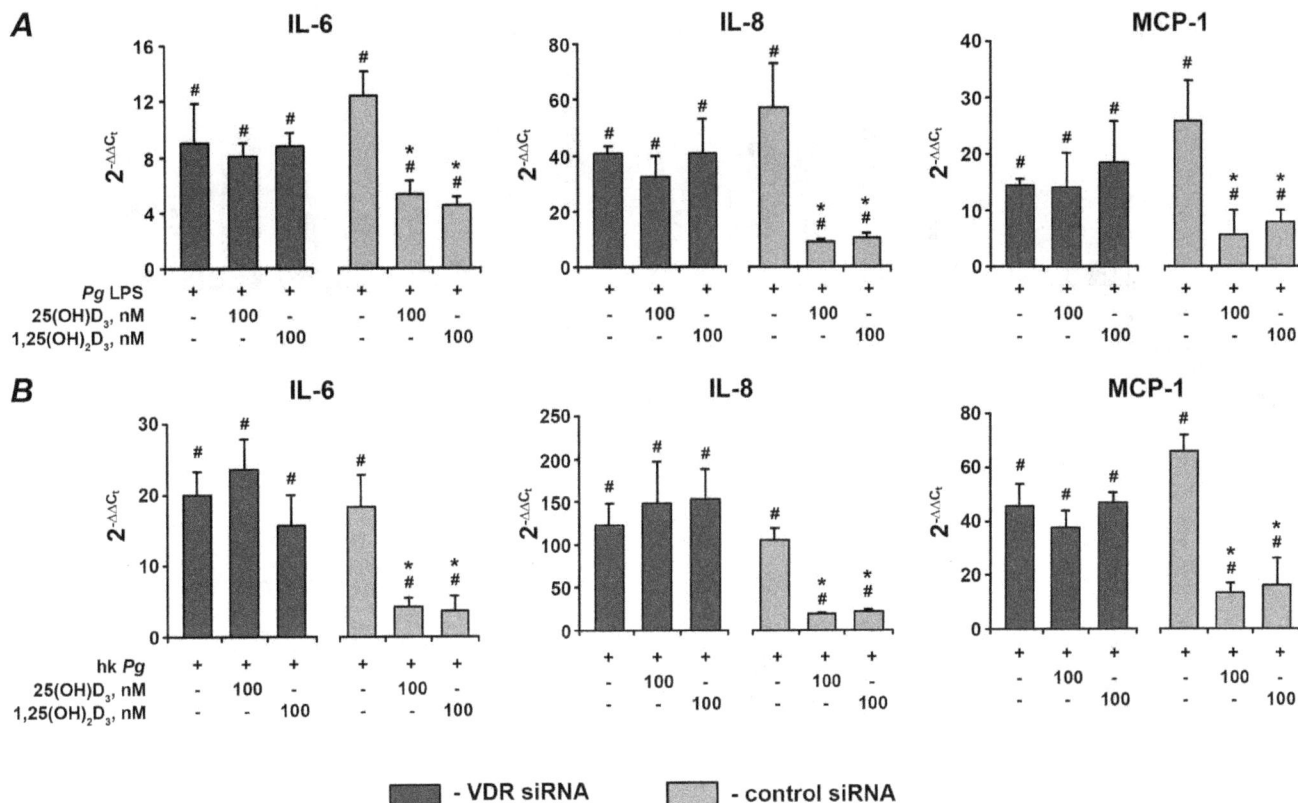

Figure 7. Effect of 25(OH)D$_3$ and 1,25(OH)$_2$D$_3$ on the gene-expression levels of pro-inflammatory mediators in hPdLF with silenced VDR in response to stimulation with *P. gingivalis* **LPS or heat-killed** *P. gingivalis.* Gene expression levels of IL-6, IL-8, and MCP-1 were measured using q-PCR in hPdLF after transfection with either VDR siRNA or control siRNA and stimulation with *P. gingivalis* LPS (A, *Pg* LPS, 1 μg/ml) or heat-killed *P. gingivalis* (B, hk *Pg*, 10^8 cells/ml) in the presence or in the absence of 25(OH)D$_3$ or 1,25(OH)$_2$D$_3$. Y-axes represent the n-fold expression levels of target gene in relation to non-stimulated cells. $^{#}$ means significantly different from control group ($2^{-\triangle\triangle Ct} = 1$). * means significantly different from cells stimulated with heat-killed *P. gingivalis* LPS or heat-killed *P. gingivalis* only.

confirmed by Ponceau S staining of the Western blot [31]. The expression levels were normalized to β-actin.

Statistical Analysis

The normal distribution of all data was tested with Kolmogorov-Smirnov test. After confirming normal distribution, the statistical differences between different groups were analysed by one-way analysis of variance (ANOVA) for repeated measures followed by t-test. All statistical analysis was performed using statistical program SPSS 19.0 (SPSS, Chicago, IL, USA). Data are expressed as mean ± S.E.M. Differences were considered to be statistically significant at $p<0.05$.

Results

Cytokine expression in hPdLF in response to stimulation with different concentrations of *P. gingivalis* LPS and heat-killed *P. gingivalis*

The response of hPdLF on the stimulation with different concentrations of *P. gingivalis* LPS (0.1–1 μg/ml) and heat-killed *P. gingivalis* (10^7–10^8 cells/ml) in comparison with that of well known pathogen *E. coli* LPS (1 μg/ml) is shown on the Figure 1. Gene expression levels of IL-6, IL-8, and MCP-1 significantly increased after stimulation with all stimuli. The increase in the expression levels of pro-inflammatory mediators in response to stimulation with 1 μg/ml of *P. gingivalis* LPS or 10^8 cells/ml of heat-killed *P. gingivalis* was similar (IL-6) or markedly higher (IL-8, MCP-1) in

comparison with that to *E. coli* LPS. Therefore, these concentrations of *P. gingivalis* LPS and heat-killed *P. gingivalis* were used in our further experiments.

Effect of vitamin D$_3$ on the gene expression of pro-inflammatory mediators in hPdLF

The effect of 25(OH)D$_3$ and 1,25(OH)$_2$D$_3$ on the gene expression levels of pro-inflammatory mediators IL-6, IL-8, and MCP-1 in hPdLF in response to stimulation with *P. gingivalis* LPS and heat-killed *P. gingivalis* is shown on the Figures 2 and 3, respectively. In commercially available cells, the expression levels of all pro-inflammatory mediators were significantly increased in response to stimulation with either *P. gingivalis* LPS or heat-killed *P. gingivalis*. Both 25(OH)D$_3$ and 1,25(OH)$_2$D$_3$ at concentrations of 10–100 nM induced a dose-dependent decrease in the *P. gingivalis* LPS- and heat-killed *P. gingivalis*-induced gene-expression levels of IL-6, IL-8, and MCP-1 ($p<0.05$).

Effect of vitamin D$_3$ on cytokines production by hPdLF in vitro

The effect of 25(OH)D$_3$ and 1,25(OH)$_2$D$_3$ on the protein content of IL-6, IL-8, and MCP-1 in conditioned media after stimulation of hPdLF cells with *P. gingivalis* LPS and heat-killed *P. gingivalis* is shown on the Figures 4 and 5, respectively. The soluble protein levels of these pro-inflammatory mediators in conditioned media were significantly increased after stimulation with either *P.*

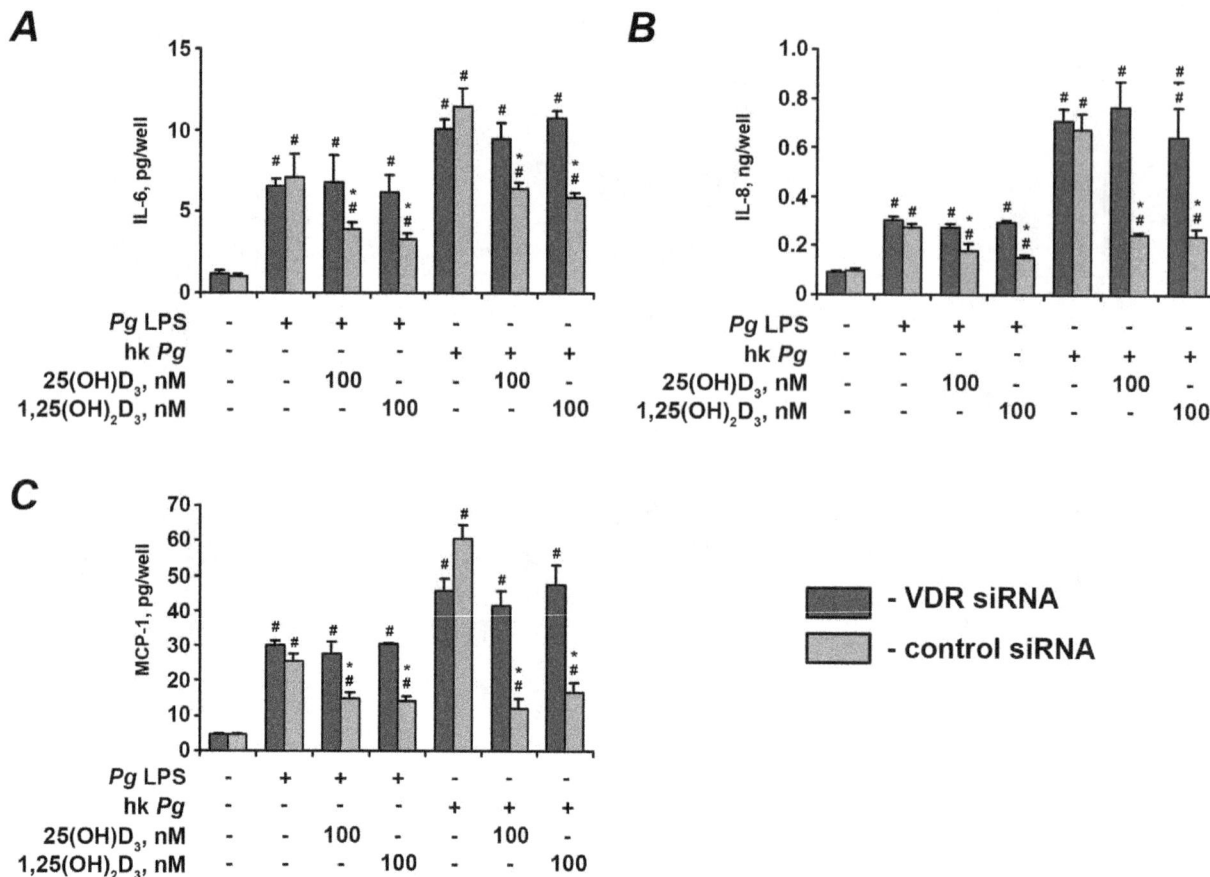

Figure 8. Effect of 25(OH)D$_3$ and 1,25(OH)$_2$D$_3$ on the production of pro-inflammatory mediators by hPdLF with silenced VDR. Cells were transfected with either VDR siRNA or control siRNA and stimulated with *P. gingivalis* LPS (*Pg* LPS, 1 µg/ml) or heat-killed *P. gingivalis* (hk *Pg*, 10^8 cells/ml) for 24 h in the presence or in the absence of 25(OH)D$_3$ or 1,25(OH)$_2$D$_3$. # means significantly different from control group (2$^{-\triangle\triangle Ct}$ = 1). * means significantly different from cells stimulated with either *P. gingivalis* LPS or heat-killed *P. gingivalis* only.

gingivalis LPS (Figure 4) or heat-killed *P. gingivalis* (Figure 5). 25(OH)D$_3$ and 1,25(OH)$_2$D$_3$ at concentrations of 10–100 nM induced dose-dependent decrease in the *P. gingivalis* LPS- and heat-killed *P. gingivalis*-induced production of IL-6, IL-8, and MCP-1.

Effect of vitamin D$_3$ on expression of pro-inflammatory mediators in hPdLF transfected with either VDR siRNA or non-silencing control siRNA

Figure 5 shows the effect of expression of VDR protein in hPdLF after transfection with either VDR siRNA or control siRNA measured by Western blot. Transfection of hPdLF with VDR siRNA resulted in significant decrease of VDR protein expression. As measured by densitometry, transfected cells expressed about 20% of VDR protein compared to non-transfected cells. Transfection of hPdLF with control siRNA did not influence VDR expression. The effect of 25(OH)D$_3$ and 1,25(OH)$_2$D$_3$ on the gene expression levels of pro-inflammatory mediators in response to stimulation with *P. gingivalis* LPS and heat-killed *P. gingivalis* in hPdLF transfected with VDR siRNA or control siRNA is shown on the Figures 6 and 7, respectively. The protein content of IL-6, IL-8, and MCP-1 in conditioned media is shown on the Figure 8. In hPdLF transfected with VDR siRNA neither 25(OH)D$_3$ nor 1,25(OH)$_2$D$_3$ were able to diminish the response to *P. gingivalis* LPS or heat-killed *P. gingivalis*. This was true for both gene expression levels of IL-6, IL-8, and MCP-1 as well as for their content in conditioned media. In hPdLF transfected with

control siRNA, both 25(OH)D$_3$ and 1,25(OH)$_2$D$_3$ diminished the production of pro-inflammatory mediators in response to stimulation with *P. gingivalis* LPS or heat-killed *P. gingivalis*.

Effect of vitamin D$_3$ on cytokines expression in primary hPdLC isolated from healthy individuals

The effect of 25(OH)D$_3$ and 1,25(OH)$_2$D$_3$ on the gene expression levels of IL-6, IL-8, and MCP-1 in primary hPdLC after stimulation with *P. gingivalis* LPS and heat-killed *P. gingivalis* is shown on the Figure 9. The content of corresponding cytokines in the conditioned media is presented on the Figure 10. Similarly to hPdLF, in primary hPdLC, both 25(OH)D$_3$ and 1,25(OH)$_2$D$_3$ induced a dose-dependent decrease in the *P. gingivalis* LPS- and heat-killed *P. gingivalis*-stimulated expression of IL-8 and MCP-1. Both forms of vitamin D$_3$ tended to diminish IL-6 production by primary hPdLC but in contrast to hPdLF this effect was not statistically significant.

Discussion

In the present study we investigated the effect of two different forms of vitamin D$_3$ 25(OH)D$_3$ and 1,25(OH)$_2$D$_3$, on the production of pro-inflammatory mediators by cells of human periodontal ligament in response to stimulation with *P. gingivalis* LPS or heat-killed *P. gingivalis*. We focused on the measurements of the expression of IL-6, IL-8, and MCP-1, which are produced by

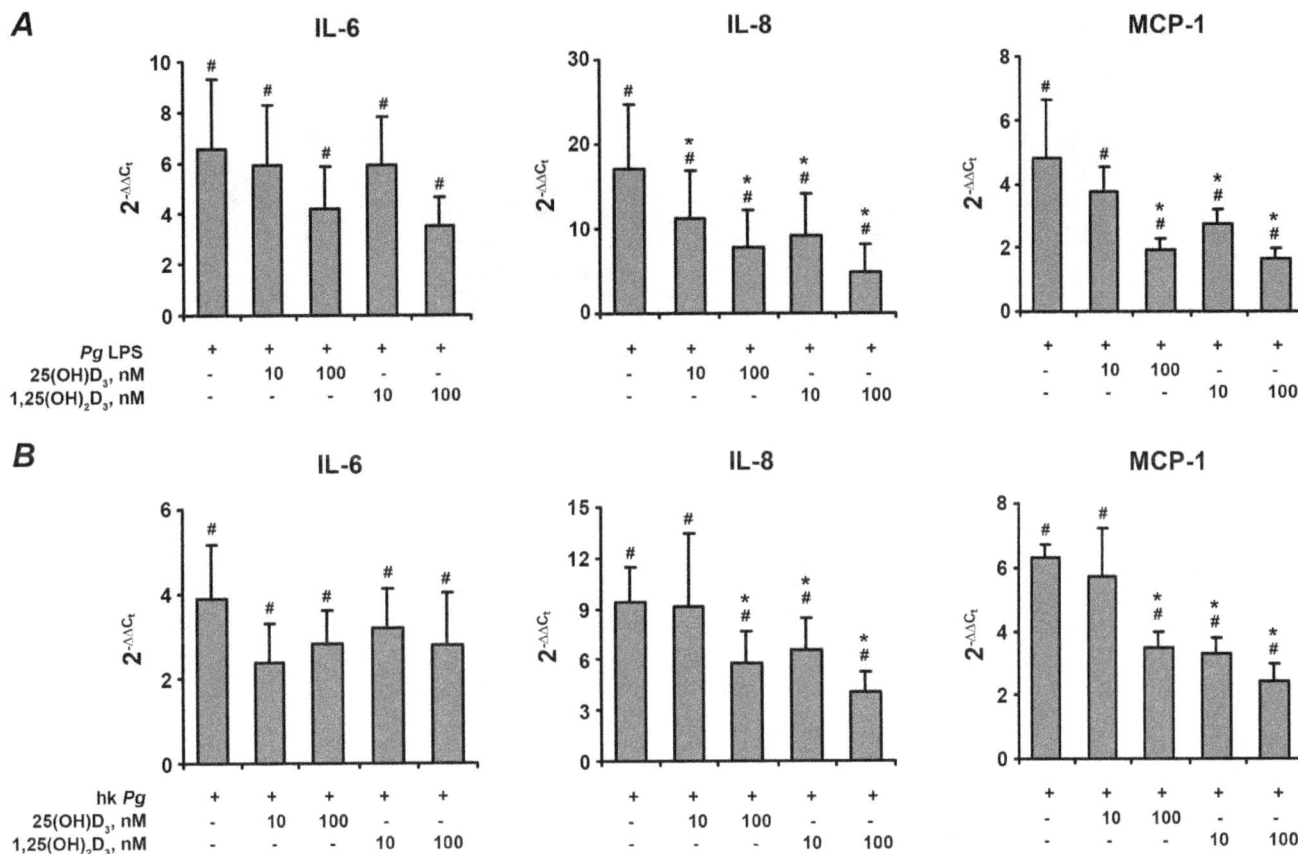

Figure 9. Effect of 25(OH)D$_3$ and 1,25(OH)$_2$D$_3$ on the gene-expression levels of pro-inflammatory mediators in primary hPdLC in response to stimulation with *P. gingivalis* LPS or heat-killed *P. gingivalis*. Cells were stimulated with *P. gingivalis* LPS (*Pg* LPS, 1 µg/ml) or heat-killed *P. gingivalis* (hk *Pg*, 10^8 cells/ml) for 24 h in the presence or in the absence of different concentrations of 25(OH)D$_3$ or 1,25(OH)$_2$D$_3$. Gene expression levels of IL-6 (A), IL-8 (B), and MCP-1 (C) were measured using q-PCR. Y-axes represent the n-fold expression levels of target gene in relation to non-stimulated cells (control). Data are presented as mean±SEM of six different donors. $^{\#}$ means significantly different from control group (2$^{-\triangle\triangle Ct}$ = 1). * means significantly different from cells stimulated with *P. gingivalis* LPS or heat-killed *P. gingivalis* only.

periodontal ligament cells and are thought to play an important role in the progression of periodontal disease. IL-6 is a pro-inflammatory cytokine, which plays a key role in acute inflammation phase and promotes bone resorption [32,33]. IL-8 and MCP-1 are chemoattractant, which induce migration of neutrophils and monocytes, respectively, to the inflammation site and promote the development of acute inflammation [34,35].

The main observation of the present study is that the production of pro-inflammatory cytokines by cells of periodontal ligament is inhibited by 25(OH)D$_3$, which is the main form of vitamin D$_3$ circulating in the blood and is commonly used for determination of vitamin D$_3$ status. The effect of 25(OH)D$_3$ was qualitatively similar to that of biologically active 1,25(OH)$_2$D$_3$. The optimal serum levels of 25(OH)D$_3$ are thought to be about 70–100 nM [36] and these levels are similar to those used in our study. 25(OH)D$_3$ is present in high amount in the gingival crevicular fluid, which is in direct proximity to periodontal ligament and its levels are increased in periodontal disease [14]. Therefore the effect of 25(OH)D$_3$ on pro-inflammatory cytokine production observed in our study is physiologically relevant. Previous studies show that hPDLCs might locally convert vitamin D$_3$ into 25(OH)D$_3$ and subsequently into 1,25(OH)$_2$D$_3$ and the expression of enzyme responsible for this conversion is influenced by some pro-inflammatory mediators [20,21]. Thus, on the one hand, the

inflammatory response of periodontal ligament is regulated by both 25(OH)D$_3$ and 1,25(OH)$_2$D$_3$ and, on the other hand, several factors involved in vitamin D$_3$ metabolism are also regulated by inflammatory stimuli by feedback mechanisms. Vitamin D$_3$ is also known to regulate osteogenic differentiation in periodontal ligament cells [37] and thus might affect the neighbouring alveolar bone. Therefore, it is plausible that vitamin D$_3$ metabolism could play an important role in the regulation of the periodontal tissue homeostasis, especially during inflammation.

The exact physiological role of vitamin D$_3$ effect on inflammatory response in periodontal ligament remains to be clarified. Decreased production of pro-inflammatory mediators by vitamin D$_3$ might reduce the ability of immune system to recognize and eliminate pathogenic microorganisms on the one hand, but also could represent a protective mechanism prohibiting local excessive pro-inflammatory response and tissue destruction on the other hand [38]. Noteworthy, the effects of vitamin D$_3$ in oral cavity are not associated only with decreased inflammatory response. Particularly, a study on human gingival epithelial cells shows that 1,25(OH)$_2$D$_3$ enhance immune response, which could lead to an increase in antibacterial activity against periodontal pathogens [39]. Periodontium is a complex tissue consisting by different cells types, which might participate in the host response to periodontal pathogens [40]. Thus, inflammatory response in various cells

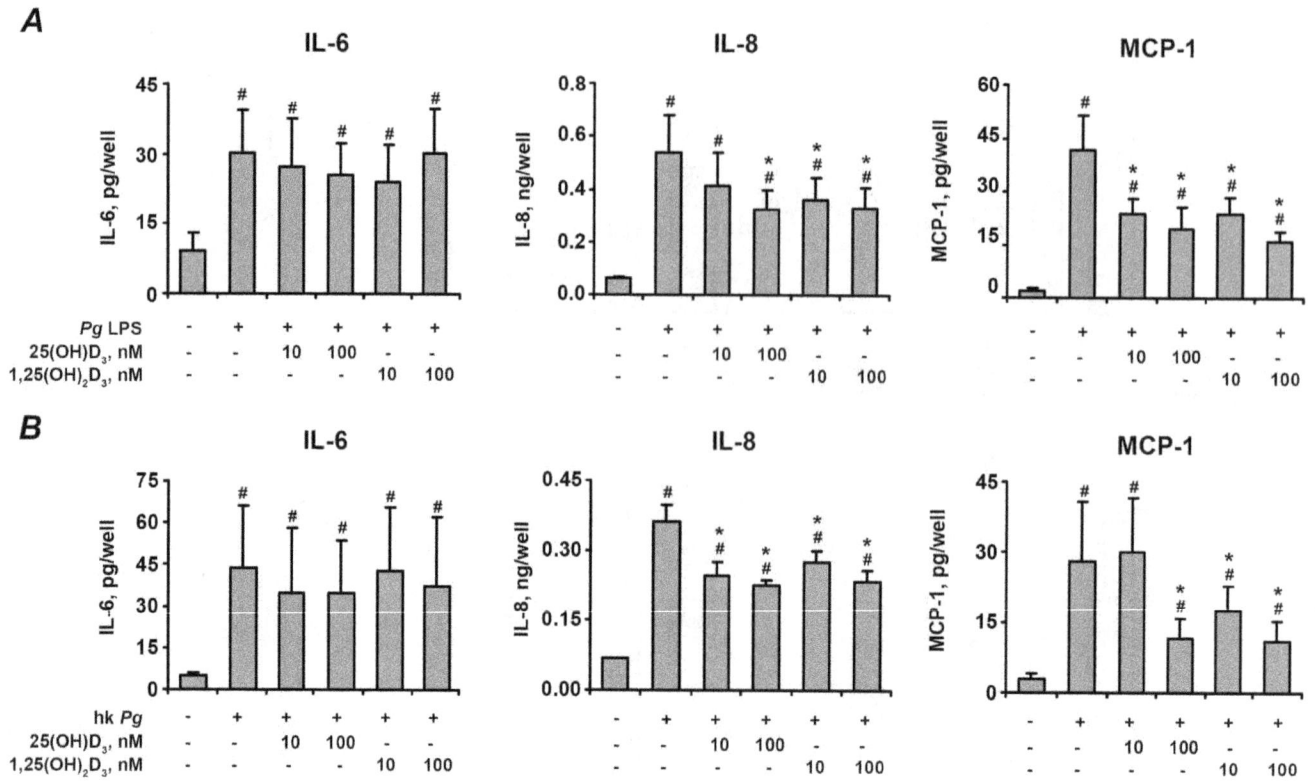

Figure 10. Effect of 25(OH)D$_3$ and 1,25(OH)$_2$D$_3$ on the production of pro-inflammatory mediators by primary hPdLC in response to stimulation with _P. gingivalis_ LPS or heat-killed _P. gingivalis_. Cells were stimulated with _P. gingivalis_ LPS (_Pg_ LPS, 1 µg/ml) or heat-killed _P. gingivalis_ (hk _Pg_, 10^8 cells/ml) for 24 h in the presence or in the absence of different concentrations of 25(OH)D$_3$ or 1,25(OH)$_2$D$_3$. The levels of IL-6 (A), IL-8 (B), and MCP-1 (C) were measured in cell supernatants using ELISA. $^{\#}$ means significantly different from control group (non stimulated cells). $*$ means significantly different from group stimulated with _P.gingivalis_ LPS or heat-killed _P. gingivalis_ only.

could be differently affected by vitamin D$_3$ and this might influence the balance between bacterial elimination and tissue destruction during progression of periodontal disease. This assumption is made based on the observations of _in vitro_ studies and further well-designed _in vivo_ animal and/or clinical studies are required to understand the role of vitamin D$_3$ in periodontitis. Since vitamin D$_3$ influences inflammatory response in periodontal tissue, it might be considered as a potential tool for periodontal therapy. Some studies show that systemic vitamin D$_3$ supplementation might have beneficial effect on periodontal health and periodontal therapy outcome [41,42,43]. Our data support the idea suggested by previous study[21], that topical application of vitamin D$_3$, particularly 25(OH)D$_3$, could be also considered as a potential tool in periodontal therapy.

We found that IL-6 production is inhibited by and 25(OH)D$_3$ and 1,25(OH)$_2$D$_3$ in commercially available hPdLF but not in primary hPdLC. The reasons for this discrepancy between isolated primary hPdLC and commercially available hPdLF are not entirely clear. Interestingly, a previous study on primary hPdLC also shows that biologically active 1,25(OH)$_2$D$_3$ inhibits IL-8 production in response to stimulation with _P. gingivalis_, but has no effect on IL-6 production [22]. One of the possible explanations of this finding could be the methodological difference in the cell isolation protocol. In the present study, similarly to study of Tang et al, primary hPdLC were isolated by tissue outgrow method, whereas commercially available hPdLF were produced by supplier's Clonetics technique. Differences in periodontal ligament cells isolation methods are known to affect some cell properties

[44]. Therefore it is possible that these changes also may lead to the modifications in cellular inflammatory responses observed in the present study. Moreover age and gender of the donor subjects may also contribute to the primary hPdLC properties [45,46].

Our data showed that the action of both 25(OH)D$_3$ and 1,25(OH)$_2$D$_3$ is mediated by VDR, because the silencing of this protein by specific siRNA resulted in abolishment of the effects of both forms of vitamin D. Therefore, regulation of expression levels of VDR in periodontal ligament cells might be important factor influencing functional properties of periodontal tissue. VDR is known to exhibit large polymorphism, which might contribute to different infectious disease [5,47]. Previous clinical studies link VDR polymorphism to the chronic and aggressive periodontitis [48,49,50]. Therefore, the possibility that VDR polymorphism contributes to the regulation of inflammatory response by vitamin D$_3$ in periodontal ligament cells cannot be excluded and requires further investigations.

Summarizing, our study shows that vitamin D$_3$ modulates inflammatory response in periodontal ligament cells through vitamin D$_3$ receptor. This finding suggests that both 1,25(OH)$_2$D$_3$ and 25(OH)D$_3$ might affect inflammatory processes in periodontal disease. The exact role of vitamin D$_3$ pathway in the progression of periodontal disease and possible therapeutic approaches in treatment or prophylaxis of periodontitis needs to be further investigated.

Acknowledgments

The authors acknowledge the help of Mrs. Phuong Quynh Nguyen and Mrs. Hedwig Rutschek (both Medical University of Vienna) for excellent technical assistance.

Author Contributions

Conceived and designed the experiments: O. Andrukhov O. Andrukhova XR-F. Performed the experiments: O. Andrukhov O. Andrukhova UH YT. Analyzed the data: O. Andrukhov O. Andrukhova UH YT XR-F. Contributed reagents/materials/analysis tools: O. Andrukhov H-PB XR-F. Wrote the paper: O. Andrukhov O. Andrukhova H-PB XR-F.

References

1. Lips P (2006) Vitamin D physiology. Prog Biophys Mol Biol 92: 4–8.
2. Jones G (2008) Pharmacokinetics of vitamin D toxicity. Am J Clin Nutr 88: 582S–586S.
3. Haussler MR, Whitfield GK, Haussler CA, Hsieh JC, Thompson PD, et al. (1998) The nuclear vitamin D receptor: biological and molecular regulatory properties revealed. J Bone Miner Res 13: 325–349.
4. Zehnder D, Bland R, Williams MC, McNinch RW, Howie AJ, et al. (2001) Extrarenal expression of 25-hydroxyvitamin d(3)-1 alpha-hydroxylase. J Clin Endocrinol Metab 86: 888–894.
5. White JH (2008) Vitamin D signaling, infectious diseases, and regulation of innate immunity. Infect Immun 76: 3837–3843.
6. Kinane DF (2001) Causation and pathogenesis of periodontal disease. Periodontol 2000 25: 8–20.
7. Holt SC, Ebersole JL (2005) Porphyromonas gingivalis, Treponema denticola, and Tannerella forsythia: the "red complex", a prototype polybacterial pathogenic consortium in periodontitis. Periodontol 2000 38: 72–122.
8. Genco RJ (1992) Host responses in periodontal diseases: current concepts. J Periodontol 63: 338–355.
9. Socransky SS, Haffajee AD, Cugini MA, Smith C, Kent RL Jr (1998) Microbial complexes in subgingival plaque. J Clin Periodontol 25: 134–144.
10. Stein SH, Livada R, Tipton DA (2013) Re-evaluating the role of vitamin D in the periodontium. J Periodontal Res.
11. Dietrich T, Joshipura KJ, Dawson-Hughes B, Bischoff-Ferrari HA (2004) Association between serum concentrations of 25–hydroxyvitamin D3 and periodontal disease in the US population. Am J Clin Nutr 80: 108–113.
12. Dietrich T, Nunn M, Dawson-Hughes B, Bischoff-Ferrari HA (2005) Association between serum concentrations of 25–hydroxyvitamin D and gingival inflammation. Am J Clin Nutr 82: 575–580.
13. Liu K, Meng H, Tang X, Xu L, Zhang L, et al. (2009) Elevated plasma calcifediol is associated with aggressive periodontitis. J Periodontol 80: 1114–1120.
14. Liu K, Meng H, Lu R, Xu L, Zhang L, et al. (2010) Initial periodontal therapy reduced systemic and local 25-hydroxy vitamin D(3) and interleukin-1beta in patients with aggressive periodontitis. J Periodontol 81: 260–266.
15. Beertsen W, McCulloch CA, Sodek J (1997) The periodontal ligament: a unique, multifunctional connective tissue. Periodontol 2000 13: 20–40.
16. Jonsson D, Nebel D, Bratthall G, Nilsson BO (2011) The human periodontal ligament cell: a fibroblast-like cell acting as an immune cell. J Periodontal Res 46: 153–157.
17. Pathirana RD, O'Brien-Simpson NM, Reynolds EC (2010) Host immune responses to Porphyromonas gingivalis antigens. Periodontol 2000 52: 218–237.
18. Scheres N, Laine ML, de Vries TJ, Everts V, van Winkelhoff AJ (2010) Gingival and periodontal ligament fibroblasts differ in their inflammatory response to viable Porphyromonas gingivalis. J Periodontal Res 45: 262–270.
19. Scheres N, Laine ML, Sipos PM, Bosch-Tijhof CJ, Crielaard W, et al. (2011) Periodontal ligament and gingival fibroblasts from periodontitis patients are more active in interaction with Porphyromonas gingivalis. J Periodontal Res 46: 407–416.
20. Liu K, Meng H, Hou J (2012) Activity of 25-hydroxylase in human gingival fibroblasts and periodontal ligament cells. PLoS ONE 7: e52053.
21. Liu K, Meng H, Hou J (2012) Characterization of the autocrine/paracrine function of vitamin D in human gingival fibroblasts and periodontal ligament cells. PLoS ONE 7: e39878.
22. Tang X, Pan Y, Zhao Y (2013) Vitamin D inhibits the expression of interleukin-8 in human periodontal ligament cells stimulated with Porphyromonas gingivalis. Arch Oral Biol 58: 397–407.
23. Jacobs C, Grimm S, Ziebart T, Walter C, Wehrbein H (2013) Osteogenic differentiation of periodontal fibroblasts is dependent on the strength of mechanical strain. Arch Oral Biol 58: 896–904.
24. Jacobs C, Walter C, Ziebart T, Grimm S, Meila D, et al. (2013) Induction of IL-6 and MMP-8 in human periodontal fibroblasts by static tensile strain. Clin Oral Investig.
25. Kumada Y, Zhang S (2010) Significant type I and type III collagen production from human periodontal ligament fibroblasts in 3D peptide scaffolds without extra growth factors. PLoS ONE 5: e10305.
26. Andrukhov O, Matejka M, Rausch-Fan X (2010) Effect of cyclosporin A on proliferation and differentiation of human periodontal ligament cells. Acta Odontol Scand 68: 329–334.
27. Kocgozlu L, Elkaim R, Tenenbaum H, Werner S (2009) Variable cell responses to P. gingivalis lipopolysaccharide. J Dent Res 88: 741–745.
28. Sekot G, Posch G, Messner P, Matejka M, Rausch-Fan X, et al. (2011) Potential of the Tannerella forsythia S-layer to delay the immune response. J Dent Res 90: 109–114.
29. Andrukhov O, Ertlschweiger S, Moritz A, Bantleon HP, Rausch-Fan X (2013) Different effects of P. gingivalis LPS and E. coli LPS on the expression of interleukin-6 in human gingival fibroblasts. Acta Odontol Scand.
30. Van Peer G, Mestdagh P, Vandesompele J (2012) Accurate RT-qPCR gene expression analysis on cell culture lysates. Sci Rep 2: 222.
31. Romero-Calvo I, Ocon B, Martinez-Moya P, Suarez MD, Zarzuelo A, et al. (2010) Reversible Ponceau staining as a loading control alternative to actin in Western blots. Anal Biochem 401: 318–320.
32. Fonseca JE, Santos MJ, Canhao H, Choy E (2009) Interleukin-6 as a key player in systemic inflammation and joint destruction. Autoimmun Rev 8: 538–542.
33. Ishimi Y, Miyaura C, Jin CH, Akatsu T, Abe E, et al. (1990) IL-6 is produced by osteoblasts and induces bone resorption. J Immunol 145: 3297–3303.
34. Baggiolini M, Dewald B, Moser B (1994) Interleukin-8 and related chemotactic cytokines—CXC and CC chemokines. Adv Immunol 55: 97–179.
35. Silva TA, Garlet GP, Fukada SY, Silva JS, Cunha FQ (2007) Chemokines in oral inflammatory diseases: apical periodontitis and periodontal disease. J Dent Res 86: 306–319.
36. Bischoff-Ferrari HA, Giovannucci E, Willett WC, Dietrich T, Dawson-Hughes B (2006) Estimation of optimal serum concentrations of 25-hydroxyvitamin D for multiple health outcomes. Am J Clin Nutr 84: 18–28.
37. Tang X, Meng H (2009) Osteogenic induction and 1,25-dihydroxyvitamin D3 oppositely regulate the proliferation and expression of RANKL and the vitamin D receptor of human periodontal ligament cells. Arch Oral Biol 54: 625–633.
38. Teng YT (2006) Protective and destructive immunity in the periodontium: Part 1—innate and humoral immunity and the periodontium. J Dent Res 85: 198–208.
39. McMahon L, Schwartz K, Yilmaz O, Brown E, Ryan LK, et al. (2011) Vitamin D-mediated induction of innate immunity in gingival epithelial cells. Infect Immun 79: 2250–2256.
40. Dixon DR, Bainbridge BW, Darveau RP (2004) Modulation of the innate immune response within the periodontium. Periodontol 2000 35: 53–74.
41. Bashutski JD, Eber RM, Kinney JS, Benavides E, Maitra S, et al. (2011) The impact of vitamin D status on periodontal surgery outcomes. J Dent Res 90: 1007–1012.
42. Garcia MN, Hildebolt CF, Miley DD, Dixon DA, Couture RA, et al. (2011) One-year effects of vitamin D and calcium supplementation on chronic periodontitis. J Periodontol 82: 25–32.
43. Miley DD, Garcia MN, Hildebolt CF, Shannon WD, Couture RA, et al. (2009) Cross-sectional study of vitamin D and calcium supplementation effects on chronic periodontitis. J Periodontol 80: 1433–1439.
44. Tanaka K, Iwasaki K, Feghali KE, Komaki M, Ishikawa I, et al. (2011) Comparison of characteristics of periodontal ligament cells obtained from outgrowth and enzyme-digested culture methods. Arch Oral Biol 56: 380–388.
45. Shu L, Guan SM, Fu SM, Guo T, Cao M, et al. (2008) Estrogen modulates cytokine expression in human periodontal ligament cells. J Dent Res 87: 142–147.
46. Krieger E, Hornikel S, Wehrbein H (2013) Age-related changes of fibroblast density in the human periodontal ligament. Head Face Med 9: 22.
47. Uitterlinden AG, Fang Y, Van Meurs JB, Pols HA, Van Leeuwen JP (2004) Genetics and biology of vitamin D receptor polymorphisms. Gene 338: 143–156.
48. Martelli FS, Mengoni A, Martelli M, Rosati C, Fanti E (2011) VDR TaqI polymorphism is associated with chronic periodontitis in Italian population. Arch Oral Biol 56: 1494–1498.
49. Brett PM, Zygogianni P, Griffiths GS, Tomaz M, Parkar M, et al. (2005) Functional gene polymorphisms in aggressive and chronic periodontitis. J Dent Res 84: 1149–1153.
50. Tanaka K, Miyake Y, Hanioka T, Arakawa M (2013) VDR gene polymorphisms, interaction with smoking and risk of periodontal disease in Japanese women: the Kyushu Okinawa maternal and child health study. Scand J Immunol 78: 371–377.

18

The Effect of Periodontal Treatment on Hemoglobin A1c Levels of Diabetic Patients

Xingxing Wang[1], Xu Han[1], Xiaojing Guo[2], Xiaolong Luo[1], Dalin Wang[1]*

1 Department of Stomatology, Changhai Hospital, The Second Military Medical University, Shanghai, China, **2** Department of Health Statistics, The Second Military Medical University, Shanghai, China

Abstract

Background: There is growing evidence that periodontal treatment may affect glycemic control in diabetic patients. And several systematic reviews have been conducted to assess the effect of periodontal treatment on diabetes outcomes. Researches of this aspect are widely concerned, and several new controlled trials have been published. The aim of this study was to update the account for recent findings.

Methods: A literature search (until the end of January 2014) was carried out using various databases with language restriction to English. A randomized controlled trial (RCT) was selected if it investigated periodontal therapy for diabetic subjects compared with a control group received no periodontal treatment for at least 3 months of the follow-up period. The primary outcome was hemoglobin A1c (HbA1c), and secondary outcomes were periodontal parameters included probing pocket depth (PPD) and clinical attachment level (CAL).

Results: Ten trials of 1135 patients were included in the analysis. After the follow-up of 3 months, treatment substantially lowered HbA1c compared with no treatment after periodontal therapy (−0.36%, 95%CI, −0.52% to −0.19%, $P<0.0001$). Clinically substantial and statistically significant reduction of PPD and CAL were found between subjects with and without treatment after periodontal therapy (PPD −0.42 mm, 95%CI: −0.60 to −0.23, $P<0.00001$; CAL −0.34 mm, 95%CI: −0.52 to −0.16, $P=0.0002$). And there is no significant change of the level of HbA1c at the 6-month comparing with no treatment (−0.30%, 95%CI, −0.69% to 0.09%, $P=0.13$).

Conclusions: Periodontal treatment leads to the modest reduction in HbA1c along with the improvement of periodontal status in diabetic patients for 3 months, and this result is consistent with previous systematic reviews. And the effect of periodontal treatment on HbA1c cannot be observed at 6-month after treatment.

Editor: Yu-Kang Tu, National Taiwan University, Taiwan

Data Availability: The authors confirm that all data underlying the findings are fully available without restriction. All relevant data are within the paper and its Supporting Information files.

Funding: These authors have no support or funding to report.

Competing Interests: The authors have declared that no competing interests exist.

* Email: Wang_Dento@163.com

Introduction

Periodontitis is a multi-factorial infectious disease of the soft tissues and bone that support the teeth [1], and it is a major cause of tooth loss in adults [2]. Periodontitis may lead to the development of a high systemic disease burden [3] and possibly affect general health [4]. It is reported that periodontitis is associate with rheumatoid arthritis [5]. cardiovascular disease [6] and even the patients in the periodontitis cohort exhibit a higher risk of developing oral cancer than those in the gingivitis cohort [7].

Diabetes mellitus is a chronic, non-communicable disease and also one of the major global public health issues [8]. The distinguishing features of diabetes mellitus type 1 and type 2 are autoimmunity and chronic low-grade inflammation, respectively [9]. A large number of studies support the point that there is an association between diabetes and periodontal disease [10]: Firstly, individuals with diabetes have a higher prevalence of periodontitis [11–13]. Nelson et al. [14] reported that the incidence of periodontitis was 2.6 times higher in subjects with diabetes than those without. Tsai et al. [11] reported that patients with poorly controlled diabetes have a 2.9 times higher risk to have sever periodontitis compared to no-diabetic subjects. Secondly, diabetes mellitus can increase the severity of periodontitis [15–17] and the severity of the periodontitis is always greater than individuals without diabetes [10,11]. And periodontitis is considered to be one of the diabetic complications [18,19].

Although strong evidence tends to support the adverse effects of diabetes on periodontitis, numerous reports indicate that periodontitis can adversely affect glycemic control in diabetics [20,21]. It is considered that this close association between periodontitis and diabetes is established on the reciprocal influence [22]. So a number of potential mechanisms for the two-way relationship between them have been proposed. It is known that periodontitis is a kind of inflammatory process which can generate localized and systemic infections, and emerging evidence implicates inflammation in the pathogenesis of type 2 diabetes [23,24]. But the exact relationship between periodontitis and diabetes remains unclear.

Some intervention studies concerning the effects of periodontal disease on glycemic control of diabetic patients report more direct evidence. Iwamoto et al. [25] showed that antimicrobial periodontal therapy can cause a significant reduction of HbA1c value in type 2 diabetic patients. Gaikwad et al. [26] also found that scaling and root planning can improve glycemic control in patients with type 2 diabetes mellitus with or without adjunctive systemic doxycycline therapy. Bharti et al. [27] gave diabetic patients with periodontitis a periodontal treatment with topical antibiotics and found that this kind of therapy protocol can improve glycemic control and elevate serum adiponectin with improvement of periodontal status in type 2 diabetic patients. However, a recent phase III randomized controlled clinical trial (RCT) with 514 patients by Engebretson et al. [28] revealed that nonsurgical periodontal therapy did not improve glycemic control in patients with type 2 diabetes.

HbA1c is related to the mean blood glucose concentration over the past 1–3 months [8], and it is also associated with an increased risk for diabetes complications [29]. So the periodic monitoring of HbA1c in diabetic patients was proposed [30]. It is considered to be a standardized measurement used to estimate the effect of diabetes treatment on control of glucose metabolism [31–33], and is widely used in trials to monitor diabetes status [34].

Several recent systematic reviews [35,36] have been conducted to assess the evidence that periodontal treatment influences the level of HbA1c. Due to several new research reports with bigger sample size, we therefore performed this meta-analysis of RCTs to evaluate the effect of periodontal treatment on glycemic control of diabetic patients.

Research Design and Methods

Search strategy

Three databases, PubMed, Embase and Cochrane Library were searched according to a method previously described by Teeuw et al. [35] and Engebretson et al. [36], using identical search criteria and terms: ((periodontal disease) OR (periodont*[Text Word]) OR (periodontitis)) AND ((diabetes[Text Word]) OR (diabet*[Text Word]) OR (diabetic*[Title]) OR (diabetic patient*[Text Word]) OR (diabetes patient[Text Word]) OR (non insulin dependent diabetes) OR (niddm[Text Word]) OR (insulin dependent diabetes[Text Word]) OR (iddm[Text Word]) OR (type 1 diabetes) OR (t1 dm) OR (type 2 diabetes) OR (t2 dm)) AND ((therapy) OR (treatment) OR (intervention)) AND ((controlled clinical trial) OR (randomized controlled trial) OR (RCT)) AND (english[Language]) until the end of the January of 2014. Additional searches were conducted in PubMed's medical subject headings with: (periodontal diseases) AND (diabetes mellitus) AND (therapeutics OR therapy OR intervention studies). Moreover, we searched the World Health Organization (http://www.who.int/triasearch) and Clinical Trials.gov (http://wwwClinicalTrials.gov.) Web sites for information on registered RCTs.

Study selection criteria

The studies to be included in the systematic review had to meet the following criteria: (1) randomized controlled trial; (2) participants over the age of 18 with both diabetes (both type 1

and type 2) and periodontitis; (3) intervention consisting of non-surgical treatment with or without adjunctive use of local drug delivery and systemic antibiotics; (4) comparator group with no periodontal treatment or delayed treatment; (5) study duration ≥ 3 months; (6) outcome consisting of mean change in HbA1c level, or pre- and post-treatment HbA1c levels.

Two independent reviewers (Xingxing Wang and Xiaolong Luo) evaluated all retrieved articles. Titles and abstracts were scanned to rule out studies that did not meet inclusion criteria. From the selected articles, the full texts were reviewed followed by a decision on their eligibility for inclusion.

Data extraction and quality assessment

Data extraction and quality assessment were independently conducted by two authors (Xingxing Wang and Xiaojing Guo) using a standardized approach, and disagreements were adjudicated by a third reviewer (Dalin Wang) after referring back to the original articles.

Data retrieved from the studies included publication details (year of publication, name of first author and country) and trial characteristics (Patients' types and treatment of diabetes, study design, sample size, interventions, follow-up duration, change of HbA1c and periodontal parameters). The quality of the included studies was assessed by Risk of Bias tool according to the Cochrane handbook for systematic reviews of interventions (Version 5.1.0) [37].

Statistical analyses

The absolute difference of HbA1c percentage in each treatment arm was recorded. When not reported, it was calculated for the intervention and the control groups by means of the formula [35]:

$$\Delta HbA1c = HbA1c_f - HbA1c_b,$$

where $HbA1c_f$ is the mean HbA1c value after treatment and $HbA1c_b$ is the mean HbA1c value before treatment. And if the standard deviation was not reported, it was obtained by the formula [35,38]:

$$SD_c = \sqrt{SD_b^2 + SD_f^2 - (2 \times Corr \times SD_b \times SD_f)}$$

Where SD_c is the standard deviation of mean change of HbA1c, SD_b is the standard deviation of mean baseline HbA1c values, SD_f is the standard deviation of mean end HbA1c values. Corr is the correlation between the baseline and end values, it was set at 0.5, consistent with the previous reviews [35,38].

For the three-arm studies, the two treatment groups or the two control groups, which were assumed to be "group 1" and "group 2", were firstly combined into a single group according to the "Cochrane handbook for systematic reviews of interventions (Version 5.1.0)" [37] and "Introduction to meta-analysis" [39].

Sample size: $N = N_1 + N_2$

Mean: $M = \dfrac{N_1 M_1 + N_2 M_2}{N_1 + N_2}$

SD: $SD =$

$$\sqrt{\dfrac{(N_1-1)SD_1^2 + (N_2-1)SD_2^2 + \dfrac{N_1 N_2}{N_1+N_2}\left(M_1^2 + M_2^2 - 2M_1 M_2\right)}{N_1 + N_2 - 1}}$$

For periodontal clinical parameters, according to the Cochrane handbook for systematic reviews of interventions (Version 5.1.0) [37]: if the value of Corr less than 0.5 is obtained, then there is no value in using change from baseline and an analysis of final values

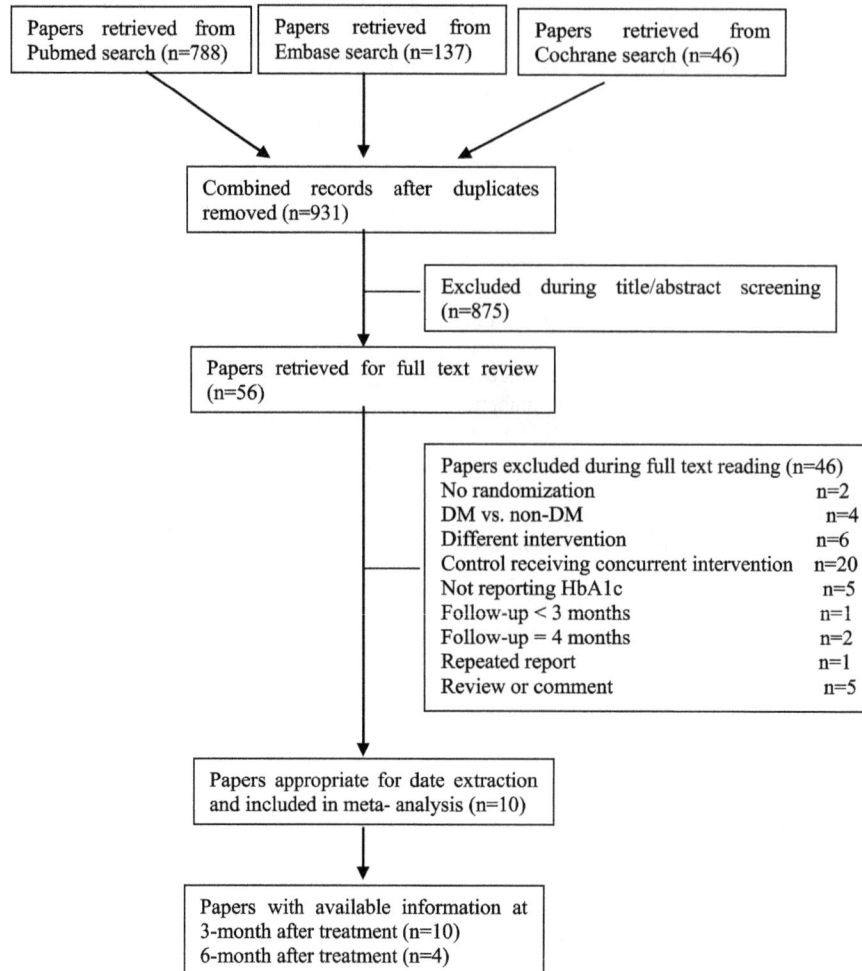

Figure 1. Flow diagram of the trials search and selection process.

will be more precise. We obtained the values of Corr by using the data extracted from Sun et al. 2011 [40] and Telgi et al. 2013 [8], and they were all less than 0.5, so we took the SD_f as the standard deviation of mean change of PPD and CAL.

The weighted mean difference (WMD) was calculated, Chi-square (χ^2) and I^2 tests were used to assess the heterogeneity of the studies included in this meta-analysis. The heterogeneity of the trials will be regarded as low-level when $P>0.10$ for the χ^2 test and $I^2<25\%$, and a fixed-effects model analysis was used to calculate a pooled effect; otherwise, a random-effects model was applied.

Forest plots showing the point estimate and confidence intervals for each study were created. Statistical significance was defined as a two-tailed $P<0.05$. All numerical data for meta-analysis were conducted using RevMan version 5.3 from the Cochrane collaboration.

Results

Study characteristics

The literature search resulted in 931 potentially relevant articles. The titles and abstracts of these articles were scanned for relevance. And the second level full text search was initiated on those remaining studies. Fifty-six potentially eligible trials were identified for full-text review, 46 of which were excluded for specific reasons listed in Figure 1. The remaining ten trials of 1135

patients (614 in the treated group and 521 in the control group) [8,28,39–46] that met the inclusion criteria were included in the meta-analysis, and the characteristics of each study were shown in Table 1. Of the ten trials, seven studies [39,41–46] were also included in the previous analysis [35,36]. Whereas two other studies [48,49] that were included in the previous systematic reviews [35,36] were excluded because their study duration were 4 months and the outcomes of the 3 months were not available.

All studies included were reported as RCTs, and the durations of the follow-up period were at least 3 months. Of the ten studies, five were of 6-month duration [28,41–43,45], but the data is not available in Katagiri et al. [43], we wrote to the author and we were not answered. And there was one study was of 9-month duration [41]. All studies described a study population having type 2 diabetes and suffering from periodontitis, and also one study included type 1 diabetes [41]. Eight studies were single centre [8,40–42,44–47], two were multi-centered [28,43]. The largest in terms of sample size of the study is Engebretson et al. [28] with 514 participants. Four trials were three-arm studies, [8,41,42,47] and three of them [41,42,47] reported two intervention groups, while the other one [8] reported two control groups. And they were combined into a single group firstly.

Overall, all included studies had different levels of bias. Six studies [28,41–43,45,46] showed a clear randomization scheme, the other four studies [8,40,44,47] did not give out sufficient

Table 1. Characteristics of included trials.

Author(s)	Country Number of subjects (tx, ctr) Single versus multicenter	HbA1c inclusion criteria Treatment in test and control group	Inclusion criteria	Periodontitis evaluation	HbAlc(%) (mean±SD) at baseline and at 3 months (mean change)	HbAlc(%) (mean±SD) at 6 months (mean change)	PPD (mm)(mean±SD), CAL (mm)(mean±SD) at baseline and at 3 months(mean change)	Number of subjects with diabetic medication at baseline Change in diabetic medication
Kiran M et al. 2005	Turkey 44DM2 (tx:22 ctr:22) single center	HbA1c 6%-8% tx:SRP+OH ctr: no treatment	not reported	PPD, CAL, GR, PI, GI, BOP	tx:7.31±0.74~6.51±0.80(-0.86) ctr:7.00±0.72~7.31±2.08(0.31)	NA	tx:PPD 2.29±0.49~1.80± 0.25(-0.49) CAL 3.19±1.13~2.80±1.03 (-0.39) ctr:PPD 2.24±0.70~2.26±0.63 (0.02) CAL 2.92±1.10~2.87±1.03(-0.05)	Diet control:3 Oral medication:30 Insulin:4 Insulin + oral:7 no change in the medication or diet
Singh S et al. 2008	India 45 DM2 (tx:15 tx2:15 ctr:15) single center	HbAlc not reported tx1:SRP TX2:SRP+ doxycycline ctr:no treatment	30% or more of the teeth examined having ≥4 mm PD	PPD, CAL, PI, GI	tx1:7.9±0.7~7.3±0.6(-0.6) tx2:8.3±0.7~7.5±0.6(-0.7) ctr:8.08±0.7~8.1±0.74(0.06)	NA	tx1:PPD 2.67±0.35~2.33± 0.35(-0.34) CAL 3.44±0.45~3.14±0.45 (-0.30) tx2: PPD 2.52±0.47~2.14±0.46 (-0.38) CAL 3.22±0.63~2.88±0.61 (-0.34) ctr:PPD 2.44±0.26~2.40±0.46 (-0.04) CAL 2.78±0.33~2.83±0.35 (0.04)	Baseline medication not reported no change in the medication or diet
Katagiri S et al. 2009	Japan 49 DM2 (tx:32 ctr:17) multicenter	HbA1c 6.5-10 tx1:SRP+ topical minocycline ctr:OH	≥11 teeth ≥2 sites with PD≥4 mm	PPD, BOP	tx:7.2±0.9~7.06* ctr:6.9±0.9~6.81	reported in a graph	tx:PPD 3.0±0.9~2.2±0.5 CAL NA ctr: PPD 2.8± 0.9~2.6±0.7 CAL NA	Diet control:3 Oral medication:27 Insulin:19 anti-diabetic drugs were not changed
Koromantzos PA et al. 2011	Greece 60DM2 (tx:30 ctr:30) single center	HbA1c 7.0%-9.9% tx:SRP+OH ctr: supragingival+OH	≥16 teeth, PD≥6 mm in≥8 sites, CAL≥5 mm, in≥2 quadrants	PPD, CAL, BOP, GI	tx:7.87±0.74~7.14±0.54* ctr:7.59±0.66~7.41±0.48	tx:(-0.72±0.93)* ctr:(-0.13±0.46)	tx:PPD NA CAL NA ctr:PPD NA CAL NA	Oral medication 48 insulin 19 change in medication reported
Sun WL et al. 2011	China 157DM2 (tx:82 ctr:75) single center	HbA1c 7.5%-9.5% tx:SRP+OH+flap when indicated+ antibiotics ctr: OH	≥20 teeth, PD>5 mm, CAL≥4 mm in ≥30% teeth or PD>4 mm, CAL>3 mm in ≥60% teeth	PPD, CAL, BI, PI	tx:8.75±0.67~8.25±0.72(-0.50±0.18) ctr:8.70±0.65~8.56±0.69(-0.14±0.12)	NA	tx:PPD 4.53±0.83~2.97± 0.78 (-1.15±0.66) CAL 4.85±1.38~4.12±0.95 (-0.73±0.51) ctr:PPD 4.49±0.85~4.28±0.81 (-0.21±0.19) CAL 4.88±1.39~4.73±1.29 (-0.15±0.13)	Diet or oral medication no medication changes

Table 1. Cont.

Author(s)	Country Number of subjects (tx, ctr) Single versus multicenter	HbA1c inclusion criteria Treatment in test and control group	Inclusion criteria	Periodontitis evaluation	HbA1c(%) (mean±SD) at baseline and at 3 months (mean change)	HbA1c(%) (mean±SD) at 6 months (mean change)	PPD (mm)(mean±SD), CAL (mm)(mean±SD) at baseline and at 3 months(mean change)	Number of subjects with diabetic medication at baseline Change in diabetic medication
Chen L et al. 2012	China 126DM2 (tx1:42 tx2:43 ctr:41) single center	HbA1c not reported tx1:SRP+subgingival debridement at 3-month tx2:SRP+ supragingival prophylaxis at 3-month ctr:no treatment+no OH	≥16 teeth, CAL≥1 mm	PPD, CAL, PI, BOP	tx1:7.31±1.23~7.30±1.50 tx2:7.29±1.55~7.43±1.53 ctr:7.25±1.49~7.59±1.54	tx1:7.09±1.34 tx2:6.87±1.12 ctr:7.38±1.57	tx:PPD 2.66±0.68~2.27± 0.50 CAL 3.57±1.31~3.28± 1.25 tx2:PPD 2.57±0.66~2.20±0.39 CAL 2.95±1.21~2.55±1.15 ctr:PPD 2.47±0.57~2.38± 0.47 CAL 3.37±1.24~ 3.29±1.23	Diet control:4 Oral medication:109 Insulin:13 no medication changes
Moeintaghavi A et al. 2012	Iran 40DM2 (tx:22 ctr:18) single center	HbA1c >7% tx: SRP+OH ctr: OH	not reported	PPD, CAL, PI, GI	tx:8.15±1.18~7.41±1.18 ctr:8.72±2.22~8.97±1.82	NA	tx:PPD 2.31±0.65~ 2.21±0.6 CAL 3.14±1.08~2.8±1.09 ctr:PPD 2.06±0.24~ 2.33±0.3 CAL 3.1±1.05~3.47±1.44	Oral medication Medical treatment unchange
Botero JE et al. 2013†	Colombia 39DM1, 66DM2(tx1:33 tx2:37 ctr:35) single center	HbA1c not reported tx1:scaling+ azithromycin tx2:scaling+placebo ctr:supragingival prophylaxis+ azithromycin	CAL≥4 mm in ≥2 interproximal sites, or PD≥5 mm in ≥2 interproximal sites	PPD, CAL, PI, BOP	tx1:7.92±1.58~±1.36(-0.8)* tx2:7.98±2.16~±1.91(-0.6) ctr:7.87±1.81~±2.48(0.2)	tx1:(-0.4) tx2:(0) ctr:(0.2)	tx1:PPD 2.7±0.6~2.3± 0.6 CAL 2.8±0.8~2.5± 0.8 tx2:PPD 2.6±0.7~ 2.5±0.5 CAL 3.1± 1.16~3.0±1.1 ctr:PPD 2.4±0.6~2.2±0.4 CAL 2.9±1.1~2.8±0.9	Baseline medication not reported change not reported
Telgi RL et al. 2013	India 60DM2 (tx:20 ctr1:20 ctr2:20) single center	HbA1c not reported tx:scaling+CHX+brush ctr1:CHX+brush ctr2:brush	PD 4-5 mm, ≥28 teeth	PPD, PI, GI	tx:7.68±0.63~7.10±0.64 (-0.58±0.27) ctr1:7.56±0.59~ 7.31±0.59(-0.25±0.14) ctr2:7.74±0.59~7.75±0.58 (0.004±0.12)	NA	tx:PPD 5.05±0.70~ 4.59±0.72(-0.46±0.26) CAL NA ctr1:PPD 5.11±0.57~4.87±0.55 (-0.25±0.11) CAL NA ctr2:PPD 5.05±0.69~ 5.03±0.69(-0.02±0.05) CAL NA	Oral medication change in medication not reported
Engebretson SP et al. 2013	USA 275DM2 (tx:240 ctr:235) multicenter	HbA1c 7%~9% tx:SRP+CHX+OH ctr:OH	PD≥5 mm in ≥2 quadrants, ≥16 teeth	PPD, CAL, PI, BOP	tx:7.84±0.65~(0.13) ctr:7.77±0.60~(0.08)	tx:(0.15) ctr:(0.09)	tx:PPD 3.3±0.6~2.8 CAL 3.5±0.8~3.2 ctr:PPD 3.3±0.7~ 3.2 CAL 3.5±0.9~3.4	No diatetes medications:11 Oral medication:244 Insulin:80 Combination:179 Changes between treatment groups were similar

PI, plaque index; GI, gingival index; PPD, probing pocket depth; CAL, clinical attachment loss; GR, gingival recession; BOP, bleeding on probing; NA, not available; CHX, chlorhexidine gluconate; OH, oral hygiene; SRP, scaling and root planning.

*reported in a graph.

†data obtained by calculation.

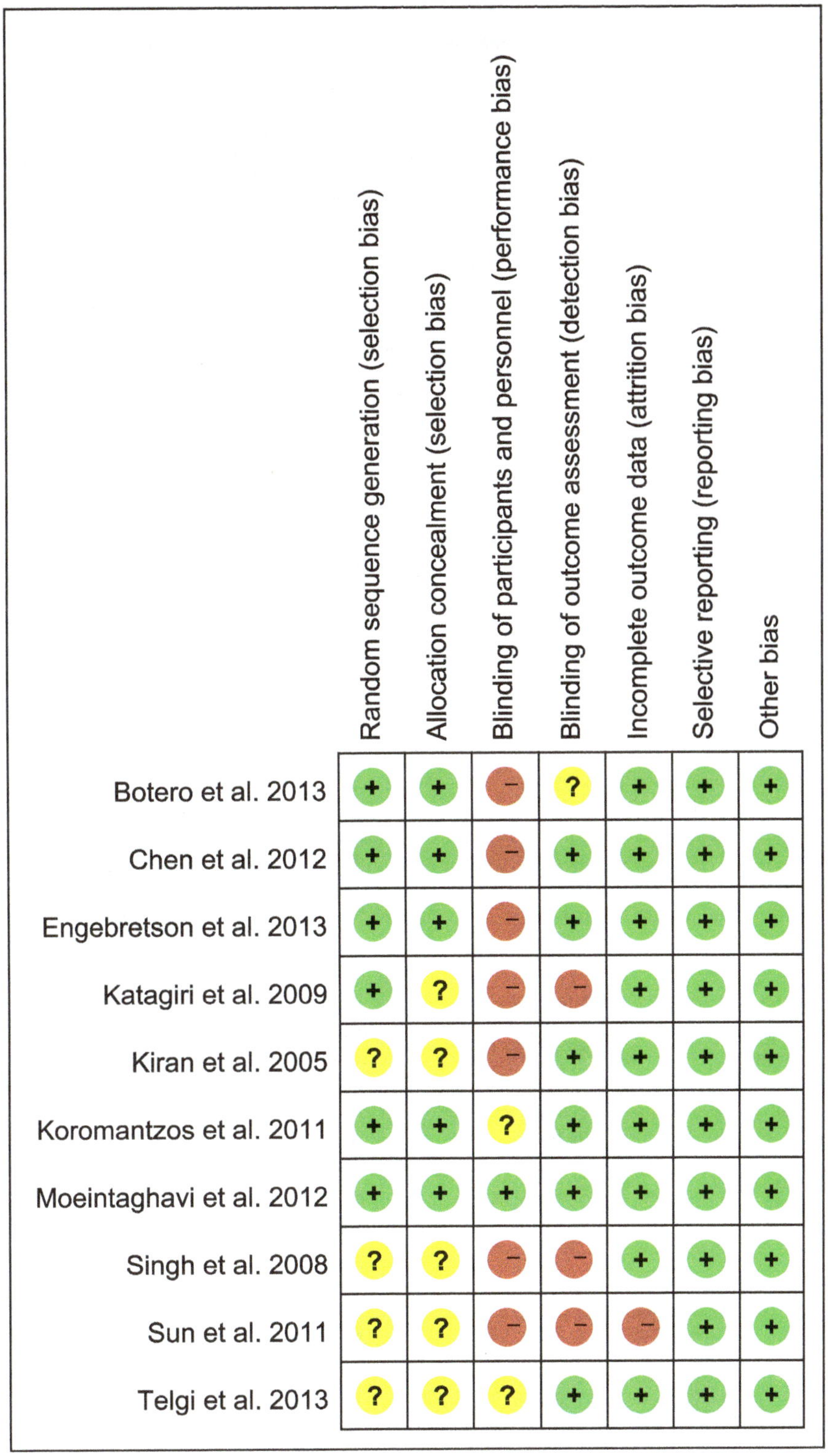

Figure 2. Judgements about each risk of bias item for each included study.

information about the generation of a randomized sequence. Concealment was inadequate in five of the included studies [8,40,43,44,47]. In one of the studies treatments were performed under the supervision of an expert [46]. Six studies were outcome assessment blinded [8,28,42,44–46]. One study [46] excluded the data of the patients who did not finish the study at the baseline. (Fig. 2, 3).

Since the heterogeneity of every outcomes was assessed and shown as P for χ^2 test and I^2, as they were shown in Fig. 4, 5–7 that all of the P<0.10 for χ^2 test and I^2>25%, so there were heterogeneity among the included trials, and a random-effects

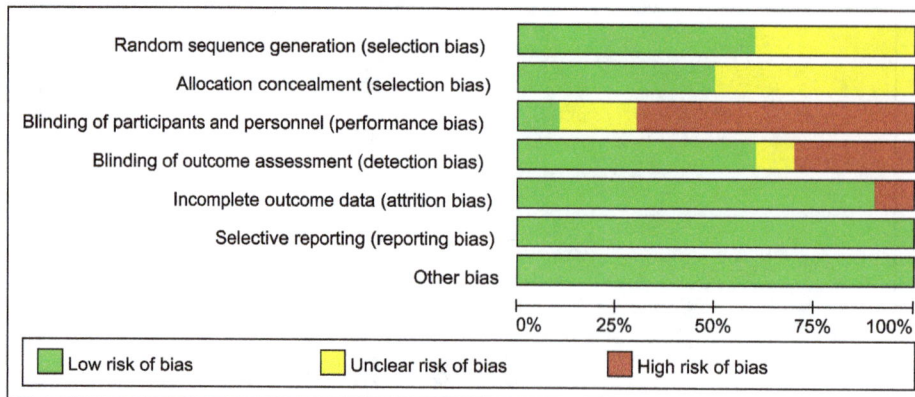

Figure 3. Each risk of bias item presented as percentages across all included studies.

model analysis was used. In addition, the results analyzed with the fixed-effects model, including the relevant forest plots (Fig. S1–S4), were provided as online supplements.

Change of HbA1c at 3-month

Data on change of HbA1c were available for analysis in 1135 patients enrolled in ten trials investigating the effect of non-surgical periodontal treatment on glycemic control of diabetic patients. The change of HbA1c for 3 months ranged from -0.86% to 0.13%, with a mean change of HbA1c from baseline of -0.36% (95%CI: -0.52%, -0.19%). As it was showed in Fig. 4, the forest plot described the effect on HbA1c in terms of mean reduction from baseline, and standard deviation, as a comparison between treatment and control groups. Nevertheless, there might be substantial heterogeneity in the change of HbA1c across studies ($P = 0.0003$, $I^2 = 71\%$). Furthermore, publication bias may exist as the funnel plot (Fig. 8) displayed an asymmetrical distribution.

Change of periodontal parameters at 3-month

Non-surgical periodontal treatment demonstrated a significant benefit on the periodontal status. Nine trials [8,28,40–44,46,47] reported the mean change of PPD in 1077 patients. The mean change of PPD from baseline to the 3-month after treatment was -0.42 mm (95%CI: -0.60, -0.23) (Fig. 5); seven trials [28,40–42,44,46,47] reported the mean change of CAL in 968 patients, and the mean change of CAL 3 months after treatment was -0.34 mm (95%CI: -0.52, -0.16) (Fig. 6).

Change of HbA1c at 6-month

Data on the change of HbA1c for 6 months in diabetic patients with periodontitis were available for 754 patients enrolled in four trials [28,41,42,45]. The change of HbA1c for 6 months ranged from -0.72% to 0.15%, and the result presented no statistical difference between the treatment and control groups (-0.30%, 95%CI: -0.69 to 0.09, $P = 0.13$), and there might be heterogeneity in the change of HbA1c for 6 months across studies ($P = 0.02$, $I^2 = 68\%$) (Fig. 7).

Treatment modalities

All treatment group interventions consisted of non-surgical periodontal therapy with or without adjunctive topical or systemic antibiotics, and/or topical antiseptics. Six trials [28,40,43–46] were two-arm studies, and four trials [8,41,42,47] were three-armed. Of the three-arm studies, Boter et al. [41] and Singh et al. [47] reported that both treatment arms received non-surgical therapy with or without adjunctive antibiotics; Chen et al. [42] reported that both treatment arms received scaling and root planning only; while in the Telgi et al. [8] study only one arm received scaling. Of the two arm studies, two studies' treatment included scaling and root planning only [44,46], Koromantzos et al. [45] treatment included scaling and root planning plus extraction of hopeless teeth, and Sun et al. [40] treatment also included flap surgery ("when indicated") and systemic Tinidazole plus ampicillin. The remaining studies included adjunctive treatment of chlorhexidine oral rinse [28] or topical use of

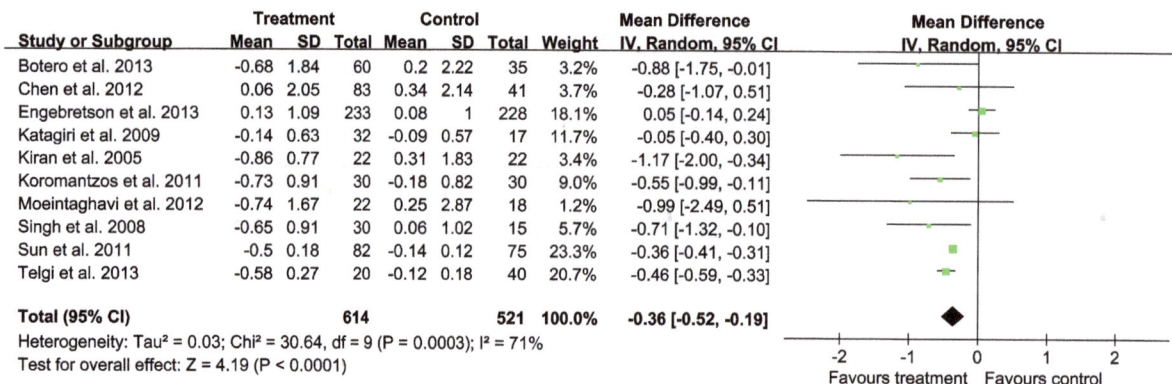

Study or Subgroup	Treatment			Control			Weight	Mean Difference IV, Random, 95% CI	Mean Difference IV, Random, 95% CI
	Mean	SD	Total	Mean	SD	Total			
Botero et al. 2013	-0.68	1.84	60	0.2	2.22	35	3.2%	-0.88 [-1.75, -0.01]	
Chen et al. 2012	0.06	2.05	83	0.34	2.14	41	3.7%	-0.28 [-1.07, 0.51]	
Engebretson et al. 2013	0.13	1.09	233	0.08	1	228	18.1%	0.05 [-0.14, 0.24]	
Katagiri et al. 2009	-0.14	0.63	32	-0.09	0.57	17	11.7%	-0.05 [-0.40, 0.30]	
Kiran et al. 2005	-0.86	0.77	22	0.31	1.83	22	3.4%	-1.17 [-2.00, -0.34]	
Koromantzos et al. 2011	-0.73	0.91	30	-0.18	0.82	30	9.0%	-0.55 [-0.99, -0.11]	
Moeintaghavi et al. 2012	-0.74	1.67	22	0.25	2.87	18	1.2%	-0.99 [-2.49, 0.51]	
Singh et al. 2008	-0.65	0.91	30	0.06	1.02	15	5.7%	-0.71 [-1.32, -0.10]	
Sun et al. 2011	-0.5	0.18	82	-0.14	0.12	75	23.3%	-0.36 [-0.41, -0.31]	
Telgi et al. 2013	-0.58	0.27	20	-0.12	0.18	40	20.7%	-0.46 [-0.59, -0.33]	
Total (95% CI)			**614**			**521**	**100.0%**	**-0.36 [-0.52, -0.19]**	

Heterogeneity: Tau² = 0.03; Chi² = 30.64, df = 9 (P = 0.0003); I² = 71%
Test for overall effect: Z = 4.19 (P < 0.0001)

Figure 4. Forest plot presenting change in HbA1c (%) at 3-month.

Study or Subgroup	treatment			Control			Weight	Mean Difference IV, Random, 95% CI
	Mean	SD	Total	Mean	SD	Total		
Botero et al. 2013	-0.22	0.56	60	-0.2	0.4	35	11.6%	-0.02 [-0.21, 0.17]
Chen et al. 2012	-0.38	0.45	85	-0.09	0.47	41	11.9%	-0.29 [-0.46, -0.12]
Engebretson et al. 2013	-0.5	0.61	233	-0.1	0.6	228	12.7%	-0.40 [-0.51, -0.29]
Katagiri et al. 2009	-0.8	0.51	32	-0.2	0.7	17	8.5%	-0.60 [-0.98, -0.22]
Kiran et al. 2005	-0.49	0.25	22	0.02	0.63	22	10.1%	-0.51 [-0.79, -0.23]
Moeintaghavi et al. 2012	-0.1	0.6	22	0.27	0.3	18	10.0%	-0.37 [-0.66, -0.08]
Singh et al. 2008	-0.36	0.4	30	-0.04	0.46	15	10.3%	-0.32 [-0.59, -0.05]
Sun et al. 2011	-1.15	0.66	82	-0.21	0.19	75	12.3%	-0.94 [-1.09, -0.79]
Telgi et al. 2013	-0.46	0.26	20	-0.14	0.14	40	12.6%	-0.32 [-0.44, -0.20]
Total (95% CI)			**586**			**491**	**100.0%**	**-0.42 [-0.60, -0.23]**

Heterogeneity: Tau² = 0.07; Chi² = 69.78, df = 8 (P < 0.00001); I² = 89%
Test for overall effect: Z = 4.46 (P < 0.00001)

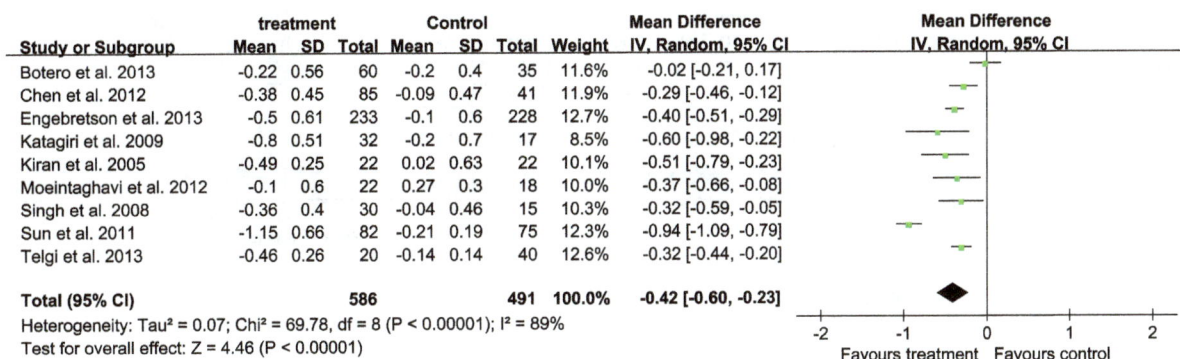

Figure 5. Forest plot presenting change in PPD (mm) at 3-month.

minocycline ointment [43]. And five trials [28,41–43,45] reported the additional supra- or subgingival debridement at the post-treatment appointment.

Discussion

There have been several excellent systematic reviews [35,36] reported about the effect of periodontal treatment on glycemic control of diabetic patients, the previous studies used for analysis in the reviews except those couldn't meet the inclusion criteria were included, and three new studies have been added. In all, ten randomized clinical trials were included in this review, with more than 3 months of follow-up period. The total number of subjects within the studies included in this review was 1135. And we could conclude from the current systematic review that non-surgical periodontal treatment for diabetic patients is beneficial in glycemic control and can reduce HbA1c levels by 0.36% 3 months after treatment, the effect at 6-month post-treatment is not obvious. It might present that non-surgical periodontal treatment may play a role on glycemic control for diabetic patient for just a period of time. But because of the difference of the treatment modalities the number of included studies is limited, the sample size is insufficient, and there is significant heterogeneity across studies, it is worthy of attention in future studies.

Although not all literature reported the related change of periodontal parameter, the available data extracted from the included studies was analyzed. The results showed that there was an overall 0.42 mm reduction in PPD and 0.34 mm reduction in CAL at 3-month post-treatment. It is generally considered that inflammation cytokines like C-reactive protein (CRP) may play an important role between diabetes and periodontitis [50], and a

meta-analysis made by Teeuw et al. [51] find that periodontal treatment can significantly reduce the level of CRP. Katagiri et al. [43] revealed that there is a relationship between the change of CRP and HbA1c level. Therefore, we believe that periodontal therapy can certainly reduce systemic inflammation by improvement of the periodontal status, then impact the glycaemic control for a period of time. And when the inflammation is under control, the effect of periodontal therapy on glycaemic control may not obvious.

It is reported that although dental prophylaxis including removal of supragingival calculus and plaque can improve periodontal health, it cannot influence HbA1c levels [52]. So we considered the group in Boter et al. [41] received removal of supragingival calculus and plaque as the control group.

High risk of bias of the included studies especially the "blinding of participants and personnel", should be explained by the fact that the intervention of the studies was periodontal treatment, such as scaling and root planning etc., while the control group without treatment, so it was difficult to mask the therapists and subjects.

Compared with the previous reports, there are some certain improvements in this study. Firstly, a phase 3, multi-center, randomized trial with a number of 514 participants was included [28]. Although the results of that trial was that non-surgical periodontal therapy did not improve glycaemic control in patients with type 2 diabetes, and was not exactly the same with this review, the difference made us to look for the reasons. Three significant reasons should be considered. One reason was that the characteristics of the participants in Engebretson et al. [28] and the previous studies were different. Although the participants were all diabetics, they were different in many aspects, such as ethnic and geographic, severity of periodontitis, compliance of the

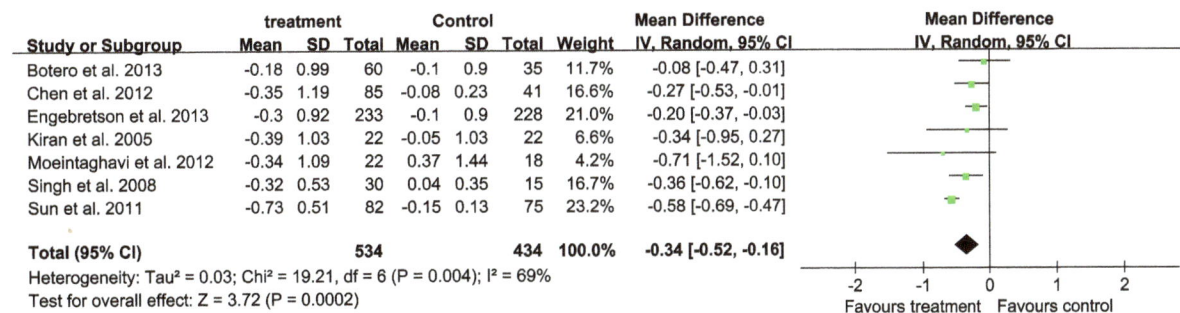

Study or Subgroup	treatment			Control			Weight	Mean Difference IV, Random, 95% CI
	Mean	SD	Total	Mean	SD	Total		
Botero et al. 2013	-0.18	0.99	60	-0.1	0.9	35	11.7%	-0.08 [-0.47, 0.31]
Chen et al. 2012	-0.35	1.19	85	-0.08	0.23	41	16.6%	-0.27 [-0.53, -0.01]
Engebretson et al. 2013	-0.3	0.92	233	-0.1	0.9	228	21.0%	-0.20 [-0.37, -0.03]
Kiran et al. 2005	-0.39	1.03	22	-0.05	1.03	22	6.6%	-0.34 [-0.95, 0.27]
Moeintaghavi et al. 2012	-0.34	1.09	22	0.37	1.44	18	4.2%	-0.71 [-1.52, 0.10]
Singh et al. 2008	-0.32	0.53	30	0.04	0.35	15	16.7%	-0.36 [-0.62, -0.10]
Sun et al. 2011	-0.73	0.51	82	-0.15	0.13	75	23.2%	-0.58 [-0.69, -0.47]
Total (95% CI)			**534**			**434**	**100.0%**	**-0.34 [-0.52, -0.16]**

Heterogeneity: Tau² = 0.03; Chi² = 19.21, df = 6 (P = 0.004); I² = 69%
Test for overall effect: Z = 3.72 (P = 0.0002)

Figure 6. Forest plot presenting change in CAL (mm) at 3-month.

Study or Subgroup	Treatment Mean	SD	Total	Control Mean	SD	Total	Weight	Mean Difference IV, Random, 95% CI
Botero et al. 2013	-0.15	1.87	60	0.2	2.01	35	14.5%	-0.35 [-1.17, 0.47]
Chen et al. 2012	-0.32	1.34	83	0.13	1.53	41	22.2%	-0.45 [-1.00, 0.10]
Engebretson et al. 2013	0.15	1.34	240	0.09	1.41	235	34.2%	0.06 [-0.19, 0.31]
Koromantzos et al. 2011	-0.72	0.93	30	-0.13	0.46	30	29.2%	-0.59 [-0.96, -0.22]
Total (95% CI)			413			341	100.0%	-0.30 [-0.69, 0.09]

Heterogeneity: Tau² = 0.10; Chi² = 9.38, df = 3 (P = 0.02); I² = 68%
Test for overall effect: Z = 1.52 (P = 0.13)

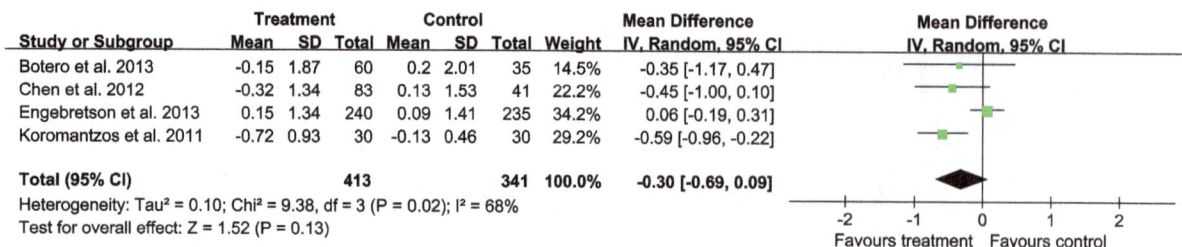

Figure 7. Forest plot presenting change in HbA1c (%) at 6-month.

participants, oral hygiene habits, etc. Especially, the concern about the treatment of diabetes was different. Only the participants enrolled in Engebretson et al. [28] were reported under the supervision of the physician for the diabetes, and the change of diabetic medicine was monitored. Six of the other studies instructed the participants not to modify the medication or diet [40,42–44,46,47], two did not reported the change of diabetic medication [8,41] and the other one [45] reported that only 13.3% for treatment group and 10% for control group participants increased their insulin dosages. It was considered that many factors, including whether the diabetic patients were under the supervision of physicians, and the different regions, the level of medical institutions (medical centers or primary clinics), and the different types that the supervisors belong to [53], can influent the level of HbA1c. So we think that the concern about the treatment of diabetes may have an impact on the outcome of the studies. Although the author disproved, Chapple et al. [54] pointed out that almost 60% patients having HbA1c level less than 8% at the baseline in Engebretson et al. Another reason was that the sample size of Engebretson et al. [28] was much more bigger than the other included studies, and the range of standard deviation of the change from baseline of HbA1c was wide. This point also increases the difficulty for us to explain the heterogeneity. When

the heterogeneity cannot be readily explained, random-effects model is one of the strategies for addressing heterogeneity according to the Cochrane handbook for systematic reviews of interventions (Version 5.1.0) [37]. So a random-effects model was used for the analysis. The other reason was that the treatment of the periodontitis was not completely the same with the other studies, this study did not use the adjunctive topical or systemic antibiotics [55,56]. Since the effect of scaling and root planning with the adjunctive topical or systemic antibiotics on reduction of HbA1c level has been shown in several studies [41,43,47], we believe that it may be a potential factor affecting the results of the study.

Secondly, the follow-up period of the studies included in this review was more than 3 months, and all of the studies reported about the HbA1c values at the 3-month after treatment. Two studies [48,49] included in the previous review reported on a 4-month follow-up outcome, and they were excluded.

Thirdly, One of the strengths of the present meta-analysis is that it takes into account the change of periodontal parameters at 3-month after treatment. It allows us to be more intuitive understanding of the effect of periodontal treatment on glycaemic control while improving periodontal status. The change of HbA1c for 6 months was also analyzed. The result can help us to

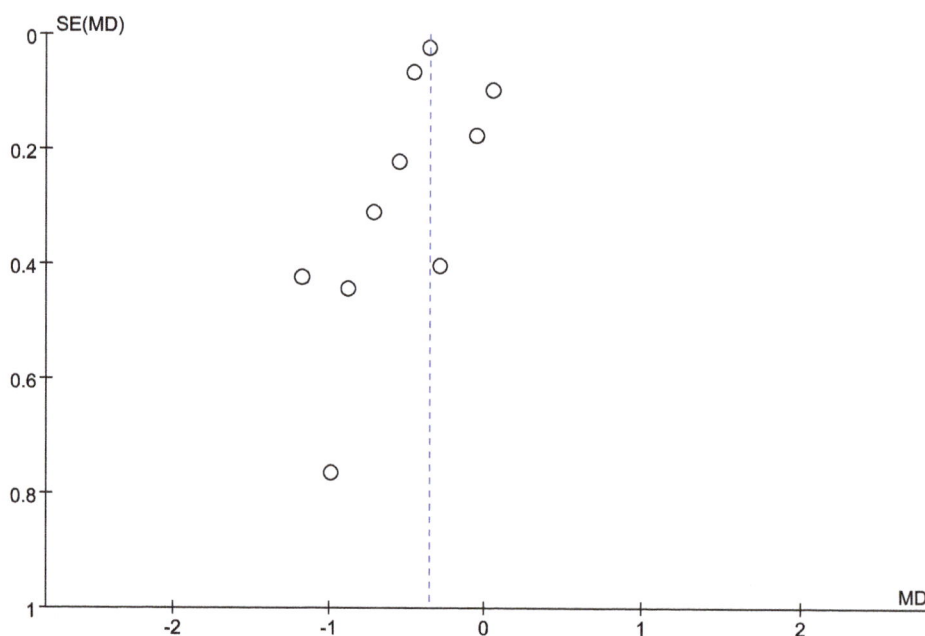

Figure 8. Funnel plot presenting change in HbA1c (%) at 3-month.

understand the long-term effect of periodontal treatment on HbA1c level in subjects with diabetes and periodontitis.

There are also several limitations to this review. The first is that the effect of periodontal treatment on glycaemic control of different type of diabetes with periodontitis cannot be analyzed in subgroups. One study [41] included participants with type 1 diabetes. But the sample size was small, and the outcomes were not reported separately, so it was analyzed as a part of treatment and control group. Another limitation is that adjunctive treatments such as: topical or systemic antibiotics and topical antiseptics were taken in many trials. And the systemic antibiotics could potentially mask the effect of scaling and root planning on HbA1c [28]. And it was not reported in this study. The other limitation of the present meta-analysis is that several studies did not reported the standard deviation of the change of HbA1c, and the data included in the analysis were obtained by calculation. The last but not the least is that only one recent trials was included in this update systemic review.

In conclusion, we demonstrate that periodontal treatment leads a reduction of HbA1c in diabetic patients with periodontitis while the improvement of periodontal status for 3 months after treatment. But the treatment may have no obvious effect on glycemic control for diabetic patient for 6 months after treatment. So physicians and dentists should carefully interpret these results when they apply them in clinical practice. And we look forward to more large randomized controlled trials with clear intervention design.

Supporting Information

Figure S1   Forest plot presenting change in HbA1c (%) at 3-month (fixed-effects model).

Figure S2   Forest plot presenting change in PPD (mm) at 3-month (fixed-effects model).

Figure S3   Forest plot presenting change in CAL (mm) at 3-month (fixed-effects model).

Figure S4   Forest plot presenting change in HbA1c (%) at 6-month (fixed-effects model).

Checklist S1   Prisma Checklist.

File S1

Flow Diagram S1

Author Contributions

Conceived and designed the experiments: W-DL W-XX. Performed the experiments: W-XX H-X L-XL W-DL. Analyzed the data: W-XX H-X G-XJ L-XL W-DL. Contributed reagents/materials/analysis tools: W-XX G-XJ. Contributed to the writing of the manuscript: W-XX H-X L-XL G-XJ W-DL.

References

1. Persson GR (2006) What has ageing to do with periodontal health and disease? Int Dent J 56: 240–249.
2. Thornton-Evans G, Eke P, Wei L, Palmer A, Moeti R, et al. (2013) Periodontitis among adults aged >/ = 30 years - United States, 2009–2010. 62 Suppl 3: 129–135.
3. Shangase SL, Mohangi GU, Hassam-Essa S, Wood NH (2013) The association between periodontitis and systemic health: an overview. Sadj 68: 8, 10–12.
4. Hung HC, Willett W, Ascherio A, Rosner BA, Rimm E, et al. (2003) Tooth loss and dietary intake. J Am Dent Assoc 134: 1185–1192.
5. Chen HH, Chen DY, Lai KL, Chen YM, Chou YJ, et al. (2013) Periodontitis and etanercept discontinuation risk in anti-tumor necrosis factor-naive rheumatoid arthritis patients: a nationwide population-based cohort study. J Clin Rheumatol 19: 432–438.
6. Holtfreter B, Empen K, Glaser S, Lorbeer R, Volzke H, et al. (2013) Periodontitis is associated with endothelial dysfunction in a general population: a cross-sectional study. PLoS One 8: e84603.
7. Wen BW, Tsai CS, Lin CL, Chang YJ, Lee CF, et al. (2013) Cancer risk among gingivitis and periodontitis patients: a nationwide cohort study. Qjm.
8. Telgi RL, Tandon V, Tangade PS, Tirth A, Kumar S, et al. (2013) Efficacy of nonsurgical periodontal therapy on glycaemic control in type II diabetic patients: a randomized controlled clinical trial. J Periodontal Implant Sci 43: 177–182.
9. Sanchez-Zamora YI, Rodriguez-Sosa M (2014) The Role of MIF in Type 1 and Type 2 Diabetes Mellitus. 2014: 804519.
10. Soskolne WA, Klinger A (2001) The relationship between periodontal diseases and diabetes: an overview. J Diabetes Res 6: 91–98.
11. Tsai C, Hayes C, Taylor GW (2002) Glycemic control of type 2 diabetes and severe periodontal disease in the US adult population. Community Dent Oral Epidemiol 30: 182–192.
12. Pucher J, Stewart J (2004) Periodontal disease and diabetes mellitus. Curr Diab Rep 4: 46–50.
13. Mealey BL, Oates TW (2006) Diabetes mellitus and periodontal diseases. J Periodontol 77: 1289–1303.
14. Nelson RG, Shlossman M, Budding LM, Pettitt DJ, Saad MF, et al. (1990) Periodontal disease and NIDDM in Pima Indians. Diabetes Care 13: 836–840.
15. Meenawat A, Punn K, Srivastava V, Meenawat AS, Dolas RS, et al. (2013) Periodontal disease and type I diabetes mellitus: Associations with glycemic control and complications. J Indian Soc Periodontol 17: 597–600.
16. Stanko P, Izakovicova Holla L (2014) Bi directional association between diabetes mellitus and inflammatory periodontal disease. A review. Biomed Pap Med Fac Univ Palacky Olomouc Czech Repub.
17. Al-Khabbaz AK (2014) Type 2 diabetes mellitus and periodontal disease severity. Oral Health Prev Dent 12: 77–82.
18. Loe H (1993) Periodontal disease. The sixth complication of diabetes mellitus. Diabetes Care 16: 329–334.
19. Mirnic J, Djuric M, Predin T, Gusic I, Petrovic D, et al. (2013) [Impact of the level of metabolic control on the non-surgical periodontal therapy outcomes in diabetes mellitus type 2 patients–clinical effects]. Srp Arh Celok Lek 141: 738–743.
20. Santacroce L, Carlaio RG, Bottalico L (2010) Does it make sense that diabetes is reciprocally associated with periodontal disease? Endocr Metab Immune Disord Drug Targets 10: 57–70.
21. Taylor GW, Borgnakke WS (2008) Periodontal disease: associations with diabetes, glycemic control and complications. Oral Dis 14: 191–203.
22. Moodley A, Wood NH, Shangase SL (2013) The relationship between periodontitis and diabetes: a brief review. Sadj 68: 260, 262–264.
23. Goldfine AB, Fonseca V, Jablonski KA, Pyle L, Staten MA, et al. (2010) The effects of salsalate on glycemic control in patients with type 2 diabetes: a randomized trial. Ann Intern Med 152: 346–357.
24. Goldfine AB, Fonseca V, Shoelson SE (2011) Therapeutic approaches to target inflammation in type 2 diabetes. Clin Chem 57: 162–167.
25. Iwamoto Y, Nishimura F, Nakagawa M, Sugimoto H, Shikata K, et al. (2001) The effect of antimicrobial periodontal treatment on circulating tumor necrosis factor-alpha and glycated hemoglobin level in patients with type 2 diabetes. J Periodontol 72: 774–778.
26. Gaikwad SP, Gurav AN, Shete AR, Desarda HM (2013) Effect of scaling and root planing combined with systemic doxycycline therapy on glycemic control in diabetes mellitus subjects with chronic generalized periodontitis: a clinical study. J Periodontal Implant Sci 43: 79–86.
27. Bharti P, Katagiri S, Nitta H, Nagasawa T, Kobayashi H, et al. (2013) Periodontal treatment with topical antibiotics improves glycemic control in association with elevated serum adiponectin in patients with type 2 diabetes mellitus. Obes Res Clin Pract 7: e129–e138.
28. Engebretson SP, Hyman LG, Michalowicz BS, Schoenfeld ER, Gelato MC, et al. (2013) The effect of nonsurgical periodontal therapy on hemoglobin A1c levels in persons with type 2 diabetes and chronic periodontitis: a randomized clinical trial. Jama 310: 2523–2532.
29. Zhang Y, Hu G, Yuan Z, Chen L (2012) Glycosylated hemoglobin in relationship to cardiovascular outcomes and death in patients with type 2 diabetes: a systematic review and meta-analysis. PLoS One 7: e42551.
30. Koenig RJ, Peterson CM, Jones RL, Saudek C, Lehrman M, et al. (1976) Correlation of glucose regulation and hemoglobin Alc in diabetes mellitus. N Engl J Med 295: 417–420.
31. Group UPDSU (1998) Intensive blood-glucose control with sulphonylureas or insulin compared with conventional treatment and risk of complications in

patients with type 2 diabetes (UKPDS 33). UK Prospective Diabetes Study (UKPDS) Group. Lancet 352: 837–853.

32. Nathan DM, Cleary PA, Backlund JY, Genuth SM, Lachin JM, et al. (2005) Intensive diabetes treatment and cardiovascular disease in patients with type 1 diabetes. N Engl J Med 353: 2643–2653.

33. Jones A, Gladstone BP, Lubeck M, Lindekilde N, Upton D, et al. (2014) Motivational interventions in the management of HbA1c levels: A systematic review and meta-analysis. Prim Care Diabetes.

34. Tricco AC, Ivers NM, Grimshaw JM, Moher D, Turner L, et al. (2012) Effectiveness of quality improvement strategies on the management of diabetes: a systematic review and meta-analysis. Lancet 379: 2252–2261.

35. Teeuw WJ, Gerdes VE, Loos BG (2010) Effect of periodontal treatment on glycemic control of diabetic patients: a systematic review and meta-analysis. Diabetes Care 33: 421–427.

36. Engebretson S, Kocher T (2013) Evidence that periodontal treatment improves diabetes outcomes: a systematic review and meta-analysis. J Periodontol 84: S153–169.

37. Higgins JPT, Green S (1996) Cochrane Handbook for Systematic Reviews of Interventions Version 5.1.0 [updated March 2011]. The Cochrane Collaboration, 2011. Available from www.cochrane-handbook.org. Control Clin Trials 17.

38. Liew AK, Punnanithinont N, Lee YC, Yang J (2013) Effect of non-surgical periodontal treatment on HbA1c: a meta-analysis of randomized controlled trials. Aust Dent J 58: 350–357.

39. Borenstein M, Hedges LV, Higgins JPT, Rothstein HR (2009) Independent Subgroups within a Study. Introduction to Meta-Analysis: John Wiley & Sons, Ltd. pp. 217–223.

40. Sun WL, Chen LL, Zhang SZ, Wu YM, Ren YZ, et al. (2011) Inflammatory cytokines, adiponectin, insulin resistance and metabolic control after periodontal intervention in patients with type 2 diabetes and chronic periodontitis. Intern Med 50: 1569–1574.

41. Botero JE, Yepes FL, Ochoa SP, Hincapie JP, Roldan N, et al. (2013) Effects of periodontal non-surgical therapy plus azithromycin on glycemic control in patients with diabetes: a randomized clinical trial. J Periodontal Res 48: 706–712.

42. Chen L, Luo G, Xuan D, Wei B, Liu F, et al. (2012) Effects of non-surgical periodontal treatment on clinical response, serum inflammatory parameters, and metabolic control in patients with type 2 diabetes: a randomized study. J Periodontol 83: 435–443.

43. Katagiri S, Nitta H, Nagasawa T, Uchimura I, Izumiyama H, et al. (2009) Multi-center intervention study on glycohemoglobin (HbA1c) and serum, high-sensitivity CRP (hs-CRP) after local anti-infectious periodontal treatment in type

2 diabetic patients with periodontal disease. Diabetes Res Clin Pract 83: 308–315.

44. Kiran M, Arpak N, Unsal E, Erdogan MF (2005) The effect of improved periodontal health on metabolic control in type 2 diabetes mellitus. J Clin Periodontol 32: 266–272.

45. Koromantzos PA, Makrilakis K, Dereka X, Katsilambros N, Vrotsos IA, et al. (2011) A randomized, controlled trial on the effect of non-surgical periodontal therapy in patients with type 2 diabetes. Part I: effect on periodontal status and glycaemic control. J Clin Periodontol 38: 142–147.

46. Moeintaghavi A, Arab HR, Bozorgnia Y, Kianoush K, Alizadeh M (2012) Non-surgical periodontal therapy affects metabolic control in diabetics: a randomized controlled clinical trial. Aust Dent J 57: 31–37.

47. Singh S, Kumar V, Kumar S, Subbappa A (2008) The effect of periodontal therapy on the improvement of glycemic control in patients with type 2 diabetes mellitus: A randomized controlled clinical trial. Int J Diabetes Dev Ctries 28: 38–44.

48. Jones JA, Miller DR, Wehler CJ, Rich SE, Krall-Kaye EA, et al. (2007) Does periodontal care improve glycemic control? The Department of Veterans Affairs Dental Diabetes Study. J Clin Periodontol 34: 46–52.

49. Yun F, Firkova EI, Jun-Qi L, Xun H (2007) Effect of non-surgical periodontal therapy on patients with type 2 diabetes mellitus. Folia Med (Plovdiv) 49: 32–36.

50. Choi YH, McKeown RE, Mayer-Davis EJ, Liese AD, Song KB, et al. (2014) Serum C-reactive Protein and Immunoglobulin G Antibodies to Periodontal Pathogens may be Effect Modifiers of Periodontitis and Hyperglycemia. J Periodontol.

51. Teeuw WJ, Slot DE, Susanto H, Gerdes VE, Abbas F, et al. (2014) Treatment of periodontitis improves the atherosclerotic profile: a systematic review and meta-analysis. J Clin Periodontol 41: 70–79.

52. Lopez NJ, Quintero A, Casanova PA, Martinez B (2013) Three-Monthly Routine Prophylaxes Improves Chronic Periodontitis Status in Type 2 Diabetes. J Periodontol.

53. Huang LY, Shau WY, Yeh HL, Chen TT, Hsieh JY, et al. (2014) A model measuring therapeutic inertia and the associated factors among diabetes patients: A nationwide population-based study in Taiwan. J Clin Pharmacol.

54. Chapple IL, Borgnakke WS, Genco RJ (2014) Hemoglobin A1c levels among patients with diabetes receiving nonsurgical periodontal treatment. Jama 311: 1919–1920.

55. Vergnes JN (2014) Hemoglobin A1c levels among patients with diabetes receiving nonsurgical periodontal treatment. Jama 311: 1920–1921.

56. Merchant AT (2014) Hemoglobin A1c levels among patients with diabetes receiving nonsurgical periodontal treatment. Jama 311: 1919.

19

Effect of Nicotine and *Porphyromonas gingivalis* Lipopolysaccharide on Endothelial Cells *In Vitro*

Na An[1,○], **Oleh Andrukhov**[2,○], **Yan Tang**[2,3], **Frank Falkensammer**[4], **Hans-Peter Bantleon**[4], **Xiangying Ouyang**[5], **Xiaohui Rausch-Fan**[2,4]*

1 Department of General Dentistry II, School and Hospital of Stomatology, Peking University, Beijing, China, 2 Division of Oral Biology, Bernhard Gottlieb School of Dentistry, Medical University of Vienna, Vienna, Austria, 3 Department of Stomatology, Xuanwu Hospital, Capital Medical University, Beijing, China, 4 Division of Orthodontics, Bernhard Gottlieb School of Dentistry, Medical University of Vienna, Vienna, Austria, 5 Department of Periodontology, School and Hospital of Stomatology, Peking University, Beijing, China

Abstract

Smoking is considered a significant risk factor for both periodontal disease and cardiovascular disease (CVD). Endothelial cells play an important role in the progression of both diseases. In the present study, we investigated *in vitro* the impact of nicotine on functional properties of human umbilical vein endothelial cells (HUVECs) stimulated with lipopolysaccharide (LPS) of periodontal pathogen *Porphyromonas gingivalis*. HUVECs were stimulated with different concentrations of nicotine (10 μM-10 mM) and/or *P. gingivalis* LPS. Expression levels of intercellular adhesion molecule-1, vascular cell adhesion molecule-1, E-selectin, monocyte chemoattractant protein 1, and interleukin-8 were measured on both gene and protein levels. Cell proliferation/viability, apoptosis, and migration were also investigated. Nicotine at a concentration of 10 mM significantly decreased *P. gingivalis* LPS-induced expression of all investigated proteins after 4 h stimulation, while lower nicotine concentrations had no significant effect on protein expression with or without *P. gingivalis* LPS. Proliferation/viability of HUVECs was also significantly inhibited by 10-mM nicotine but not by lower concentrations. Migration of HUVECs was significantly decreased by nicotine at concentrations of 1–10 mM. Nicotine at a concentration similar to that observed in the serum of smokers had no significant effect on the functional properties of HUVECs. However, high concentrations of nicotine, similar to that observed in the oral cavity of smokers, inhibited the inflammatory response of HUVECs. This effect of nicotine might be associated with decreased gingival bleeding indices in smoking periodontitis patients.

Editor: Michael Glogauer, University of Toronto, Canada

Funding: This work was supported by Ministry of Science and Technology of China under contract International Science & Technology Cooperation Program Foundation Nr.1019. The funders had no role in study design, data collection and analysis, decision to publish or preparation of the manuscript.

Competing Interests: The authors have declared that no competing interests exist.

* E-mail: xiaohui.rausch-fan@meduniwien.ac.at

○ These authors contributed equally to this work.

Introduction

Periodontitis is a chronic inflammatory disease which is caused by bacterial infection and leads to the destruction of periodontal tissues and resorption of alveolar bone. It is initiated by the accumulation of gram-negative bacteria in the dental biofilm [1]. Several gram-negative bacteria, such as *Porphyromonas gingivalis* (*P. gingivalis*), *Treponema denticola*, and *Tannerella forsythia*, are thought to be the primary etiological agents associated with periodontal disease [2]. Nowadays, it is widely accepted that there is an association between periodontal disease and cardiovascular disease (CVD), though no causative relationship between these diseases has been observed [3].

It is well recognized that tobacco smoking is a major risk factor for both periodontitis and CVD [3]. Smoking periodontitis patients exhibit greater bone loss, greater attachment loss, and deeper periodontal pockets than nonsmokers [4]. At the same time, smoking periodontitis patients have lower gingival bleeding indices compared to non-smoking patients, which is supposedly due to dysfunction of gingival vasculature [5,6]. There is also strong evidence indicating that smoking causes injury to the vascular endothelium, leading to endothelial dysfunction and initiating the pathogenesis of atherosclerosis [7–9]. Thus, the impact of smoking on both periodontitis and CVD seems to be largely associated with its effect on endothelial cells (ECs). ECs underlie the inner surface of blood vessels and play an important role in the progression of both diseases. In particular, ECs are shown to mediate leukocyte infiltration into periodontal tissue during periodontitis [10,11]. Endothelial dysfunction is considered to be the first inflammatory change of the vascular endothelium leading to arteriosclerosis [7]. The function of ECs in the inflammation process is associated with the production of several cytokines and adhesion molecules which regulate the migration of leukocytes toward the inflammatory area [12].

Nicotine is a major component of tobacco smoke and one of its most pharmacologically active agents. Park et al show that nicotine at concentrations similar to those found in habitual smokers does not induce any morphological changes in ECs but does enhance functional changes such as cellular proliferation, migration, and angiogenesis *in vitro* [13]. Heeschen et al suggest that nicotine enhances cellular proliferation, migration, and angiogenesis by stimulating nicotinic receptors in vascular ECs [14]. An *in vitro* study by Villablanca mentions that nicotine at concentrations observed in habitual smokers stimulates DNA synthesis and proliferation in vascular ECs, whereas higher nicotine concentrations might have cytotoxic effects [15]. Previous studies have also shown that the major periodontal pathogen *P. gingivalis* and/or its lipopolysaccharide (LPS) can activate the expression of adhesion molecules in ECs, which might then be involved in the progression of both periodontitis and CVD [16–18]. However, the influence of nicotine on the response of ECs to periodontal pathogens is still unknown. Therefore, in the present study, we investigated the influence of nicotine on cell proliferation, migration, and on the expression of several pro-inflammatory cytokines in ECs with and without stimulation with *P. gingivalis* LPS.

Materials and Methods

Cell culture

Commercially available human umbilical vein endothelial cells (HUVECs, Technoclone, Austria) were grown in endothelial cell medium (ECM) supplemented with 100 U/ml penicillin, 100 μg/ml streptomycin, 0.25 μg/ml fungizone, 2 mM L-glutamine, 5 U/ml heparin, 30–50 μg/ml endothelial cell growth supplement, and 20% fetal calf serum (FCS)¶. Cells were cultured in culture flasks coated with 0.2% gelatine at 37°C in a humidified atmosphere of 5% CO_2 and 95% air. All experiments were performed using cells between the third and sixth passage and were repeated in triplicate.

Commercially available ultrapure *P. gingivalis* LPS (Invivogene, San Diego, CA, USA) was used in the present study. As reported by another study [19], LPS preparations were free from contaminating lipoproteins.

Cell proliferation/viability

MTT assay was used for determining cell proliferation/viability. For each experiment, 2×10^4 cells were added to each well in standard 24-well gelatin-coated tissue culture plates and stimulated with different concentrations of nicotine and/or *P. gingivalis* LPS. After incubation for 4 h, 24 h, 48 h, and 72 h, a 5 mg/ml concentration of 3-(4,5-dimethylthiazol-2-yl)-2,5-diphenyl-tetrazolium bromide (MTT solution, Sigma, St-Louis, USA) in PBS was added to each well, and culture plates were incubated at 37°C for 4 h. The medium was removed, and 500 μl dimethylsulfoxide (DMSO) was added to each well followed by a 5-min incubation on a shaker. Finally, 100 μl of each cultured solution was transferred to a separate 96-well plate, and the optical density (OD) was measured at 570 nm with an ELISA Reader (SpectraMax Plus 384, Molecular Devices, USA).

Production of pro-inflammatory mediators by HUVECs

HUVECs were seeded in gelatin-coated 6-well tissue culture plates at a density of 5×10^5 cells per well in 3 ml of ECM. After 24 h, the culture medium was replaced by ECM medium containing 5% FCS, and cells were stimulated with different concentrations of nicotine (10^{-5}-10^{-2} M) in the presence or absence of *P. gingivalis* LPS (1 μg/ml) for 4–72 h. Non-stimulated cells were used as a negative control. After stimulation, the gene-expression levels of intercellular adhesion molecule-1 (ICAM-1), vascular cell adhesion molecule-1 (VCAM-1), E-selectin, interleukin-8 (IL-8), and monocyte chemoattractant protein-1 (MCP-1) were analyzed by real-time PCR. In addition, the cell surface expression levels of ICAM-1, VCAM-1, and E-selectin as well as the quantities of IL-8 and MCP1 protein in conditioned media were analyzed by flow cytometry and ELISA, respectively.

Real-time PCR (qPCR) was performed as described previously [20–22]. Isolation of total cellular mRNA and its subsequent transcription into cDNA was performed using the TaqMan Gene Expression Cells-to-CT kit (Ambion/Applied Biosystems, Foster City, USA). Real-time PCR was performed on an Applied Biosystems Step One Plus real-time PCR system using TaqMan gene expression assays (all from Applied Biosystems, Foster City, USA) with the following ID numbers: ICAM-1: Hs00164932_m1, VCAM-1: Hs00365486_m1, E-selectin: Hs00174057_m1, IL-8: Hs00174103_m1, MCP-1: Hs00234140_m1. Triplicate qPCR reactions were prepared for each sample. During the reaction run, the point at which the PCR product was first detected above a fixed threshold (cycle threshold (CT)) was recorded for each sample. Data were presented as the relative amount of mRNA in one sample versus a control (fold change) using the formula $2^{(-\Delta\Delta CT)}$, meaning we used the difference between the CT of a gene of interest and the CT of the housekeeping gene GAPDH for one sample (ΔCT) and then compared this value to that of the calibrator (control) sample ($\Delta\Delta CT$).

Analysis of the cell surface expression levels of adhesion molecules in HUVECs was performed using a flow cytometer (FACSCalibur, BD Bioscience, CA, USA) [21]. Cells were stained with one of the following monoclonal antibodies conjugated with phycoerythrin (all from eBioscience, San-Diego, CA, USA): mouse anti-human ICAM-1 antibody (Cat. Nr. 12-0549), mouse anti-human VCAM-1 antibody (Cat. Nr. 12-1069), mouse anti-human E-selectin antibody (Cat. Nr. 12-0627), and isotype control antibody (Cat. Nr. 12-4714). Cell counting was limited by 10,000 events.

Commercially available ELISA kits (Hoelzel Diagnostika, Cologne, Germany) were used for measurements of IL-8 (Cat. Nr. 950050192) and MCP-1 (Cat. Nr. BOS-EK0441) levels in the conditioned medium. The samples were diluted by a ratio of 1:20 and 1:5 for the measurements of IL-8 and MCP-1, respectively.

Quantification of apoptosis in HUVECs by flow cytometry

HUVECs were seeded in 6-well plates and stimulated with nicotine as described above for 4-72 h. After incubation, apoptosis was detected using the Annexin V-FITC Apoptosis Detection Kit I (BD Biosciences, San Jose, CA) according to the manufacturer's protocol. Cells were stained with both annexin V and propidium iodide to detect early and late apoptosis, respectively. The cells were washed twice after staining and acquired by a flow cytometer (FACSCalibur, BD Bioscience, CA, USA). Cell counting was limited by 10,000 events. The proportion of apoptotic and viable cells was quantified using CellQuest Software (BD Bioscience, CA, USA). The standard error of the mean was calculated from four independent trials.

Migration assay

Cell migration was assessed in a 48-well microchemotaxis chamber (Neuroprobe, Gaithersburg, MD, USA) on a polycarbonate filter with 8-μm pore size, as described previously [23]. The chamber consisted of acrylic top and bottom plates, each containing 48 matched wells. Top and bottom plates were separated by a polycarbonate filter with 8-μm pore size (Neuroprobe, Gaithersburg, MD, USA). Twenty-six microliters of serum-free medium containing different concentrations of nicotine and/or *P. gingivalis* LPS were filled in wells of the bottom plate. Subsequently, the bottom plate was covered with a filter, and the top plate was applied so that each well corresponded to that of the bottom plate. A cell suspension containing 1×10^4 cells in 50 μL of serum-free medium was added to each well of the top plate, and the whole chamber was incubated at 37°C in humidified air with

5% CO_2 for 8 h. After incubation, cells on the upper surface of the filter were removed over the wiper blade, and the filters were then fixed with methanol and stained with Hemacolor for microscopy (Merck, Darmstadt, Germany). The cells that migrated across the filter were counted under a light microscope at high-power magnification (x100) to measure transmigration in each well. Four fields were counted in each well, and the total number was calculated. Four wells were used for each group, and experiments were repeated in triplicate.

Statistical analysis

All experiments were performed in triplicate. A one-way analysis of variance (ANOVA) with Tukey's HSD test was performed to assess the significance. Values of $p < 0.05$ were considered statistically significant. All data analysis was performed using specific software (SPSS 19.0, SPSS Inc., Chicago, IL, USA).

Results

Effect of nicotine and *P. gingivalis* LPS on proliferation/viability of HUVECs

The effect of nicotine at concentrations of 10 µM-10 mM on the proliferation/viability of HUVECs in the presence or absence of *P. gingivalis* LPS, as measured by MTT assay after 4, 24, 48, and 72 h of stimulation, is shown in Figure 1. Nicotine at a concentration of 10 mM significantly inhibited proliferation/viability of HUVECs after 4 h of stimulation. Microscopic observation revealed that after stimulation with 10-mM nicotine for 24–72 h, most cells were detached from the well bottom, and therefore no parameters were measured in these groups. No significant effects were observed at nicotine concentrations of 10 µM-1 mM for any of the stimulation time points. In all groups, except those stimulated with 10-mM nicotine, the proliferation/viability continuously increased with time. *P. gingivalis* LPS at a concentration of 1 µg/ml did not affect the proliferation/viability of HUVECs at any of the stimulation time points.

Figure 2 shows the proportion of viable cells after stimulation with different nicotine concentrations and/or *P. gingivalis* LPS for 4, 24, and 72 h. Viable cells were determined as those which were negative for annexin V and propidium iodide. The proportion of viable cells was not affected by nicotine at concentrations of 10 µM-1 mM at any of the stimulation time points. This was true both in the presence and in the absence of *P. gingivalis* LPS. After 4 h of stimulation with 10-mM nicotine, the proportion of viable cells was significantly lower compared to that of the control group ($p < 0.05$).

Effect of nicotine on the expression of pro-inflammatory mediators in HUVECs

Figure 3 shows the effect of nicotine on the mRNA expression levels of different pro-inflammatory mediators after stimulation for 4, 24, and 72 h. Nicotine at concentration of 10 µM-1 mM had no significant effect on the gene expression levels of ICAM-1 (Fig. 3A), VCAM-1 (Fig. 3B), E-selectin (Fig. 3C), MCP-1 (Fig. 3D), or IL-8 (Fig. 3E) at any of the stimulation time points. Similarly, no significant change in the expression of any of the pro-inflammatory mediators in HUVECs were observed after stimulation with 10-mM nicotine for 4 h.

The effect of nicotine on the *P. gingivalis* LPS-induced mRNA and protein expression of pro-inflammatory mediators in HUVECs is shown in Figures 4 and 5, respectively. The largest increase in the mRNA expression levels of ICAM-1 (Fig. 4A), VCAM-1 (Fig. 4B), E-selectin (Fig. 4C), MCP-1 (Fig. 4D), and IL-8 (Fig.4E) was observed after 4 h of stimulation with 1 µg/ml of *P. gingivalis*, whereas the response was substantially diminished after 24 and 72 h of stimulation. Similarly, the largest surface expression levels of ICAM-1 (Fig. 5A), VCAM-1 (Fig. 5B), and E-selectin (Fig. 5C) were observed after 4 h of stimulation. The quantity of MCP-1 and IL-8 in conditioned media (Figs 5D and 5E, respectively) was continuously increased with stimulation time. Nicotine at a concentrations of 10 mM induced a significant decrease of *P. gingivalis* LPS-induced mRNA and protein expression levels of ICAM-1, VCAM-1, MCP-1, and IL-8 after 4 h of stimulation. *P. gingivalis* LPS-induced surface expression of E-selectin was significantly decreased by 10 mM after 4 h of stimulation, whereas the mRNA expression level of E-selectin was not affected. Nicotine at concentrations of 10 µM-1 mM had no significant effect on the *P. gingivalis* LPS-induced expression of pro-inflammatory mediators at any of the stimulation time points.

Effect of nicotine on HUVEC migration

Figure 6 shows the number of HUVECs that migrated through the 8-µm polycarbonate membrane in the presence or absence of nicotine at concentrations of 10 µM-10 mM and/or *P. gingivalis* LPS. The number of migrated HUVECs was significantly decreased by nicotine at concentrations of 1–10 mM in a dose dependent manner ($p < 0.05$). This was observed both in the presence and the absence of *P. gingivalis* LPS. *P. gingivalis* LPS induced a significant decrease in the number of migrated cells ($p < 0.05$).

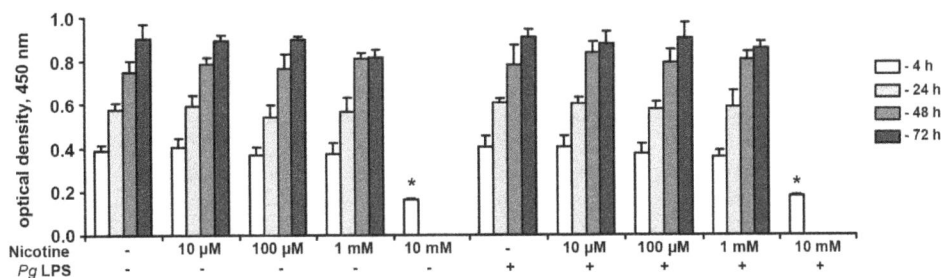

Figure 1. Effect of nicotine and *P. gingivalis* LPS on the proliferation/viability of HUVECs. HUVECs were stimulated with nicotine (10 µM-10 mM) and/or *P. gingivalis* LPS, and the proliferation/viability was measured after 4, 24, 48, and 72 h using the MTT assay. The y-axis represents mean ±SD values of optical densities measured at 450 nm from four wells of one representative experiment. * – significantly lower compared to control group, $p < 0.05$.

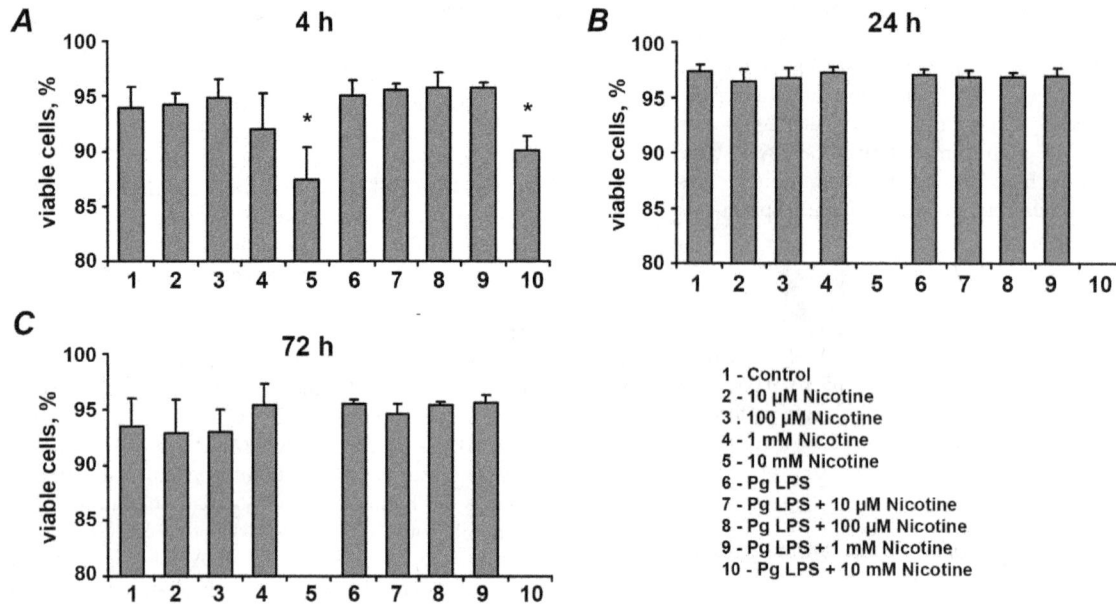

Figure 2. Effect of nicotine and *P. gingivalis* LPS on the proportion of viable HUVECs. HUVECs were stimulated with nicotine (10 µM-10 mM) and/or *P. gingivalis* LPS, and the proportion of viable cells was measured using a flow cytometry apoptosis assay after 4 (A), 24 (B), and 72 (C) h. Viable cells were those negative for annexin V and propidium iodide. Data are presented as mean ±SD of three independent experiments. * – significantly lower compared to control group, p<0.05.

Discussion

In the present *in vitro* study, we evaluated the effect of nicotine on EC properties under normal and inflammatory conditions. We found that nicotine at concentrations of 10 µM-1 mM had no effect on the proliferation/viability of HUVECs, as measured by MTT assay. At these nicotine concentrations, the proliferation/viability of HUVECs gradually increased with time, suggesting that cells proliferated during the observation period. However, 10-mM nicotine substantially inhibited the proliferation/viability of HUVECs after 4 h of stimulation; after stimulation for longer than 24 h, no viable cells were observed. Thus, it seems that 10-mM nicotine has a cytotoxic effect on HUVECs. Many previous studies also reported that nicotine at high concentrations inhibits EC proliferation and is cytotoxic. However, quantitative differences in estimating the toxicity of nicotine concentrations exist between studies. In particular, a recent study showed that the proliferation/viability of HUVECs is inhibited by nicotine at concentrations higher than 400 µg/ml (~2.5 mM) [24], which is generally in agreement with our data. In contrast, another study showed that HUVEC proliferation measured by cell count is inhibited by as little as 0.1-µM nicotine [13]. A study on calf ECs showed that cell proliferation measured by DNA synthesis is inhibited by nicotine at concentrations higher than 1 µM [15]. Interestingly, lower nicotine concentrations (<1 µM) might also stimulate proliferation of different ECs [13,15,25]. The difference in the experimental conditions, particularly initial cell seeding densities, could help explain the variable results of different studies. In particular, a recent study showed that HUVEC proliferation depends highly on the cell seeding density, and even a small increase of cell density might inhibit proliferation [26]. The diversity of nicotine effects might also be explained by the fact that ECs express a variety of nicotinic acetylcholine receptors which might differently regulate various cellular functions [27].

We further investigated the effect of nicotine on the expression of several factors associated with inflammation, namely ICAM-1,

VCAM-1, E-selectin, MCP-1, and IL-8, in the presence and absence of *P. gingivalis* LPS, which was used to model the conditions of periodontal inflammation. An increased expression of adhesion molecules in ECs is tightly associated with the progression of atherosclerosis [28]. In particular, E-selectin mediates the "rolling" of leukocytes along the endothelium, which is the reversible first interaction between endothelial and immune cells, whereas ICAM-1 and VCAM-1 are involved in the firm attachment of leukocytes to the endothelium and trans-endothelial migration [29]. MCP-1 and IL-8 are chemoattractants that induce the migration of neutrophils and monocytes, respectively, to the site of inflammation and promote the development of acute inflammation [30,31]. In this study, nicotine had no effect on the expression of any pro-inflammatory mediators in the absence of *P. gingivalis* LPS. A recent study showed that nicotine at concentrations of 100 µg/ml (~0.62 mM) had no effect on the on the production of IL-8 by HUVECs and slightly inhibited MCP-1 production [24]. Another study found that mRNA expression levels of VCAM-1 in human coronary artery ECs were slightly increased by a factor of about 1.6 in response to stimulation with 10-µM nicotine [32]. Finally, the surface expression of ICAM-1 and VCAM-1 in HUVECs was slightly increased by stimulation with 10-µM nicotine [33]. Thus, it might be concluded that the expression of pro-inflammatory mediators in HUVECs is only slightly—if at all—influenced by nicotine.

Stimulation of HUVECs with *P. gingivalis* LPS resulted in a significant increase in the expression of all pro-inflammatory mediators. This was observed at both mRNA and protein levels and is in agreement with previous reports [16–19,22,34]. The maximal response to *P. gingivalis* LPS was observed 4 h after stimulation, which is also in agreement with previous studies showing that maximal response of ECs to LPS is usually within several hours after stimulation [16,35–37]. It should be also considered that, at the late stages, the autocrine response of HUVECs to produce cytokines might play an important role and interfere with the reaction to LPS. We found that nicotine in

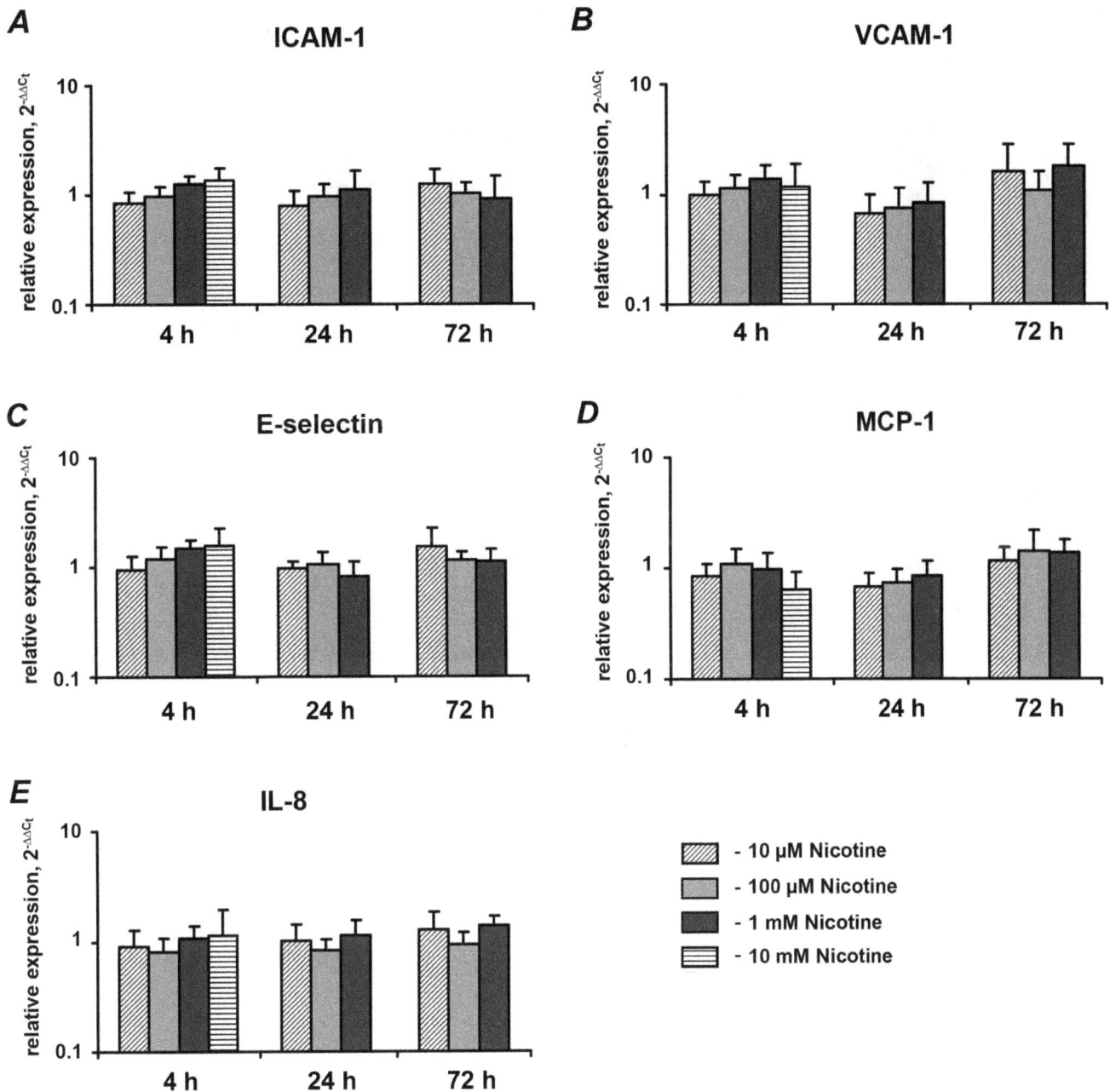

Figure 3. Effect of nicotine on the expression of pro-inflammatory mediators in HUVECs. HUVECs were stimulated with nicotine (10 μM-10 mM), and the expression levels of ICAM-1 (A), VCAM-1 (B), E-selectin (C), MCP-1 (D), and IL-8 (E) were measured by qPCR. GAPDH was used as endogenous control gene. Each value represents mean ±SEM of three independent assays. Non-stimulated HUVECs were used as a control (= 1). The expression levels of pro-inflammatory mediators were not analyzed after stimulation with 10-mM nicotine for 24 and 72 h because the cells were not viable.

concentrations of 10 μM-1 mM did not influence the response of HUVECs to *P. gingivalis* LPS. However, nicotine at a concentration of 10 mM significantly decreased the expression of pro-inflammatory mediators induced by *P. gingivalis* LPS stimulation, which could be related to nicotine cytotoxicity. Interestingly, no significant effect of 10-mM nicotine on the expression of adhesion molecules was found in the absence of *P. gingivalis* LPS stimulation (Fig. 3). Therefore, one can assume that nicotine could influence pro-inflammatory pathways in HUVECs, which are activated upon *P. gingivalis* LPS stimulation. The effect of nicotine on the

inflammatory response in HUVECs was also previously investigated. Patton et al showed that pre-incubation of human coronary artery ECs with 1-μM nicotine reduced the expression of IL-8 and MCP-1 in response to LPS [38]. Similarly, Saeed et al showed that nicotine in micromolar concentrations inhibited the expression of ICAM-1 in human microvascular ECs in response to stimulation with tumor necrosis factor α [39]. In contrast to these studies, we observed that only millimolar concentrations of nicotine were able to diminish inflammatory response of HUVECs to LPS. The reason for this discrepancy is not clear. Theoretically, it could be

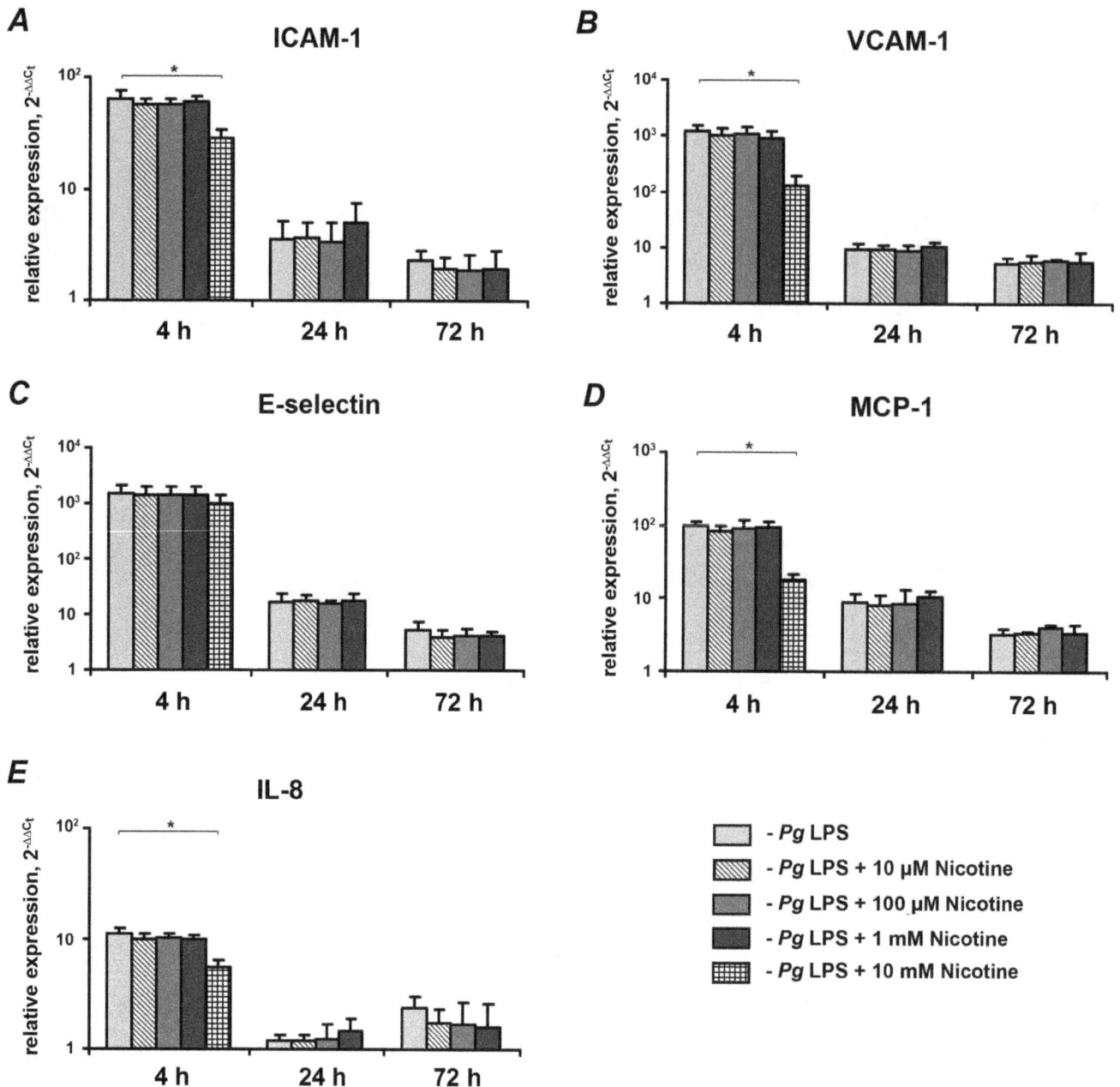

Figure 4. Effect of nicotine on the *P. gingivalis* LPS-induced mRNA expression of pro-inflammatory mediators in HUVECs. HUVECs were stimulated by *P. gingivalis* LPS in the presence or absence of nicotine (10 μM–10 mM), and the expression levels of ICAM-1 (A), VCAM-1 (B), E-selectin (C), MCP-1 (D), and IL-8 (E) were measured by qPCR after 4, 24, and 72 h. GAPDH was used as endogenous control gene. Each value represents mean ±SEM of three independent assays. Non-stimulated HUVECs were used as a control (= 1). All proteins exhibited significantly higher mRNA expression levels after stimulation with *P. gingivalis* LPS compared to the control group (p<0.05). The expression levels of pro-inflammatory mediators were not analyzed after stimulation with 10-mM nicotine for 24 and 72 h because the cells were not viable. * – significantly different between groups, p<0.05.

due to heterogeneity in the expression of nicotine receptors in different ECs [27], but this question needs to be investigated further.

Migration of ECs is an important process involved in angiogenesis and wound healing. We found that nicotine at concentrations of 1–10 mM inhibited EC migration in the presence and absence of *P. gingivalis*. The inhibitory effect of 10-mM nicotine on HUVEC migration could be at least partially explained by nicotine cytotoxicity. However, 1-mM nicotine was

not cytotoxic as it did not affect HUVEC viability and apoptosis. Previous studies reported that nicotine at a concentration of about 1 μM stimulated EC migration [13,40,41]. Another study showed that nicotine at a concentration of 20 μg/ml (~123.2 μM) had no effect on EC migration [42], which is in agreement with our observations. We can thereby conclude that the effect of nicotine on EC migration depends on its concentration.

Nicotine is the major component of tobacco smoke, and its presence in the body fluids of smokers is significantly increased

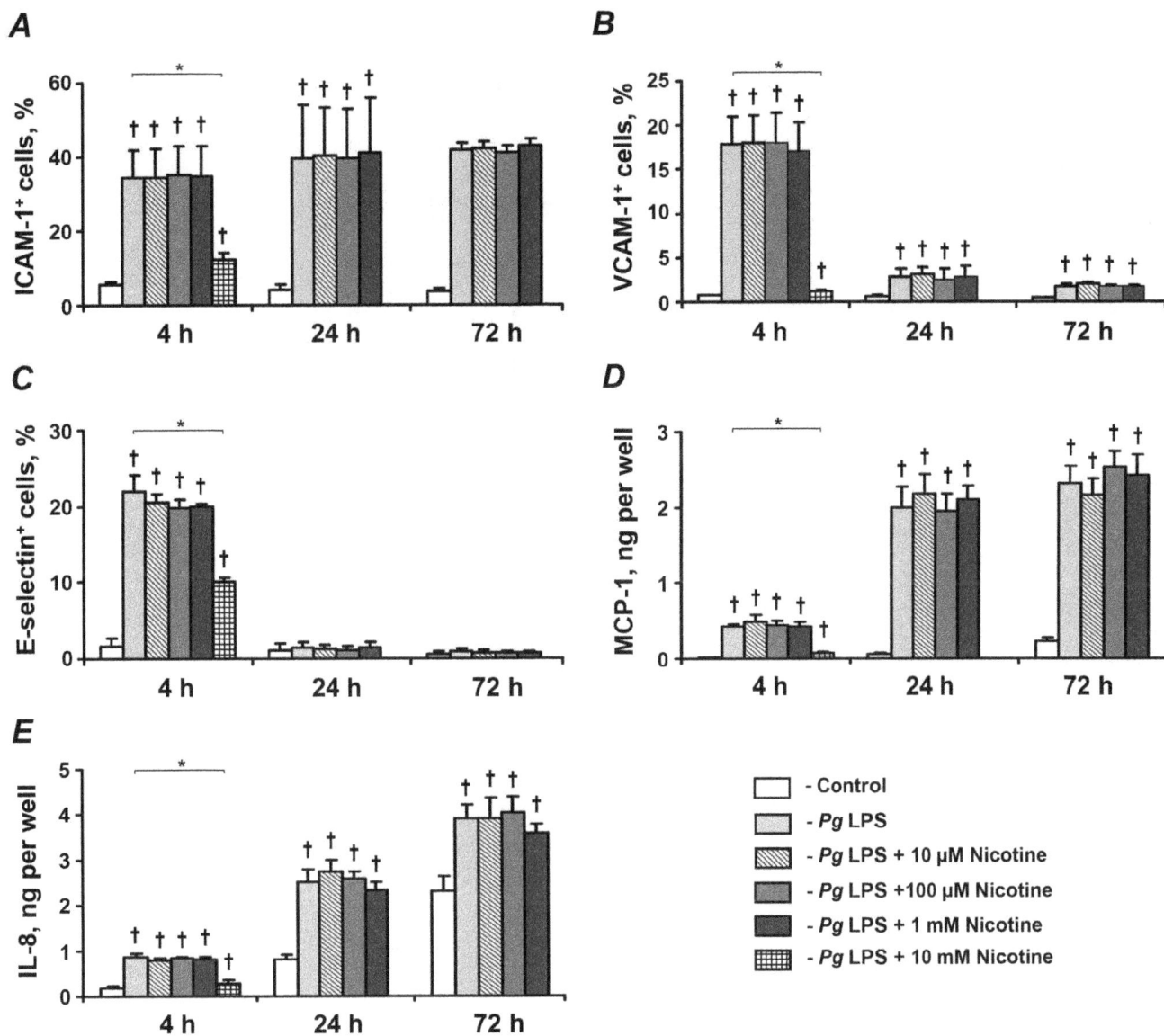

Figure 5. Effect of nicotine on the *P. gingivalis* LPS-induced protein expression of pro-inflammatory mediators in HUVECs. HUVECs were stimulated by *P. gingivalis* LPS in the presence or absence of nicotine (10 µM–10 mM) for 4, 24, and 72 h. After stimulation, the surface expression levels of ICAM-1 (A), VCAM-1 (B), and E-selectin (C) were measured by flow cytometry, and the quantity of MCP-1 (D) and IL-8 (E) in conditioned media was measured by ELISA. Each value represents mean ±SD of three independent assays. Non-stimulated HUVECs were used as a control. The protein expression levels of pro-inflammatory mediators were not analyzed after stimulation with 10-mM nicotine for 24 and 72 h because the cells were not viable. * – significantly different between groups, p<0.05. † – significantly higher compared to controls, p<0.05.

compared to non-smokers. Previous studies showed that the serum levels of nicotine in smokers achieve near a 1-µM concentration [43]. In contrast, nicotine levels in the saliva of smokers may reach millimolar concentrations [44]. Similar nicotine levels were also assumed to be in respiratory system tissues of smokers [45]. Our study showed that inhibition of HUVEC proliferation, migration, and inflammatory response is induced by millimolar concentrations of nicotine. Therefore, it seems that the effects described in the present study might be physiologically important for the oral cavity but not as much on the systemic level.

A decrease of EC proliferation and migration *in vitro* might suggest less vascularization and impaired wound healing *in vivo*, which is supported by numerous clinical studies (for review, see [46]). For mimicking inflammation *in vitro*, we stimulated

HUVECs with *P. gingivalis* LPS. Under these conditions, nicotine in millimolar concentrations attenuated the inflammatory response of HUVECs. A decreased release of chemoattractants MCP-1 and IL-8 following nicotine stimulation might be associated with a decreased requirement to attract leukocytes to sites of inflammation. Similarly, a decreased expression of adhesion molecules ICAM-1, VCAM-1, and E-selectin might be associated with decreased infiltration into the periodontal tissue. Thus, our data suggest that nicotine might decrease periodontal inflammation *in vivo*. This is supported by clinical studies showing that smoking periodontal patients have a decreased inflammatory response and gingival bleeding compared to non-smoking patients (for review, see [47,48]).

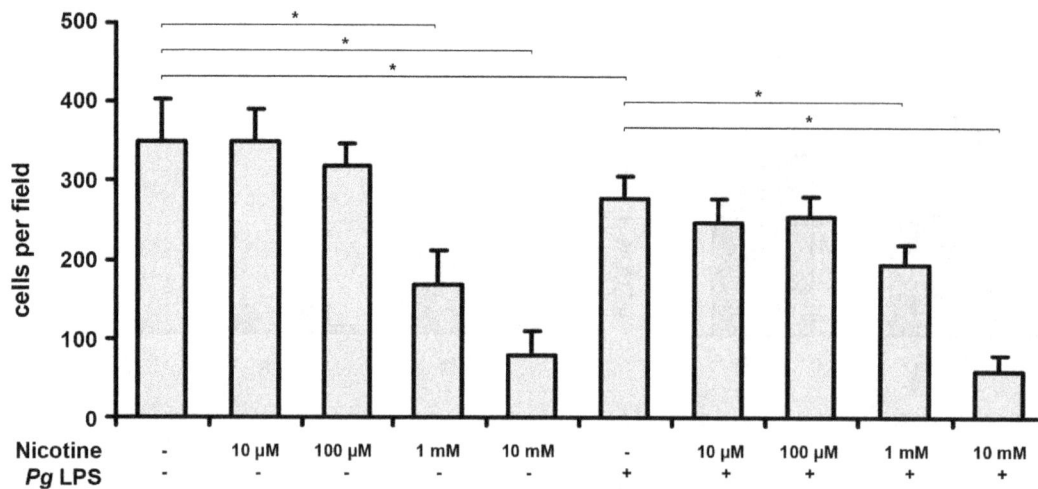

Figure 6. Effect of nicotine and *P. gingivalis* LPS on HUVEC migration measured in the microchemotaxis chamber. HUVEC migration through a polycarbonate membrane with pore size of 8 μm over 8 h was assessed in a 48-well microchemotaxis chamber. The y-axis represents mean ±SD of cells per microscope field of four different wells of one representative experiment. * – significantly different between groups, $p < 0.05$.

In conclusion, our data show that the functional properties of ECs are affected by millimolar concentrations of nicotine, which are similar to that observed in the oral cavity of smokers. In contrast, micromolar concentrations of nicotine, which are usually present in the serum of smokers, had no influence on the functional properties of ECs. Nicotine at millimolar concentrations inhibited proliferation and migration of ECs as well as their response to periodontal pathogens. These effects of nicotine might be associated with decreased bleeding indices observed in smoking periodontitis patient.

References

Acknowledgments

The authors would like to thank Mrs. Nguyen Phuong Quynh and Mrs. Hedwig Rutschek (both Medical University of Vienna) for excellent technical assistances.

Author Contributions

Conceived and designed the experiments: NA OA XR. Performed the experiments: NA OA YT. Analyzed the data: NA OA FF XO XR. Contributed reagents/materials/analysis tools: HB XR. Wrote the paper: NA OA FF HB XO XR.

1. Socransky SS, Haffajee AD, Cugini MA, Smith C, Kent RL Jr. (1998) Microbial complexes in subgingival plaque. J Clin Periodontol 25: 134–144.
2. Socransky SS, Haffajee AD (1992) The bacterial etiology of destructive periodontal disease: current concepts. J Periodontol 63: 322–331.
3. Lockhart PB, Bolger AF, Papapanou PN, Osinbowale O, Trevisan M, et al. (2012) Periodontal disease and atherosclerotic vascular disease: does the evidence support an independent association?: a scientific statement from the American Heart Association. Circulation 125: 2520–2544.
4. Johnson GK, Guthmiller JM (2007) The impact of cigarette smoking on periodontal disease and treatment. Periodontol 2000 44: 178–194.
5. Bergstrom J, Persson L, Preber H (1988) Influence of cigarette smoking on vascular reaction during experimental gingivitis. Scand J Dent Res 96: 34–39.
6. Mavropoulos A, Brodin P, Rosing CK, Aass AM, Aars H (2007) Gingival blood flow in periodontitis patients before and after periodontal surgery assessed in smokers and non-smokers. J Periodontol 78: 1774–1782.
7. Ross R (1999) Atherosclerosis—an inflammatory disease. N Engl J Med 340: 115–126.
8. Pepine CJ (1998) Clinical implications of endothelial dysfunction. Clin Cardiol 21: 795–799.
9. Quyyumi AA (1998) Endothelial function in health and disease: new insights into the genesis of cardiovascular disease. Am J Med 105: 32S–39S.
10. Moughal NA, Adonogianaki E, Thornhill MH, Kinane DF (1992) Endothelial cell leukocyte adhesion molecule-1 (ELAM-1) and intercellular adhesion molecule-1 (ICAM-1) expression in gingival tissue during health and experimentally-induced gingivitis. J Periodontal Res 27: 623–630.
11. Gemmell E, Walsh LJ, Savage NW, Seymour GJ (1994) Adhesion molecule expression in chronic inflammatory periodontal disease tissue. J Periodontal Res 29: 46–53.
12. Paoletti R, Gotto AM Jr., Hajjar DP (2004) Inflammation in atherosclerosis and implications for therapy. Circulation 109: III20–26.
13. Park YJ, Lee T, Ha J, Jung IM, Chung JK, et al. (2008) Effect of nicotine on human umbilical vein endothelial cells (HUVECs) migration and angiogenesis. Vascul Pharmacol 49: 32–36.
14. Heeschen C, Weis M, Cooke JP (2003) Nicotine promotes arteriogenesis. J Am Coll Cardiol 41: 489–496.
15. Villablanca AC (1998) Nicotine stimulates DNA synthesis and proliferation in vascular endothelial cells in vitro. J Appl Physiol 84: 2089–2098.
16. Khlgatian M, Nassar H, Chou HH, Gibson FC 3rd, Genco CA (2002) Fimbria-dependent activation of cell adhesion molecule expression in Porphyromonas gingivalis-infected endothelial cells. Infect Immun 70: 257–267.
17. Nakamura N, Yoshida M, Umeda M, Huang Y, Kitajima S, et al. (2008) Extended exposure of lipopolysaccharide fraction from Porphyromonas gingivalis facilitates mononuclear cell adhesion to vascular endothelium via Toll-like receptor-2 dependent mechanism. Atherosclerosis 196: 59–67.
18. Honda T, Oda T, Yoshie H, Yamazaki K (2005) Effects of Porphyromonas gingivalis antigens and proinflammatory cytokines on human coronary artery endothelial cells. Oral Microbiol Immunol 20: 82–88.
19. Kocgozlu L, Elkaim R, Tenenbaum H, Werner S (2009) Variable cell responses to P. gingivalis lipopolysaccharide. J Dent Res 88: 741–745.
20. Andrukhov O, Andrukhova O, Hulan U, Tang Y, Bantleon HP, et al. (2014) Both 25-hydroxyvitamin-d3 and 1,25-dihydroxyvitamin-d3 reduces inflammatory response in human periodontal ligament cells. PLoS ONE 9: e90301.
21. Andrukhov O, Steiner I, Liu S, Bantleon HP, Moritz A, et al. (2013) Different effects of Porphyromonas gingivalis lipopolysaccharide and TLR2 agonist Pam3CSK4 on the adhesion molecules expression in endothelial cells. Odontology.
22. Andrukhov O, Ertlschweiger S, Moritz A, Bantleon HP, Rausch-Fan X (2013) Different effects of P. gingivalis LPS and E. coli LPS on the expression of interleukin-6 in human gingival fibroblasts. Acta Odontol Scand.
23. Qu Z, Laky M, Ulm C, Matejka M, Dard M, et al. (2010) Effect of Emdogain on proliferation and migration of different periodontal tissue-associated cells. Oral Surg Oral Med Oral Pathol Oral Radiol Endod 109: 924–931.
24. Allam E, Delacruz K, Ghoneima A, Sun J, Windsor L (2012) Effects of tobacco on cytokine expression from human endothelial cells. Oral Dis 19: 660–665.
25. Li XW, Wang H (2006) Non-neuronal nicotinic alpha 7 receptor, a new endothelial target for revascularization. Life Sci 78: 1863–1870.
26. Heng BC, Bezerra PP, Preiser PR, Law SK, Xia Y, et al. (2011) Effect of cell-seeding density on the proliferation and gene expression profile of human umbilical vein endothelial cells within ex vivo culture. Cytotherapy 13: 606–617.

27. Wu JC, Chruscinski A, De Jesus Perez VA, Singh H, Pitsiouni M, et al. (2009) Cholinergic modulation of angiogenesis: role of the 7 nicotinic acetylcholine receptor. J Cell Biochem 108: 433–446.

28. Libby P (2000) Changing concepts of atherogenesis. J Intern Med 247: 349–358.

29. Lusis AJ (2000) Atherosclerosis. Nature 407: 233–241.

30. Baggiolini M, Dewald B, Moser B (1994) Interleukin-8 and related chemotactic cytokines—CXC and CC chemokines. Adv Immunol 55: 97–179.

31. Silva TA, Garlet GP, Fukada SY, Silva JS, Cunha FQ (2007) Chemokines in oral inflammatory diseases: apical periodontitis and periodontal disease. J Dent Res 86: 306–319.

32. Zhang S, Day I, Ye S (2001) Nicotine induced changes in gene expression by human coronary artery endothelial cells. Atherosclerosis 154: 277–283.

33. Albaugh G, Bellavance E, Strande L, Heinburger S, Hewitt CW, et al. (2004) Nicotine induces mononuclear leukocyte adhesion and expression of adhesion molecules, VCAM and ICAM, in endothelial cells in vitro. Ann Vasc Surg 18: 302–307.

34. Nassar H, Chou HH, Khlgatian M, Gibson FC 3rd, Van Dyke TE, et al. (2002) Role for fimbriae and lysine-specific cysteine proteinase gingipain K in expression of interleukin-8 and monocyte chemoattractant protein in Porphyromonas gingivalis-infected endothelial cells. Infect Immun 70: 268–276.

35. Takahashi Y, Davey M, Yumoto H, Gibson FC 3rd, Genco CA (2006) Fimbria-dependent activation of pro-inflammatory molecules in Porphyromonas gingivalis infected human aortic endothelial cells. Cell Microbiol 8: 738–757.

36. Eppihimer MJ, Russell J, Anderson DC, Wolitzky BA, Granger DN (1997) Endothelial cell adhesion molecule expression in gene-targeted mice. Am J Physiol 273: H1903–1908.

37. Lubos E, Mahoney CE, Leopold JA, Zhang YY, Loscalzo J, et al. (2010) Glutathione peroxidase-1 modulates lipopolysaccharide-induced adhesion molecule expression in endothelial cells by altering CD14 expression. Faseb J 24: 2525–2532.

38. Patton GW, Powell DA, Hakki A, Friedman H, Pross S (2006) Nicotine modulation of cytokine induction by LPS-stimulated human monocytes and coronary artery endothelial cells. Int Immunopharmacol 6: 26–35.

39. Saeed RW, Varma S, Peng-Nemeroff T, Sherry B, Balakhaneh D, et al. (2005) Cholinergic stimulation blocks endothelial cell activation and leukocyte recruitment during inflammation. J Exp Med 201: 1113–1123.

40. Park HS, Cho K, Park YJ, Lee T (2011) Chronic nicotine exposure attenuates proangiogenic activity on human umbilical vein endothelial cells. J Cardiovasc Pharmacol 57: 287–293.

41. Ng MK, Wu J, Chang E, Wang BY, Katzenberg-Clark R, et al. (2007) A central role for nicotinic cholinergic regulation of growth factor-induced endothelial cell migration. Arterioscler Thromb Vasc Biol 27: 106–112.

42. Snajdar RM, Busuttil SJ, Averbook A, Graham DJ (2001) Inhibition of endothelial cell migration by cigarette smoke condensate. J Surg Res 96: 10–16.

43. Russell MA, Jarvis M, Iyer R, Feyerabend C (1980) Relation of nicotine yield of cigarettes to blood nicotine concentrations in smokers. Br Med J 280: 972–976.

44. Feyerabend C, Higenbottam T, Russell MA (1982) Nicotine concentrations in urine and saliva of smokers and non-smokers. Br Med J (Clin Res Ed) 284: 1002–1004.

45. Seow WK, Thong YH, Nelson RD, MacFarlane GD, Herzberg MC (1994) Nicotine-induced release of elastase and eicosanoids by human neutrophils. Inflammation 18: 119–127.

46. Chambrone L, Chambrone D, Pustiglioni FE, Chambrone LA, Lima LA (2009) The influence of tobacco smoking on the outcomes achieved by root-coverage procedures: a systematic review. J Am Dent Assoc 140: 294–306.

47. Rivera-Hidalgo F (2003) Smoking and periodontal disease. Periodontol 2000 32: 50–58.

48. Heasman L, Stacey F, Preshaw PM, McCracken GI, Hepburn S, et al. (2006) The effect of smoking on periodontal treatment response: a review of clinical evidence. J Clin Periodontol 33: 241–253.

20

Analysis of Interleukin-8 Gene Variants Reveals Their Relative Importance as Genetic Susceptibility Factors for Chronic Periodontitis in the Han Population

Nan Zhang[1]*, Yuehong Xu[2], Bo Zhang[3], Tianxiao Zhang[5], Haojie Yang[7], Bao Zhang[6], Zufei Feng[6], Dexing Zhong[4]

1 Department of Dentistry, the First Affiliated Hospital, College of Medicine, Xi'an Jiaotong University, Xi'an, China, 2 Key Laboratory of Environment and Genes Related to Diseases, College of Medicine, Xi'an Jiaotong University, Xi'an, China, 3 School of Life Science and Technology, Xi'an Jiaotong University, Xi'an, China, 4 School of Electronic and Information Engineering, Xi'an Jiaotong University, Xi'an, China, 5 Department of Psychiatry, Washington University in Saint Louis, Saint Louis, Missouri, United States of America, 6 Key Laboratory of National Ministry of Health for Forensic Sciences, College of Medicine, Xi'an Jiaotong University, Xi'an, China, 7 The Second Department of Orthopedics, the Second Affiliated Hospital, College of Medicine, Xi'an Jiaotong University, Xi'an, China

Abstract

Interleukin (IL)-8, an important chemokine that regulates the inflammatory response, plays an important role in periodontitis. Previous studies indicate that certain IL-8 gene polymorphisms are associated with periodontitis susceptibility in some populations. However, the literature is somewhat contradictory, and not all IL-8 polymorphisms have been examined, particularly in Han Chinese individuals. The aim of this study was to investigate the association of every IL-8 SNP with chronic periodontitis in Han Chinese individuals. We analyzed 23 SNPs with minor allele frequency (MAF)≥0.01, which were selected from 219 SNPs in the NCBI dbSNP and preliminary HapMap data analyses from a cohort of 400 cases and 750 controls from genetically independent Han Chinese individuals. Single SNP, haplotype and gender-specific associations were performed. We found that rs4073 and rs2227307 were significantly associated with chronic periodontitis. Further haplotype analysis indicated that a haplotype block (rs4073-rs2227307-rs2227306) that spans the promoter and exon1 of IL-8 was highly associated with chronic periodontitis. Additionally, the ATC haplotype in this block was increased 1.5-fold in these cases. However, when analyzing the samples by gender, no significant gender-specific associations in IL-8 were observed, similar to the results of haplotype association analyses in female and male subgroups. Our results provide further evidence that IL-8 is associated with chronic periodontitis in Han Chinese individuals. Furthermore, our results confirm previous reports suggesting the intriguing possibilities that IL-8 plays a role in the pathogenesis of chronic periodontitis and that this gene may be involved in the etiology of this condition.

Editor: Salomon Amar, Boston University, United States of America

Funding: This research was totally supported by China Postdoctoral Science Foundation Funded Project (No. T70927 and M532029), Shaanxi Province Postdoctoral Science Foundation Funded Project (No. 201318420005), Ph.D. Programs Foundation of Ministry of Education of China (No. 2013021120078), Fundamental Research Funds for the Central Universities (No. 08142024 and 08143003) and National Natural Science Foundation of China (No. 61105021). The funding sources had no role in the design of this study, the collection, analysis and interpretation of data, the writing of the report, or the decision to submit the paper for publication.

Competing Interests: The authors have declared that no competing interests exist.

* Email: 111-zhangnan@163.com

Introduction

Oral Gram-negative bacteria trigger periodontitis, which produces an inflammatory response in a susceptible host [1]. Individual variations in the host's immune response, which are influenced by environmental and genetic characteristics, account for the predisposition, initiation and progression of periodontitis [2]. Environmental factors, such as hormones, diabetes and drugs, modify preexisting periodontal conditions [3]. Among these factors, tobacco use is one of the main risk factors for periodontitis, because tobacco affects the oral environment, gingival vasculature, inflammatory and immunological responses, as well as the healing potential of periodontal connective tissues [4–6]. Furthermore, increasing evidence suggests that genetic factors are important risk factors for predicting the susceptibility to chronic periodontitis [7].

Several studies have investigated the role of genes and their variants (polymorphisms) in host responses to chronic periodontitis and the progression of this disease [8–11]. In some situations, genetic polymorphisms may change protein's function or expression, altering innate and adaptive immunity, which might affect disease outcomes [12]. Genetic polymorphisms may also be protective against this disease [13]. Furthermore, the immune response of patients affected by periodontitis has been widely investigated, focusing on cytokine production and its association with chronic periodontitis [14–16]. Genetic susceptibility to chronic periodontitis has also been studied, focusing on immune system genes, such as interleukin-8 (IL-8). The IL-8 gene, which is located on chromosome 4q12-q13, encodes the IL-8 protein. This protein is the most potent chemokine studied to date, and it is responsible for inducing chemotaxis, which is the directed migration of cells to a site of inflammation [17]. This chemokine

Table 1. Demographic characteristics and clinical parameters of chronic periodontitis and controls.

	Chronic periodontitis (n = 400)	Controls (n = 750)
Gender (male/female)	200/200	375/375
Range of age (years)	28–62	27–60
Mean age (years)	50.46±9.14	50.32±8.27
PD (mm)	5.52±0.26	NA
CAL (mm)	5.58±0.45	NA
BOP (%)	48.06±13.43	NA

is important for regulation of the inflammatory response and for its ability to recruit and activate acute inflammatory cells. IL-8 is also mediates the activation and migration of neutrophils, which are the first line of defense against periodontopathic bacteria, which migrate from the peripheral blood into the tissues [18]. Moreover, IL-8 is produced early in the inflammatory response, and its presence persists for a long period of time [19].

While association studies provide a promising approach for studying the genetics of complex diseases, such as schizophrenia [20–23], identifying individual candidate genes/variants for disease risk is also important. Previous studies indicate the association between IL-8 SNPs and periodontitis compared with healthy controls. Some studies suggest that SNPs within IL-8 are associated with susceptibility to periodontitis [24–28], whereas other studies failed to demonstrate associations between periodontitis and IL-8 polymorphisms [29,30]. The association between IL-8 and chronic periodontitis has not been systematically investigated in the Han Chinese population. Despite evidence of a significant association within some populations, the contribution of IL-8 to periodontitis and its potential mechanisms of action in periodontitis remain to be elucidated. Therefore, an exploration of possible association between IL-8 polymorphisms and periodontitis is necessary among genetically independent populations. To confirm the association of IL-8 with chronic periodontitis, we performed an association study for IL-8 with chronic periodontitis in Han Chinese individuals. Additionally, this study provides further information regarding the use of IL-8 polymorphisms as markers of susceptibility to periodontal disease.

Materials and Methods

Patients and controls

This study was designed as a case-controlled study. The study group was composed of 1150 individuals, ranging from 27–62 years of age. It took almost one year (June 2012 to April 2013) to complete sample collection. All of the subjects were unrelated Han Chinese individuals randomly selected from the Shaanxi Province, with no migration history within the previous 3 generations. Additionally, all participants were of a similar socio-economic level, which is important because there is a strong association between low socio-economic status and a higher risk of periodontal disease [31]. All enrolled individuals answered a questionnaire to obtain information regarding dental history, family history of periodontal disease, cigarette smoking habits and general health. All of the subjects were required to have at least 10 teeth, be in good general health and be free of oral soft tissue abnormalities or severe dental caries, except for the presence of chronic periodontitis. Patients who reported the following characteristics were excluded from the study: use of orthodontic appliances, chronic anti-inflammatory drugs or immunosuppressive chemotherapy, antibiotics within the previous 3 months, chronic inflammatory diseases, a history of diabetes mellitus, hepatitis, HIV infection, nephritis, bleeding or autoimmune disorders, diseases with severe commitment of the immune function, current pregnancy or breastfeeding. Other authors have previously used these exclusion criteria [32–35]. Because tobacco is associated with increased clinical attachment loss (CAL) and supports alveolar bone loss, it represents an important risk factor for the initiation and progression of periodontal disease [3,36–38]. The individuals enrolled in this study were all nonsmokers (never smoked before).

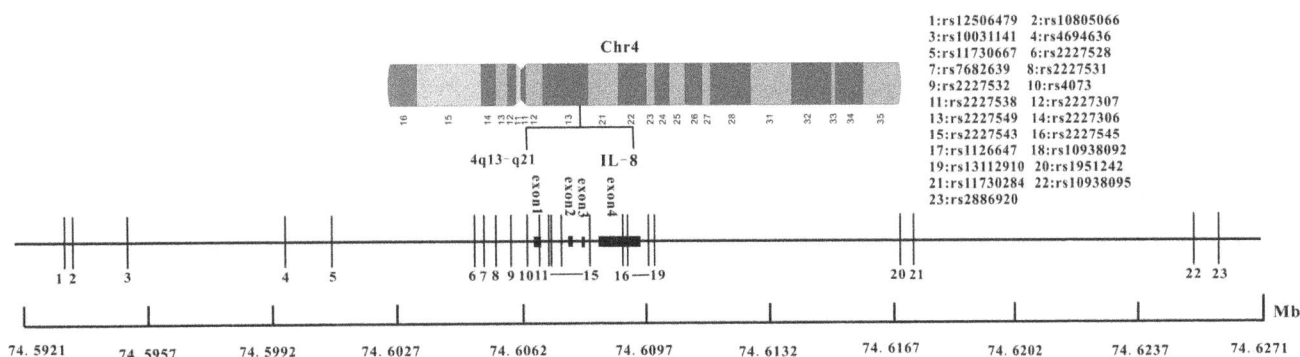

Figure 1. Distribution of the 23 SNPs across the IL-8 gene selected for the association analysis and their relationship with gene exons.

Individuals were categorized into the control and chronic periodontitis groups.

The healthy control group did not have signs of any periodontal disease at the time of sample collection and did not have a history of previous periodontal disease as determined by a lack of sites with probing depth (PD) >3 mm and the absence of gingival recession, CAL, and bleeding on probing (BOP). The 750 blood samples from periodontally healthy Han Chinese subjects were obtained randomly, which represented the controlled population (375 males and 375 females, aged 27 to 60 years with a mean age of 50.32±8.27 years; Table 1).

Patients with chronic periodontitis often presented an amount of destruction consistent with the amount of microbial deposits, presence of subgingival calculus, probable association with local predisposing factors and a slow to moderate rate of progression. All of the chronic periodontitis subjects were previously diagnosed with moderate or severe chronic periodontal disease. Diagnosis of chronic periodontitis (CP) was established clinically and by X-ray verification, according to the criteria of the American Academy of Periodontal Disease (AAP, 1999) [39], presence of chronic gingivorrhagia, bleeding on probing, clinical attachment loss, and horizontal or vertical loss of alveolar bone. In all patients, the degree of clinical attachment loss was defined using confirmed periodontal probe. Patients with probing depths greater than 5 mm, CAL greater than 4 mm, and some degree of gingival recession and tooth mobility were chosen. This clinical form is most prevalent in adults, but its occurrence may be present in younger individuals [40]. This patient group was composed of 400 subjects (200 males and 200 females, aged 28 to 62 years with a mean age of 50.46±9.14 years; Table 1) that were recruited from the inpatient and outpatient clinical services at the First Affiliated Hospital of Xi'an Jiaotong University, the second Affiliated Hospital of Xi'an Jiaotong University and the Stomatology Hospital of Xi'an Jiaotong University.

This study was approved by the Xi'an Jiaotong University Ethics Committee. All participants completed written informed consent forms. Data related to the participants are described in Table 1.

SNP selection and genotyping

IL-8 polymorphisms were identified using the National Center for Biotechnology Information single nucleotide polymorphism database, and 209 SNPs were identified. For the first screen of the most common SNPs in Han Chinese chronic periodontitis patients, a MAF≥0.01 was used as the cut-off. Based on these criteria, we selected 14 SNPs in IL-8 (rs2227528, rs7682639, rs2227531, rs2227532, rs4073, rs2227538, rs2227307, rs2227549, rs2227306, rs2227543, rs2227545, rs1126647, rs10938092 and rs13112910). Next, we then searched for all SNPs with minor allele frequencies (MAF)≥0.01 between 20 kb upstream and 20 kb downstream of IL-8 in the HapMap HCB database using Haploview [41], which identified 9 SNPs (rs12506479, rs10805066, rs10031141, rs46946336, rs11730667, rs1951242, rs11730284, rs10938095 and rs2886920). Therefore, we selected 23 SNPs in the 45 kb region containing IL-8 (Fig. 1).

Patients and controls were mixed on the same plates using a double-blind procedure. Plasma samples were stored at −20°C. Genomic DNA was isolated from peripheral blood leukocytes according to the manufacturer's protocol (Genomic DNA kit, Axygen Scientific Inc., California, USA), and DNA samples were stored at −20°C for SNP analysis. SNP genotyping was performed using the Sequenom MassARRAY platform with iPLEX GOLD chemistry (Sequenom, San Diego, CA, USA), according to the manufacturer's protocol. Polymerase chain reaction (PCR) prim-

Table 2. Allele and genotype frequency of single SNP association analysis.

SNP Makers	Allele Freq. (%)		p-value[1]	Genotype Freq. (%)			p-value[1]	H-W E p value	OR[2] 95%CI	Dominant	Recessive	Co-dominant
rs4073	A	T		AA	AT	TT						
Case	318(39.8)	482(60.2)	*0.028251*	71(17.7)	177(44.2)	152(38.1)	*0.014604*	0.121	1.207 (1.014-1.437)	0.702	*0.004*	0.547
Control	668(44.5)	833(55.5)		140(18.7)	387(51.6)	223(29.7)		0.222				
rs2227307	G	T		GG	GT	TT						
Case	282(35.2)	518(64.8)	*0.003455*	44(11.1)	193(48.2)	163(40.7)	*0.008132*	0.258	1.312 (1.098-1.567)	*0.007*	*0.021*	*0.035*
Control	623(41.5)	877(58.5)		127(16.9)	369(49.2)	254(33.9)		0.716				
rs2227306	C	T		CC	CT	TT						
Case	574(71.8)	226(28.2)	0.063353	209(52.3)	156(39.0)	35(8.7)	0.119011	0.460	1.195 (0.990-1.443)	0.538	0.063	0.977
Control	1020(68.0)	480(32.0)		344(45.9)	332(44.2)	74(9.9)		0.669				

OR: odds ratio; CI: confidence interval.
[1]P values of the normal chi-square statistics from Monte Carlo stimulation using CLUMP (T1), and significant p values are in italic bold.
[2]OR refers to risk allele odds ratio in cases and controls.

Table 3. Results of logistic regression analysis for susceptibility to chronic periodontitis.

Characteristics of subjects		Case	Control	OR	95%CI	p-value
Age				1.292	1.168–1.435	*0.002*
Gender	Male	200(34.78%)	375(65.22%)	Reference		
	Female	200(34.78%)	375(65.22%)	1.003	0.832–1.375	0.974
rs4073 TT carriage	Non-carriers	248(32.00%)	527(68.00%)	Reference		
	Carriers	152(40.53%)	223(59.47%)	1.451	1.196–1.628	*0.017*
rs2227307 T allele carriage	Non-carriers	44(25.73%)	127(74.27%)	Reference		
	Carriers	356(36.36%)	623(63.64%)	1.597	1.206–1.985	*0.029*
rs2227307 TT carriage	Non-carriers	237(32.33%)	496(67.67%)	Reference		
	Carriers	163(39.09%)	254(60.91%)	1.328	0.863–1.794	0.081
rs2227307 GT carriage	Non-carriers	207(35.20%)	381(64.80%)	Reference		
	Carriers	193(34.34%)	369(65.66%)	0.959	0.721–1.288	0.163

OR: odds ratio; CI: confidence interval.
Significant p values are in italic bold.

ers and locus-specific extension primers were designed using MassARRAY Assay Design software package (v. 3.1). 50 nanograms of DNA template were used in each multiplexed PCR well. PCR products were treated with shrimp alkaline phosphatase (USB, Cleveland, OH, USA) prior to use in the iPLEX GOLD primer extension reaction. Single base extension products were desalted with SpectroCLEAN resin (Sequenom), and 10 nL of the desalted product was spotted onto a 384-format SpectroCHIP using the MassARRAY Nanodispenser. Mass determination was performed with a MALDI-TOF mass spectrometer, and MassARRAY Typer 4.0 software was employed for data acquisition. The final genotype call rate of each SNP was greater than 96% and the overall genotyping call rate was 98.1%, confirming the reliability of further statistical analyses.

Statistical analysis and power analysis

Hardy–Weinberg equilibrium (HWE) for each SNP was assessed using GENEPOP v4.0. Allelic and genotypic association tests were performed using CLUMP v2.4 with 10,000 simulations, and this program employed an empirical Monte Carlo test of significance through simulation. To control for possible confounding effects, age and gender were used as independent variables in a multiple logistic regression analysis for adjustment by commercially available software (Statistical Package for Social Sciences, version 16.0 for windows, SPSS Inc., Chicago, IL, USA). The D' values for each pair of markers were calculated using the software program 2LD [42]. Haplotype frequencies were estimated using GENECOUNTING v2.2, which computes maximum-likelihood

estimates of haplotype frequencies from unknown phase data using an expectation–maximization algorithm [43]. The significance of a haplotypic association with chronic periodontitis was evaluated using a likelihood ratio test, followed by permutation testing that compared the estimated haplotype frequencies in patients and controls [43,44]. Differences were considered significant when the p value was less than 0.05. For haplotype analyses, the global p value was based on a comparison of the frequency distribution of all possible combinations of haplotypes among patients and controls. Furthermore, we performed power calculations for case–control genetic association analyses using PGA v2.0 [45]. Our sample size can detect SNP and haplotype associations with 91% and 85% power, respectively, at a false positive rate of 5%, and a presumed minimum odds ratio (OR) of 1.5.

Results

In total, 23 SNPs in the 45 kb region containing IL-8 were genotyped in 400 cases and 750 controls. The allele and genotype frequencies of all in case and control SNPs, including the results of the HWE test, are shown in Table 2 and Table S1. All SNPs were highly polymorphic in both cases and controls, with the exception of 7 SNPs (rs2227528, rs7682639, rs2227531, rs2227532, rs2227538, rs2227549 and rs2227545) in IL-8, and all SNPs were in HWE in both groups. First, we conducted a single SNP association analysis. When all of the samples were considered, we observed a significant association for rs4073 (p = 0.028251; OR = 1.207; 95% CI 1.014–1.437), and rs2227307

Table 4. Estimation of LD between each pair of loci within IL-8.

	rs4073	rs2227307	rs2227306	rs2227543	rs1126647
rs4073	-	0.743	0.322	0.028	0.015
rs2227307	0.916	-	0.321	0.039	0.022
rs2227306	0.924	0.981	-	0.097	0.098
rs2227543	0.257	0.322	0.331	-	0.099
rs1126647	0.222	0.284	0.347	0.369	-

D'-value are shown below the subtraction sign, and r^2-value are shown above the subtraction sign.

Table 5. Haplotypes frequency and association analysis.

Haplotype				Genecounting (frequency %)				
ID	SNP6	SNP7	SNP8	Case	Control	p-value[1]	correction[2]	Global p[3]
HAP1	T	T	C	40.3	39.4	0.692		<0.001
HAP2[4]	A	T	C	20.3	15.6	*0.005*	*0.039*	
HAP3[4]	A	G	T	10.6	18.2	*<0.001*	*<0.001*	
HAP4	T	G	T	13.4	10.3	*0.028*	0.227	
HAP5	A	G	C	7.02	8.75	0.147		
HAP6	T	G	C	4.15	4.28	0.872		

Significant p-values are in italic bold. Common Haplotypes are shown, if frequency more than 2.5%.
[1]Based on 10000 permutations.
[2]Corrected by Bonferroni.
[3]Based on comparison of frequency distribution of all haplotypes for the combination of SNPs.
[4]Haplotypes in italics are the significant ones in the study.

(p = 0.003455; OR = 1.312; 95% CI 1.098–1.567). Genotype association analyses for the two SNPs suggested a similar pattern with a significant p value (p = 0.014604, p = 0.008132, respectively). Because we observed significant associations for rs4073 in the recessive model (p = 0.004) and rs2227307 in the dominant, recessive and co-dominant models (p = 0.007, 0.021 and 0.035, respectively) (Table 2), a multiple logistic regression analysis was used for rs4073 in the recessive model and used for rs2227307 in the dominant, recessive and co-dominant models to evaluate the associations of alleles or genotypes with chronic periodontitis susceptibility, while adjusting for modifying factors, such as subject age and gender, to control for possible confounding effects (Table 3). A significant association was observed between age and chronic periodontitis (p = 0.002), while gender was not associated with chronic periodontitis (Table 3). The rs4073 TT genotype and rs2227307 T allele were identified as significant risk factors for chronic periodontitis after adjustment for age and gender (OR = 1.451, 95% CI = 1.196–1.628, P = 0.017; OR = 1.597, 95% CI = 1.206–1.985, P = 0.029; respectively) (Table 3).

Table 4 presents the results of LD tests (noted as D′ and r²) between pairs of SNP markers within IL-8 for the respective control groups. According to these results, LD (D′>0.8) was observed in the five-SNP linkage disequilibrium estimation. When combining the allele frequency data with the LD, the associated SNPs, rs4073 and rs2227307, were detected in the same LD block as rs2227306 (D′>0.8 between them, Table 4). Next, we performed the haplotypic association analysis of the LD block mentioned above (Table 5). Tests of the common three-marker haplotype (frequency >0.025) association for rs4073, rs2227307, and rs2227306 indicated a significant association between these SNPs and chronic periodontitis (p<0.001, global permutation). Some haplotypes of these three SNPs were significantly associated with chronic periodontitis. For example, HAP2 (ATC) was significantly associated with chronic periodontitis, and its frequency increased nearly 1.5-fold in cases (corrected p = 0.039). Due to higher frequencies in the controls, HAP3 (AGT) may provide a protective effect with nearly a 1.8-fold prevalence in controls (corrected p<0.001) (Table 5).

To examine whether gender would play a key role in the association, we analyzed our data by separating females and males according to the above results. Neither rs4073 nor rs2227307 displayed gender-specific associations with chronic periodontitis (Table 6). Moreover, haplotype association analyses were similar to the single-SNP analysis results, revealing no gender-specific association in females or males (Table 7).

Discussion

IL-8 is a chemokine related to the initiation and amplification of acute inflammatory responses and the chronic inflammatory process [46]. The purpose of this study was to explore the relationship between all SNPs within the IL-8 gene and chronic periodontitis in Han Chinese individuals. In this study, we present evidence for the association of markers that are mapped to the 45 kb region of IL-8 gene with chronic periodontitis. We identified a significant association in the region between rs4073 and rs2227306, and several lines of evidence suggest that the observed association is unlikely to be an artifact. First, both the single SNP and the haplotype-based association analyses support the association. Second, population stratification is an unlikely explanation because all of our samples are from the same geographical region. Lastly, similar results were obtained from other genetically independent populations in previous studies [25,26,28,47], reaffirming the observed association.

In association studies, it is critical to identify common risk variants in different populations. To examine whether common risk variants exist in genetically independent populations, we compared our results with those of previous studies. Individual differences in interleukins levels can be attributed to gene polymorphisms, especially when these polymorphisms are located within exons or promoters. The common rs4073 A/T polymorphism in the IL-8 promoter influences the production and expression of IL-8. The rs4073 A allele increases IL-8 production both in vitro and in vivo [48,49]. Lee et al. [49] reported that the presence of the rs4073 T allele of IL-8 exerts a 2–5-fold higher transcriptional activity than the rs4073 A allele. Two additional studies evaluated the association of the IL-8 rs4073 A/T polymorphism and periodontitis, but contradictory results were obtained [25,50]. Kim et al. [29] found no association between the genotype distribution and allele frequency of this gene and chronic periodontitis in the Brazilian population. In contrast, Andia et al. [25] discovered a significant association between the IL-8 rs4073 A/T polymorphism and chronic periodontitis in Brazilian nonsmokers, with a higher frequency of the A allele in the disease group compared to the control group. The results of our study do not agree with these studies. We found that the A allele of rs4073 displayed a tendency to be lower in cases compared to controls in

Table 6. Allele and genotype association analysis in female and male.

Marks		Allele frequency (%)		p value[1]	Genotype frequency (%)			H-W E p value	p value[1]	OR[2], 95%CI	p value		
											Dominant	Recessive	Co-dominant
rs4073		A	T		AA	AT	TT						
Female	Case	157(39.3)	243(60.7)	0.110589	34(17.1)	89(44.4)	77(38.5)	0.327	0.103541	1.223	0.735	0.066	0.711
	Control	331(44.1)	419(55.9)		68(18.1)	195(52.0)	112(29.9)	0.290		(0.955–1.565)			
Male	Case	161(40.3)	239(59.7)	0.126923	37(18.3)	88(44.0)	75(37.7)	0.226	0.139648	1.192	0.838	0.054	0.633
	Control	337(44.9)	413(55.1)		72(19.3)	192(51.2)	111(29.5)	0.501		(0.932–1.525)			
rs2227307		G	T		GG	GT	TT						
Female	Case	142(35.5)	258(64.5)	*0.035592*	25(12.5)	92(46.0)	83(41.5)	0.950	0.111624	1.309	*0.045*	0.881	0.238
	Control	314(41.9)	436(58.1)		67(17.9)	180(48.0)	128(34.1)	0.784		(1.018–1.682)			
Male	Case	140(34.9)	260(65.1)	*0.044555*	19(9.7)	101(50.4)	80(39.9)	0.123	0.063942	1.316	*0.031*	0.127	0.070
	Control	308(41.1)	442(58.9)		60(15.9)	189(50.4)	126(33.7)	0.427		(1.023–1.693)			
rs2227306		C	T		CC	CT	TT						
Female	Case	290(72.5)	110(27.5)	0.191898	105(52.5)	80(40.0)	15(7.5)	0.965	0.398158	1.196	0.522	0.183	0.794
	Control	516(68.8)	234(31.2)		175(46.7)	166(44.2)	34(9.1)	0.567		(0.914–1.564)			
Male	Case	284(71.1)	116(28.9)	0.186387	104(52.1)	76(38.0)	20(9.9)	0.287	0.273542	1.195	0.803	0.113	0.774
	Control	504(67.2)	246(32.8)		169(45.1)	166(44.2)	40(10.7)	0.959		(0.917–1.557)			

OR: odds ratio; CI: confidence interval.

Significant p values are in italic bold. CI: confidence interval; OR: odds ratio.

[1]P values of the normal chi-square statistics from Monte Carlo stimulation using CLUMP (T1), and significant p values are in italic bold.

[2]OR refers to risk allele odds ratio in cases and controls.

Table 7. Haplotypes frequency and association analysis in female and male.

Haplotype	Female		Male		p value[1]		
	Case	Control	Case	Control	Female	Male	All
Frequency (%)							
rs4073- rs2227307- rs2227306			Global-p value <*0.001*				
ATC	21.2	16.4	19.4	14.8	*0.042*	*0.041*	*0.039*
AGT	11.3	18.1	9.65	18.5	*<0.001*	*<0.001*	*<0.001*

[1]Based on 10000 permutations, and significant p values are in italic bold.

the Han Chinese population. Collectively, the consistency between these studies in different ethnic populations provides strong evidence that the rs4073 polymorphism in the IL-8 gene may be involved in chronic periodontitis susceptibility. Additionally, we also observed other differences among these studies. Rs2227307 had a significant allelic and genotypic association with chronic periodontitis in our analysis; however, only genotypic association data were similar to that reported by Scarel-Caminaga et al. [28]. To evaluate potential confounding effects that could cause bias in this association study of chronic periodontitis, important factors known to influence the pathogenesis of chronic periodontitis were assessed by multiple logistic regression analysis. Multiple logistic regression analysis revealed that age was associated with chronic periodontitis (Table 3). Regarding age, an important risk factor for periodontitis, Grossi et al. (1995) observed an OR = 2.6 (95% CI: 1.75–3.83) for the age group 35–44 years and an OR = 24.08 (95% CI: 15.93–36.29) for the age group 65–74 years, which are similar to the results of our study (Table 3) [51]. There is evidence that both the prevalence and severity of chronic periodontitis increase with increasing age [52]. However, the age effect could conceivably represent the cumulative effect of prolonged exposure to other risk factors [53].

The ability to draw conclusions regarding associations based on the analysis of individual SNPs is limited [54]. Therefore, to obtain stronger statistical evidence, we performed a haplotype analysis. Haplotype analysis uses additional information regarding the linkage between typed markers. The results of haplotype frequency estimation for three-SNP combinations (rs4073-rs2227307-rs2227306) indicated significant associations with chronic periodontitis (p<0.001, global permutation). The frequency of the ATC haplotype was 20.3% in cases and 15.6% in controls, demonstrating that individuals with ATC were almost 1.5 times more likely to develop chronic periodontitis than individuals carrying other haplotypes. This result was consistent with that reported by Scarel-Caminaga et al. [28]. However, a protective haplotype, AGT, which was almost 1.8 times more prevalent in controls than in cases, displayed a significant positive association with chronic periodontitis in our studies. Additionally, no gender-specific associations were observed in single SNP or haplotype analyses.

Genetic backgrounds vary among ethnic populations; therefore, differences in the results among these studies might be the result of ethnic differences and the genetic heterogeneity that existing in the IL-8 gene, despite some similarities in general association patterns. Nevertheless, our results should be validated in other populations or with a larger sample size in this population. This validation is required because the statistically significant results could occur by chance, and because the associations were not significant after an adjustment for multiple testing, despite remaining significant after 10,000 permutation tests. In addition, SNPs and haplotype structures can vary amongst different ethnic groups. Therefore, our data should be interpreted with caution, as the combination of these polymorphisms with others in different genes may also be important to define the role of these polymorphisms in the pathogenesis of chronic periodontitis.

A major limitation of the current study was that we did not perform further replication analyses for the possible risk of the SNPs identified in the study due to the lack of another cohort of patients and controls. However, as a replication study to confirm the previous studies and providing further evidence for the association of IL-8 with chronic periodontitis, our study did not appear extremely heterogeneous, and it could be considered reasonable and reliable. Additionally, although we selected subjects with no migration history within the previous three generations to control population stratification caused by genetic factors, we did not focus on other possible factors leading to population stratification; thus, we cannot completely rule out hidden stratification interference. Therefore, our findings should be considered preliminary. Given that the pathomechanism of chronic periodontitis includes further cytokines, chemokines, and pattern-associated molecules, additional follow-up studies are required to find possible causal variants. Ideally, these studies will involve the use of more sophisticated techniques of genetic investigation, such as DNA microarrays, to better understand the involvement of genetic factors in chronic periodontitis. Additionally, it is important to investigate the interaction of host genetics with clinical parameters and the immune response because chronic periodontitis is a complex disease, and the interaction of different factors has been insufficiently evaluated.

In recent years, particular interest has been given to investigating functional polymorphisms in candidate genes for disease association. The expression levels of a protein may be modulated by genetic polymorphisms in regulatory regions of the gene, mainly the promoter region [55]. Considering that some IL-8 polymorphisms were previously reported to be associated with higher IL-8 production and that a significantly higher level of this protein was found in the gingival crevicular fluid from patients with periodontitis [56], we hypothesize that the genetic differences between individuals in relation to IL-8 production may somehow predispose them to periodontal disease. The significantly associated SNPs identified in our study are not randomly distributed over the gene. Rather, these SNPs in the promoter and intron 1 are in the same LD block spanning the promoter and exon 1 of IL-8. Therefore, the significant associations in our study may be of interest for future studies. First, there is a cluster of significantly associated SNPs that span the promoter and exon 1 of IL-8, indicating a region of interest that might harbor functionally relevant variants. Second, we provide additional data in agreement with the previously reported IL-8 polymorphisms that are associated with chronic periodontitis susceptibility. To remedy the

mentioned shortcomings, we will try to observe the effects of these polymorphisms on periodontal systemic therapy in future studies.

In summary, our work provides supportive evidence for the association of IL-8 with chronic periodontitis. To our knowledge, this is the first study to demonstrate all SNPs between 20 kb upstream and 20 kb downstream of the IL-8 gene with chronic periodontitis in the Han Chinese population. Moreover, as an intriguing new insight into the pathogenesis of chronic periodontitis, we also confirmed previous reports suggesting that this gene plays an important role in the etiology of this condition. Because chronic periodontitis is multifactorial in nature, involving interactions between genes, the environment and lifestyle, genetic periodontal risk assessments may be valuable in developing preventive, diagnostic and therapeutic strategies against the incidence and progression of this condition. Given the complex patterns of findings from association studies focusing on chronic periodontitis and its underlying genetic heterogeneity, further inquiries and wider replications are required, particularly within different ethnic samples.

Acknowledgments

We thank all of the donors for their assistance in accessing collections and their advice and comments during the preparation of this paper.

Author Contributions

Conceived and designed the experiments: NZ. Performed the experiments: NZ DXZ HJY. Analyzed the data: YHX TXZ Bo Zhang. Contributed reagents/materials/analysis tools: Bao Zhang ZFF. Wrote the paper: NZ.

References

1. Schenkein HA (2006) Host responses in maintaining periodontal health and determining periodontal disease. Periodontol 2000 40: 77–93.
2. Bartold PM (2006) Periodontal tissues in health and disease: introduction. Periodontol 2000 40: 7–10.
3. Kinane DF, Peterson M, Stathopoulou PG (2006) Environmental and other modifying factors of the periodontal diseases. Periodontol 2000 40: 107–119.
4. Erdemir EO, Duran I, Haliloglu S (2004) Effects of smoking on clinical parameters and the gingival crevicular fluid levels of IL-6 and TNF-alpha in patients with chronic periodontitis. J Clin Periodontol 31: 99–104.
5. Palmer RM, Wilson RF, Hasan AS, Scott DA (2005) Mechanisms of action of environmental factors–tobacco smoking. J Clin Periodontol 32 Suppl 6: 180–195.
6. Gautam DK, Jindal V, Gupta SC, Tuli A, Kotwal B, et al. (2011) Effect of cigarette smoking on the periodontal health status: A comparative, cross sectional study. J Indian Soc Periodontol 15: 383–387.
7. Dutra WO, Moreira PR, Souza PE, Gollob KJ, Gomez RS (2009) Implications of cytokine gene polymorphisms on the orchestration of the immune response: lessons learned from oral diseases. Cytokine Growth Factor Rev 20: 223–232.
8. Gera I, Vari M (2009) [Genetic background of periodontitis. Part II. Genetic polymorphism in periodontal disease. A review of literature]. Fogorv Sz 102: 131–140.
9. Laine ML, Loos BG, Crielaard W (2010) Gene polymorphisms in chronic periodontitis. Int J Dent 2010: 324719.
10. Loos BG, John RP, Laine ML (2005) Identification of genetic risk factors for periodontitis and possible mechanisms of action. J Clin Periodontol 32 Suppl 6: 159–179.
11. Nikolopoulos GK, Dimou NL, Hamodrakas SJ, Bagos PG (2008) Cytokine gene polymorphisms in periodontal disease: a meta-analysis of 53 studies including 4178 cases and 4590 controls. J Clin Periodontol 35: 754–767.
12. Kinane DF, Hart TC (2003) Genes and gene polymorphisms associated with periodontal disease. Crit Rev Oral Biol Med 14: 430–449.
13. Kornman KS, di Giovine FS (1998) Genetic variations in cytokine expression: a risk factor for severity of adult periodontitis. Ann Periodontol 3: 327–338.
14. Ferreira SB Jr, Trombone AP, Repeke CE, Cardoso CR, Martins W Jr, et al. (2008) An interleukin-1beta (IL-1beta) single-nucleotide polymorphism at position 3954 and red complex periodontopathogens independently and additively modulate the levels of IL-1beta in diseased periodontal tissues. Infect Immun 76: 3725–3734.
15. Kamma JJ, Giannopoulou C, Vasdekis VG, Mombelli A (2004) Cytokine profile in gingival crevicular fluid of aggressive periodontitis: influence of smoking and stress. J Clin Periodontol 31: 894–902.
16. Trombone AP, Cardoso CR, Repeke CE, Ferreira SB Jr, Martins W Jr, et al. (2009) Tumor necrosis factor-alpha −308G/A single nucleotide polymorphism and red-complex periodontopathogens are independently associated with increased levels of tumor necrosis factor-alpha in diseased periodontal tissues. J Periodontal Res 44: 598–608.
17. Remick DG (2005) Interleukin-8. Critical Care Medicine 33(12 Suppl.): S466–467.
18. Marshall JC (2005) Neutrophils in the pathogenesis of sepsis. Critical Care Medicine 33(12 Suppl.): S502–504.
19. Deforge LE, FantonE JC, Kenney JS, Remick DJ (1992) Oxygen radical scavengers selectively inhibit interleukin 8 production in human whole blood. Journal of Clinical Investigation 90(5): 2123–2129.
20. Guan FL, Zhang C, Wei SG, Zhang HB, Gong XM, et al. (2012) Association of PDE4B polymorphisms and schizophrenia in Northwestern Han Chinese. Human Genetics 131(7): 1047–1056.
21. Guan FL, Wei SG, Feng JL, Zhang C, Xing B, et al. (2012) Association study of a new schizophrenia susceptibility locus of 10q24.32-33 in a Han Chinese population. Schizophrenia Research, 138(1): 63–68.
22. Guan FL, Wei SG, Zhang C, Zhang HB, Zhang B, et al. (2013) A population-based association study of 2q32.3 and 8q21.3 loci with schizophrenia in Han Chinese. Journal of Psychiatric Research 47(6): 712–717.
23. Guan FL, Zhang B, Yan TL, Li L, Liu F, et al. (2014) MIR137 gene and target gene CACNA1C of miR-137 contribute to schizophrenia susceptibility in Han Chinese. Schizophrenia Research 152(1): 97–104.

24. Amaya MP, Criado L, Blanco B, Gomez M, Torres O, et al. (2013) Polymorphisms of pro-inflammatory cytokine genes and the risk for acute suppurative or chronic nonsuppurative apical periodontitis in a Colombian population. Int Endod J 46: 71–78.

25. Andia DC, de Oliveira NF, Letra AM, Nociti FH Jr, Line SR, et al. (2011) Interleukin-8 gene promoter polymorphism (rs4073) may contribute to chronic periodontitis. J Periodontol 82: 893–899.

26. Kim YJ, Viana AC, Curtis KM, Orrico SR, Cirelli JA, et al. (2010) Association of haplotypes in the IL-8 gene with susceptibility to chronic periodontitis in a Brazilian population. Clin Chim Acta 411: 1264–1268.

27. Li G, Yue Y, Tian Y, Li JL, Wang M, et al. (2012) Association of matrix metalloproteinase (MMP)-1, 3, 9, interleukin (IL)-2, 8 and cyclooxygenase (COX)-2 gene polymorphisms with chronic periodontitis in a Chinese population. Cytokine 60: 552–560.

28. Scarel-Caminaga RM, Kim YJ, Viana AC, Curtis KM, Corbi SC, et al. (2011) Haplotypes in the interleukin 8 gene and their association with chronic periodontitis susceptibility. Biochem Genet 49: 292–302.

29. Kim YJ, Viana AC, Curtis KM, Orrico SR, Cirelli JA, et al. (2009) Lack of association of a functional polymorphism in the interleukin 8 gene with susceptibility to periodontitis. DNA Cell Biol 28: 185–190.

30. Andia DC, Letra A, Casarin RC, Casati MZ, Line SR, et al. (2012) Genetic analysis of the IL-8 gene polymorphism (rs4073) in generalized aggressive periodontitis. Arch Oral Biol.

31. Albandar JM, Rams TE (2002) Risk factors for periodontitis in children and young persons. Periodontol 2000 29: 207–222.

32. Fan WH, Liu DL, Xiao LM, Xie CJ, Sun SY, et al. (2011) Coronary heart disease and chronic periodontitis: is polymorphism of interleukin-6 gene the common risk factor in a Chinese population? Oral Dis 17: 270–276.

33. Moreira PR, de Sa AR, Xavier GM, Costa JE, Gomez RS, et al. (2005) A functional interleukin-1 beta gene polymorphism is associated with chronic periodontitis in a sample of Brazilian individuals. J Periodontal Res 40: 306–311.

34. Nibali L, Madden I, Franch Chillida F, Heitz-Mayfield L, Brett P, et al. (2011) IL6 −174 genotype associated with Aggregatibacter actinomycetemcomitans in Indians. Oral Dis 17: 232–237.

35. Scarel-Caminaga RM, Trevilatto PC, Souza AP, Brito RB, Camargo LE, et al. (2004) Interleukin 10 gene promoter polymorphisms are associated with chronic periodontitis. J Clin Periodontol 31: 443–448.

36. Apatzidou DA, Riggio MP, Kinane DF (2005) Impact of smoking on the clinical, microbiological and immunological parameters of adult patients with periodontitis. J Clin Periodontol 32: 973–983.

37. Bergstrom J (2004) Tobacco smoking and chronic destructive periodontal disease. Odontology 92: 1–8.

38. Kornman KS (2005) Diagnostic and prognostic tests for oral diseases: practical applications. J Dent Educ 69: 498–508.

39. Armitage GC (1999) Development of a classification system for periodontal diseases and conditions. Ann Periodontol 4: 1–6.

40. Highfield J (2009) Diagnosis and classification of periodontal disease. Aust Dent J 54 Suppl 1: S11–26.

41. Barrett JC, Fry B, Maller J, Daly MJ (2005) Haploview: analysis and visualization of LD and haplotype maps. Bioinformatics 21: 263–265.

42. Zhao JH (2004) 2LD, GENECOUNTING and HAP: Computer programs for linkage disequilibrium analysis. Bioinformatics 20: 1325–1326.

43. Curtis D, Knight J, Sham PC (2006) Program report: GENECOUNTING support programs. Ann Hum Genet 70: 277–279.

44. Zhao JH, Lissarrague S, Essioux L, Sham PC (2002) GENECOUNTING: haplotype analysis with missing genotypes. Bioinformatics 18: 1694–1695.

45. Menashe I, Rosenberg PS, Chen BE (2008) PGA: power calculator for case-control genetic association analyses. BMC Genet 9: 36.

46. Campa D, Hung RJ, Mates D, Zaridze D, Szeszenia-Dabrowska N, et al. (2005) Lack of association between −251 TNA polymorphism of IL8 and lung cancer risk. Cancer Epidemiol Biomarkers Prev 14: 2457–2458.

47. Corbi SC, Anovazzi G, Finoti LS, Kim YJ, Capela MV, et al. (2012) Haplotypes of susceptibility to chronic periodontitis in the Interleukin 8 gene do not influence protein level in the gingival crevicular fluid. Arch Oral Biol 57: 1355–1361.

48. Taguchi A, Ohmiya N, Shirai K, Mabuchi N, Itoh A, et al. (2005) Interleukin-8 promoter polymorphism increases the risk of atrophic gastritis and gastric cancer in Japan. Cancer Epidemiol Biomarkers Prev 14: 2487–2493.

49. Lee WP, Tai DI, Lan KH, Li AF, Hsu HC, et al. (2005) The −251T allele of the interleukin-8 promoter is associated with increased risk of gastric carcinoma featuring diffuse-type histopathology in Chinese population. Clin Cancer Res 11: 6431–6441.

50. Cipollone F, Toniato E, Martinotti S, Fazia M, Iezzi A, et al. (2004) A polymorphism in the cyclooxygenase 2 gene as an inherited protective factor against myocardial infarction and stroke. JAMA 291: 2221–2228.

51. Grossi SG, Genco RJ, Machtei EE, Ho AW, Koch G, et al. (1995) Assessment of risk for periodontal disease. II. Risk indicators for alveolar bone loss. J Periodontol 66: 23–29.

52. Borrell LN, Papapanou PN (2005) Analytical epidemiology of periodontitis. J Clin Periodontol 32 Suppl 6: 132–158.

53. Papapanou PN, Lindhe J, Sterrett JD, Eneroth L (1991) Considerations on the contribution of ageing to loss of periodontal tissue support. J Clin Periodontol 18: 611–615.

54. Korostishevsky M, Kaganovich M, Cholostoy A, Ashkenazi M, Ratner Y, et al. (2004) Is the G72/G30 locus associated with schizophrenia? single nucleotide polymorphisms, haplotypes, and gene expression analysis. Biol Psychiatry 56: 169–176.

55. Stern DL (2000) Evolutionary biology. The problem of variation. Nature 408: 529–531.

56. Tsai CC, Ho YP, Chen CC (1995) Levels of interleukin-1 beta and interleukin-8 in gingival crevicular fluids in adult periodontitis. J Periodontol 66: 852–859.

21

Endocannabinoids and Inflammatory Response in Periodontal Ligament Cells

Burcu Özdemir[1,2]*, Bin Shi[2,5], Hans Peter Bantleon[3], Andreas Moritz[4], Xiaohui Rausch-Fan[2,3], Oleh Andrukhov[2]*

1 Department of Periodontology, Faculty of Dentistry, Gazi University, Ankara, Turkey, 2 Division of Oral Biology, Bernhard Gottlieb School of Dentistry, Medical University, Vienna, Austria, 3 Division of Orthodontics, Bernhard Gottlieb School of Dentistry, Medical University, Vienna, Austria, 4 Division of Conservative Dentistry, Periodontology and Prophylaxis, Bernhard Gottlieb School of Dentistry, Medical University, Vienna, Austria, 5 Department of Oral Surgery, First Affiliated Hospital of Fujian Medical University, Fuzhou, China

Abstract

Endocannabinoids are associated with multiple regulatory functions in several tissues. The main endocannabinoids, anandamide (AEA) and 2-arachidonylglycerol (2-AG), have been detected in the gingival crevicular fluid of periodontitis patients, but the association between periodontal disease or human periodontal ligament cells (hPdLCs) and endocannabinoids still remain unclear. The aim of the present study was to examine the effects of AEA and 2-AG on the proliferation/viability and cytokine/chemokine production of hPdLCs in the presence/absence of *Porphyromonas gingivalis* lipopolysaccharide (*P. gingivalis* LPS). The proliferation/viability of hPdLCs was measured using 3,4,5-dimethylthiazol-2-yl-2,5-diphenyl tetrazolium bromide (MTT)-assay. Interleukin-6 (IL-6), interleukin-8 (IL-8), and monocyte chemotactic protein-1 (MCP-1) levels were examined at gene expression and protein level by real-time PCR and ELISA, respectively. AEA and 2-AG did not reveal any significant effects on proliferation/viability of hPdLCs in the absence of *P. gingivalis* LPS. However, hPdLCs viability was significantly increased by 10–20 µM AEA in the presence of *P. gingivalis* LPS (1 µg/ml). In the absence of *P. gingivalis* LPS, AEA and 2-AG did not exhibit any significant effect on the expression of IL-8 and MCP-1 expression in hPdLCs, whereas IL-6 expression was slightly enhanced by 10 µM 2-AG and not affected by AEA. In *P.gingivalis* LPS stimulated hPdLCs, 10 µM AEA down-regulated gene-expression and protein production of IL-6, IL-8, and MCP-1. In contrast, 10 µM 2-AG had an opposite effect and induced a significant up-regulation of gene and protein expression of IL-6 and IL-8 (P<0.05) as well as gene-expression of MCP-1 in *P. gingivalis* LPS stimulated hPdLCs. Our data suggest that AEA appears to have an anti-inflammatory and immune suppressive effect on hPdLCs' host response to *P.gingivalis* LPS, whereas 2-AG appears to promote detrimental inflammatory processes. In conclusion, AEA and 2-AG might play an important role in the modulation of periodontal inflammation.

Editor: Rajesh Mohanraj, Faculty of Medicine & Health Sciences, United Arab Emirates

Funding: This work was supported by the authors' institution, Bernhard Gottlieb School of Dentistry, Medical University of Vienna and by Ministry of Science and Technology of China under contract International Science & Technology Cooperation Program foundation (Nr. 1019). The funders had no role in study design, data collection and analysis, decision to publish or preparation of the manuscript.

Competing Interests: The authors have declared that no competing interests exist.

* Email: cburcu@gazi.edu.tr (BO); oleh.andrukhov@meduniwien.ac.at (OA)

Introduction

Endocannabinoid receptor ligands, also known as endocannabinoids are an emerging class of arachidonic acid derivates that activate cannabinoid receptors [1]. Expressions of major cannabinoid receptors, CB1 and CB2, have been documented in various immune cells and tissues [2,3]. Anandamide (AEA) and 2-arachidonoylglycerol (2-AG) are major endocannabinoids, which behave as partial and full agonists at CB1 and CB2 receptors, respectively [1]. Endocannabinoids are known to be produced by various cell types, including endothelial cells, osteoblasts and osteoclasts [4–6].

The endocannabinoid (EC) system is strongly associated with an infection- or inflammation-related immune response [2,3,7]. Endocannabinoids are reported to modulate the proliferation and apoptosis of T- and B-lymphocytes, inflammatory cytokine production, and immune cell activation and migration [2,8,9]. The accumulating data on the EC system's regulation of the immune response also identifies the EC system as a new therapeutic target for many diseases [2,3,7].

Periodontitis is a chronic inflammatory processes that occur in the periodontium in response to bacterial accumulations (dental plaque) on the teeth [10]. In periodontitis, tissue destruction is a result of an excessive inflammatory response, caused by the interaction of periodontal pathogenic bacteria with the host [11]. One of the major periodontal pathogens is *Porphyromonas gingivalis* (*P. gingivalis*), which belongs to the red complex group of bacteria [12]. Since the EC system is recognized to modulate immune response, an association between the EC system and periodontal inflammation is possible, but remains largely unknown.

To date, only limited number of studies have been examined the association between periodontal disease and the EC system [13–18]. Anandamide (AEA) and 2-arachidonoylglycerol (2-AG) were detected in the gingival crevicular fluid (GCF) of periodontitis patients [13], but not in periodontally healthy individuals [14]. Moreover, AEA levels appeared to decrease significantly in periodontitis patients after periodontal surgery, whereas 2-AG levels remained virtually unchanged [13]. *In vitro* studies show that AEA reduces the production of pro-inflammatory mediators induced by *P. gingivalis* lipopolysaccharide (LPS) in human gingival fibroblasts [14] and promotes the proliferation of these cells [13]. Animal studies have shown that AEA and its synthetic analog methanandamide diminish the inflammatory response in experimentally induced periodontitis [16,17]. However, the exact role of endocannabinoid system in pathogenesis of periodontal disease remains largely unknown.

Human periodontal ligament cells (hPdLCs) are one of the essential elements for the homeostasis of the periodontal ligament, connecting the cementum to the alveolar bone. Along with various other cell types of periodontium, hPdLCs may be involved in the host response to periodontitis [19]. hPdLCs respond to *P. gingivalis* or its components by initiating an inflammatory response, including the expression and production of proinflammatory cytokines and chemokines, as shown both at the mRNA and protein levels [20–22]. hPdLC model stimulated with *P. gingivalis* LPS is widely used for simulating the *in vivo* conditions such as those found in diseased periodontal sites [18,23]. The CB2 receptor is expressed in hPdLCs and its specific agonist is shown to attenuate inflammatory response to LPS [18]. However, it is not known how endocannabinoids AEA and 2-AG might influence the response of hPdLCs to periodontal pathogens.

In the present study, in order to determine the impact of AEA and 2-AG on the host response of human primary hPdLCs, the production of pro-inflammatory mediators, such as interleukin (IL)-6, IL-8, and MCP-1 in hPdLCs in response to stimulation with *P. gingivalis* LPS was examined.

Materials and Methods

Ethic Statement

Protocol for primary human periodontal ligament cells isolation was approved by the Ethics Committee of the Medical University of Vienna. Patients were informed in details before the surgical procedures and gave their written agreement.

Cell Culture and Reagents

The hPdLCs were isolated from erupted third molars extracted from three healthy donors as described previously [24]. In addition, primary commercially available human periodontal ligament cells (Lonza, Switzerland) were used. None of the donors were smokers. hPdLCs were cultured in Dulbecco's modified Eagle's medium (DMEM, Gibco, Invitrogen, Wien, Austria) supplemented with fetal bovine serum (FBS, 10%), 50 µg/mL streptomycin, and 100 U/mL penicillin at 37°C under humidified atmosphere of 5% CO_2 and 95% air. The hPdLCs from the third to fifth passages in culture were used.

Ultrapure LPS from *P. gingivalis* (Invivogen, California, USA) and single lots of AEA and 2-AG (both, Sigma-Aldrich Co, St. Louis, MO, USA) were used in the study. The AEA oil form was dissolved in 96% ethanol to a concentration of 10 mM. This stock solution was further diluted in 1% FCS containing DMEM to AEA concentrations of 0.1 to 20 µM. Therefore, the working solution with 20 µM AEA contained 0.192% ethanol. No effect of ethanol at this concentration on any parameters investigated was

found. The 2-AG acetonitrile form stock solution was further diluted in 1% fetal calf serum (FCS) containing DMEM to 2-AG concentrations of 0.1 to 20 µM.

Cell proliferation/viability

Cells were seeded in 48-well microplates (TPP, Trasadingen, Switzerland) at the density of 2×10^4 cells in 300 µL of DMEM supplemented with 1% FCS with different amounts of AEA and 2-AG in the presence or absence of *P. gingivalis* LPS (1 µg/ml) and incubated for 24 h. After incubation 50 µl of 3,4,5-dimethylthiazol-2-yl-2,5-diphenyl tetrazolium bromide (MTT) reagent (5 mg/ml) (Sigma-Aldrich Co, St. Louis, MO, USA) were added to each well and cells were additionally incubated at 37°C for 2 hours. Subsequently, the media were discarded and 300 µL dimethylsulfoxide was added to each well, followed by 5 min incubation on a shaker. The absorbance was measured at 570 nm using a microplate reader (Molecular Devices, Sunnyvale, CA, USA).

Measurements of cytokine production by hPdLCs

hPdLCs were seeded in 24-well plates at a density of 5×10^4 cells/well in 500 µl of DMEM supplemented with 10% FCS. After 24 hours, the media were replaced by DMEM supplemented with 1% FBS and the hPdLCs were incubated by AEA/2-AG (1–10 µM) and/or *P. gingivalis* LPS (1 µg/ml). After 24 h incubation, the gene expression levels of IL-6, IL-8, and MCP-1 in the hPdLCs and the content of the corresponding protein in conditioned media were determined by qPCR and ELISA, respectively.

The mRNA expression levels of pro-inflammatory mediators were determined as described in previous studies [25,26]. Isolation of mRNA and transcription into cDNA was performed using the TaqMan Gene Expression Cells-to-CT[TM] kit (Ambion/Applied Biosystems, Foster City, CA, USA) according to the manufacturer's instructions. qPCR was performed on an ABI StepOnePlus device (Applied Biosystems, Foster City, CA, USA) in paired reactions using the TaqMan gene expression assays (Applied Biosystems, Foster City, CA, USA) with the following ID numbers: IL-6, Hs00985639_m1; IL-8, Hs00174103_m1; MCP-1, Hs00234140_m1; β-actin, Hs99999903_m1. qPCR reactions were performed in triplicate in 96-well plates using the following thermocycling conditions: 95°C for 10 min; 40 cycles, each for 15 s at 95°C and at 60°C for 1 min. The point at which the PCR product was first detected above a fixed threshold (cycle threshold, C_t), was determined for each sample. Changes in the expression of target genes were calculated using the $2^{-\Delta\Delta Ct}$ method, where $\Delta\Delta C_t = (C_t^{target} - C_t^{\beta\text{-actin}})_{sample} - (C_t^{target} - C_t^{\beta\text{-actin}})_{control}$, taking an untreated sample as a control.

Commercially available ELISA kits (Hoelzel Diagnostika, Cologne, Germany) were used for measurements of IL-6, IL-8, and MCP-1 levels in the conditioned medium. For measurement of IL-6 samples were not diluted, whereas for measurements of IL-8 and MCP-1 samples were diluted 1:10 and 1:5, respectively.

Statistical analysis

After confirming normal distribution with the Kolmogorov-Smirnov test, the statistical differences between different groups were analysed by one-way analysis of variance (ANOVA) for repeated measures followed LSD post-hoc test. All statistical analysis was performed using the statistical program SPSS 19.0 (SPSS, Chicago, IL, USA). Data are expressed as mean ± s.e.m. Differences were considered to be statistically significant at p< 0.05.

Results

Effect of Endocannabinoids on Proliferation/Viability of hPdLCs

The influence AEA and 2-AG in the concentrations of 0.1–20 µM on the proliferation/viability of hPdLCs after 24 hours of treatment is shown on the Figure 1. Neither AEA nor 2-AG exhibited significant effect on the proliferation/viability of hPDLC in the absence of *P. gingivalis* LPS. AEA in concentration of 10–20 µM induced a significant increase of hPdLCs proliferation/viability in the presence of *P. gingivalis* LPS (1 µg/ml). No effect of 2-AG on the proliferation/viability of hPDLCs in the presense of *P. gingivalis* LPS was observed.

Effect of Endocannabinoids on Gene Expression of Pro-Inflammatory Mediators of HPdLCs

The effects of AEA and 2-AG on gene-expression levels of IL-6, IL-8, and MCP-1 in hPdLCs are summarized in Figure 2. Treatment of hPdLCs with AEA in concentration of 1–10 µM did not result in any significant effect on the gene expression levels of IL-6, IL-8, and MCP-1. Similarly, treatment of hPdLCs with 2-AG in concentration of 1–10 µM din not exhibit any significant effect on the gene expression levels of IL-8 and MCP-1. Treatment of hPdLCs with 10 µM 2-AG resulted in a significant increase of IL-6 gene expression level, whereas no significant changes were observed after treatment with 1 µM 2-AG.

Effect of AEA on pro-inflammatory mediators levels in hPdLCs stimulated by *P. gingivalis* LPS

In next series of experiments, we investigated the effect of AEA on the hPdLCs response to *P. gingivalis* LPS. *P. gingivalis* LPS induced a significant increase of the expression of IL-6, IL-8, and MCP-1 on both gene and protein levels (p<0.05). 10 µM AEA induced a significant decrease of *P. gingivalis* LPS stimulated IL-6, IL-8 and MCP-1 gene expression levels (Fig. 3A, p<0.05). In agreement with qPCR data, 10 µM AEA induced a significant decrease in the content of IL-6, IL-8, and MCP-1 in the conditioned media (Fig. 3B, p<0.05). AEA in concentration 1 µM had no significant effect on the response of hPdLCs to *P. gingivalis* LPS.

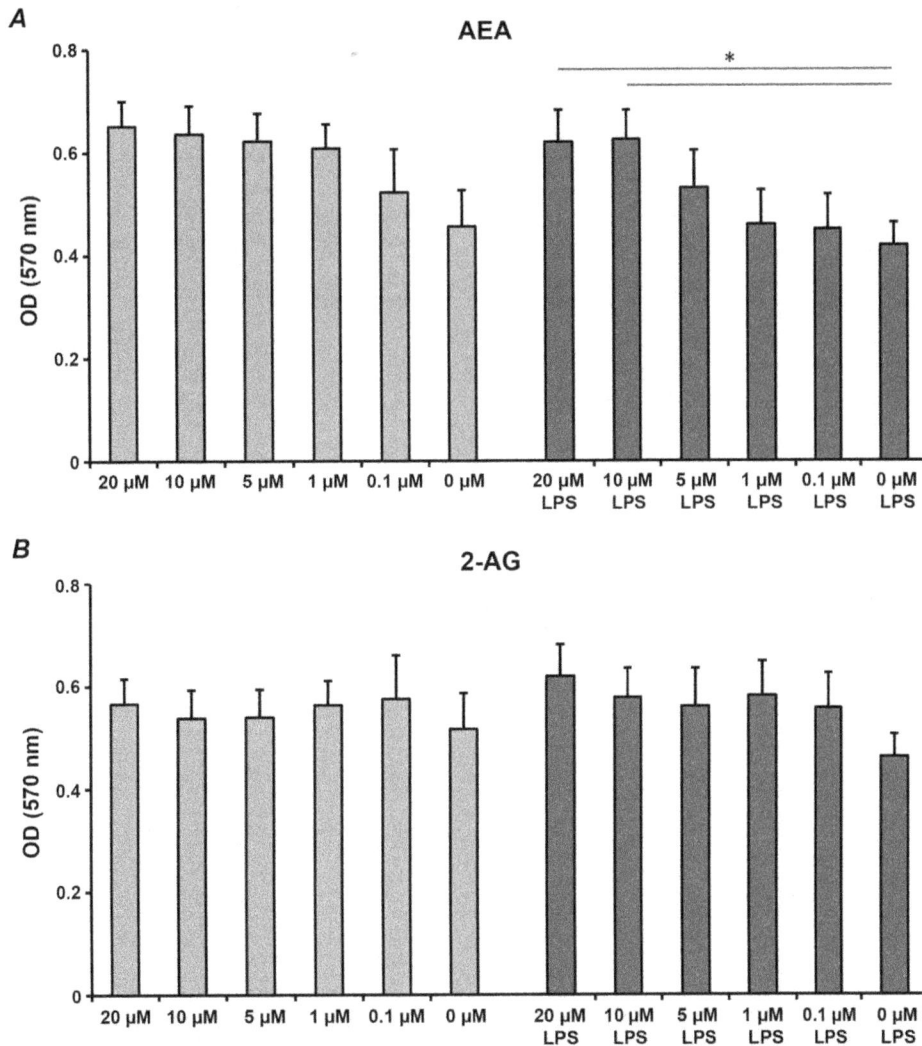

Figure 1. The effects of endocannabinoids on proliferation/viability of hPdLCs. hPdLCs were stimulated by different concentrations of AEA (A) or 2-AG (B) in the presence or in the absence of *P. gingivalis* LPS (1 µg/ml) for 24 h and the proliferation/viability was measured by the MTT method. Cells stimulated with DMEM supplemented by 1% FCS were used as a control (Co). The Y-axis represents mean ± s.e.m. of optical densities measured at 570 nm in 4 independent experiments. *Means were significantly different between groups (P<0.05).

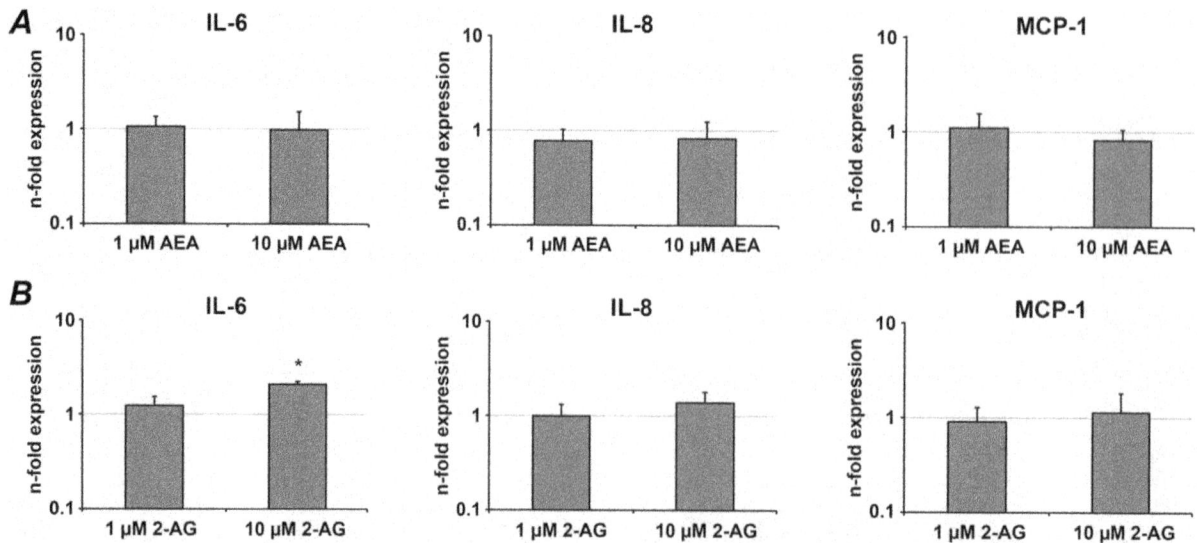

Figure 2. The effect of endocannabinoids on the expression of pro-inflammatory mediators in hPdLCs. hPdLCs were stimulated with AEA (A) or 2-AG (B) and the expression of pro-inflammatory mediators IL-6, IL-8, and MCP-1 was measured by real-time PCR. Changes in gene expression were calculated by $2^{-\Delta\Delta Ct}$ method, taking non-stimulated cells as a reference ($2^{-\Delta\Delta Ct} = 1$) and β-actin as a house-keeping gene. Each value represents the mean ± s.e.m of 4 independent experiments. *Means were significantly compared to the control group and tested with analysis of variance (P<0.05).

Effect of 2-AG on pro-inflammatory mediators levels in hPdLCs stimulated by *P. gingivalis* LPS

In last series of experiments, we investigated the effect of 2-AG on *P. gingivalis* LPS induced response in hPdLCs. 10 μM 2-AG induced a significant increase of *P. gingivalis* LPS stimulated IL-6, IL-8 and MCP-1 gene expression levels (Fig. 4A, p<0.05), whereas no significant effect of 1 μM 2-AG was observed. Measurements of proteins content in the conditioned media showed that the *P. gingivalis* LPS stimulated IL-6 and IL-8

production by hPdLCs were significantly increased by 1–10 μM 2-AG in a concentration-dependent manner (Fig. 4B, p<0.05). In contrast, no significant effect of 2-AG on *P.gingivalis* LPS induced MCP-1 production by hPdLCs was observed (Fig. 4B, p>0.09).

Discussion

To our knowledge, this study is the first to evaluate the effects of the endocannabinoids AEA and 2-AG on the production of pro-inflammatory by hPdLCs. In particular, we investigated the effect

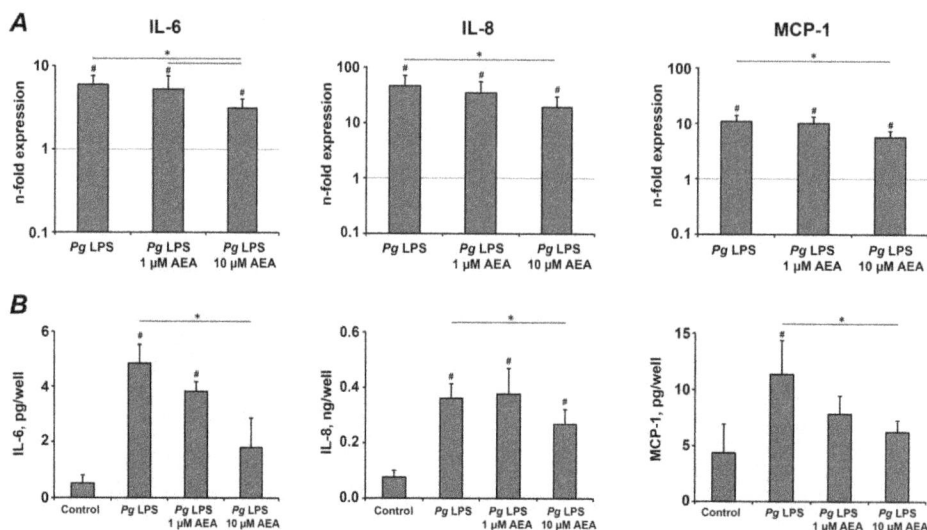

Figure 3. The effect of AEA on the production of pro-inflammatory mediators in hPdLCs in response to stimulation with *P. gingivalis* LPS. hPdLC were stimulated with *P. gingivalis* LPS in the presence or in the absence of AEA for 24 h, and the production of pro-inflammatory mediators was measured on gene and protein levels by real-time PCR (A) and ELISA (B) respectively. A – Changes in the gene expression levels of IL-6, IL-8, and MCP-1 calculated by $2^{-\Delta\Delta Ct}$ method taking non-stimulated cells as a reference ($2^{-\Delta\Delta Ct} = 1$) and β-actin as a house-keeping gene. B – Content of pro-inflammatory mediators in the conditioned media measured by ELISA. Each value represents the mean ± s.e.m of 4 independent experiments. #Means were significantly compared to the control group, and tested with analysis of variance (P<0.05). *Means were significantly different between groups, tested with analysis of variance (P<0.05).

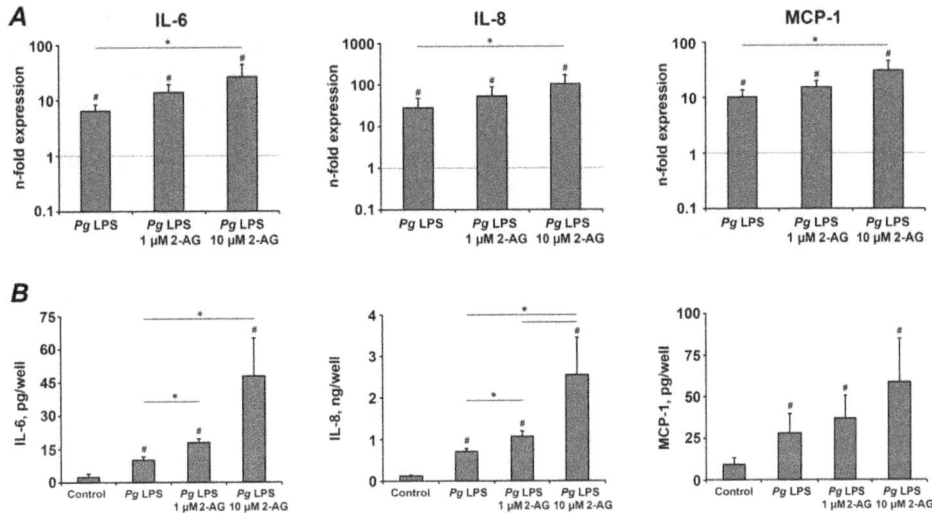

Figure 4. The effect of 2-AG on the production of pro-inflammatory mediators in hPdLCs in response to stimulation with *P. gingivalis* LPS. hPdLC were stimulated with *P. gingivalis* LPS in the presence or in the absence of 2-AG for 24 h and the production of pro-inflammatory mediators was measured on gene and protein levels by real-time PCR (A) and ELISA (B) respectively. A – Changes in the gene expression levels of IL-6, IL-8, and MCP-1 calculated by $2^{-\Delta\Delta Ct}$ method taking non-stimulated cells as a reference ($2^{-\Delta\Delta Ct} = 1$) and β-actin as a house-keeping gene. B – Content of pro-inflammatory mediators in the conditioned media measured by ELISA. Each value represents the mean ± s.e.m of 4 independent experiments. #Means were significantly compared to control group, tested with analysis of variance (P<0.05). *Means were significantly different between groups, tested with analysis of variance (P<0.05).

of endocannabinoids on proliferation/viability as well as on the production of IL-6, IL-8, and MCP-1 by hPdLCs. IL-6 is a multifunctional pro-inflammatory cytokine that plays a significant role in inflammation and also stimulates osteoclastogenesis and bone destruction in chronic inflammatory diseases such as periodontitis [27]. One of the most important chemotactic factors for polymorphonuclear leukocytes (PMNLs) is IL-8 [28], which is also produced by hPdLCs, and its levels have been shown to increase in the presence of *P. gingivalis* LPS [29]. MCP-1 chemokine is a chemo-attractant for macrophages and their precursors, monocytes, and a small subset of lymphocytes [30]. Earlier, GCF MCP-1 levels were associated with periodontitis [31].

AEA and 2-AG are reported to have different effects on the proliferation/viability of different cell types [13,14,32]. In the present study we used MTT assay, which detects the activity of the mitochondria respiratory chain and is considered as a measure for proliferation of viable cells [33]. Our current data suggests that AEA or 2-AG in concentrations of up to 20 μM did not have significant effects on the proliferation/viability of hPdLCs in the absence of *P. gingivalis* LPS (Fig. 1). However, in the presence of *P. gingivalis* LPS AEA induced a significant increase in hPdLCs proliferation viability. This increase could be associated with activation of CB1 and CB2 receptors. Previous study on human gingival fibroblasts show that AEA as well as specific agomists of CB1 and CB2 receptors induce an increase in cell proliferation [13]. Another study shows that *P. gingivalis* LPS at high concentrations (10 μg/ml) stimulates proliferation of hPdLCs [34]. In our study we used *P. gingivalis* LPS in lower concentration (1 μg/ml) but it can be assumed that the increase in proliferation/viability might be due to cumulative effect of LPS and AEA.

Our results revealed that AEA has suppressive effects on the pro-inflammatory mediators production triggered by *P. gingivalis* LPS. 10 μM AEA significantly reduced the gene-expression levels of all investigated pro-inflammatory mediators, as well as their

levels in conditioned media. A similar effect of AEA on the inflammatory response is also found in other cell types. Particularly, the production of IL-6, IL-8, and MCP-1 is shown to be significantly reduced by 10 μM AEA in *P. gingivalis* LPS stimulated human gingival fibroblasts [14]. The production of IL-6 by murine macrophages in response to *Escherichia coli* LPS stimulation is shown to be significantly reduced by 10–30 μM AEA [35]. The effect of AEA on the production of pro-inflammatory mediators is concentration-dependent: 1 μM AEA did not exhibit any significant effect on the response of hPdLCs to *P. gingivalis* LPS stimulation. This finding is in agreement with a previous study reporting no significant effects of 1 μM AEA on MCP-1 production of HL-60 cells with or without stimulation by *E. coli* LPS [36].

2-AG stimulation induced an increase of the *P. gingivalis* LPS stimulated production of pro-inflammatory mediator by hPdLCs. 10 μM 2-AG caused a significant increase of IL-6 and IL-8 gene expression levels and protein release by hPdLCs. Moreover, the content of IL-6 and IL-8 in hPdLCs conditioned media were also increased also by 1 μM 2-AG. The gene-expression levels of MCP-1 after stimulation with *P. gingivalis* were significantly increased in the presence of 10 μM 2-AG but no significant differences was observed on protein level. The differences between qPCR and ELISA experiments observed in our study could be due to the fact that qPCR measurements reflect gene expression levels exactly after 24 h treatment, whereas amount of protein in conditioned media reflect accumulation during whole treatment period. Studies on other cells controversially describe the effect of 2-AG on inflammatory response. Stimulation of human promyelocytic leukemia cells with 1 μM 2-AG alone or together with 100 ng/ml of *E. coli* LPS were reported to increase IL-8 and MCP-1 levels significantly [36]. Contrariwise, 3–30 μM 2-AG was reported to inhibit LPS induced IL-6 production in murine J774 macrophages in a concentration-dependent manner [35].

Present data revealed that AEA has no substantial influence on the expression of pro-inflammatory mediators in the absence of *P.*

gingivalis LPS stimulation. We also did not find any significant effect of 2-AG on the expression of IL-8 and MCP-1 in hPdLCs without *P. gingivalis* LPS stimulation. In contrast, 2-AG itself induced a significant increase of IL-6 gene expression in hPdLCs. However, this effect was rather small compared to that of *P. gingivalis* LPS response itself and to the 2-AG induced augmentation of the *P. gingivalis* response. These observations suggest that endocannabinoids are probably not able to induce pro-inflammatory response themselves, but rather affect some pro-inflammatory signalling pathways in hPdLCs and modulate inflammatory response of these cells.

Cytokine production by hPdLCs upon LPS stimulation is thought to play an important role in the progression of periodontal disease. In our experiments, stimulation of hPdLCs with *P. gingivalis* LPS resulted in the increase of IL-6, IL-8, and MCP-1 expression. However, some quantitative differences in the production of pro-inflammatory mediators upon *P. gingivalis* LPS treatment were observed (see, Figure 3 and 4). There are several reasons, which can underlie these differences. First, hPdLC in culture are supposed to consist of several subpopulations [19]. Second, large inter-individual heterogeneity in hPdLCs response to *P. gingivalis* exists [21]. Third, properties of hPdLCs might be changed with passaging [37]. Nevertheless, it is unlikely that these quantitative differences in hPdLCs response to *P. gingivalis* LPS might influence the conclusion of our study on the effect of AEA and 2-AG on IL-6, IL-8, and MCP-1.

So far not much clinical data has been published about endocannabinoids in periodontology. AEA and 2-AG were detected in the GCF of periodontitis patients [13,14]. Kozono et al. examined the role of the EC system in periodontal wound healing by GCF analysis of patients with periodontitis before and after periodontal surgery, and demonstrated that AEA levels significantly increased 3 days after periodontal surgery in GCF, whereas 2-AG levels did not change significantly [13]. Our present results suggest that both endocannabinoids AEA and 2-AG have significant effects on the regulation of host response from hPdLCs triggered by *P. gingivalis* LPS. While neither endocannabinoid had an important effect on cell proliferation/viability of hPdLCs, it was interesting to see that they seemed to have opposite effects on IL-6, IL-8 and MCP-1 levels of *P. gingivalis* LPS induced hPdLCs. Immune response in periodontitis is aimed to destroy and eliminate periodontal pathogen, but excessive response leads to host tissue destruction [38]. Regulation of cytokine production by endocannabinoids might play an important role in the balancing between bacterial clearance and tissue destruction in periodontal disease. Our data reveals that AEA may have an anti-inflamma-

tory and immune suppressive effect on host defense of *P. gingivalis* LPS induced hPdLCs, whereas 2-AG seems to support inflammatory processes. Regulatory mechanisms beyond these opposite effects on cytokine and chemokine production still remain unknown. Moreover, it has also been stated that stressful or pathological inducements affect the EC system within a certain tissue in more than just one way, and end up with more than just one functional result depending on the nature and duration of this inducement [39].

The reasons why AEA and 2-AG exert opposite effects on LPS-induced production of pro-inflammatory cytokines in hPdLCs are not entirely clear. Both AEA and 2-AG are described as agonists for both CB1 and CB2 receptors [1,40]. However, there are conflicting results about their affinity to these receptors [1]. In addition, AEA but not 2-AG is known to activate transient receptor potential vanilloid type-1 receptor (TRPV1) [41]. Recent study shows that this receptor is expressed in hPdLC and might be activated by AEA [42]. Moreover, ablation of TRPV1 in mice results in exacerbated inflammatory response during endotoxic shock [43], which also suggests the role of this receptor in LPS-induced signaling. Therefore, it could be hypothesized that activation of TRPV1 by AEA can underline reduced inflammatory response of hPdLC upon stimulation with *P. gingivalis* LPS.

The endocannabinoid system is one of the most important signalling systems that has been discovered within the last few decades, and many researchers are currently focused on it for developing new treatment strategies for many disease and pathological conditions [39]. We still assume that, in the near future, regulation of the endocannabinoid system might play a role in the management of periodontal disease. Further studies, clinical as well as experimental, are needed to understand the balance between AEA and 2-AG and their exact roles in periodontal inflammation and regeneration.

Acknowledgments

The authors would like to thank Mrs. Nguyen Phuong Quynh and Mrs. Hedwig Rutschek (both Medical University of Vienna) for excellent technical assistances.

Author Contributions

Conceived and designed the experiments: BÖ XRF OA. Performed the experiments: BÖ OA. Analyzed the data: BÖ BS XRF OA. Contributed reagents/materials/analysis tools: BÖ HPB AM XRF OA. Contributed to the writing of the manuscript: BÖ BS HPB AM XRF OA.

References

1. Kreitzer FR, Stella N (2009) The therapeutic potential of novel cannabinoid receptors. Pharmacol Ther 122: 83–96.
2. Klein TW, Newton C, Larsen K, Lu L, Perkins I, et al. (2003) The cannabinoid system and immune modulation. J Leukoc Biol 74: 486–496.
3. Croxford JL, Yamamura T (2005) Cannabinoids and the immune system: potential for the treatment of inflammatory diseases? J Neuroimmunol 166: 3–18.
4. Bab I, Ofek O, Tam J, Rehnelt J, Zimmer A (2008) Endocannabinoids and the regulation of bone metabolism. J Neuroendocrinol 20 Suppl 1: 69–74.
5. Ridge FL, Cameron GA, Ross RA, Rogers MJ. (2007) Endocannabinoids are produced by bone cells and stimulate bone resorption in vitro. Calcif Tissue Int.
6. Opitz CA, Rimmerman N, Zhang Y, Mead LE, Yoder MC, et al. (2007) Production of the endocannabinoids anandamide and 2-arachidonoylglycerol by endothelial progenitor cells. FEBS Lett 581: 4927–4931.
7. Tanasescu R, Constantinescu CS (2010) Cannabinoids and the immune system: an overview. Immunobiology 215: 588–597.
8. Pandey R, Mousawy K, Nagarkatti M, Nagarkatti P (2009) Endocannabinoids and immune regulation. Pharmacol Res 60: 85–92.

9. Cencioni MT, Chiurchiu V, Catanzaro G, Borsellino G, Bernardi G, et al. (2010) Anandamide suppresses proliferation and cytokine release from primary human T-lymphocytes mainly via CB2 receptors. PLoS One 5: e8688.
10. Loesche WJ, Grossman NS (2001) Periodontal disease as a specific, albeit chronic, infection: diagnosis and treatment. Clin Microbiol Rev 14: 727–752, table of contents.
11. Genco RJ (1992) Host responses in periodontal diseases: current concepts. J Periodontol 63: 338–355.
12. Socransky SS, Haffajee AD, Cugini MA, Smith C, Kent RL, Jr. (1998) Microbial complexes in subgingival plaque. J Clin Periodontol 25: 134–144.
13. Kozono S, Matsuyama T, Biwasa KK, Kawahara K, Nakajima Y, et al. (2010) Involvement of the endocannabinoid system in periodontal healing. Biochem Biophys Res Commun 394: 928–933.
14. Nakajima Y, Furuichi Y, Biswas KK, Hashiguchi T, Kawahara K, et al. (2006) Endocannabinoid, anandamide in gingival tissue regulates the periodontal inflammation through NF-kappaB pathway inhibition. FEBS Lett 580: 613–619.
15. Qian H, Zhao Y, Peng Y, Han C, Li S, et al. (2010) Activation of cannabinoid receptor CB2 regulates osteogenic and osteoclastogenic gene expression in human periodontal ligament cells. J Periodontal Res 45: 504–511.

16. Rettori E, De Laurentiis A, Zorrilla Zubilete M, Rettori V, Elverdin JC (2012) Anti-inflammatory effect of the endocannabinoid anandamide in experimental periodontitis and stress in the rat. Neuroimmunomodulation 19: 293–303.

17. Ossola CA, Surkin PN, Pugnaloni A, Mohn CE, Elverdin JC, et al. (2012) Long-term treatment with methanandamide attenuates LPS-induced periodontitis in rats. Inflamm Res 61: 941–948.

18. Qian H, Yi J, Zhou J, Zhao Y, Li Y, et al. (2013) Activation of cannabinoid receptor CB2 regulates LPS-induced pro-inflammatory cytokine production and osteoclastogenic gene expression in human periodontal ligament cells. Open Journal of Stomatology 3: 44–51.

19. Jonsson D, Nebel D, Bratthall G, Nilsson BO (2011) The human periodontal ligament cell: a fibroblast-like cell acting as an immune cell. J Periodontal Res 46: 153–157.

20. Pathirana RD, O'Brien-Simpson NM, Reynolds EC (2010) Host immune responses to Porphyromonas gingivalis antigens. Periodontol 2000 52: 218–237.

21. Scheres N, Laine ML, de Vries TJ, Everts V, van Winkelhoff AJ (2010) Gingival and periodontal ligament fibroblasts differ in their inflammatory response to viable Porphyromonas gingivalis. J Periodontal Res 45: 262–270.

22. Andrukhov O, Andrukhova O, Hulan U, Tang Y, Bantleon HP, et al. (2014) Both 25-hydroxyvitamin-d3 and 1,25-dihydroxyvitamin-d3 reduces inflammatory response in human periodontal ligament cells. PLoS ONE 9: e90301.

23. Rizzo A, Bevilacqua N, Guida L, Annunziata M, Romano Carratelli C, et al. (2012) Effect of resveratrol and modulation of cytokine production on human periodontal ligament cells. Cytokine 60: 197–204.

24. Andrukhov O, Matejka M, Rausch-Fan X (2010) Effect of cyclosporin A on proliferation and differentiation of human periodontal ligament cells. Acta Odontol Scand 68: 329–334.

25. Andrukhov O, Ertlschweiger S, Moritz A, Bantleon HP, Rausch-Fan X (2013) Different effects of P. gingivalis LPS and E. coli LPS on the expression of interleukin-6 in human gingival fibroblasts. Acta Odontol Scand.

26. An N, Andrukhov O, Tang Y, Falkensammer F, Bantleon HP, et al. (2014) Effect of nicotine and porphyromonas gingivalis lipopolysaccharide on endothelial cells in vitro. PLoS One 9: e96942.

27. Nibali L, Fedele S, D'Aiuto F, Donos N (2012) Interleukin-6 in oral diseases: a review. Oral Dis 18: 236–243.

28. Baggiolini M, Clark-Lewis I (1992) Interleukin-8, a chemotactic and inflammatory cytokine. FEBS Lett 307: 97–101.

29. Morandini AC, Chaves Souza PP, Ramos-Junior ES, Brozoski DT, Sipert CR, et al. (2013) Toll-like receptor 2 knockdown modulates interleukin (IL)-6 and IL-8 but not stromal derived factor-1 (SDF-1/CXCL12) in human periodontal ligament and gingival fibroblasts. J Periodontol 84: 535–544.

30. Graves DT (1999) The potential role of chemokines and inflammatory cytokines in periodontal disease progression. Clin Infect Dis 28: 482–490.

31. Kurtis B, Tuter G, Serdar M, Akdemir P, Uygur C, et al. (2005) Gingival crevicular fluid levels of monocyte chemoattractant protein-1 and tumor necrosis factor-alpha in patients with chronic and aggressive periodontitis. J Periodontol 76: 1849–1855.

32. Czifra G, Szollosi AG, Toth BI, Demaude J, Bouez C, et al. (2012) Endocannabinoids regulate growth and survival of human eccrine sweat gland-derived epithelial cells. J Invest Dermatol 132: 1967–1976.

33. Mosmann T (1983) Rapid colorimetric assay for cellular growth and survival: application to proliferation and cytotoxicity assays. J Immunol Methods 65: 55–63.

34. Jonsson D, Nebel D, Bratthall G, Nilsson BO (2008) LPS-induced MCP-1 and IL-6 production is not reversed by oestrogen in human periodontal ligament cells. Arch Oral Biol 53: 896–902.

35. Chang YH, Lee ST, Lin WW (2001) Effects of cannabinoids on LPS-stimulated inflammatory mediator release from macrophages: involvement of eicosanoids. J Cell Biochem 81: 715–723.

36. Kishimoto S, Kobayashi Y, Oka S, Gokoh M, Waku K, et al. (2004) 2-Arachidonoylglycerol, an endogenous cannabinoid receptor ligand, induces accelerated production of chemokines in HL-60 cells. J Biochem 135: 517–524.

37. Itaya T, Kagami H, Okada K, Yamawaki A, Narita Y, et al. (2009) Characteristic changes of periodontal ligament-derived cells during passage. J Periodontal Res 44: 425–433.

38. Teng YT (2006) Protective and destructive immunity in the periodontium: Part 1–innate and humoral immunity and the periodontium. J Dent Res 85: 198–208.

39. Di Marzo V (2008) Targeting the endocannabinoid system: to enhance or reduce? Nat Rev Drug Discov 7: 438–455.

40. Idris AI, Ralston SH (2010) Cannabinoids and bone: friend or foe? Calcif Tissue Int 87: 285–297.

41. Zygmunt PM, Petersson J, Andersson DA, Chuang H, Sorgard M, et al. (1999) Vanilloid receptors on sensory nerves mediate the vasodilator action of anandamide. Nature 400: 452–457.

42. Sooampon S, Manokawinchoke J, Pavasant P (2013) Transient receptor potential vanilloid-1 regulates osteoprotegerin/RANKL homeostasis in human periodontal ligament cells. J Periodontal Res 48: 22–29.

43. Wang Y, Wang DH (2013) TRPV1 ablation aggravates inflammatory responses and organ damage during endotoxic shock. Clin Vaccine Immunol 20: 1008–1015.

22

Functional Diversity of the Microbial Community in Healthy Subjects and Periodontitis Patients Based on Sole Carbon Source Utilization

Yifei Zhang[1]◑, Yunfei Zheng[2]◑, Jianwei Hu[1], Ning Du[1], Feng Chen[1]*

1 Central Laboratory, School of Stomatology, Peking University, Beijing, P. R. China, **2** Department of Periodontology, School of Stomatology, Peking University, Beijing, P. R. China

Abstract

Chronic periodontitis is one of the most common forms of biofilm-induced diseases. Most of the recent studies were focus on the dental plaque microbial diversity and microbiomes. However, analyzing bacterial diversity at the taxonomic level alone limits deeper comprehension of the ecological relevance of the community. In this study, we compared the metabolic functional diversity of the microbial community in healthy subjects and periodontitis patients in a creative way—to assess the sole carbon source utilization using Biolog assay, which was first applied on oral micro-ecology assessment. Pattern analyses of 95-sole carbon sources catabolism provide a community-level phenotypic profile of the microbial community from different habitats. We found that the microbial community in the periodontitis group had greater metabolic activity compared to the microbial community in the healthy group. Differences in the metabolism of specific carbohydrates (e.g. β-methyl-D-glucoside, stachyose, maltose, D-mannose, β-methyl-D-glucoside and pyruvic acid) were observed between the healthy and periodontitis groups. Subjects from the healthy and periodontitis groups could be well distinguished by cluster and principle component analyses according to the utilization of discriminate carbon sources. Our results indicate significant difference in microbial functional diversity between healthy subjects and periodontitis patients. We also found Biolog technology is effective to further our understanding of community structure as a composite of functional abilities, and it enables the identification of ecologically relevant functional differences among oral microbial communities.

Editor: Michael Glogauer, University of Toronto, Canada

Funding: This work was supported by grants 81300880 and 81200762 from National Natural Science Foundation of China, and by funding from Peking University School of Stomatology (PKUSS20110301). The funders had no role in study design, data collection and analysis, decision to publish, or preparation of the manuscript.

Competing Interests: The authors have declared that no competing interests exist.

* E-mail: moleculecf@gmail.com

◑ These authors contributed equally to this work.

Introduction

Periodontal disease is one of the most common adult diseases, leading to disorders of the supporting structures of the teeth, including the gingivae, periodontal ligaments, and supporting alveolar bone. The accumulation of plaque around the gingival margin triggers gingivitis [1,2]. Once the homeostasis of microbial diversity within the plaque is lost, gingivitis leads to periodontitis [3,4].

Attempts have been made to compare the microbial diversity in patients with periodontitis and healthy subjects [4–7]. Socransky *et al.* (1998) reported that the "orange complex," consisting of Gram-negative, anaerobic species such as *Prevotella intermedia* and *Fusobacterium nucleatum*, was associated with periodontitis, whereas the "red complex," consisting of periodontal pathogens such as *Porphyromonas gingivalis*, *Tannerella forsythia*, and *Treponema denticola*, is detected as the disease worsens [3,8]; Using the Human Oral Microbe Identification Microarray, Colombo *et al.* (2009) detected more species in patients with periodontal disease compared to those without disease.[9]; Using 16S pyrosequencing, Griffen *et al.* (2012) found that community diversity was higher in periodontal disease subjects [10]; Abusleme *et al.* (2013) reported that the shifts in community structure from health to periodontitis are characterized by the emergence of newly dominant taxa without replacement of primary health-associated species [11]. However, these studies merely focused on the taxonomic structure of communities, and thus provided limited insight into the ecological relevance of microbial community structure. Because changes in bacterial types do not necessarily change the function of a community [12], the phenetic status of the microbial community should be considered when the microflora are studied.

Analyses of phenetic characteristics such as microbial metabolism allow for deeper insight into microbial community structure. First, metabolic processes represent a key component in determining the virulence properties of oral pathogens [13,14]. Furthermore, the development of food chains between bacteria and endogenous nutrient metabolism would enhance the diversity of the microflora, which plays a key role in maintaining homeostasis within a microbial community [15]. For example, frequent carbohydrate consumption increases the levels of mutans streptococci and lactobacilli but decreases *Streptococcus sanguinis* levels [16], Aggressive periodontitis appears to be associated with a loss of colonization by *S. sanguinis* [17]. Grenier and Mayrand

(1986) also reported that the nutritional relationships among oral bacteria could explain the mechanisms favoring bacterial succession in periodontal sites [18].

The sole carbon source utilization (SCSU) patterns of microbial samples determined using the Biolog assay (Biolog Inc., Hayward, CA, USA) [19] could be used as a functionally based measure for classifying heterotrophic microbial communities. The Biolog assay for community analysis involves outgrowth of the entire microbiota ecosystem on multiple carbon substrates. Each well contains tetrazolium violet and a minimal amount of proprietary growth media. Color produced from the reduction of tetrazolium violet is used as an indicator of respiration. Commercially available microplates allow for the simultaneous testing of 95 separate carbon sources such that the metabolic response patterns of microbial communities from different habitats can be compared [20–23]. Anderson *et al.* first analyzed the metabolic similarity of experimental dental plaque biofilms [24]. However, the metabolism or activities of the microflora in periodontitis patients and healthy subjects has not been reported.

Here we used Biolog technology to compare the microbial functional diversity between patients with chronic periodontitis and healthy controls to further our knowledge of the ecological basis of periodontal disease.

Materials and Methods

Subjects and sample collection

Plaque samples were collected from 11 patients who had been diagnosed with generalized chronic periodontitis (according to the international Classification of Periodontal Diseases in 1999: more than 30% of sites with a pocket depth >4 mm, inter-proximal attachment loss of >3 mm, bleeding on probing, and radiographic evidence of alveolar bone loss; course >6 weeks) and 12 controls that had been defined as "periodontally healthy" by a licensed periodontist. The following inclusion criteria were used: at least 18 years of age, a minimum of six natural teeth in every quadrant, an absence of other oral diseases such as caries or mucosal disease, and good systemic health. The exclusion criteria were professional periodontal therapy in the 6 months before enrollment, antibiotic use for any purpose within 1 month before entering the study, and smoking. For inclusion in the healthy group, subjects were required to have no clinical signs of inflammation, including redness, swelling, or bleeding on probing, and no pockets with a probing depth >3 mm.

Supragingival and subgingival plaque around the gingival margin was collected 2–3 h after a meal. To avoid salivary contamination, the sample collection sites (≤1 mm above the gingival margin for supragingival plaque collection, and ≤3 mm below the gingival margin for subgingival plaque collection) were isolated with cotton rolls and gently air-dried. Pooled plaque samples were carefully taken from 16 teeth (2 premolars and 2 molars in each quadrant, but not wisdom teeth) of each subject using a scaler and stored in phosphate-buffered saline (PBS; 0.01 M, pH = 7.2–7.4) (Biotop, Huangshang City, China) on ice.

The study protocol was approved by the Institutional Review Board (IRB) of Peking University School and Hospital of Stomatology (Beijing, China) (approval number: PKUSSIRB-2012063). Participants have provided their written informed consent to participate in this study, and the consent procedure was also approved by the IRB of Peking University School and Hospital of Stomatology.

Biolog assays. The collected plaque samples were re-suspended in 11 ml of PBS (0.01 M, pH = 7.2–7.4) and vortexed thoroughly for 60 s. Each plaque suspension was inoculated into

Biolog anaerobic-negative (AN) microplates (Biolog Inc.) at 100 μl per well. The Biolog AN plates contained 95 sole carbon sources and a blank well with water only (Table S1 in File S1). The initial optical densities (ODs) of the plaque suspensions were measured before inoculation.

The plates were incubated in a 5% CO_2 incubator at 37°C for up to 4 days. The OD at 590 nm (OD_{590}) in each well was recorded every 24 h using a Biolog microstation and associated software (Biolog OmniLog version 4.1).

Data analyses

Reactions were interpreted as positive or negative using Biolog OmniLog software. Positive wells found in at least 50% of subjects in the healthy and periodontitis groups were defined as core utilized carbon sources.

The overall metabolic activity for a microbial community in the Biolog plates was expressed as average well color development (AWCD) and calculated as follows:

$$AWCD = \sum_{i=1}^{n} \frac{c_i}{n}$$

Where C is the corrected OD value (obtained by subtracting the OD of the control well from that of each experimental well to correct for the background activity) in each well and n is the number of substrates (n = 95). If the result was negative, the OD would be deemed to be zero. An independent *t*-test was performed on the measurement data to compare the mean differences in AWCD between the periodontal disease group and healthy group over 4 days.

Richness and evenness were determined using the Shannon index [25], while dominance was determined using the Simpson index [26]. To avoid negative values with the Simpson index, the control-corrected OD was multiplied by 1000.

To avoid artificial differences (differences caused by varying initial OD values of the plaque suspensions, rather than by the pattern of carbon source consumption) between the communities, we standardized the corrected OD value as proposed previously [19,27] by dividing each corrected OD value by the AWCD of the plate. Differently exploited carbon sources were measured based on standardized OD values using independent *t*-tests and Pearson's correlation [27] (SPSS Statistics version 17.0).

The relationships between the healthy and periodontitis groups based on discriminative carbon sources were determined using cluster analyses (Cluster 3.0, Java TreeView, version 1.1.3) and principle component analyses (PCAs) (Canoco, version 4.5).

Results

Functional diversity in the healthy and periodontitis groups

The demographic and clinical characteristics of the subjects are described in Table 1. The initial OD value of the inoculum was higher in the periodontitis group compared to the healthy group, which reflects the greater amount of accumulated plaque in the periodontitis group. Compared to the healthy group, the periodontitis group yielded greater metabolic responses. Significant differences in the overall rate of color development (AWCD) between the healthy and periodontitis groups were noted during the linear increase stage of inoculation (i.e., the first 24 h in Fig. 1). The curves then presented an asymptotic nature during later incubation periods. No significant difference was found between

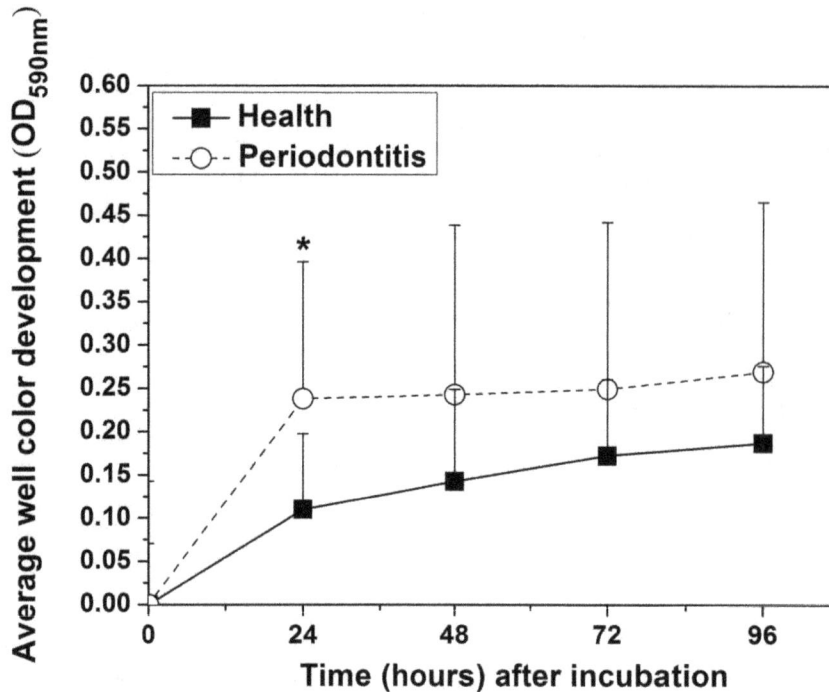

Figure 1. Color development (AWCD) with incubation time in the healthy and periodontitis groups (* indicates a significant difference).

the Shannon indices of diversity between the healthy and periodontitis groups ($p>0.05$, t-test; Table 2). The periodontitis group had a significantly higher Simpson diversity index value than the healthy group at 72 and 96 h after incubation ($p<0.05$, t-test) (Table 2).

Core positive carbon sources utilized by the microbial community in healthy subjects and periodontitis patients

Despite varying intensity levels, a total of 31 carbon sources were positive in most subjects ($\geq 50\%$) in the healthy or periodontitis group after 96 h incubation, which was defined as core positive carbon sources (Fig. 2). Six of these were found in all subjects: D-fructose, maltose, D-raffinose, maltotriose, D-mannose, and sucrose. Another five sources were present in most healthy subjects, whereas the remaining 17 were preferentially associated with periodontitis (Fig. 2). The periodontitis group harbored more core positive carbon sources than the healthy group (Fig. 2).

Table 1. Demographic and clinical characteristics of the subjects.

Parameter	Healthy subjects	Periodontitis patients	p-value
No. of subjects	12	11	
Age (years)	34.6±7.1	34.9±12.5	NS[a]
Missing teeth	None	None	—
Smoker	None	None	—
Women (%)	50	54.5	NS[b]
Percentage of sites with a PD (%):			
>6 mm	0	27.3	
4–6 mm	0	54.5	
<4 mm	100	18.2	
OD$_{630}$ of plaque suspension	0.04±0.028	0.08±0.03	0.003[a]

[a]Independent t-tests
[b]Chi-square tests
NS: not significant
PD: pocket depth
Quantitative data are presented as the mean±standard deviation (SD); categorical data are presented as percentages.

Table 2. Diversity indices of the periodontally healthy and diseased groups during incubation (mean±SD, $p<0.05$).

Index		Healthy subjects	Periodontitis patients	*p*-value
Shannon	24 h	3.98±0.45	4.08±0.23	0.52
	48 h	3.84±0.37	3.95±0.36	0.44
	72 h	3.77±0.35	3.99±0.40	0.16
	96 h	3.81±0.31	3.95±0.32	0.31
Simpson	24 h	47±22	51±12	0.27
	48 h	37±18	47±18	0.10
	72 h	32±13	50±19	**0.025**
	96 h	33±12	45±15	**0.025**

Correlation between healthy status and carbon source utilization patterns

Analyses of 95-sole carbon source utilization patterns showed 14, 8, 11, and 8 significantly different ($p<0.05$) carbon sources between the two groups at 24, 48, 72, and 96 h, respectively (Table S2 in File S1). Of these, five core positive carbon sources

were identified at different time points (Fig. 3): β-methyl-D-glucoside and stachyose were identified at 24 h, maltose and D-mannose were identified at 72 h, and β-methyl-D-glucoside and pyruvic acid at 96 h.

To identify correlations between the pattern of carbon source consumption and healthy status, cluster analyses of 23 subjects from each group were performed based on 14 discriminative carbon sources, which distinguished the healthy group (H) from the diseased group (D) at 24 h (Fig. 4). Our results suggest that the 23 samples could be classified into two groups: 8 of the 12 samples from the healthy group were classified as cluster one, while the 11 samples from the diseased group were classified as cluster two, which coincided with the clinical classification according to the diagnosis. However, certain pairs of samples from different groups were closely associated, such as samples H07 and D04 (Fig. 4). Additionally, the data indicate that some of the samples in the healthy group were similar to those in the diseased group (e.g., H04, H07, H08, and H12) (Fig. 4).

PCAs were performed to identify those carbon sources with key roles in difference between groups at 24 h. We maintained four PCs in the subsequent analysis because they accounted for more than 75% of the total eigenvalue sum (Table 3). Our PCA plots show that PC1 and PC2 accounted for 38.9 and 15% of the total variance, respectively (Fig. 5). Subsequent *t*-tests for the PCs indicated significant differences ($p<0.05$) between the two groups

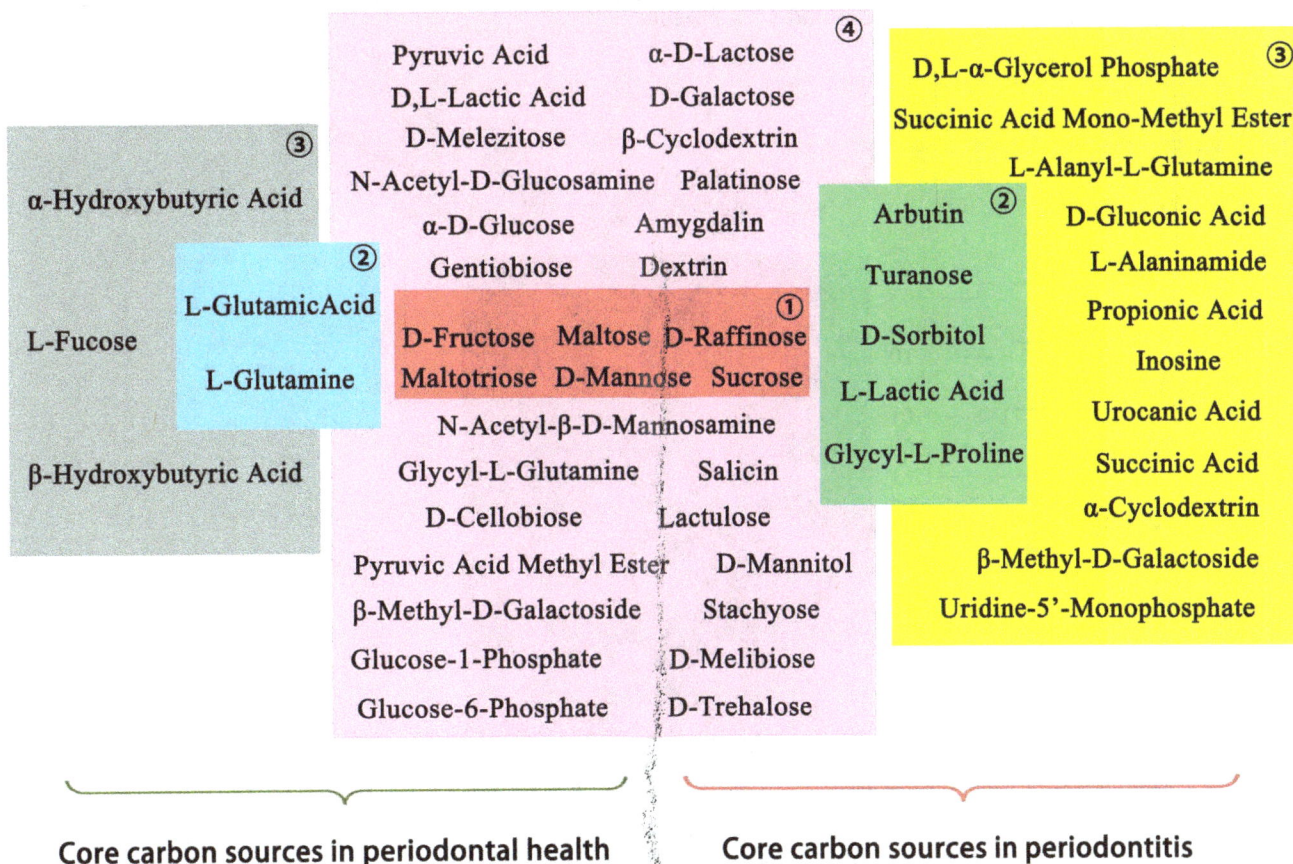

Core carbon sources in periodontal health   Core carbon sources in periodontitis

Figure 2. Core positive carbon sources in the healthy subjects and periodontitis patients. Inner box (numbered with 1), positive carbon sources found in all subjects (100%); middle boxes (numbered with 2), present in 71–99% of subjects from each group (H: healthy, P: periodontitis); outer boxes (numbered with 3), present in 50–70% of subjects from the healthy and periodontitis groups; middle box (numbered with 4), positive carbon sources present in at least 50% of subjects in both the healthy and periodontitis groups.

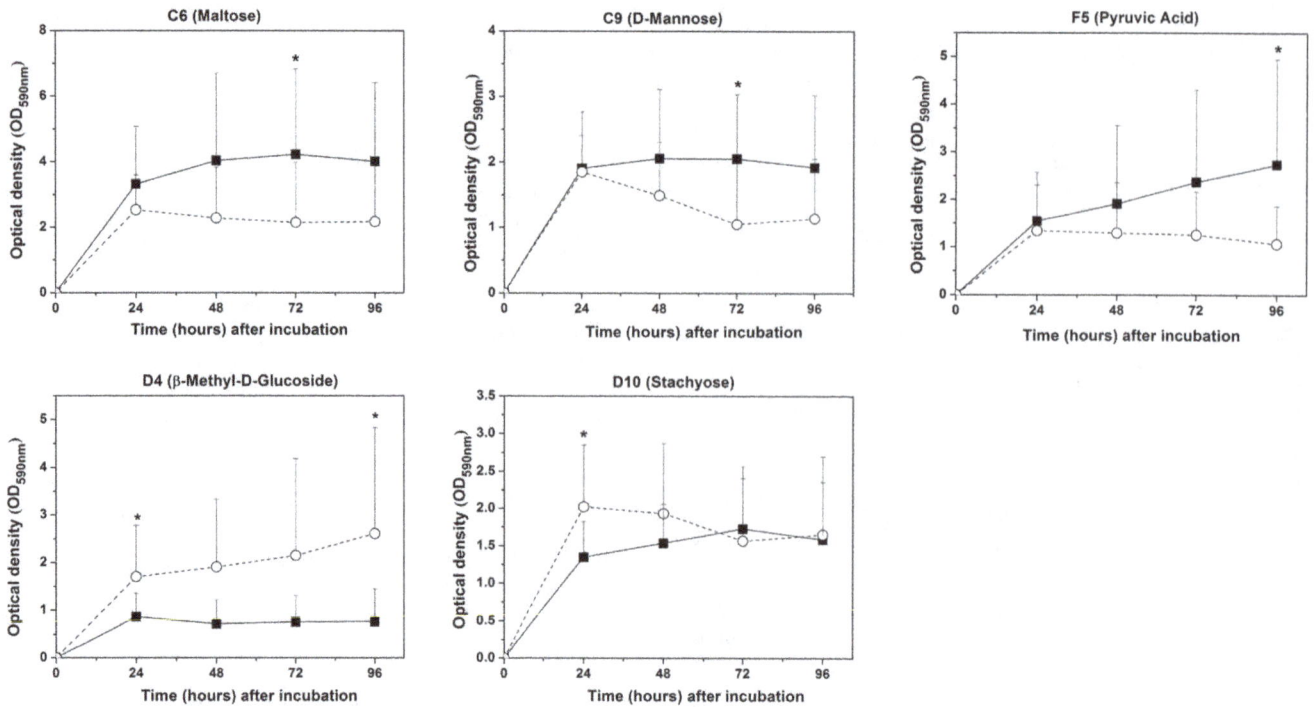

Figure 3. Catabolic kinetics according to inoculation time for discriminative core positive carbon sources (* indicates a significant difference) in the healthy (—■—) and periodontitis (--○--) groups.

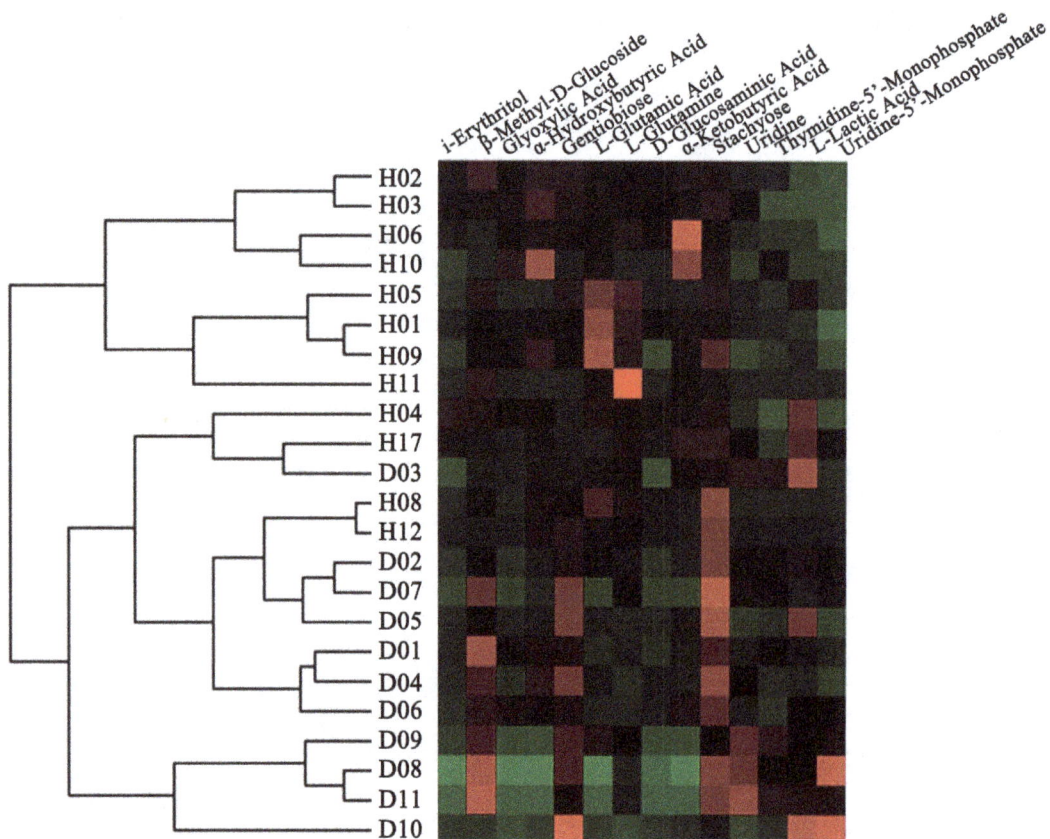

Figure 4. Cluster analyses of 23 clinical plaque samples from healthy (H) and diseased (D) subjects based on standardized OD values of the discriminative carbon sources at 24 h.

on PC1 (Table 3) and identified the carbon sources that best described these differences: E5 (glyoxylic acid), E6 (α-hydroxybutyric acid), E9 (α-ketobutyric acid), and B9 (D-glucosaminic acid) were identified most positively by their PC1 scores, whereas H12 (uridine-5'-monophosphate), H10 (uridine), and H11 (thymidine-5'-monophosphate) were identified most negatively by their PC1 scores (Table 4). The utilization patterns of each microbial community were compared by principal component analysis (PCAs) of the 24 h absorption data. Microbial community samples from different subjects served as objects and the absorbance values of carbon source utilization as variables (Fig.5). It is possible to identify the substrates which contribute to the separation of each sample plot on the ordination biplot (Fig. 5).

Discussion

Plaque around the gingival margin, with its toxic products, stimulates gingival tissue directly and leads to tissue destruction, likely causing periodontal disease [28]. Thus, in this study, we focused on plaque around the gingival margin from patients with periodontitis and orally healthy individuals to determine whether there were functional differences between the two groups. Because many of the anaerobic bacteria isolated from deep subgingival sites are proteolytic and asaccharolytic [28], deeper sampling (>3 mm) would not be optimal because these organisms may not be responsive to the substrates.

Comparisons of overall color development between groups were dependent on both the density and composition of the inoculum: samples with a denser microbial community would produce more effective reactions on the premise that a larger percentage of

Table 3. *t*-tests for PCs extracted from 14 discriminative carbon sources at 24 h (*p*<0.05).

	Healthy subjects	Periodontitis patients	*p*-value
PC1	1.69±1.13	−1.85±1.74	<0.001
PC2	−2.98±1.89	0.33±0.78	0.32
PC3	0.23±0.92	−0.26±1.58	0.38
PC4	0.10±1.03	−0.11±1.43	0.68

microorganisms are able to utilize the substrate. However, in this study, we did not achieve equivalent inoculum densities by dilution or concentration of the samples despite performing functional tests on the original community. The microbial community in the periodontitis patients was more metabolically active than that in the orally healthy individuals, indicating that both the amount and composition of plaque around the gingival margin accounted for the functional diversity. Thus, we confirmed the importance of plaque control in the initial therapy of periodontal disease. In addition, we normalized the raw color response data to the AWCD to account for different inoculum densities.

Analyses of sole carbon source consumption levels indicated differences in the metabolism of specific carbohydrates between the healthy and periodontitis groups. Differences in carbon source utilization are related to the color response in a given well, which is related to the number of microorganisms that are able to utilize the substrate within that well. Increased color development in

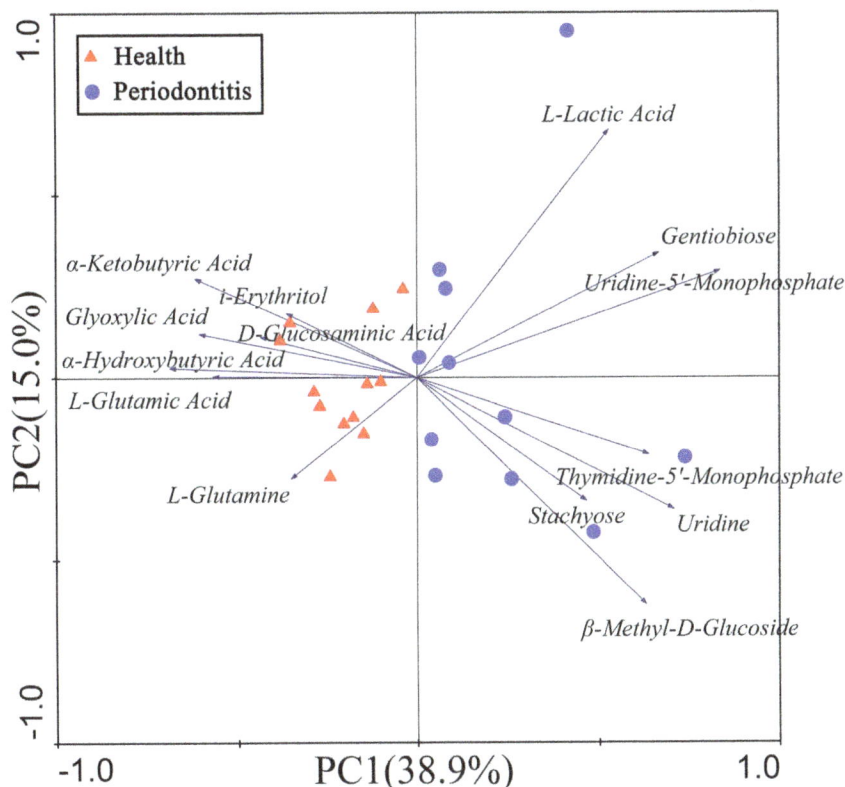

Figure 5. Ordination biplot of principal component analyses of the substrate utilization patterns of the microbial communities in the healthy and periodontitis groups using Biolog AN plate assays. Arrows indicate the directions and relative importance (arrow lengths) of the 14 substrates variables.

Table 4. Substrates with high correlation coefficients ($|r| > 0.6$) for PC1 in a PCA of substrate utilization patterns among microbial communities from periodontally healthy and diseased groups.

	r	*p*-value
E5 (Glyoxylic acid)	0.78	<0.001
E6 (α-Hydroxybutyric acid)	0.76	<0.001
E9 (α-Ketobutyric acid)	0.73	<0.001
H12 (Uridine-5′-monophosphate)	−0.72	<0.001
B9 (D-Glucosaminic acid)	0.66	0.001
H10 (Uridine)	−0.65	0.001
H11 (Thymidine-5′-monophosphate)	−0.64	0.001

certain response wells suggests that the inoculum contained a larger number of microorganisms able to utilize the substrate. The lag phase in color development in a single well (Fig. 2) indicates that a longer period of growth would produce a sufficient density of stained cells; a smaller percentage of microorganisms in the inoculum able to utilize the substrate may be reflected at later incubations times. This could explain the variety of discriminating sole carbon sources at different incubation times (Table S2 in File S1). Moreover, the patterns are a reflection of functional potential rather than *in situ* functional ability because growth plays an important role in this assay.

Cluster analyses were carried out based on the utilization of the discriminative carbon sources at 24 h because the most significant differences in sole carbon source consumption levels were obtained at this phase (linear increase; Fig. 2). In the present study, cluster analyses were used to describe the associations between healthy status and sole carbon source consumption level. Here, we hypothesized that closely associated samples possess similar community-level metabolic functions. This classification further improved the metabolic discrimination of specific carbohydrates between healthy subjects and periodontitis patients, and periodontal health or disease could be distinguished using Biolog AN plates. Furthermore, certain samples in the healthy group were closely associated with those in the disease group. This suggests that the disease-associated metabolic pattern was also found in the healthy subjects. The presence of disease-associated function might be prognostic for future disease in the absence of disease symptoms.

PCA revealed the carbon sources that contributed most to the diversity; it is well established that the biomass and diversity of the microbial community in supragingival and subgingival plaque around the gingival margin are distinguished by the consumption of substrates. In our study, the periodontitis patients resulted in a larger biomass accumulation of the microbial community (indicated by initial OD value) and remarkable changes in its diversity (indicated by AWCD). The close links between the biomass and diversity of the microbial community and the periodontal health status can be reflected by the carbon sources metabolism in plaque samples.

Because oral microbial communities may be dominated by <1000 species-level taxa [10,29], evaluation of the dominant functional characteristics may be more accurate and efficient for classifying and characterizing microbial community structure [9]. Our findings suggest that periodontitis communities result from ecological shifts in community structure [11] as well as shifts in

metabolic function. Despite differences in plaque amounts between the healthy subjects and periodontitis patients, most carbon sources utilized in the periodontitis group were also utilized by the healthy group, albeit at varying sole carbon source consumption levels. However, more carbon sources dominated in the periodontitis group compared to the healthy group. The core microbiome has already been defined in healthy individuals and periodontitis patients [6,11]; nevertheless, it may not be adequate to interpret functional shifts. Different bacterial types would have the same function; for example, both *Streptococcus* spp. and *Neisseria* spp. can utilize sucrose. Conversely, different species in the same genera could have different metabolic functions. *Streptococcus mutans* is able to utilize mannitol but *Streptococcus mitis* cannot. Clearly, the concept of core microbial ecology may be better defined with community function measurements rather than taxonomic structure or membership.

The Shannon index is used extensively in the measurement of taxonomic diversity and community structure [30]. However, using the Shannon index to characterize functional microbial diversity may be questionable [31]. In this study, richness was defined as the total number of carbon substrates utilized while evenness was defined as the equability of substrate utilization between all utilized substrates [31]. The Biolog carbon substrate richness and evenness did not vary between the healthy subjects and periodontitis patients. Other variables that can affect microbial diversity such as differences in the dominant species may have contributed to the higher Simpson index in the periodontitis group at later incubation stages, which coincided with the higher number of core positive carbon sources in the periodontitis group. Although carbon source utilization profiles are not a direct representation of bacterial growth, the Biolog substrate catabolic responses for the microbial communities exhibited a lag phase (before 24 h, data not shown), an exponential phase, and a stationary phase, similar to bacterial growth curves. This nonlinearity has important implications for the interpretation of the disparate catabolic kinetics patterns of different carbon sources (as depicted in Fig. 2) and the single fixed-time readings of community Biolog responses.

Microbial community in our oral cavity is not constant, and would be easily affected by environmental factors such as temperature, pH value and so on. Thus analyzing the microbial diversity in a fixed-time point would be a misleading in our comprehension. In our study, the changes in community metabolism according to time had been well demonstrated by Biolog assay (indicated by AWCD and Simpson index), reflecting the changes in community structure.

One limitation of Biolog technology is that it cannot detect microorganisms that do not make use of the carbon sources on the Biolog microplate. Additionally, the response to substrate catabolism requires an effective quantity and activity of the microbial community in the tested samples. Nevertheless, Biolog technology was found to be an effective assay to rapidly visualize community structure as a composite of functional abilities or potential, and it enables the identification of ecologically relevant functional differences among oral microbial communities. Our study showed a distinguishing characteristic of carbonate metabolism, which may provide a potential adjuvant method for the diagnosis of periodontitis. More importantly, certain carbohydrates should be avoided in the diet according to your suggestion, which might prevent susceptible individuals from developing periodontitis.

Supporting Information

File S1   Table S1 & S2. Table S1. Carbon-sources pattern of the Biolog AN microplate. Table S2 Discriminative carbon sources between health (H) group and periodontitis group (P) based on standardized OD values ($p<0.05$).

Author Contributions

Conceived and designed the experiments: Y. Zhang FC. Performed the experiments: Y. Zhang Y. Zheng. Analyzed the data: Y. Zhang JH FC. Contributed reagents/materials/analysis tools: Y. Zheng JH ND. Wrote the paper: Y. Zhang. Obtained biospecimen: Y. Zheng.

References

1. Loe H, Theilade E, Jensen SB (1965) Experimental gingivitis in man. J Periodontol 36:177–187.
2. Theilade E, Wright WH, Jensen SB, Loe H (1966) Experimental gingivitis in man. II. A longitudinal clinical and bacteriological investigation. J. Periodont. Res. 1: 1–13.
3. Socransky SS, Haffajee AD, Cugini MA, Smith C, Kent RL Jr (1998) Microbial complexes in subgingival plaque. J Clin Periodontol 25: 134–144.
4. Moore WE, Moore LV (1994) The bacteria of periodontal diseases. Periodontol 2000 5: 66–77.
5. Aas JA, Paster BJ, Stokes LN, Olsen I, Dewhirst FE (2005) Defining the normal bacterial flora of the oral cavity. J Clin Microbiol 43: 5721–5732.
6. Bik EM, Long CD, Armitage GC, Loomer P, Emerson J, et al. (2010) Bacterial diversity in the oral cavity of 10 healthy individuals. Isme Journal 4: 962–974.
7. Zhang S-M, Tian F, Huang Q-F, Zhao Y-F, Guo X-K, et al. (2011) Bacterial diversity of subgingival plaque in 6 healthy Chinese individuals. Exp Ther Med 2: 1023–1029.
8. Socransky SS, Haffajee AD (2005) Periodontal microbial ecology. Periodontol 2000 38: 135–187.
9. Colombo APV, Boches SK, Cotton SL, Goodson JM, Kent R, et al. (2009) Comparisons of Subgingival Microbial Profiles of Refractory Periodontitis, Severe Periodontitis, and Periodontal Health Using the Human Oral Microbe Identification Microarray. J Periodontol 80: 1421–1432.
10. Griffen AL, Beall CJ, Campbell JH, Firestone ND, Kumar PS, et al. (2012) Distinct and complex bacterial profiles in human periodontitis and health revealed by 16S pyrosequencing. Isme Journal 6: 1176–1185.
11. Abusleme L, Dupuy AK, Dutzan N, Silva N, Burleson JA, et al. (2013) The subgingival microbiome in health and periodontitis and its relationship with community biomass and inflammation. Isme Journal 7: 1016–1025.
12. White DC, Findlay RH (1988) Biochemical markers for measurement of predation effects on the biomass, community structure, nutritional status, and metabolic activity of microbial biofilms. Hydrobiologia 159: 119–132.
13. Shah HN, Seddon SV, Gharbia SE (1989) Studies on the virulence properties and metabolism of pleiotropic mutants of Porphyromonas gingivalis (Bacteroides gingivalis) W50. Oral Microbiol Immunol 4: 19–23.
14. Mazumdar V, Snitkin ES, Amar S, Segre D (2009) Metabolic network model of a human oral pathogen. J Bacteriol 191: 74–90.
15. Marsh PD (1994) Microbial ecology of dental plaque and its significance in health and disease. Adv Dent Res 8: 263–271.
16. Minah GE, Solomon ES, Chu K (1985) The association between dietary sucrose consumption and microbial population shifts at six oral sites in man. Arch Oral Biol 30: 397–401.
17. Stingu CS, Eschrich K, Rodloff AC, Schaumann R, Jentsch H (2008) Periodontitis is associated with a loss of colonization by Streptococcus sanguinis. J Med Microbiol 57: 495–499.
18. Grenier D, Mayrand D (1986) Nutritional relationships between oral bacteria. Infect Immun 53: 616–620.
19. Garland JL, Mills AL (1991) Classification and characterization of heterotrophic microbial communities on the basis of patterns of community-level sole-carbon-source utilization. Appl Environ Microbiol 57: 2351–2359.
20. Haack SK, Garchow H, Klug MJ, Forney LJ (1995) Analysis of factors affecting the accuracy, reproducibility, and interpretation of microbial community carbon source utilization patterns. Appl Environ Microbiol 61: 1458–1468.
21. Schutter M, Dick R (2001) Shifts in substrate utilization potential and structure of soil microbial communities in response to carbon substrates. Soil Biol Biochem 33: 1481–1491.
22. Rusznyak A, Vladar P, Molnar P, Reskone MN, Kiss G, et al. (2008) Cultivable bacterial composition and BIOLOG catabolic diversity of biofilm communities developed on Phragmites australis. Aquatic Botany 88: 211–218.
23. Fisk MC, Ruether KF, Yavitt JB (2003) Microbial activity and functional composition among northern peatland ecosystems. Soil Biol Biochem 35: 591–602.
24. Anderson SA, Sissons CH, Coleman MJ, Wong L (2002) Application of carbon source utilization patterns to measure the metabolic similarity of complex dental plaque biofilm microcosms. Appl. Environ. Microbiol. 68: 5779–5783.
25. Staddon WJ, Duchesne LC, Trevors JT (1997) Microbial diversity and community structure of postdisturbance forest soils as determined by sole-carbon-source utilization patterns. Microbial Ecology 34: 125–130.
26. Kuhn I, Austin B, Austin DA, Blanch AR, Grimont PAD, et al. (1996) Diversity of Vibrio anguillarum isolates from different geographical and biological habitats, determined by the use of a combination of eight different typing methods. Syst Appl Microbiol 19: 442–450.
27. Glimm E, Heuer H, Engelen B, Smalla K, Backhaus H (1997) Statistical comparisons of community catabolic profiles. J Microbiol Methods 30: 71–80.
28. Marsh PD, Martin MV (2009) Oral Microbiology. United Kingdom: Elsevier. 63 p.
29. Dewhirst FE, Chen T, Izard J, Paster BJ, Tanner ACR, et al. (2010) The Human Oral Microbiome. J Bacteriol 192: 5002–5017.
30. Krebs CJ (1994) Ecology: The Experimental Analysis of Distribution and Abundance. New York: Harper Collins College Publishers. 514p.
31. Derry AM, Staddon WJ, Trevors JT (1998) Functional diversity and community structure of microorganisms in uncontaminated and creosote-contaminated soils as determined by sole-carbon-source-utilization. World J Microbiol Biotechnol 14: 571–578.

23

Involvement of Trigeminal Transition Zone and Laminated Subnucleus Caudalis in Masseter Muscle Hypersensitivity Associated with Tooth Inflammation

Kohei Shimizu[1,3]*, Kunihito Matsumoto[2,3], Noboru Noma[4,5], Shingo Matsuura[1], Kinuyo Ohara[1], Hiroki Komiya[1], Tetsuro Watase[1], Bunnai Ogiso[1,3], Yoshiyuki Tsuboi[6,7], Masamichi Shinoda[6,7], Keisuke Hatori[1,3], Yuka Nakaya[4], Koichi Iwata[6,7,8]

1 Department of Endodontics, Nihon University School of Dentistry, Tokyo, Japan, **2** Department of Radiology, Nihon University School of Dentistry, Tokyo, Japan, **3** Divisions of Advanced Dental Treatment, Dental Research Center, Nihon University School of Dentistry, Tokyo, Japan, **4** Department of Oral Diagnosis, Nihon University School of Dentistry, Tokyo, Japan, **5** Divisions of Clinical Research, Dental Research Center, Nihon University School of Dentistry, Tokyo, Japan, **6** Department of Physiology, Nihon University School of Dentistry, Tokyo, Japan, **7** Division of Functional Morphology, Dental Research Center, Nihon University School of Dentistry, Tokyo, Japan, **8** Division of Applied System Neuroscience Advanced Medical Research Center, Nihon University Graduate School of Medical Science, Tokyo, Japan

Abstract

A rat model of pulpitis/periapical periodontitis was used to study mechanisms underlying extraterritorial enhancement of masseter response associated with tooth inflammation. Periapical bone loss gradually increased and peaked at 6 weeks after complete Freund's adjuvant (CFA) application to the upper molar tooth pulp (M1). On day 3, the number of Fos-immunoreactive (IR) cells was significantly larger in M1 CFA rats compared with M1 vehicle (veh) rats in the trigeminal subnucleus interpolaris/caudalis transition zone (Vi/Vc). The number of Fos-IR cells was significantly larger in M1 CFA and masseter (Mass) capsaicin applied (M1 CFA/Mass cap) rats compared with M1 veh/Mass veh rats in the contralateral Vc and Vi/Vc. The number of phosphorylated extracellular signal-regulated kinase (pERK)-IR cells was significantly larger in M1 CFA/ Mass cap and M1 veh/Mass cap rats compared to Mass-vehicle applied rats with M1 vehicle or CFA in the Vi/Vc. Pulpal CFA application caused significant increase in the number of Fos-IR cells in the Vi/Vc but not Vc on week 6. The number of pERK-IR cells was significantly lager in the rats with capsaicin application to the Mass compared to Mass-vehicle treated rats after pulpal CFA- or vehicle-application. However, capsaicin application to the Mass did not further affect the number of Fos-IR cells in the Vi/Vc in pulpal CFA-applied rats. The digastric electromyographic (d-EMG) activity after Mass-capsaicin application was significantly increased on day 3 and lasted longer at 6 weeks after pulpal CFA application, and these increase and duration were significantly attenuated by i.t. PD98059, a MEK1 inhibitor. These findings suggest that Vi/Vc and Vc neuronal excitation is involved in the facilitation of extraterritorial hyperalgesia for Mass primed with periapical periodontitis or acute pulpal-inflammation. Furthermore, phosphorylation of ERK in the Vi/Vc and Vc play pivotal roles in masseter hyperalgesia after pulpitis or periapical periodontitis.

Editor: Theodore J. Price, University of Texas at Dallas, United States of America

Funding: This study was supported in part by Research grants from Sato and Uemura Funds from Nihon University School of Dentistry, and Grant from Dental Research Center, Nihon University School of Dentistry; Nihon University multidisciplinary research grant and Individual Research Grant; a Grant from the Ministry of Education, Culture, Sports, Science and Technology to promote multi-disciplinary research Projects (KAKENHI (Grant-in-Aid for Young Scientist (B)) # 21791868 and # 23792192 to KS, # 22792021 to MS, KAKENHI (Challenging Exploratory Research) #24659832 to KI); grants from the Ministry of Education, Culture, Sports, Science, Technology to promote multidisciplinary research projects "Brain Mechanisms for Cognition, Memory and Behavior" and "Translational Research Network on Orofacial Neurological Disorders" at Nihon University. The funders had no role in study design, data collection and analysis, decision to publish, or preparation of the manuscript.

Competing Interests: The authors have declared that no competing interests exist.

* Email: shimizu.kouhei01@nihon-u.ac.jp

Introduction

Orofacial persistent pain following trigeminal nerve injury or orofacial inflammation is known to cause various motor as well as sensory disorders in the orofacial regions such as mastication or swallowing dysfunction [1]. Orofacial dysesthesia is known as the secondary hyperalgesia often associated with pulpitis and/or periapical periodontitis [2], suggesting that oral and craniofacial organs are target regions for ectopic pain following intraoral inflammation. Furthermore, it has been reported that the chronic orofacial pain associated with pulpitis and/or periapical peri-odontitis is one of the most frequent referred pain in the orofacial region, and pulpitis or periapical periodontitis is also known to be involved in the referred pain in various intraoral structures [3,4]. Referred pain in non-inflamed orofacial areas associated with pulpitis or periapical periodontitis is often accounted for misdiagnosis or inappropriate clinical treatment. Thus, it is very important to understand the mechanisms underlying orofacial-referred pain associated with pulpitis or periapical periodontitis to develop appropriate diagnosis and treatment of these patients.

The spinal trigeminal subnucleus caudalis (Vc) has been known as a key nucleus to relay tooth pulp afferent inputs to the higher central nervous system, and a large number of nociceptive neurons in the Vc are activated by orofacial noxious stimulation as well as tooth pulp stimulation [5,6]. Electrical stimulation of the tooth pulp produces Fos protein expression in many neurons in the transition zone between the subnucleus interpolaris (Vi) and Vc (Vi/Vc) and the caudal Vc and upper cervical cord [5]. These two areas are thought to play differential roles in processing noxious information from the tooth pulp as well as orofacial skin or muscles [7,8]. It has been reported that Vi/Vc and Vc have a role to process masseter muscle pain [9]. Furthermore, many neurons in these two areas are also known to receive noxious as well as non-noxious inputs from the orofacial regions [7,10]. Therefore, it is highly possible that nociceptive neurons in the Vi/Vc and Vc enhance their firings following pulpitis or periapical periodontitis and play a role in orofacial cutaneous and/or Mass nociception as well as processing tooth pulp or periapical inputs. We hypothesized therefore that Vi/Vc and Vc neurons are involved in masseter muscle hypersensitivity associated with tooth pulp and periapical inflammation.

Extracellular signal-regulated protein kinase (ERK) is a member of mitogen-activated protein kinase family that can be activated by calcium influx within 10 min after noxious stimulation [11]. Phosphorylated ERK-immunoreactive (pERK-IR) cells are known to be distributed in Vc with somatotopic organization, and the number of pERK-IR cells increased in an intensity-dependent manner in the Vc [12]. Previous studies indicated that C-fiber but not A-fiber stimulation accelerates ERK phosphorylation in dorsal root ganglion and spinal dorsal horn (SDH) neurons [13]. These findings indicate that ERK phosphorylation in Vc neurons could be a reliable indicator of neuronal activation following noxious stimulation of the orofacial regions.

Fos-IR cells have been widely used as a marker of neuronal activation in the SDH following noxious stimulation [14]. Fos expression could be detected 0.5–1 hour after noxious stimulation and lasts for 2–3 hours after stimulation. Recently, we have also reported that many pERK-IR cells show Fos-IR in Vc neurons following noxious mechanical stimulation of the periodontal tissues [15], suggesting that ERK phosphorylation is followed by Fos protein expression after noxious stimulation.

To clarify the central mechanisms underlying Mass hypersensitivity associated with pulpitis or periapical periodontitis following CFA application to the tooth pulp, we studied ERK phosphorylation and Fos expression in Vi/Vc and Vc neurons in tooth pulp- or periapical inflamed rats.

Materials and Methods

This study was approved by the Animal Experimentation Committee at the Nihon University (Animal protocol AP10D001). All surgery and animal care were conducted in accordance with the National Institutes of Health Guide for the Care and Use of Laboratory Animals and the guidelines for Institutional Animal Care, and the guidelines of the International Association for the Study of Pain [16]. Male Sprague-Dawley rats (n = 152) weighing 250–450 g were used in this study. The rats were housed under 12 h light/dark cycle conditions and had free access to food and water except during the test period. To minimize animal suffering, the number of animals used was based on the minimum required for statistically valid results. Immunohistochemical and Electrophysiological analysis were carried out in a blind manner.

Pulpal or periapical inflammation

Rats were lightly anesthetized with 2% isoflurane (Mylan, Canonsburg, PA), then deeply anesthetized with intraperitoneal

(i.p.) application of sodium pentobarbital (50 mg/kg; Schering Plough, Whitehouse Station, NJ), and placed on a warm mat (37°C) in a dorsal recumbent position. To allow for application of CFA (n = 4, Sigma-Aldrich, 50% CFA was diluted in saline) or vehicle (n = 4, isotonic physiological saline) to the right maxillary first molar (M1) tooth pulp, the rats' mouth was gently opened and the dental pulp was exposed by means of low-speed dental drill with a round tungsten carbide bur (No. 1-4: JOTA, Tokyo) under water cooling. CFA or vehicle was applied to the tooth pulp by a small piece of dental paper point (diameter, 0.15 mm; length, 1.5 mm; PIERCE ABSORBENT POINTS, #15) soaked with CFA or vehicle. After CFA or vehicle application with dental points, the cavity was tightly sealed with dental cement (GC Fuji I, Tokyo). The bone loss around the tooth apex was evaluated using in vivo Micro X-ray CT System R_mCT (R_mCT, Rigaku, Tokyo). There were no any abnormal animal behaviors such as grooming, locomotion and feeding. The rats did not lose weight during experimental period.

The sagittal CT images for tooth apex were obtained at 300 μm intervals, and then the bone loss around tooth apex was drawn using Neurolucida (Micro-Brightfield Inc., Colchester, VT). The drawn images were integrated and 3D image of the periapical bone loss was constructed. The change in the volume was calculated by the Neuroexplore software (Micro-Brightfield Inc., Colchester, VT). Furthermore, on day 3 or week 6 after CFA application to upper molar tooth pulp, rats were anesthetized with sodium pentobarbital (80 mg/kg, i.p.) and perfused with 4% paraformaldehyde. Maxillar bone and M1 were removed and decalcified overnight and 15 mm serial sections were cut. Then sections were stained with hematoxylin and eosin and coverslipped.

pERK and Fos immunohistochemistries

For double immunofluorescence histochemistry for pERK and NeuN, sections were rinsed in PBS, 10% normal goat serum in PBS for 1 h, and then incubated in rabbit antiphospho-p44/42 MAP Kinase Antibody (1:200, Cell Signaling Technology) for 72 h at room temperature. Then the sections were incubated in mouse anti-neuronal nuclei monoclonal Antibody (1:500, Chemicon, Temicula, CA) for 2 h at room temperature. Next, the sections were incubated in Alexa Fluor 488 anti-rabbit IgG (1:200 in 0.01 M PBS; Invitrogen, Paisley) and in Alexa Fluor 568 anti-mouse IgG (1:200 in 0.01 M PBS; Invitrogen) for 2 h at room temperature. After rinsing with 0.01 M PBS, sections were coverslipped in mounting medium (Thermo Fisher Scientific, Fremont, CA) and examined under a fluorescence microscope and analyzed using a BZ-9000 system (Keyence, Osaka).

At 3 days and 6 weeks after CFA or vehicle application to M1 (n = 6 each), rats were deeply anesthetized with 2% isoflurane, and a 26 G needle with a Hamilton syringe was inserted into the ipsilateral Mass. After 30 min rest period, capsaicin was applied to the ipsilateral Mass, and at 5 minutes after capsaicin application, rats were transcardially perfused with isotonic saline followed by a fixative containing 4% paraformaldehyde in 0.1 M phosphate buffer (pH 7.4). The whole brain including medulla and upper cervical cord was removed and post-fixed in the same fixative for 3 days at 4°C. The tissues were then transferred to 20% sucrose (w/v) in 0.01 M phosphate-buffered saline (PBS) for several days for cryoprotection. Thirty-micron-thick sections were cut with a freezing microtome, and every fourth section was collected in PBS. Free-floating tissue sections were washed in PBS and rinsed in 1% hydrogen peroxide with 0.75% Triton X-100 (Sigma, St. Louis, MO) in PBS for 1 hour. After washing in PBS, the sections were incubated in 10% normal goat serum in PBS, and then incubated in polyclonal rabbit anti-Fos antibody (c-Fos ab-5, 1:5,000 dilution; Oncogene, Cambridge, MA) for overnight at 4°C. Next, the sections were incubated in biotinylated goat anti-rabbit IgG (1:600; Vector Labs, Burlingame, CA) for 2 h at room temperature. After washing in PBS, the sections were incubated in peroxidase-conjugated avidin-biotin complex (1:100; ABC, Vector Labs) for 2 h at room temperature. After washing in 0.05 M Tris Buffer (TB), the sections were incubated in 0.035% 3,3-diaminobenzidine-tetra HCl (DAB, Sigma, St. Louis, MO), 0.2% nickel ammonium sulfate and 0.05% peroxide in 0.05 M TB (pH 7.4). After washing in PBS and incubated in 10% normal horse serum in PBS, the sections reacted with Fos antibody were incubated in mouse anti-phospho-p44/42 MAP Kinase Antibody (pERK, 1 1000, Cell Signaling Technology) for 72 h at 4°C. The following immunohistochemical procedures were similar to those of c-Fos immunohistochemistry. The reaction products of biotinylated horse anti-mouse antiserum and avidin-conjugated horseradish peroxidase were visualized with 0.035% DAB and 0.05% hydrogen peroxide without nickel.

The sections were washed in PBS, serially mounted on gelatin-coated slides, dehydrated in alcohols and cover slipped. The pERK-IR, Fos protein-IR and double-labeled neurons were drawn under the light microscope using Neurolucida drawing tube. The neurons stained with DAB as brown in the nuclei and cytoplasm were determined as pERK-IR cells. The neurons stained with DAB as black in the nuclei were determined as Fos-IR cells. The number of pERK-IR, Fos protein-IR neurons was counted from every 8th section. The total number of IR neurons from 3 of every 8th section was calculated, and the mean number of those cells (3 sections/rat) was obtained from each animal.

Digastric electromyographic recording after capsaicin application into the Mass

On day 3 or week 6 after CFA or vehicle application to the M1 tooth pulp (n = 6 each), rats were anesthetized with 2% isoflurane and a pair of bipolar wire electrodes (enamel-coated stainless steel wire, inter-polar distance: 5 mm) was inserted into the digastric muscle on the side ipsilateral to the tooth. After that, a 26G needle connected with a Hamilton syringe was gently inserted into the ipsilateral Mass.

The digastric electromyographic (d-EMG) activity was continuously monitored before, during and after the application of capsaicin, dissolved in 100% ethanol and 7% Tween 80 in saline (3 μM, 100 μl), into the Mass. Before capsaicin application, baseline of d-EMG activity was monitored for 20 min, and d-EMG activity was continuously monitored for an additional 20 min. Then, the d-EMG activity was amplified, rectified and integrated, and the area under the curve of d-EMG activity was calculated by the Spike 2 software (CED, Cambridge). The area under the curve of d-EMG activity was measured for every 1 min before and after capsaicin application, and mean d-EMG activity was calculated in each time period. The calculated d-EMG value more than 2 standard deviation of the baseline after capsaicin application was selected and evaluated.

PD98059 administration

Rats were anesthetized with 2% isoflurane and placed in a stereotaxic apparatus. After a midline skin incision, an opening was made in the caudal part of the skull with a dental drill to insert intrathecally (i.t.) a soft polyethylene tube (PE45, ID, 0.58 mm; OD, 0.96 mm; Natsume, Tokyo, Japan) [17]. The tube was connected to a mini-osmotic pump (Alzet model 2001, Alzet, Cupertino, CA, USA; total volume, 200 μL) filled with the drug and embedded subcutaneously in the dorsal portion of the body.

Thus, the MEK1 inhibitor PD98059 was intrathecally applied for 7 days (1.0 μL/h). The dosage and duration of the drug (0.1 μg/μL) for pump infusion was chosen primarily based on previous reports [18–21]. For the rats with periapical periodontitis, CFA was applied into the M1 at 35 days before PD98059 or saline administration, and then capsaicin was applied to the Mass on 7 days after PD98059 administration. For the rats with pulpitis, CFA was applied into the M1 at 4 days after PD98059 or saline administration, and then capsaicin was applied into the Mass at 3 days after CFA application. The d-EMG activity was continuously monitored before and after capsaicin application (n = 6 each).

For pERK and Fos immunohistochemistries, capsaicin was applied into the Mass in CFA-treated rats on day 7 after PD98059 or saline administration (n = 6 each). At 5 minutes after capsaicin application, the rats were perfused, and the pERK and Fos immunohistochemistries were performed.

All subsequent d-EMG recording and staining steps and counting analysis were the same as described above. All d-EMG recording and immunohistochemical experiments were conducted on animals without any obvious neurological deficits. Also, the Alzet pump was removed at the end of each experiment, and the amount of the drug remaining in the pump was checked. If there was still residual drug in the pump, the data from that rat were excluded from the final analysis.

Statistical analysis

Data were expressed as mean ± SEM. Statistical analyses were performed by Student's t-test, one-way or two-way repeated-measures analysis of variance (ANOVA) followed by Turkey or Dunnet test appropriately. A value of $p < 0.05$ was considered as significant.

Results

1. The effect of CFA on tooth and periapical tissues

The application of CFA to the M1 tooth pulp induced inflammation in the tooth pulp on day 3 and in the periapical tissues on week 6 (Fig. 1). The detail tooth structures of M1 were indicated in Fig. 1A–C. In naive rats or the rats with CFA application to the M1 tooth pulp on day 3, periapical bone loss was not observed (Fig. 1A, B), indicating that the CFA-induced inflammation is limited within the pulp or at the apex region of the tooth. The periapical bone loss was clearly detected at 3 weeks after CFA application to the pulp, as shown by formation of granuloma in the periapical periodontitis (Fig. 1C–I). The bone loss was gradually increased and peaked at 6 weeks after CFA application (Fig. 1J). The volume of bone loss measured by 3D micro-CT imaging analysis software was significantly greater in CFA-treated rats compared with vehicle-treated rats from 3 weeks after CFA application (p < 0.05, Fig. 1J).

2. Change in d-EMG activities following tooth pulp or periapical inflammation

We observed significant increase in the d-EMG activity within 1 min after capsaicin application into the Mass in pulpal CFA-applied rats (p < 0.01, Fig. 2A, B). On the other hand, the duration of d-EMG activities after pulpal-CFA or pulpal-vehicle application was about 2 minutes, and no significant difference was observed between CFA and vehicle groups (Fig. 2C).

The d-EMG activities elicited by capsaicin application into the Mass at 6 weeks after pulpal-CFA application were shown in Fig. 2D. Compared with the pulpal-vehicle applied rats, the d-EMG activity was significantly increased (Fig. 2E) and the duration of the d-EMG activity was significantly lasted (Fig. 2F)

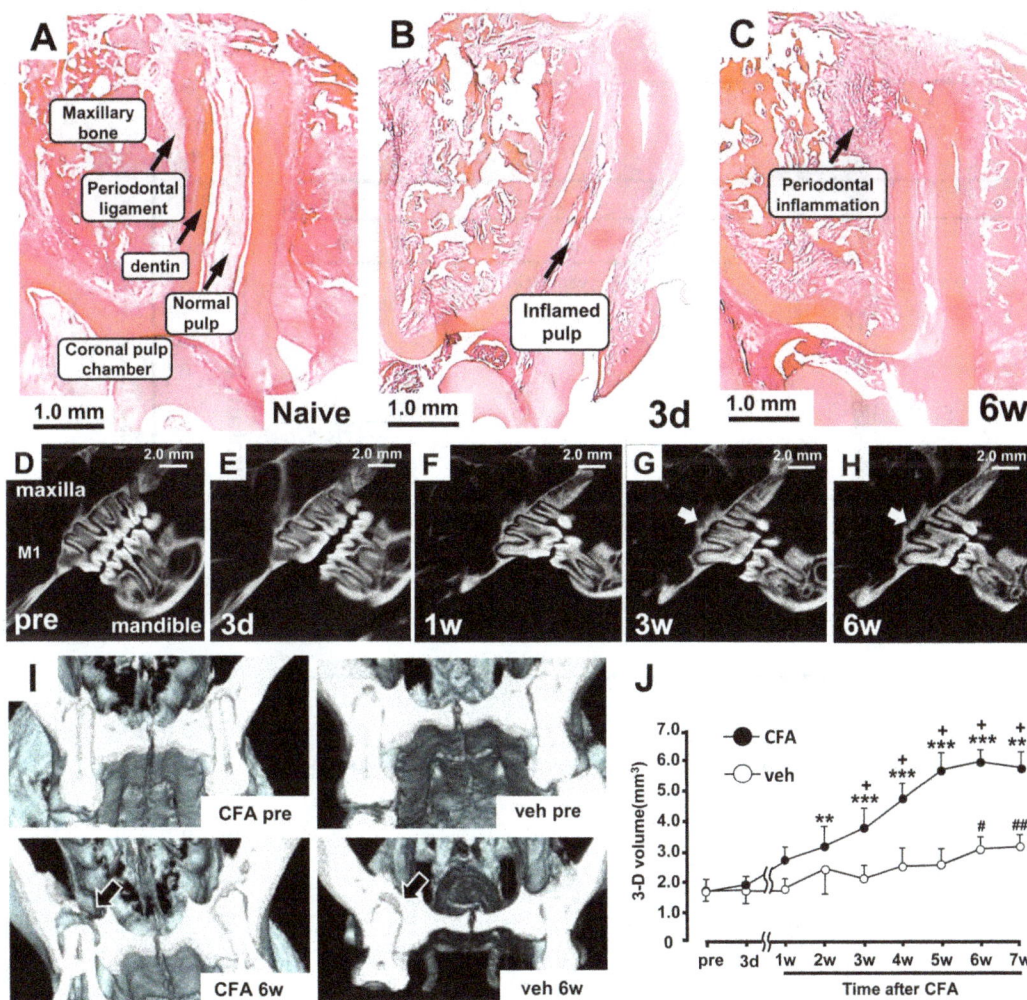

Figure 1. The change in the apical periapical tissues after CFA application to M1 tooth pulp. A, B and C: Photomicrographs of periapical tissues of the naive rats (A) and the rats on day 3 (B) and week 6 (C) after CFA application to the pulp. D–H: Lateral views of 3D X-lay photographs of periapical tissues of pre-CFA application (D), on day 3 (E), on 1 week (F), 3 week (G) and 6 week (H) after CFA application. I: Sagittal views of X-lay micro-CT images of the periapical tissues before and at 6 week after CFA or vehicle application. J: Time course change in the size of the bone loss at the periapical tissues after CFA application to the M1 pulp (n = 4 each). Solid arrows in A-C indicate detail tooth and periapical structures. White arrows in G and H, and black arrow in I indicate periapical bone loss. veh: vehicle in this and following figures. *: Pre vs. post (CFA), #: Pre vs. post (veh), +: CFA vs. veh, +, #: p<0.05, ##, **: p<0.01, ***: p<0.001.

after capsaicin application into the Mass at 6 weeks after pulpal CFA application.

3. pERK-IR and Fos-IR cells and Rostral-caudal distribution in Vi/Vc or Vc

To examine the effect of M1 pulpitis or periapical periodontitis on the neuronal excitability, the ERK phosphorylation and Fos expression were studied in Vi/Vc and Vc neurons following unilateral capsaicin application into the Mass. A number of pERK-IR cells in the Vi/Vc and Vc induced by capsaicin at 3 days or 6 weeks after pulpal CFA application were double-stained with NeuN, a neuronal marker (Fig. 3A–C). However, some of the pERK-positive cells lacked NeuN staining. These results suggest that ERK phosphorylation occurs in grail cells as well as neurons. A large number of pERK-IR and Fos-IR cells were observed in the ventral portion of the Vi/Vc and in the dorsal portion of the Vc after capsaicin application into the Mass on day 3 or week 6 after CFA application into the M1 tooth pulp (Fig. 3G and 4A). Though we observed a few cells double-stained (Fig. 3F) with Fos

(Fig. 3D) and pERK (Fig. 3E) antibodies, there are no double-stained cells in the Vi/Vc and Vc.

Rostral-caudal distribution of pERK-IR and Fos-IR cells in the medulla and upper cervical spinal cord were shown in Fig. 3G, H and Fig. 4A and B. A large number of pERK-IR and Fos-IR cells were observed in the Vi/Vc and Vc following capsaicin application into the ipsilateral Mass on day 3 or week 6 after pulpal CFA application (Fig. 3H and 4B). The total number of cells in Vc and Vi/Vc region indicated by red squares in Fig. 3H and 4B were calculated and the results of statistical analysis were shown in Fig. 3I and Fig. 4C, respectively. Blank indicate a lack of significant difference. The total number of pERK- or Fos-IR cells in the Vi/Vc or Vc in each group was compared respectively (Fig. 3I and Fig. 4C).

On day 3 (Fig. 3I), the number of Fos-IR cells was significantly larger in M1 CFA/Mass veh and M1 CFA/Mass cap rats compared to M1 veh/Mass cap rats in the ipsilateral Vi/Vc. The number of Fos-IR cells was significantly larger in M1 CFA/Mass

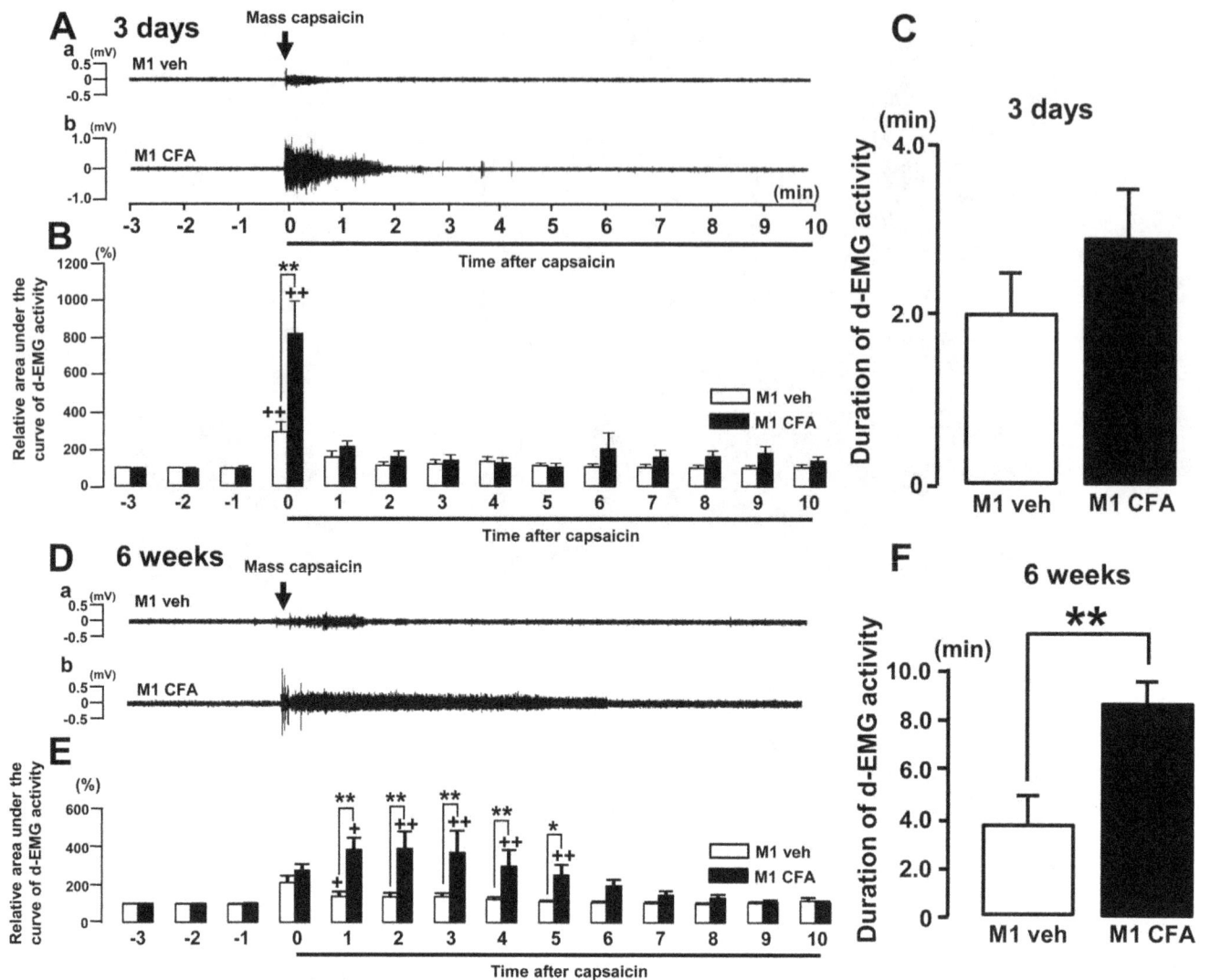

Figure 2. The d-EMG activities after tooth pulp or periapical inflammation. The capsaicin was applied into the Mass in the rats with CFA or vehicle application to the tooth pulp on day 3 and week 6. A: The d-EMG activity following capsaicin application into the Mass in the rats with pulpal-vehicle or pulpal-CFA application on day 3. B: Relative d-EMG activity following capsaicin application into the Mass in the rats with pulpal-vehicle or pulpal-CFA application. C: Mean duration of d-EMG activity following capsaicin application into the Mass in the rats with pulpal-vehicle or pulpal-CFA application. D: The d-EMG activity following capsaicin application into the Mass in the rats with pulpal-vehicle or pulpal-CFA application on week 6. E: Relative d-EMG activity following capsaicin application into the Mass in the rats with pulpal-vehicle or pulpal-CFA application. F: Mean duration of d-EMG activity following capsaicin application into the Mass in the rats with pulpal-vehicle or pulpal-CFA application. +: vs. −1 min, *: veh vs. CFA, +, *: $p < 0.05$, ++, **: $p < 0.01$.

capsaicin rats compared to M1 veh/Mass veh rats in the contralateral Vi/Vc and Vc.

Furthermore, the numbers of pERK-IR cells was significantly larger in M1 veh/Mass cap and M1 CFA/Mass cap rats compared to M1 veh/Mass veh rats and M1 CFA/Mass veh in the ipsilateral Vi/Vc or Vc, respectively. In the contralateral side to injections, the number of pERK-IR cells was significantly larger in M1 veh/Mass cap compared to M1 CFA/Mass veh in the Vi/Vc.

On week 6 (Fig. 4C), the number of Fos-IR cells was significantly larger in M1 CFA/Mass veh or M1 CFA/Mass cap rats compared to M1 veh/Mass cap rats in the ipsilateral Vi/Vc, respectively. The number of pERK-IR cells was also significantly larger in M1 CFA/Mass cap rats compared to M1 veh/Mass veh, M1 veh/Mass cap or M1 CFA/Mass veh rats in the ipsilateral Vi/Vc. Furthermore, the number of pERK-IR cells was significantly

larger in M1 veh/Mass cap or M1 CFA/Mass cap rats compared to M1 CFA/Mass veh rats in the ipsilateral Vc. In the contralateral side to M1 injections, the number of pERK-IR cells was significantly larger in M1 CFA/Mass cap compared to M1 CFA/Mass veh in the Vi/Vc.

4. Comparison of pERK-IR and Fos-IR cells on day 3 and week 6

To examine the difference for the expression of pERK-IR and Fos-IR cells on day 3 and week 6, the ERK phosphorylation and Fos expression were studied in Vi/Vc and Vc neurons following unilateral saline or capsaicin application into the Mass.

In the rats with saline application into the Mass, the number of Fos-IR cells was significantly larger in M1 veh/Mass veh rats in the ipsilateral Vi/Vc or in M1 CFA/Mass veh rats in the ipsi- and

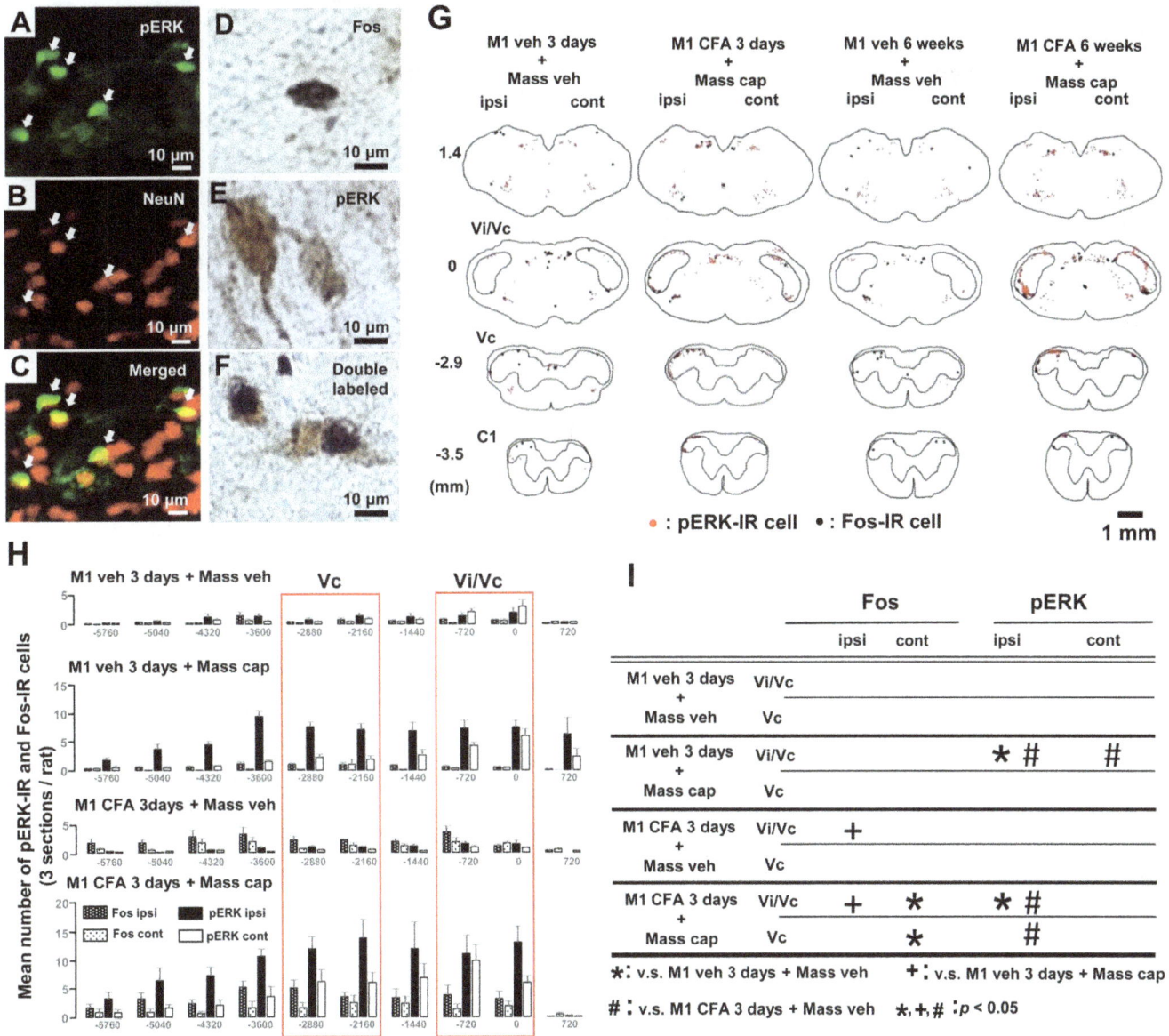

Figure 3. Photomicrographs and Rostral-caudal distribution for pERK-IR cells and Fos-IR cells after tooth pulp inflammation in Vi/Vc and Vc. A: pERK-IR cells. B: NeuN-IR cells. C: A merged with B. D: Fos-IR cell stained with nickel-conjugated DAB. E: pERK-IR cell stained with DAB. F: double stained cells (black: Fos-IR, brown: pERK-IR). G: Neurolucida drawings of pERK-IR (red and triangle dots) and Fos-IR cells (black and round dots) in the Vi/Vc and Vc. H: Rostral-caudal distribution of pERK-IR and Fos-IR cells in the Vi/Vc and Vc. I: *, + and # signs indicate significant expression of pERK-IR or Fos-IR cells compared to each region in M1 veh/Mass veh, M1 veh/Mass cap and M1 CFA/Mass veh on day 3, respectively. Arrows in A indicate pERK-IR cells, those in B indicate NeuN-IR cells and those in C are pERK-IR cells merged with NeuN-IR cells. The negative numbers on the left in G indicate the distance caudal to the obex (0 mm). cap: capsaicin, veh: vehicle, ipsi: ipsilateral, cont: contralateral.

contralateral Vi/Vc and ipsilateral Vc on week 6 compared to those in M1 veh/Mass veh rats on day 3 (p<0.05). The number of pERK-IR cells was also significantly larger in M1 CFA/Mass veh rats on week 6 compared to M1 veh/Mass veh on day 3, M1 veh/Mass veh on week 6 or M1 CFA/Mass veh rats on day 3 in the ipsilateral Vi/Vc (p<0.05).

In the rats with capsaicin application into the Mass, the number of Fos-IR cells was significantly larger in M1 CFA/Mass cap rats on week 6 compared to M1 veh/Mass cap rats on day 3 or M1 veh/Mass cap rats on week 6 in the ipsilateral Vi/Vc (p<0.05).

5. The effect of PD98059 in the Vi/Vc and Vc neurons

We further examined the effect of MEK1 inhibitor PD98059-pretreatment for the Mass hypersensitivity in the rats with M1 pulpitis or periapical periodontitis. We observed significant decrease in the d-EMG activity within 1 minute after capsaicin application into the Mass in the PD98059 i.t.-pretreated rats compared with saline i.t.-pretreated rats on day 3 after M1 CFA application (p<0.01, Fig. 5A, B).

On the other hand, the durations of d-EMG activities after capsaicin application were about 2 minutes, and no significant difference was observed between PD98059- or saline-pretreated rats on day 3 after M1 CFA application (Fig. 5C).

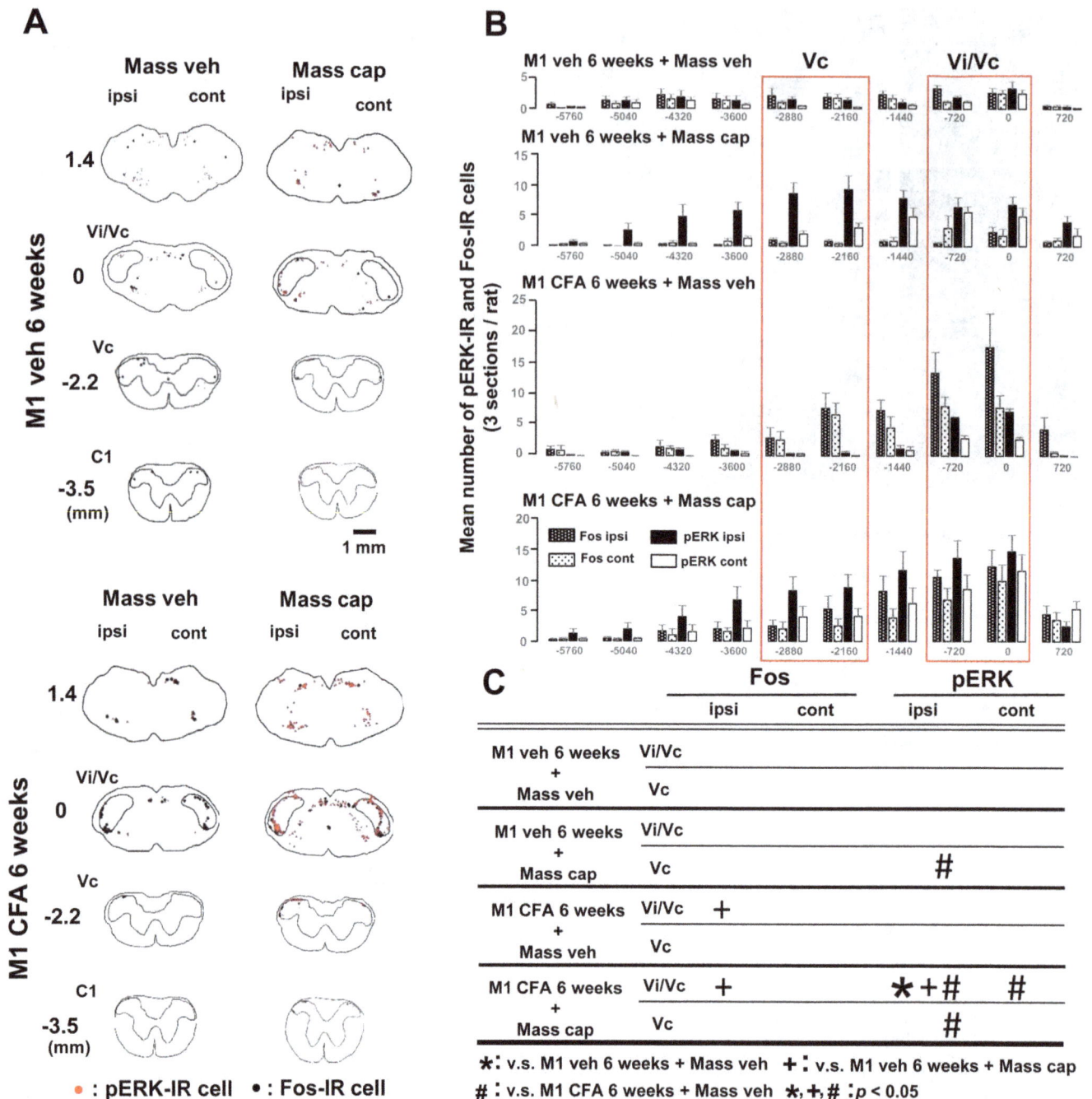

Figure 4. Rostral-caudal distribution for pERK-IR cells and Fos-IR cells after periapical inflammation in Vi/Vc and Vc. The capsaicin was applied into the Mass in the rats with CFA or vehicle application to the tooth pulp on week 6. A and B: Neurolucida drawings (A) and Rostral-caudal distribution (B) of pERK-IR and Fos-IR cells in the Vi/Vc and Vc. C: *, + and # signs indicate significant expression of pERK-IR or Fos-IR cells compared to each region in M1 veh/Mass veh, M1 veh/Mass cap and M1 CFA/Mass veh on day 3, respectively.

We observed significant attenuation in the d-EMG activity within 2 minute after capsaicin application into the Mass in the PD98059 i.t.-pretreated rats compared with saline i.t.-pretreated rats on week 6 after M1 CFA application (p<0.01, Fig. 5D, E).

Furthermore, the mean duration of d-EMG activities after capsaicin application was significantly decreased in the PD98059-pretreated rats compared with saline-pretreated rats on 6 week after M1 CFA application (p<0.01, Fig. 5F).

To examine the effect of PD98059 on ERK phosphorylation caused by M1 pulpitis or periapical periodontitis, the change in the

number of ERK-IR cells following pretreatment with PD98059 was studied in Vi/Vc and Vc following capsaicin application into the Mass (Fig. 6A and B).

On day 3 and week 6, the number of pERK-IR cells after Mass-capsaicin application was significantly decreased following PD98059 i.t. administration compared to saline i.t. administration in the ipsilateral Vi/Vc and Vc of the M1 CFA rats. Furthermore, the number of Fos-IR cells was not altered after the pretreatment of PD98059 or saline on day 3 or week 6 in the rats with M1 CFA/Mass cap (Fig. 6C).

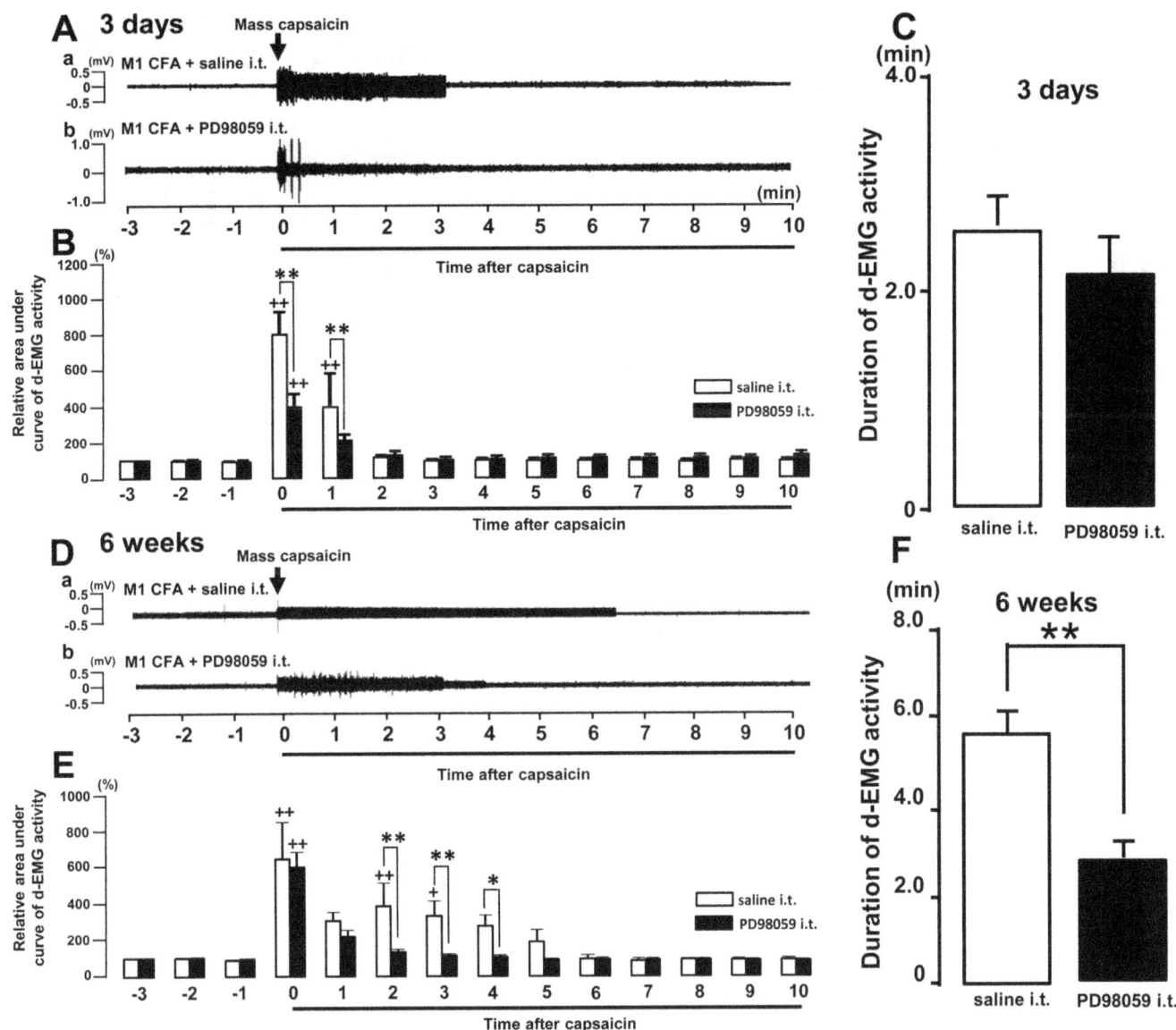

Figure 5. The effect of PD98059 on the d-EMG activities after tooth pulp or periapical inflammation. The capsaicin was applied into the Mass after pretreatment of PD98059 in the rats with M1 CFA application on day 3 and week 6. A: The d-EMG activity following capsaicin application into the Mass after pretreatment of PD98059 or saline in the rats with M1 CFA application on day 3. B: Relative d-EMG activity following capsaicin application into the Mass after pretreatment with PD98059 or saline in the rats with M1 CFA application. C: Mean duration of d-EMG activity following capsaicin application into the Mass after pretreatment with PD98059 or saline in the rats with M1 CFA application. D: The d-EMG activity following capsaicin application into the Mass after pretreatment of PD98059 or saline in the rats with M1 CFA application on week 6. E: Relative d-EMG activity following capsaicin application into the Mass after pretreatment with PD98059 or saline in the rats with M1 CFA application. C: Mean duration of d-EMG activity following capsaicin application into the Mass after pretreatment of PD98059 or saline in the rats with M1 CFA application. +: vs. −1 min, *: saline i.t. vs. PD98059 i.t., +,*: p<0.05., ++, **: p<0.01.

Discussion

Periapical inflammation frequently causes referred pain in the orofacial cutaneous tissue and/or muscle as well as tooth pulp [22]. It is well known that inflammation within the tooth pulp often extends into the periapical tissues after pulpal inflammation, resulting in pulpal necrosis and periapical inflammation. At the early stage of periapical inflammation, severe persistent pain occurs in the apex region of the tooth [23]. Eventually, periapical pain could change its' quality from an acute to a chronic state. Chronic periapical pain is dull and persistent, lasts for a long period, and also causes referred pain in the orofacial skin and/or

muscles. The orofacial referred pain originated from the periapical inflammation is difficult to diagnose and treat [3]. Despite increasing necessity of the clarification of the pathogenesis for the odontogenic referred pain in the orofacial region, it is still unclear on the mechanisms underlying extraterritorial orofacial persistent pain associated with periapical inflammation. In the present study, therefore, we examined the excitability of the Vi/Vc and Vc neurons in a rat model of experimental pulpitis/periodontitis and its' involvement in the enhancement of d-EMG activity.

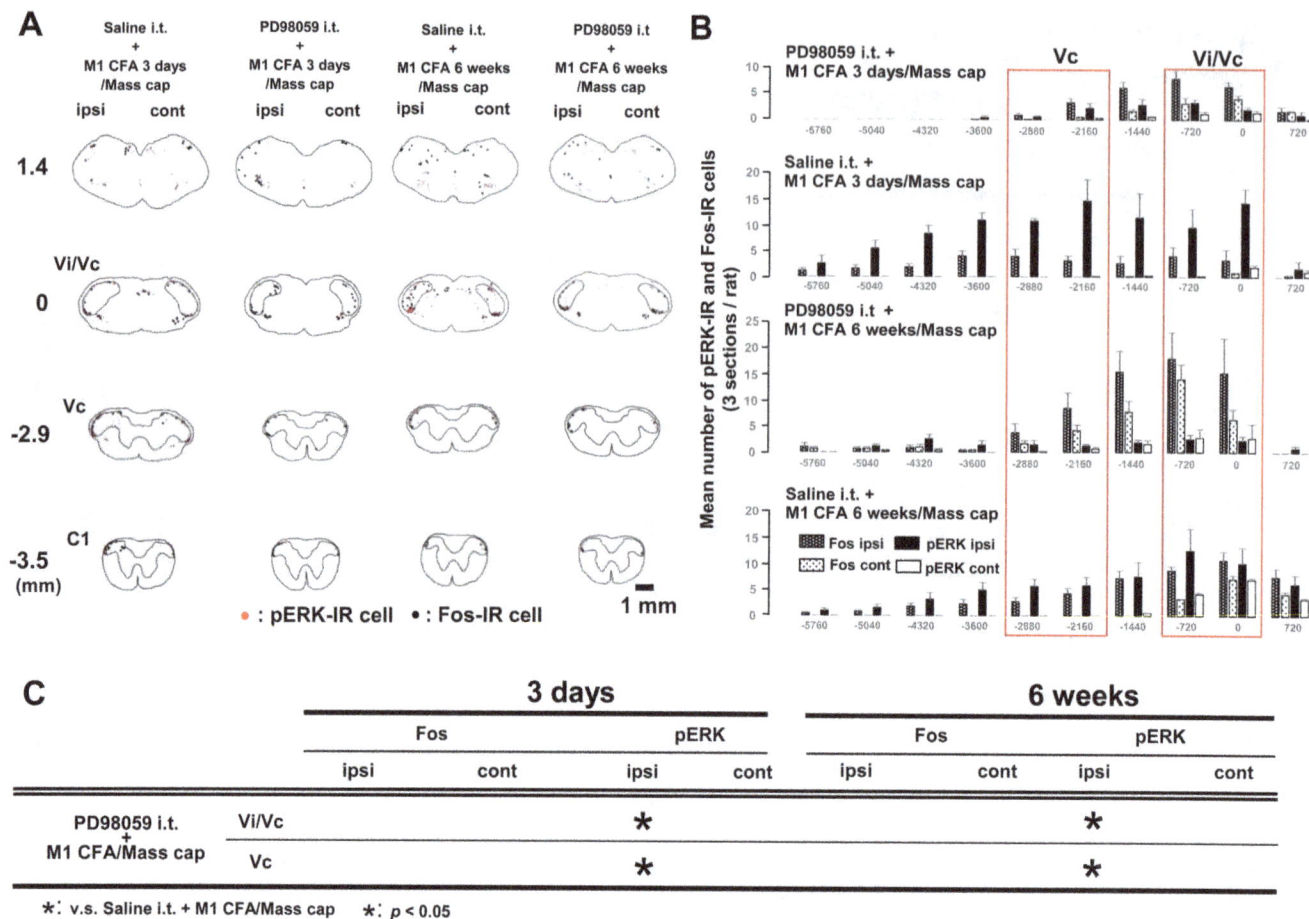

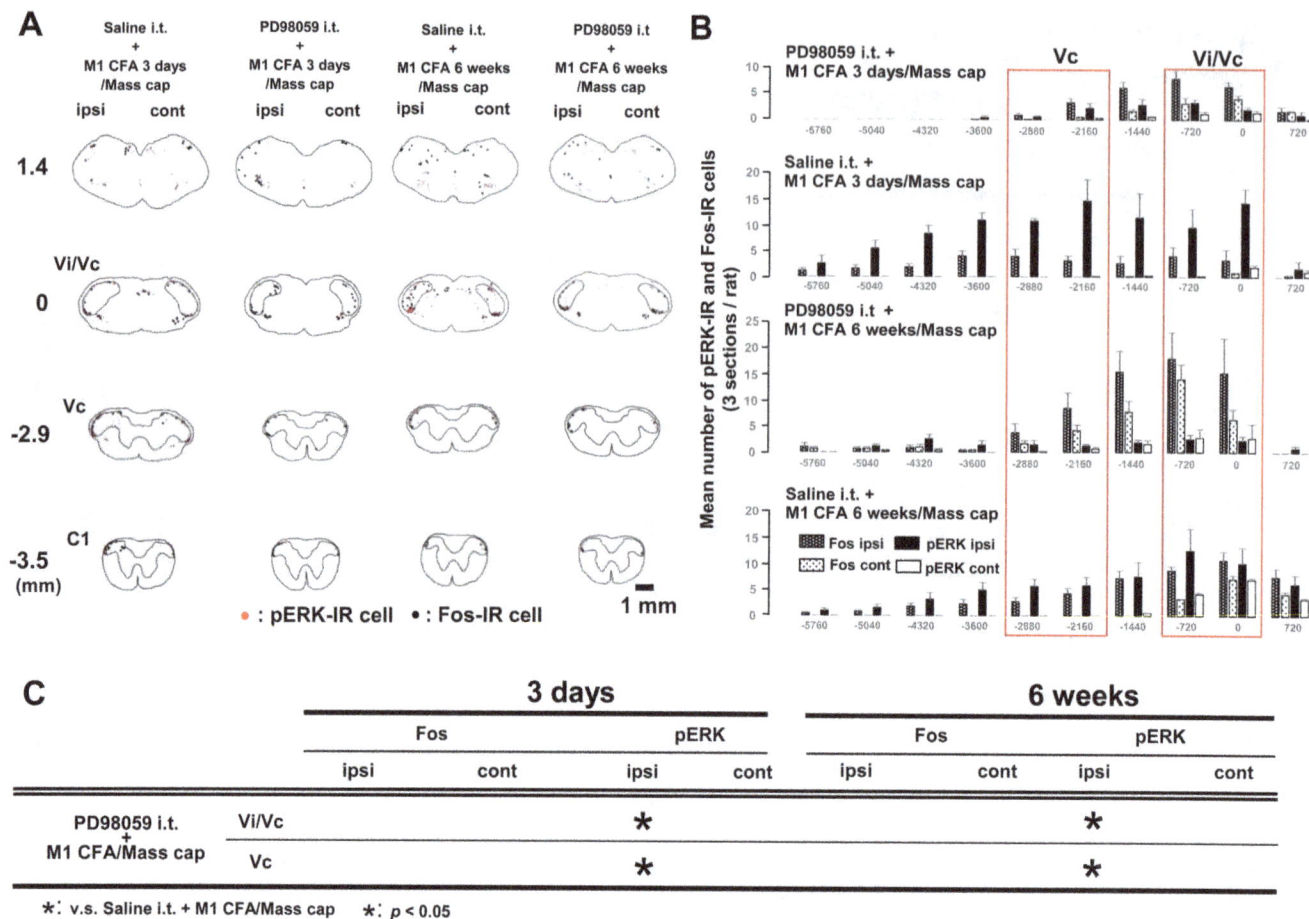

Figure 6. The effect of PD98059 on ERK phosphorylation in Vi/Vc and Vc neurons after tooth pulp or periapical inflammation. The capsaicin was applied into the Mass after PD98059 i.t. administration in the rats with M1 CFA on day 3 or week 6. A and B: Neurolucida drawings (A) and Rostral-caudal distribution (B) of pERK-IR and Fos-IR cells in the Vi/Vc and Vc. C: * indicates significant decrease in the number of pERK-IR or Fos-IR cells. Each region in each model was compared with M1 CFA/Mass cap rats with saline i.t. on day 3 or week 6, respectively.

1. Rat model of periapical inflammation

It is well known that periapical bone loss is observed during development of the periapical inflammation, suggesting that the periapical bone loss could be one of the reliable indicators for the periapical inflammation [24]. Thus, we analyzed the time-course change in the bone loss using X-ray micro-CT imaging to quantify the periapical inflammation. The advantage of this technique is that the size of bone loss can be measured in same rats throughout the experimental period. Periapical bone loss was detected at 3 weeks after pulpal application of CFA, and the largest bone loss was observed at 6 weeks after CFA application to the pulp, indicating that chronic phase characterized by lesion stabilization was commenced from 6 weeks after CFA application. The time-course of bone loss we observed in this study is similar to that of previous study [24], suggesting that this model can be used as a reliable animal model with experimental periodontitis following long lasting pulpal inflammation.

2. Changes in the Vi/Vc and Vc neuronal activities following pulpal or periapical inflammation

The d-EMG activity elicited by noxious stimulation is known as a good indicator of the noxious responses in the trigeminal system [25]. We observed significant increase in the d-EMG activity after capsaicin application into the Mass on day 3 and week 6 after pulpal-CFA or pulpal-vehicle application. Furthermore, the d-EMG activity elicited by Mass-capsaicin application was significantly higher in M1 CFA-applied rats compared with M1-vehicle applied rats. The number of Fos-IR cells in the Vi/Vc was significantly larger in M1 CFA applied rats compared with M1 vehicle-applied rats on day 3 and week 6. On the other hand, ERK phosphorylation in the Vi/Vc and/or Vc neurons significantly increased in Mass-capsaicin applied rats compared with Mass-vehicle applied rats both in pulpal CFA- or vehicle applied rats. These indicate that noxious stimulus to the Mass induces the enhancement of noxious responses in the orofacial region following pulpal or periapical inflammation. It is strongly suggested that the increase in d-EMG activities and pERK expression in Vi/Vc and Vc neurons are the result of enhancement of Vi/Vc and/or Vc neuronal activities following pulpal or periapical inflammation. Taken together, the EMG activities and pERK expression were significantly enhanced after capsaicin application into the Mass on day 3 and week 6 after pulpal CFA application, suggesting that pathogenesis of pulpal or periapical inflammation might induce pain hypersensitivity in remote organs or tissues in the orofacial region.

We also observed that the duration of EMG activity was significantly longer at 6 weeks after pulpal CFA application compared with that of pulpal vehicle application. The enhancement of EMG activity and the increased duration were significantly reversed following i.t. administration of PD98059. These results indicate that periapical inflammation may induce and maintain pain hypersensitivity in the remote organs or tissues in orofacial region, whereas pulpal inflammation may only induce pain hypersensitivity. Furthermore, the ERK phosphorylation in Vi/Vc and Vc neurons has a pivotal role in the maintenance and/ or modulation of pain processing in remote regions after tooth pulp or periapical inflammation.

3. Involvement of the Vi/Vc and Vc neurons in Mass hypersensitivity

Fos protein expression in SDH neurons following noxious stimulation of the peripheral structures is known to be caused 1–2 hours and lasted 24 hours after noxious stimulation [26], and therefore Fos protein expression in SDH neurons is thought to be a good marker of the excitation of nociceptive neurons [27]. The ventral portion of the Vi/Vc is known to have a various functions in trigeminal nociception [28]. Many Vi/Vc neurons are known to express Fos-IR products following CFA application into the Mass or noxious stimulation of the cornea [29,30]. Many of them were also observed on both sides of the Vi/Vc following unilateral noxious stimulation.

It has been reported that the number of pERK-IR cells increases unilaterally in the Vc following increase in noxious stimulus intensity [31]. In the trigeminal system, ERK can be phosphorylated in a large number of dorsal horn neurons in the Vc and C1-C2 within 5 min after noxious stimulation to various orofacial regions; these pERK-IR neurons are somatotopically organized in Vc and C1-C2, and the number of pERK-IR neurons increases following increases in the noxious stimulus intensity [12,20], indicating that ERK phosphorylation in Vc and C1-C2 neurons is a reliable marker of excitable neurons following orofacial noxious stimulation.

We observed that pERK expression was significantly enhanced after capsaicin application into the Mass both in M1 CFA- and

vehicle-applied rats compared with Mass-vehicle applied rats in both Vi/Vc and Vc on day 3 and week 6. Furthermore, on day 3 after pulpal application, we observed a large number of Fos-IR cells in the bilateral Vi/Vc in pulpal CFA-applied rats. Meanwhile, on week 6 after pulpal-CFA application, we observed a large number of Fos-IR cells just in the ipsilateral Vi/Vc in pulpal CFA-applied rats, and the number of them was also significantly larger in CFA-applied rats compared with vehicle-applied rats. These findings suggest that nociceptive neurons in the Vi/Vc and Vc may have important roles for orofacial pain hypersensitivity associated with tooth pulp inflammation and periapical inflammation.

Furthermore, we could not observe significant change in the number of Fos-IR cells in these two areas between Mass-capsaicin and vehicle applied rats, suggesting that Fos expression may be mainly due to the CFA application to the tooth pulp but not Mass-capsaicin application.

Conclusions

The present findings revealed that the Vi/Vc and Vc neurons was involved in the enhancement of Mass nociception under acute pulpal-inflamed state as well as chronic periapical inflammation, suggesting that nociceptive neurons in these areas are involved in pain hypersensitivity for orofacial muscle associated with acute pulpal and chronic periapical inflammation.

Author Contributions

Conceived and designed the experiments: KS. Performed the experiments: KS KM NN SM KO KH KD TW HK YT. Analyzed the data: KS KM NN SM KO YN YT. Contributed reagents/materials/analysis tools: BO. Wrote the paper: KS KI. Contributed to discussion and reviewed/edited the manuscript: MS KI BO.

References

1. Ertekin C, Secil Y, Yuceyar N, Aydogdu I (2004) Oropharyngeal dysphagia in polymyositis/dermatomyositis. Clin Neurol Neurosurg 107: 32–37.
2. Grushka M, Sessle BJ (1984) Applicability of the McGill Pain Questionnaire to the differentiation of 'toothache' pain. Pain 19: 49–57.
3. Bender IB (2000) Pulpal pain diagnosis–a review. J Endod 26: 175–179.
4. Wright EF (2008) Pulpalgia contributing to temporomandibular disorder-like pain: a literature review and case report. J Am Dent Assoc 139: 436–440.
5. Iwata K, Takahashi O, Tsuboi Y, Ochiai H, Hibiya J, et al. (1998) Fos protein induction in the medullary dorsal horn and first segment of the spinal cord by tooth-pulp stimulation in cats. Pain 75: 27–36.
6. Sessle BJ (1987) The neurobiology of facial and dental pain: present knowledge, future directions. J Dent Res 66: 962–981.
7. Sessle BJ, Hu JW, Amano N, Zhong G (1986) Convergence of cutaneous, tooth pulp, visceral, neck and muscle afferents onto nociceptive and non-nociceptive neurones in trigeminal subnucleus caudalis (medullary dorsal horn) and its implications for referred pain. Pain 27: 219–235.
8. Shimizu K, Asano M, Kitagawa J, Ogiso B, Ren K, et al. (2006) Phosphorylation of Extracellular Signal-Regulated Kinase in medullary and upper cervical cord neurons following noxious tooth pulp stimulation. Brain Res 1072: 99–109.
9. Wang H, Wei F, Dubner R, Ren K (2006) Selective distribution and function of primary afferent nociceptive inputs from deep muscle tissue to the brainstem trigeminal transition zone. J Comp Neurol 498: 390–402.
10. Amano N, Hu JW, Sessle BJ (1986) Responses of neurons in feline trigeminal subnucleus caudalis (medullary dorsal horn) to cutaneous, intraoral, and muscle afferent stimuli. J Neurophysiol 55: 227–243.
11. Shoda E, Kitagawa J, Suzuki I, Nitta-Kubota I, Miyamoto M, et al. (2009) Increased phosphorylation of extracellular signal-regulated kinase in trigeminal nociceptive neurons following propofol administration in rats. J Pain 10: 573–585.
12. Noma N, Tsuboi Y, Kondo M, Matsumoto M, Sessle BJ, et al. (2008) Organization of pERK-immunoreactive cells in trigeminal spinal nucleus caudalis and upper cervical cord following capsaicin injection into oral and craniofacial regions in rats. J Comp Neurol 507: 1428–1440.
13. Dai Y, Iwata K, Fukuoka T, Kondo E, Tokunaga A, et al. (2002) Phosphorylation of extracellular signal-regulated kinase in primary afferent neurons by noxious stimuli and its involvement in peripheral sensitization. J Neurosci 22: 7737–7745.
14. Harris JA (1998) Using c-fos as a neural marker of pain. Brain Res Bull 45: 1–8.
15. Hasegawa M, Kondo M, Suzuki I, Shimizu N, Sessle BJ, et al. (2012) ERK is involved in tooth-pressure-induced Fos expression in Vc neurons. J Dent Res 91: 1141–1146.
16. Zimmermann M (1983) Ethical guidelines for investigations of experimental pain in conscious animals. Pain 16: 109–110.
17. Terayama R, Omura S, Fujisawa N, Yamaai T, Ichikawa H, et al. (2008) Activation of microglia and p38 mitogen-activated protein kinase in the dorsal column nucleus contributes to tactile allodynia following peripheral nerve injury. Neuroscience 153: 1245–1255.
18. Gasparini F, Lingenhohl K, Stoehr N, Flor PJ, Heinrich M, et al. (1999) 2-Methyl-6-(phenylethynyl)-pyridine (MPEP), a potent, selective and systemically active mGlu5 receptor antagonist. Neuropharmacology 38: 1493–1503.
19. Honda K, Kitagawa J, Sessle BJ, Kondo M, Tsuboi Y, et al. (2008) Mechanisms involved in an increment of multimodal excitability of medullary and upper cervical dorsal horn neurons following cutaneous capsaicin treatment. Mol Pain 4: 59.
20. Honda K, Noma N, Shinoda M, Miyamoto M, Katagiri A, et al. (2011) Involvement of peripheral ionotropic glutamate receptors in orofacial thermal hyperalgesia in rats. Mol Pain 7: 75.
21. Kobayashi A, Shinoda M, Sessle BJ, Honda K, Imamura Y, et al. (2011) Mechanisms involved in extraterritorial facial pain following cervical spinal nerve injury in rats. Mol Pain 7: 12.
22. Sessle BJ (1978) Oral-facial pain: old puzzles, new postulates. Int Dent J 28: 28–42.
23. Morse DR (1977) Immunologic aspects of pulpal-periapical diseases. A review. Oral Surg Oral Med Oral Pathol 43: 436–451.
24. Stashenko P, Yu SM, Wang CY (1992) Kinetics of immune cell and bone resorptive responses to endodontic infections. J Endod 18: 422–426.

25. Sunakawa M, Chiang CY, Sessle BJ, Hu JW (1999) Jaw electromyographic activity induced by the application of algesic chemicals to the rat tooth pulp. Pain 80: 493–501.

26. Hunt SP, Pini A, Evan G (1987) Induction of c-fos-like protein in spinal cord neurons following sensory stimulation. Nature 328: 632–634.

27. Williams S, Evan GI, Hunt SP (1990) Changing patterns of c-fos induction in spinal neurons following thermal cutaneous stimulation in the rat. Neuroscience 36: 73–81.

28. Ren K, Dubner R (2011) The role of trigeminal interpolaris-caudalis transition zone in persistent orofacial pain. Int Rev Neurobiol 97: 207–225.

29. Bereiter DA, Hathaway CB, Benetti AP (1994) Caudal portions of the spinal trigeminal complex are necessary for autonomic responses and display Fos-like immunoreactivity after corneal stimulation in the cat. Brain Res 657: 73–82.

30. Imbe H, Dubner R, Ren K (1999) Masseteric inflammation-induced Fos protein expression in the trigeminal interpolaris/caudalis transition zone: contribution of somatosensory-vagal-adrenal integration. Brain Res 845: 165–175.

31. Ji RR, Baba H, Brenner GJ, Woolf CJ (1999) Nociceptive-specific activation of ERK in spinal neurons contributes to pain hypersensitivity. Nat Neurosci 2: 1114–1119.

24

Synergistic Anti-Inflammatory Activity of the Antimicrobial Peptides Human Beta-Defensin-3 (hBD-3) and Cathelicidin (LL-37) in a Three-Dimensional Co-Culture Model of Gingival Epithelial Cells and Fibroblasts

Telma Blanca Lombardo Bedran[1], Márcia Pinto Alves Mayer[2], Denise Palomari Spolidorio[3], Daniel Grenier[4]*

1 Department of Oral Diagnosis and Surgery, Araraquara Dental School, State University of São Paulo, São Paulo, Brazil, **2** Department of Microbiology, Institute of Biomedical Sciences, University of São Paulo, São Paulo, Brazil, **3** Department of Physiology and Pathology, Araraquara Dental School, State University of São Paulo, São Paulo, Brazil, **4** Oral Ecology Research Group, Faculty of Dentistry, Université Laval, Quebec City, QC, Canada

Abstract

Given the spread of antibiotic resistance in bacterial pathogens, antimicrobial peptides that can also modulate the immune response may be a novel approach for effectively controlling periodontal infections. In the present study, we used a three-dimensional (3D) co-culture model of gingival epithelial cells and fibroblasts stimulated with *Aggregatibacter actinomycetemcomitans* lipopolysaccharide (LPS) to investigate the anti-inflammatory properties of human beta-defensin-3 (hBD-3) and cathelicidin (LL-37) and to determine whether these antimicrobial peptides can act in synergy. The 3D co-culture model composed of gingival fibroblasts embedded in a collagen matrix overlaid with gingival epithelial cells had a synergistic effect with respect to the secretion of IL-6 and IL-8 in response to LPS stimulation compared to fibroblasts and epithelial cells alone. The 3D co-culture model was stimulated with non-cytotoxic concentrations of hBD-3 (10 and 20 µM) and LL-37 (0.1 and 0.2 µM) individually and in combination in the presence of *A. actinomycetemcomitans* LPS. A multiplex ELISA assay was used to quantify the secretion of 41 different cytokines. hBD-3 and LL-37 acted in synergy to reduce the secretion of GRO-alpha, G-CSF, IP-10, IL-6, and MCP-1, but only had an additive effect on reducing the secretion of IL-8 in response to *A. actinomycetemcomitans* LPS stimulation. The present study showed that hBD-3 acted in synergy with LL-37 to reduce the secretion of cytokines by an LPS-stimulated 3D model of gingival mucosa. This combination of antimicrobial peptides thus shows promising potential as an adjunctive therapy for treating inflammatory periodontitis.

Editor: Jürgen Harder, University Hospital Schleswig-Holstein, Campus Kiel, Germany

Funding: This study was supported by the Canadian Institutes of Health Research and the Laboratoire de Contrôle Microbiologique de l'Université Laval. The funders had no role in study design, data collection and analysis, decision to publish, or preparation of the manuscript.

Competing Interests: The authors have declared that no competing interests exist.

* Email: daniel.grenier@greb.ulaval.ca

Introduction

Periodontitis is a multifactorial chronic inflammatory disease of polymicrobial origin that causes the destruction of the tooth-supporting tissues, including the periodontal ligament and alveolar bone [1]. A limited number of Gram-negative, mostly anaerobic bacteria that colonize the subgingival sites and activate the host immune response have been associated with this disease [2]. More specifically, *Aggregatibacter actinomycetemcomitans* is considered to be a key etiological agent of aggressive periodontitis [3]. The lipopolysaccharide (LPS) of *A. actinomycetemcomitans* is a major virulence factor that can promote adhesion to oral cells and can activate the host immune response, resulting in the secretion of large amounts of pro-inflammatory cytokines, including interleukin-6 (IL-6) and interleukin-8 (IL-8) that contribute to the destruction of periodontal tissues [4–6].

Epithelial cells and fibroblasts are the predominant cells of periodontal tissues and serve as a first line of defense against periodontopathogens. They act as a mechanical barrier against bacterial invasion in addition to secreting different classes of inflammatory mediators and tissue-destructive enzymes in response to pathogen stimulation. When the immune and inflammatory responses do not stop the progression of the periodontal infection, uncontrolled secretion of cytokines occurs, leading to chronic inflammation and periodontal tissue destruction [7]. For instance, higher levels of IL-8 and monocyte chemo-attractant protein 1 (MCP-1) have been found in gingival crevicular fluid (GCF) from periodontitis sites than in GCF from healthy control sites, while their levels decrease after periodontal treatments [8–12].

Traditional scaling and root planing remain the "gold standard" for the treatment of periodontitis. However, some patients do not respond adequately to this conventional therapy and require adjunctive antimicrobials. Given that many bacteria have developed resistance to antibiotics, new strategies need to be developed for adjunctive therapies [13]. Antimicrobial peptides (AMPs) are small cationic molecules of the innate immune response with a broad activity spectrum against pathogens, including those associated with periodontitis [14]. Gingival epithelial cells have been reported to secrete several AMPs either constitutively or in response to an infection [14,15]. LL-37 and human β-defensin (hBD-3) are the most important AMPs found in humans. CAP18 is the only member of the cathelicidin family found in humans. The C-terminal of CAP18 is proteolytically cleaved to generate LL-37, a 37-amino-acid peptide beginning with two leucine residues [16,17]. hBD-3 is an important defensin in the oral cavity and is expressed in response to bacterial invasion [15,18]. Both hBD-3 and LL-37 have a broad activity spectrum and have been detected in GCF and saliva [19–22]. Some studies have reported a marked reduction in the amounts of hBD-3 and LL-37 in gingival crevicular fluid during periodontitis, which could be related to the ability of certain periodontopathogens to proteolytically inactivate the peptides or down-regulate their expression [23–25].

hBD-3 and LL-37 show antimicrobial activity against a broad range of oral Gram-positive and Gram-negative bacteria [26,27]. These positively charged cationic peptides bind to the negatively charged bacterial membrane components leading to the formation of pores and cell lysis [28–30]. In addition to exert antimicrobial activity, both peptides modulate the immune response [31]. hBD-3 and LL-37 can neutralize the inflammatory potential of LPS by binding directly to LPS or by preventing the binding of LPS to host cell receptors, thus blocking the cell signaling pathway triggered by TLR ligands [32–34]. Walters et al. [35] showed that LL-37 reduces cytokine secretion by LPS-stimulated human whole blood and proposed that this peptide should be considered for use in adjunctive periodontal treatments. By acting on the two etiological components of periodontitis, i.e., periodontopathogens and the inflammatory response, hBD-3 and LL-37 are very attractive candidates for adjunctive periodontal treatments.

Previous studies have shown that hBD-3 and LL-37 may work in association with other antimicrobial agents to enhance their antibacterial activities [36–38]. More specifically, Chen et al. [39] reported that hBD-3 and LL-37 work in synergy to inhibit the growth of *Staphylococcus aureus*. This may be related to the fact that hBD-3 and LL-37 are able to act on different cell targets. In this study, we hypothesized that synergistic interactions between hBD-3 and LL-37 may also exist in regard to reduction of LPS-induced inflammatory response of host cells. Consequently, we used an in vitro three-dimensional (3D) co-culture model of gingival epithelial cells and fibroblasts stimulated with *A. actinomycetemcomitans* LPS to determine the effect of cell interactions on cytokine secretion and to investigate the synergistic anti-inflammatory activities of hBD-3 and LL-37.

Materials and Methods

Antimicrobial peptides and LPS preparation

The synthetic hBD-3 (H-GIINTLQKYYCRVRGGR-CAVLSCLPKEEQIGKCSTRGRKCCRRKK-OH) and LL-37 (H-LLGDFFRKSKEKIGKEFKRIVQRIKDFLRNLVPRTES-OH) peptides were from Biomatik (Cambridge, ON, Canada). They were dissolved in sterile UltraPure DNase/RNase-free distilled water (Life Technologies Inc., Burlington, ON, Canada) at a concentration of 1 mM and were stored at $-20°C$ until used. *A. actinomycetemcomitans* (ATCC 29522) LPS was isolated using the protocol previously described by Darveau and Hancock [40].

Stock solutions (1 mg/mL) prepared in sterile distilled water were stored at $-20°C$ until used.

Cultivation of gingival epithelial cells and fibroblasts

The immortalized human gingival epithelial cell line OBA-9 [41], which was kindly provided by M. Mayer (Department of Microbiology, Institute of Biomedical Sciences, University of São Paulo, São Paulo, Brazil), was cultured in keratinocyte serum-free medium (K-SFM; Life Technologies Inc.) containing insulin, epidermal growth factor, fibroblast growth factor, and 100 μg/mL of penicillin G-streptomycin. The primary human gingival fibroblast cell line HGF-1 (ATCC CRL-2014) was purchased from the American Type Culture Collection (ATCC) (Manassas, VA, USA) and was cultured in Dulbecco's modified Eagle's medium (DMEM) supplemented with 4 mM L-glutamine (Hy-Clone Laboratories, Logan, UT, USA), 10% heat-inactivated fetal bovine serum (FBS), and 100 μg/mL of penicillin G-streptomycin. Both cell lines were incubated at 37°C in a 5% CO_2 atmosphere until they reached confluence.

Preparation of the three-dimensional (3D) co-culture model

A 3D co-culture model composed of gingival fibroblasts embedded in a collagen matrix overlaid with gingival epithelial cells was prepared according to the protocol described by Gursoy et al. [42], with slight modifications. Preliminary assays allowed to determine the incubation times to be used to obtain fibroblast and epithelial cell differentiation with a cell confluence of approximately 80%. A commercial bovine type I collagen solution (95–98%; PureCol, Advanced BioMatrix, Tucson, AZ, USA) was mixed with DMEM (10X) (Sigma-Aldrich Canada, Oakville, ON, Canada) on ice to obtain a final collagen concentration of 76–78%. The pH was adjusted to 7. Confluent HGF-1 cells were detached by gentle trypsinization (0.05% trypsin-EDTA; Gibco-BRL, Grand Island, NY, USA). The trypsin was then inactivated by adding DMEM +10% FBS. The cells were harvested by centrifugation (500×g for 5 min) and were suspended at a density of 5×10^5 cells/mL in the collagen solution described above. The collagen cell suspension was placed in the wells of 6-well tissue culture plates (2 mL/well; 2.5-mm-thick) (Sarstedt, Newton, NC, USA). The collagen gel was allowed to solidify for 2 h at 37°C under aerobic conditions, and the plates were then incubated for a further 10 h at 37°C in a 5% CO_2 atmosphere. The OBA-9 cells were detached by gentle trypsinization (5 min) (TrypLE Express; Life Technologies Inc.) at 37°C. The trypsin was then inactivated by adding 0.3 mg/mL of trypsin inhibitor, and the cells were harvested by centrifugation (500×g for 5 min) and suspended in fresh K-SFM medium. Aliquots (2 mL) of OBA-9 cells were seeded on top of the collagen-fibroblast gels at a density of 1×10^6 cell/mL. The 3D co-culture model (Figure 1) was incubated overnight at 37°C in a 5% CO_2 atmosphere to allow cell adhesion prior to stimulation.

Comparative analysis of LPS-induced IL-6 and IL-8 secretion by the 3D co-culture model and the individual cell lines

The 3D co-culture model was stimulated with *A. actinomyce-temcomitans* LPS (1 μg/mL) for 24 h at 37°C in a 5% CO_2 atmosphere. Unstimulated cells (individually and in co-culture) were used as controls. The supernatants were collected, centrifuged (3000×g for 10 min at 4°C), and then stored at $-20°C$ until used for the IL-6 and IL-8 assays. After a 24-h incubation, the co-culture model, the collagen-fibroblast gel, and the epithelial cells

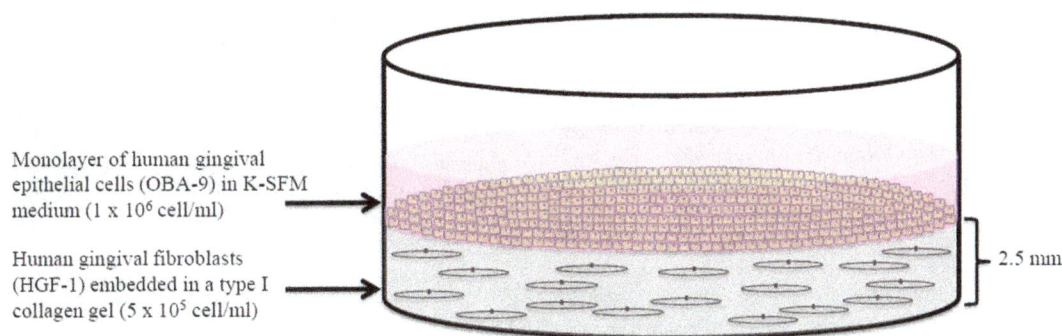

Monolayer of human gingival epithelial cells (OBA-9) in K-SFM medium (1×10^6 cell/ml)

Human gingival fibroblasts (HGF-1) embedded in a type I collagen gel (5×10^5 cell/ml)

2.5 mm

Figure 1. Schematic representation of the 3D co-culture model. The model is composed of gingival fibroblasts (HGF-1) embedded in a collagen matrix overlaid with gingival epithelial cells (OBA-9) and is a modification of the model described by Gursoy et al. [42].

were visualized by inverted phase-light microscopy. Commercial enzyme-linked immunosorbent assay (ELISA) kits (eBioscence, Inc., San Diego, CA, USA) were used to quantify the IL-6 and IL-8 concentrations in the culture supernatants according to the manufacturer's protocols. The absorbance at 450 nm (A_{450}) was recorded using a microplate reader with the wavelength correction set at 570 nm. Assays were performed in triplicate in two independent experiments and the means ± standard deviations were calculated.

Stimulation of the 3D co-culture model

The 3D co-culture model was pre-treated for 2 h with hBD-3 (10 and 20 µM) or LL-37 (0.1 and 0.2 µM), or both, prior to being stimulated with *A. actinomycetemcomitans* LPS (1 µg/mL) for 24 h at 37°C in a 5% CO_2 atmosphere. These concentrations of hBD-3 and LL-37 were selected based on preliminary assays in the 3D co-culture model that showed that such amounts of antimicrobial peptides were not cytotoxic and provided a moderate anti-inflammatory effect (data not shown). Co-cultures not pre-treated with hBD-3 or LL-37 and not stimulated with LPS were used as controls. The supernatants were collected, centrifuged (1000 ×g for 5 min at 4°C), and stored at −20°C until used. Assays were performed in triplicate.

Determination of the viability of the OBA-9 and HGF-1 cell lines

We determined the effect of hBD-3, LL-37, and *A. actinomycetemcomitans* LPS, individually and in combination, on the viability of the OBA-9 and HGF-1 cells. Briefly, HGF-1 and OBA-9 cells (1×10^4 cells/well) were seeded in the wells of a 96-well microplate (0.1 mL/well) (Sarstedt) and were incubated for 4 h at 37°C in a 5% CO_2 atmosphere to allow cell adhesion. The culture medium was then aspirated, and the cells were pre-treated for 2 h with hBD-3 (5, 10, 20, 40 µM) and/or LL-37 (0.05, 0.1, 0.2, 0.5, 1, 5 µM) prior to adding 1 µg/mL of *A. actinomycetemcomitans* LPS. The cells were incubated for an additional 24 h at 37°C in a 5% CO_2 atmosphere. A colorimetric MTT cell viability assay (Roche Diagnostics, Mannheim, Germany) using 3-[4,5-diethylthiazol-2-yl]-2,5-diphenyltetrazolium bromide as the substrate was performed according to the manufacturer's protocol. Untreated control cells were assigned a value of 100%, and all the other conditions were compared to the control. Results are expressed as means ± standard deviations of duplicate assays from two independent experiments.

Determination of cytokine secretion using multiplex ELISA assays

Samples of the 3D co-culture model subjected to the various treatments were sent to Eve Technologies (Calgary, AB, Canada, http://www.evetechnologies.com) for multiplex ELISA analyses. Eve Technologies uses the Bio-Plex Suspension Array System to quantify 41 different cytokines, chemokines, and growth factors (Human 41-Plex Discovery Assay): epidermal growth factor (EGF), C-C motif chemokine 11 (Eotaxin-1), basic fibroblast growth factor (FGF-2), FMS-like tyrosine kinase 3 ligand (Flt3l), chemokine (C-X3-C motif) ligand 1 (Fractalkine), granulocyte colony-stimulating factor (G-CSF), granulocyte-macrophage colony-stimulating factor (GM-CSF), CXC-chemokine ligand 1 (GRO-α), interferon alpha 2 (IFN-α2), interferon gamma (IFNγ), interleukin-1 alpha (IL-1α), interleukin-1 beta (IL-1β), interleukin-1 receptor antagonist (IL-1ra), interleukin-2 (IL-2), interleukin-3 (IL-3), interleukin-4 (IL-4), interleukin-5 (IL-5), interleukin-6 (IL-6), interleukin-7 (IL-7), interleukin-8 (IL-8), interleukin-9 (IL-9), interleukin-10 (IL-10), interleukin-12B (IL-12B), interleukin-12 (p70) [IL-12 (p70)], interleukin-13 (IL-13), interleukin-15 (IL-15), interleukin 17A (IL-17A), interferon-γ inducible protein 10 (IP-10), monocyte chemo-attractant protein 1 (MCP-1), monocyte-specific chemokine 3 (MCP-3), C-C motif chemokine 22 (MDC), macrophage inflammatory protein 1α (MIP-1α), macrophage inflammatory protein 1β (MIP-1β), platelet-derived growth factor AA (PDGF-AA), platelet-derived growth factor AB/BB (PDGF-AB/BB), regulated on activation, normal T cell expressed and secreted (RANTES), soluble CD40 ligand (sCD40L), transforming growth factor alpha (TGF-α), tumor necrosis factor alpha (TNF-α), tumor necrosis factor beta (TNF-β), and vascular endothelial growth factor A (VEGF-A).

Data analysis

To determine the synergistic inhibitory effect of hBD-3 and LL-37 on cytokine secretion following stimulation of the 3D co-culture model with *A. actinomycetemcomitans* LPS, the sums of the inhibition values of each peptide were compared with the values of both compounds used in combination. Experiments were carried out a minimum of three times to ensure reproducibility. The means ± SD from a representative experiment are presented. Differences between the means were analyzed for statistical significance using a one-way ANOVA. Statistical significance was set at $p < 0.05$.

Results

The HGF-1 gingival fibroblast cells (Figure 2A), OBA-9 gingival epithelial cells (Figure 2B), and the 3D co-culture model composed of both cell types were observed by light microscopy. Given the density and close proximity of epithelial cells and fibroblasts in the 3D co-culture model, several interactions between the two cells types are likely to occur.

Preliminary experiments showed that the treatment of the gingival fibroblasts and epithelial cells with 1 µg/mL of *A. actinomycetemcomitans* LPS had no cytotoxic effect (data not shown). To determine whether the interactions between the two cell types modified the response to LPS stimulation, the secretion of IL-6 and IL-8 by each cell type and by the 3D co-culture model was determined by ELISA. While the stimulation of the fibroblasts with LPS did not significantly increase IL-6 and IL-8 secretion, the stimulation of the epithelial cells with LPS resulted in the secretion of higher amounts of both cytokines compared to the unstimulated cells (Figure 3). More specifically, the secretion of IL-6 and IL-8 by epithelial cells increased by 97% and 120%, respectively, in the presence of LPS. Interestingly, the LPS-stimulated 3D co-culture model had a synergistic response with respect to the secretion of IL-6 and IL-8 compared to that of the individual cell types (Figure 3), secreting 475 pg/mL of IL-6 and 756 pg/mL of IL-8 compared to 239 pg/mL and 496 pg/mL, respectively, by the

individual cell lines. No synergistic effect was observed in the absence of LPS stimulation (Figure 3).

Prior to investigating the anti-inflammatory potential of hBD-3 and LL-37 in the 3D co-culture model, we determined their effect on the viability of LPS-stimulated gingival epithelial cells and gingival fibroblasts. None of the concentrations of hBD-3 (5, 10, 20, and 40 µM) and LL-37 (0.05, 0.1, 0.2, 0.5, 1, and 5 µM) tested had a significant effect on the viability of either cell type (Figure 4A). We then determined the effect of combinations of concentrations of hBD-3 (10 and 20 µM) and LL-37 (0.05, 0.1, 0.2, 0.5, and 1 µM) on cell viability. None of the combinations of hBD-3 and LL-37 had a cytotoxic effect on the OBA-9 and HGF-1 cells (Figure 4B). The viability of the 3D co-culture model was also not affected by hBD-3 and LL-37 (data not shown).

The LPS-stimulated 3D co-culture model was then used to investigate the anti-inflammatory properties of hBD-3 (10 and 20 µM) and LL-37 (0.1 and 0.2 µM) alone and in combination. The concentrations of 41 cytokines, chemokines, and growth factors in the cell-free culture supernatants were assayed using a multiplex ELISA assay. Only G-CSF, GRO-α, IP-10, IL-6, IL-8, and MCP-1 were detected in the culture supernatants. *A. actinomycetemcomitans* LPS significantly increased the secretion of G-CFS (36-fold), GRO-α (8-fold), IP-10 (20-fold), IL-6 (10-fold), IL-8 (20-fold), and MCP-1 (5-fold) by the 3D co-culture model compared to the unstimulated control (Figure 5). In the absence of

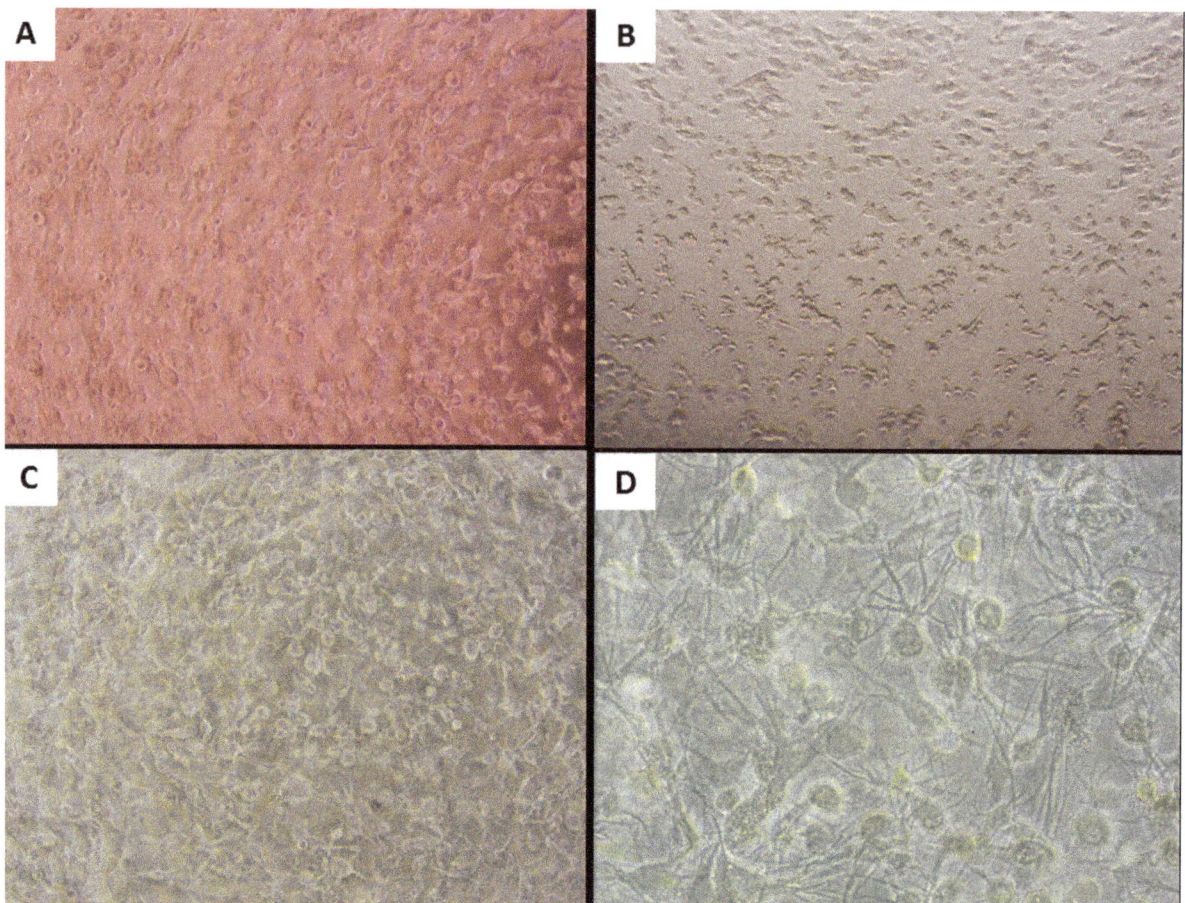

Figure 2. Light microscopic observations of the individual cell lines and the 3D co-culture model. A: Collagen-gingival fibroblast (HGF-1) gel; B: Gingival epithelial cells (OBA-9) seeded on the collagen gel; C and D: 3D co-culture model composed of gingival fibroblasts embedded in a collagen matrix overlaid with gingival epithelial cells. The epithelial cells, fibroblasts, and 3D co-culture model were stimulated with *A. actinomycetemcomitans* LPS (1 µg/mL) for 24 h at 37°C in a 5% CO$_2$ atmosphere. Panels A, B, and C (4× magnification). Panel D (10× magnification).

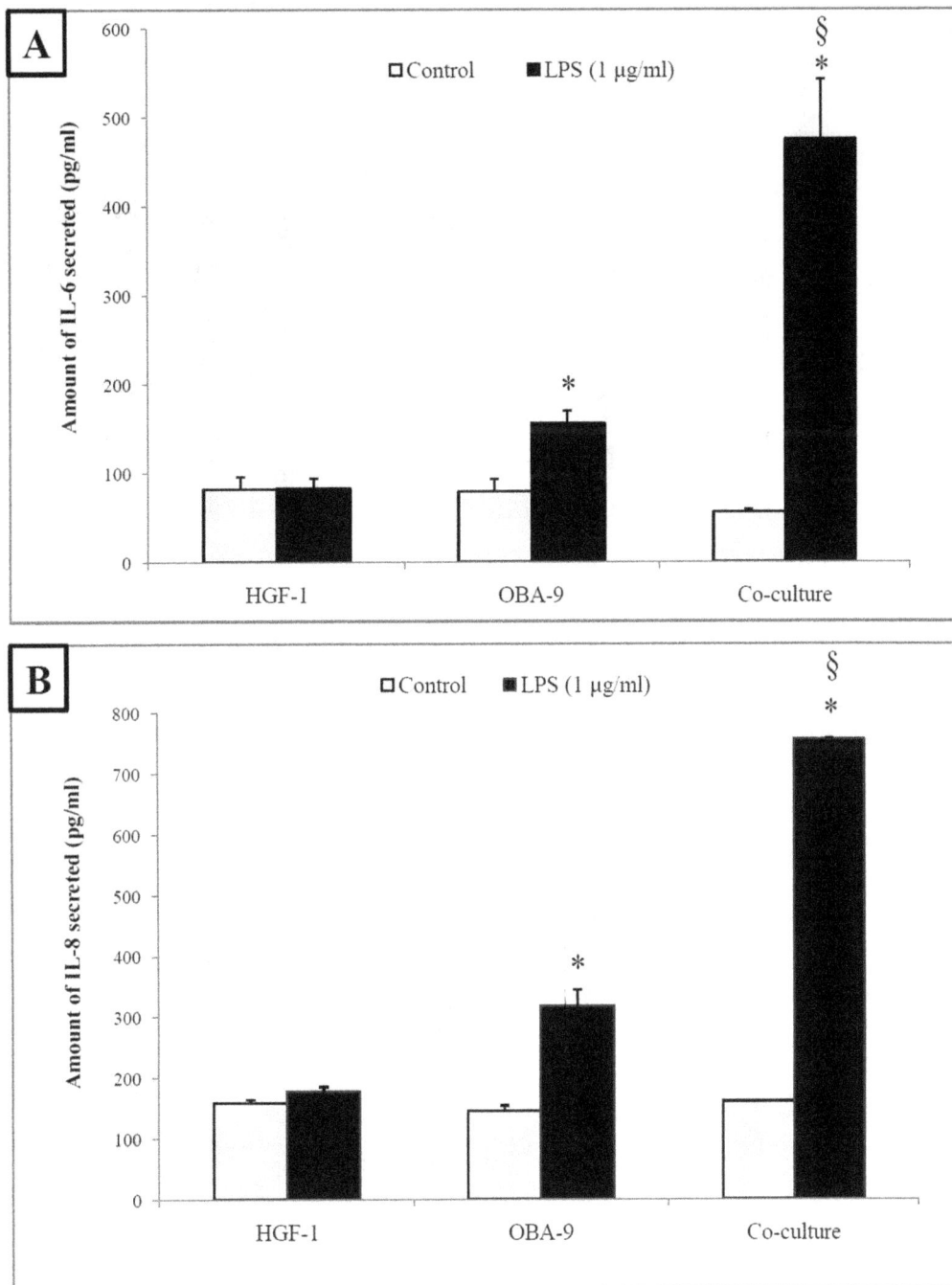

Figure 3. Amount of IL-6 (A) and IL-8 (B) secreted by gingival fibroblasts (HGF-1), gingival epithelial cells (OBA-9), and the 3D co-culture model in the absence and presence of *A. actinomycetemcomitans* **LPS (1 μg/mL).** Results are expressed as means ± standard deviation of triplicate assays from two independent experiments. *, $p < 0.05$: significantly different from the control cells without LPS stimulation for the individual cell lines and the 3D co-culture model; §, $p < 0.05$: synergistic effect of the cells in the 3D co-culture model compared to the individual cell lines.

LPS stimulation, hBD-3 and LL-37 did not induce any secretion of the above factors (data not shown). While the secretion of the cytokines was significantly reduced by 10 and 20 μM hBD-3 and by 0.1 and 0.2 μM LL-37 alone, only the secretion of GRO-α and IP-10 was significantly reduced by all the concentrations of hBD-3 and LL-37 tested following the stimulation of the 3D co-culture model with LPS. hBD-3 (20 μM) and LL-37 (0.1 μM) in combination synergistically inhibited the secretion of five of the six cytokines (G-CSF, GRO-α, IP-10, IL-6, and MCP-1) by the LPS-stimulated 3D co-culture model (Figure 5). All the concentrations of hBD-3 and LL-37 tested in combination had a synergistic inhibitory effect on the secretion of G-CSF. None of the concentrations of hBD-3 and LL-37 tested in combination had a synergistic inhibitory effect on the secretion of IL-8.

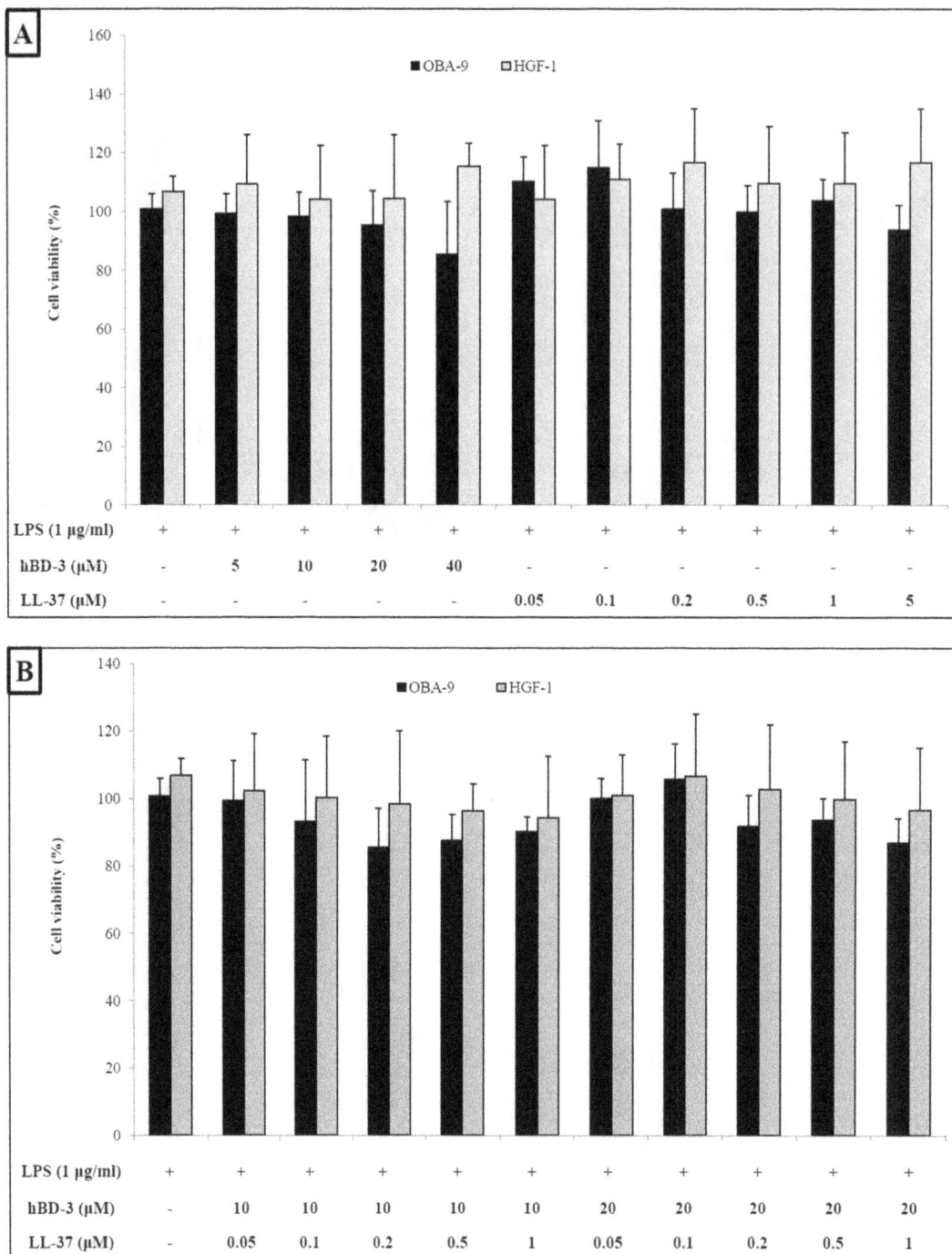

Figure 4. Effect of hBD-3 and LL-37 alone (A) and in combination (B) on the viability of LPS-stimulated gingival fibroblasts (HGF-1) and gingival epithelial cells (OBA-9). Untreated cells were assigned a value of 100%. All the other stimulations were compared to the control. Results are expressed as means ± standard deviation of duplicate assays from two independent experiments. No statistical significance was observed using ANOVA.

Discussion

Previous studies have shown that hBD-3 and LL-37 display anti-inflammatory activity in monocultures of fibroblasts, monocytes, macrophages, and periodontal ligament cells [43–46]. In this study, we investigated for the first time the anti-inflammatory activities of hBD-3 and LL-37, individually and in association, in a 3D co-culture model of gingival epithelial cells and fibroblasts, the two main cell types of the periodontium. Cytokine secretion by the co-culture model was induced by *A. actinomycetemcomitans* LPS based on a previous study showing that among LPS isolated from a number of periodontopathogens, the one of *A. actinomycetemcomitans* induced the highest pro-inflammatory response [47].

The 3D co-culture model is advantageous in that it takes interactions between gingival epithelial cells and fibroblasts into consideration. It has previously been shown that gingival

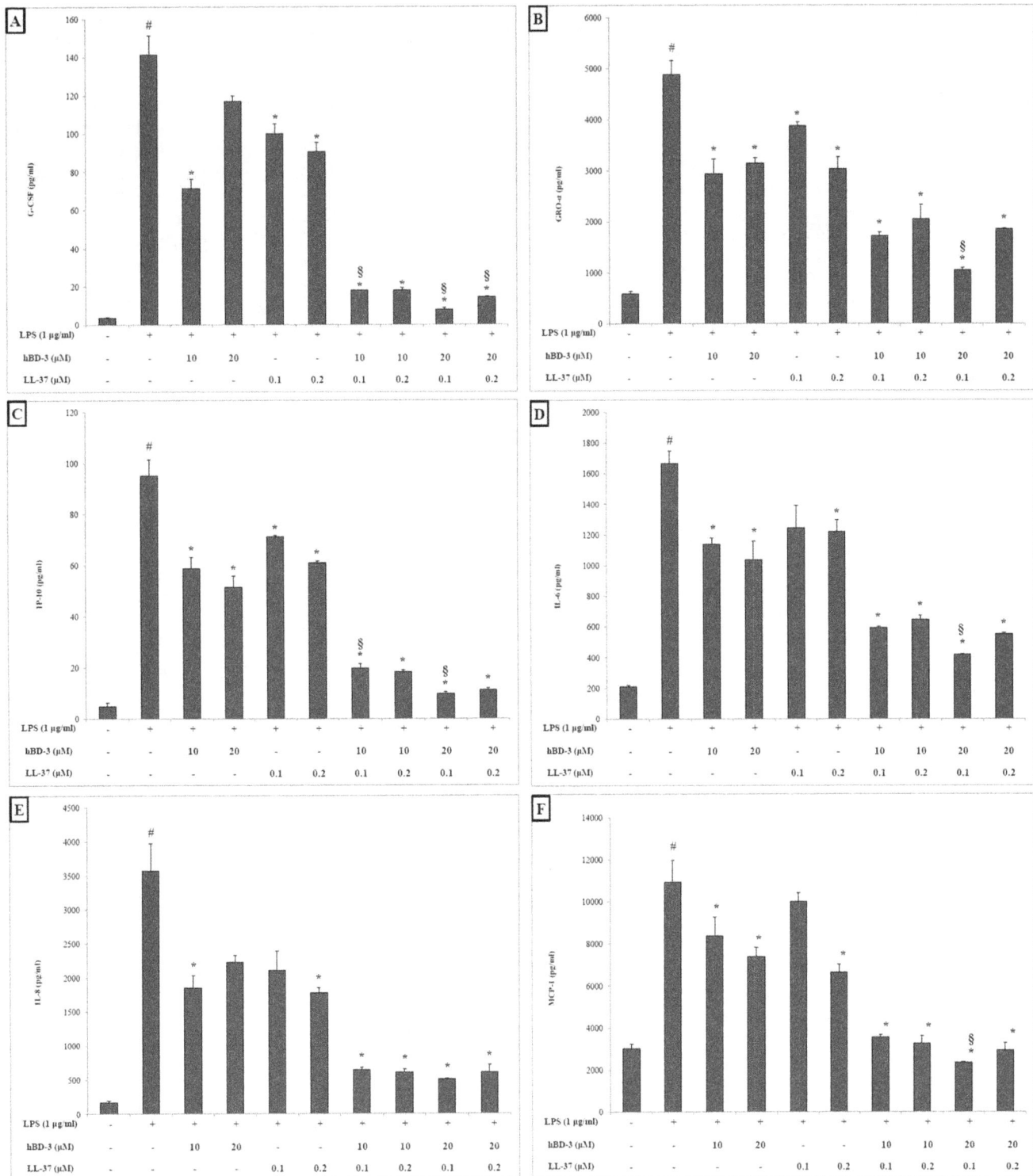

Figure 5. Effect of hBD-3 and LL-37 alone and in combination on the secretion of G-CFS (A), GRO-α (B), IP-10 (C), IL-6 (D), IL-8 (E), and MCP-1 (F) by the LPS-stimulated 3D co-culture model. Results are expressed as means ± standard deviation of triplicate assays from two independent experiments. #, significantly higher than the unstimulated (LPS) negative control ($p<0.01$); *, significantly lower than the untreated (hBD-3, LL-37) positive control ($p<0.05$); §, synergistic effect of the peptides; significantly lower than the sum of the inhibitory values of each peptide alone ($p<0.05$) compared to the two peptides in combination.

fibroblasts stimulate the proliferation of keratinocytes, while keratinocytes induce the expression of specific fibroblast genes [48,49]. Gron et al. [50] reported that cultivating oral fibroblasts and keratinocytes together increases the secretion of keratinocyte and hepatocyte growth factors, thus modulating the proliferation and migration of the junctional epithelium. Interactions between gingival fibroblasts and epithelial cells were also observed in our study as evidenced by the fact that the amounts of IL-6 and IL-8 secreted by the LPS-stimulated 3D co-culture model are significantly higher than the amounts secreted by the individual cell lines.

There has been growing interest in recent years in the synergistic antimicrobial and anti-inflammatory properties of various compounds, more particularly because many diseases, including periodontitis, have a multifactorial etiology. During periodontitis, periodontopathogens activate the host inflammatory response, resulting in the secretion of pro-inflammatory mediators, which in turn modulate the destruction of tooth-supporting tissues [7]. Compounds such as AMPs that possess both antimicrobial and anti-inflammatory properties may be potential alternatives to antibiotics in adjunctive therapies for treating periodontitis [51]. In addition to their antimicrobial properties, some AMPs can modulate the immune response and can bind directly to LPS, preventing the binding of LPS to the CD14 receptor and thus inhibiting the secretion of some pro-inflammatory cytokines [32,52]. Some AMPs can also bind to LPS when it is already bound to macrophage receptors [53]. While a wide variety of human AMPs have been identified, cathelicidins and defensins are the two most thoroughly characterized families. LL-37 is the only member of cathelicidin family present in humans and is produced by several cell types, including epithelial cells, monocytes, and natural killer cells [17,54,55]. In addition to have antibacterial activity, it also possesses a broad range of immuno-modulatory effects that allow it to interact with host cell membrane receptors and to inhibit the interaction between these receptors and pathogens [17,54,55]. Defensins are found in humans, animals, and plants, and can interact with and disrupt the lipid membranes of microbial pathogens inducing bacterial lysis [29]. More specifically, hBD-3 is expressed by epithelial cells, and has also been shown to possess anti-inflammatory properties [14,15,21].

hBD-3 and LL-37 were selected to investigate their anti-inflammatory synergistic effect in the 3D co-culture model for several reasons. First, since these antimicrobial peptides belong to different families, we hypothesized that they are more likely to act in synergy given that hBD-3 modulates the immune response by binding to the TLR4 receptor, that LL-37 can bind to the TLR1/2 and TLR4 receptors [34,45]. Second, hBD-3 is the predominant defensin in the oral cavity and is produced and stored by cells in the gingival epithelium [56–58]. Lastly, many investigators have reported that hBD-3 and LL-37 possess anti-inflammatory properties [43–46], although the peptides were tested individually. Pingel et al. [59] reported that hBD-3 can significantly decrease the secretion of IL-6, IL-10, GM-CSF, and TNF-α by human myeloid dendritic cells stimulated with recombinant *Porphyromonas gingivalis* hemagglutinin B (rHagB), while Semple et al. [45] showed that hBD-3 inhibits the secretion of TNF-α and IL-6 by macrophages stimulated with *Escherichia coli* LPS. LL-37 is a potent LPS-neutralizing peptide [52,53] and strongly suppresses *E. coli* LPS- and *P. gingivalis* LPS-induced IL-6, IL-8, and CXCL 10 secretion by gingival fibroblasts [60]. In addition, Lee et al. [32] recently reported that LL-37 suppresses the pro-inflammatory activities of LPS from *Prevotella intermedia* and *Tannerella forsythia* in both monocytes and gingival fibroblasts.

We investigated the effect of hBD-3 and LL-37, individually and in combination, on cytokine secretion by the 3D co-culture model of gingival epithelial cells and fibroblasts stimulated with A. *actinomycetemcomitans* LPS. This model provides a better interpretation of the inflammatory process since it takes into consideration the possible synergistic effect mediated by cell interactions on cytokine secretion. The 3D co-culture model

secreted higher levels of MCP-11, GRO-α, IL-6, and IL-8 and, to a lesser extent, IP-10 and G-CSF in response to A. *actinomyce-temcomitans* LPS. All of these molecules may contribute in different ways to the progression of periodontitis. As reported by Sager et al. [61], GRO-α induces an intense inflammatory response when injected into mice, contributing to the degradation of the extracellular matrix and promoting leukocyte infiltration. Kurtis et al. [9] reported that the concentration of MCP-1 in the GCF from diseased sites is significantly higher than in the GCF from healthy sites. Moreover, IL-6 and IL-8 are important inflammatory mediators secreted by macrophages, fibroblasts, and epithelial cells and are found in high concentrations in inflamed gingival and periodontal tissues [62–64]. Almasri et al. [65] reported that gingival fibroblasts stimulated with *P. gingivalis* LPS secrete more GRO-α, IL-6, IL-8, and MCP-1 than unstimulated controls, which is in agreement with our results.

Our results showed that 10 μM hBD-3 and 0.2 μM LL-37 alone significantly reduce the secretion of G-CSF, GRO-α, IL-6, IL-8, IP-10, and MCP-1 by the 3D co-culture model in response to LPS. In addition to the anti-inflammatory property of each peptide alone, the combination of 20 μM hBD-3 and 0.1 μM LL-37 synergistically reduced the secretion of GM-SCF, GRO-α, IL-6, IP-10, and MCP-1 in response to LPS. However, the combination of hBD-3 and LL-37 only had an additive effect on reducing the secretion of IL-8 at all the concentrations tested compared to the 3D co-culture model. To the best of our knowledge, no study has reported that a combination of AMPs can exert a synergistic anti-inflammatory effect. However, Semple et al. [45] showed that the association of hBD-3 with 8-bromoadenosine-cAMP (8Br-cAMP), a membrane permeable cAMP analogue, reduces the secretion of TNF-α by mouse macrophages (RAW 264.7) more than hBD-3 or 8Br-cAMP alone. Semple et al. [45] concluded that hBD-3 acts through toll-like receptor 4 (TLR4) while evidence has been brought that LL-37 acts through both TLR4 and TLR1/2 [66]. The combination of the two peptides used in this study may thus be more effective in reducing pro-inflammatory cytokine secretion because they act through different signaling pathways.

It is still unclear whether hBD-3 and LL-37 are pro-inflammatory or anti-inflammatory. hBD-3 may behave like LL-37, which is a multifunctional modulator of the immune response and which is pro-inflammatory at high concentrations and anti-inflammatory activity at lower concentrations [67]. This may explain why hBD-3 at low concentrations (10 μM) was able to reduce the production of G-CSF and IL-8, although at higher concentration (20 μM) hBD-3 was not able to significantly reduce the production of those cytokines (Figure 5).

In summary, the 3D co-culture model used in the present study takes into consideration the interactions that may occur between different cell types (epithelial cells and fibroblasts) and thus mimics the in vivo condition more accurately compared to individual cell types. The 3D co-culture model produced a synergistic increase in the secretion of IL-6 and IL-8 following A. *actinomycetemcomitans* LPS stimulation compared to the individual cell lines. In addition, while hBD-3 and LL-37 both displayed anti-inflammatory activity when applied individually to the model, they acted in synergy when applied together. This suggests that the combination of the two AMPs could be a valuable strategy for replacing antibiotics in adjunctive therapies for the treatment of periodontitis. Further studies are required to investigate the effect of hBD-3 and LL-37 in vivo.

Synergistic Anti-Inflammatory Activity of the Antimicrobial Peptides Human Beta...

223

Author Contributions

Conceived and designed the experiments: TBLB MPAM DPS DG. Performed the experiments: TBLB. Analyzed the data: TBLB MPAM DPS DG. Contributed reagents/materials/analysis tools: DG. Wrote the paper: TBLB MPAM DPS DG.

References

1. Loesche WJ, Grossman NS (2001) Periodontal disease as a specific, albeit chronic, infection: diagnosis and treatment. Clin Microbiol Rev 14: 727–752.
2. Socransky SS, Haffajee AD (2005) Periodontal microbial ecology. Periodontol 2000 38: 135–187.
3. Slots J, Ting M (1999) *Actinobacillus actinomycetemcomitans* and *Porphyromonas gingivalis* in human periodontal disease: occurrence and treatment. Periodontol 2000 20: 82–121.
4. Fives-Taylor PM, Meyer DH, Mintz KP, Brissette C (1999) Virulence factors of *Actinobacillus actinomycetemcomitans*. Periodontol 2000 20: 136–167.
5. Madeira MF, Queiroz-Junior CM, Cisalpino D, Werneck SM, Kikuchi H, et al. (2013) MyD88 is essential for alveolar bone loss induced by *Aggregatibacter actinomycetemcomitans* lipopolysaccharide in mice. Mol Oral Microbiol 28: 415–424.
6. Yoshimura A, Hara Y, Kaneko T, Kato I (1997) Secretion of IL-1β, TNF-α, IL-8 and IL-1ra by human polymorphonuclear leukocytes in response to lipopolysaccharides from periodontopathic bacteria. J Periodont Res 32: 279–286.
7. Yucel-Lindberg T, Båge T (2013) Inflammatory mediators in the pathogenesis of periodontitis. Expert Rev Mol Med 5: 1–22.
8. Gamonal J, Acevedo A, Bascones A, Jorge O, Silva A (2001) Characterization of cellular infiltrate, detection of chemokine receptor CCR5 and interleukin-8 and RANTES chemokines in adult periodontitis. J Periodont Res 36: 194–203.
9. Kurtiş B, Tüter G, Serdar M, Akdemir P, Uygur C, et al. (2005) Gingival crevicular fluid levels of monocyte chemoattractant protein-1 and tumor necrosis factor-alpha in patients with chronic and aggressive periodontitis. J Periodontol 76: 1849–1855.
10. Liu RK, Cao CF, Meng HX, Gao Y (2001) Polymorphonuclear neutrophils and their mediators in gingival tissues from generalized aggressive periodontitis. J Periodontol 72: 1545–1553.
11. Pradeep AR, Daisy H, Hadge P, Garg G, Thorat M (2009) Correlation of gingival crevicular fluid interleukin-18 and monocyte chemoattractant protein-1 levels in periodontal health and disease. J Periodontol 80: 1454–1461.
12. Thunell DH, Tymkiw KD, Johnson GK, Joly S, Burnell KK, et al. (2010) A multiplex immunoassay demonstrates reductions in gingival crevicular fluid cytokines following initial periodontal therapy. J Periodont Res 45: 148–152.
13. Giannobile WV (2008) Host-response therapeutics for periodontal diseases. J Periodontol 79: 1592–1600.
14. Gorr SU (2009) Antimicrobial peptides of the oral cavity. Periodontol 2000 51: 152–180.
15. Gursoy UK, Kononen E (2012) Understanding the roles of gingival beta-defensins. J Oral Microbiol 4: 1–10.
16. Cederlund A, Gudmundsson GH, Agerberth B (2011) Antimicrobial peptides important in innate immunity. FEBS J 278: 3942–3951.
17. Durr UH, Sudheendra US, Ramamoorthy A (2006) LL-37, the only human member of the cathelicidin family of antimicrobial peptides. Biochim Biophys Acta 1758: 1408–1425.
18. Vankeerberghen A, Nuytten H, Dierickx K, Quirynen M, Cassiman J-J, et al. (2005) Differential induction of human beta-defensin expression by periodontal commensals and pathogens in periodontal pocket epithelial cells. J Periodontol 76: 1293–1303.
19. Bachrach G, Chaushu G, Zigmond M, Yefenof E, Stabholz A, et al. (2006) Salivary LL-37 secretion in individuals with Down syndrome is normal. J Dent Res 85: 933–936.
20. Chung WO, Dommisch H, Yin L, Dale BA (2007) Expression of defensins in gingiva and their role in periodontal health and disease. Curr Pharm Des 213: 3073–3083.
21. Gorr SU (2012) Antimicrobial peptides in periodontal innate defense. Front Oral Biol 15: 84–98.
22. Tao R, Jurevic RJ, Coulton KK, Tsutsui MT, Roberts MC, et al. (2005) Salivary antimicrobial peptide expression and dental caries experience in children. Antimicrob Agents Chemother 49: 3883–3883.
23. Carlisle MD, Srikantha RN, Brogden KA (2009) Degradation of alpha- and beta-defensins by culture supernatants of *Porphyromonas gingivalis* strain 381. J Innate Immun 1: 118–122.
24. Ji S, Kim Y, Min BM, Han SH, Choi Y (2007) Innate immune responses of gingival epithelial cells to nonperiodontopathic and periodontopathic bacteria. J Periodont Res 42: 503–510.
25. Maisetta G, Brancatisano FL, Esin S, Campa M, Batoni G (2011) Gingipains produced by *Porphyromonas gingivalis* ATCC 49417 degrade human β-defensin 3 and affect peptide's antibacterial activity in vitro. Peptides 32: 1073–1077.
26. Joly S, Maze C, McCray PB Jr, Guthmiller JM (2004) Human β-defensins 2 and 3 demonstrate strain-selective activity against oral microorganisms. J Clin Microbiol 42: 1024–1029.
27. Komatsuzawa H, Ouhara K, Kawai T, Yamada S, Fujiwara T, et al. (2007) Susceptibility of periodontopathogenic and cariogenic bacteria to defensins and potential therapeutic use of defensins in oral diseases. Curr Pharm Des 13: 3084–3095.
28. Scott MG, Yan H, Hancock RE (1999) Biological properties of structurally related alpha-helical cationic antimicrobial peptides. Infect Immun 67: 2005–2009.
29. Brandenburg LO, Merres J, Albrecht LJ, Varoga D, Pufe T (2012) Antimicrobial peptides: multifunctional drugs for different applications. Polymers 4: 539–560.
30. Sochacki KA, Barns KJ, Bucki R, Weisshaar JC (2011) Real-time attack on single *Escherichia coli* cells by the human antimicrobial peptide LL-37. Proc Natl Acad Sci 108: 77–81.
31. McCormick TS, Weinberg A (2010) Epithelial cell-derived antimicrobial peptides are multifunctional agents that bridge innate and adaptive immunity. Periodontol 2000 54: 195–206.
32. Lee SH, Jun HK, Lee HR, Chung CP, Choi BK (2010) Antibacterial and lipopolysaccharide (LPS)-neutralising activity of human cationic antimicrobial peptides against periodontopathogens. Int J Antimicrob Agents 35: 138–145.
33. Golec M (2007) Cathelicidin LL-37: LPS-neutralizing, pleiotropic peptide. Ann Agric Environ Med 14: 1–4.
34. Into T, Inomata M, Shibata K, Murakami Y (2010) Effect of the antimicrobial peptide LL-37 on Toll-like receptors 2-, 3- and 4- triggered expression of IL-6, IL-8 and CXCL10 in human gingival fibroblasts. Cell Immunol 264: 104–109.
35. Walters SM, Dubey VS, Jeffrey NR, Dixon DR (2010) Antibiotic-induced *Porphyromonas gingivalis* LPS release and inhibition of LPS-stimulated cytokines by antimicrobial peptides. Peptides 31: 1649–1653.
36. Maisetta G, Batoni G, Esin S, Luperini F, Pardini M, et al. (2003) Activity of human β-defensin 3 alone or combined with other antimicrobial agents against oral bacteria. Antimicrob Agents Chemother 47: 3349–3351.
37. Midorikawa K, Ouhara K, Komatsuzawa H, Kawai T, Yamada S, et al. (2003) *Staphylococcus aureus* susceptibility to innate antimicrobial peptides, β-defensins and CAP18, expressed by human keratinocytes. Infect Immun 71: 3730–3739.
38. Nagaoka I, Hirota S, Yomogida S, Ohwada A, Hirata M (2000) Synergistic actions of antibacterial neutrophil defensins and cathelicidins. Inflamm Res 49: 73–79.
39. Chen X, Niyonsaba F, Ushio H, Okuda D, Nagaoka I, et al. (2005) Synergistic effect of antibacterial agents human β-defensins, cathelicidin LL-37 and lysozyme against *Staphylococcus aureus* and *Escherichia coli*. J Dermatol Sci 40: 123–132.
40. Darveau RP, Hancock RE (1983) Procedure for isolation of bacterial lipopolysaccharides from both smooth and rough *Pseudomonas aeruginosa* and *Salmonella typhimurium* strains. J Bacteriol 155: 831–838.
41. Kusumoto Y, Hirano H, Saitoh K, Yamada S, Takedachi M, et al. (2004) Human gingival epithelial cells produce chemotactic factors interleukin-8 and monocyte chemoattractant protein-1 after stimulation with *Porphyromonas gingivalis* via toll-like receptor 2. J Periodontol 75: 370–379.
42. Gursoy UK, Pöllänen M, Könönen E, Uitto VJ (2012) A novel organotypic dento-epithelial culture model: effect of *Fusobacterium nucleatum* biofilm on β-defensin-2, -3, and LL-37 expression. J Periodontol 83: 242–247.
43. Jönsson D, Nilsson BO (2012) The antimicrobial peptide LL-37 is anti-inflammatory and proapoptotic in human periodontal ligament cells. J Periodont Res 47: 330–335.
44. Lee SH, Baek DH (2012) Antibacterial and neutralizing effect of human β-defensins on *Enterococcus faecalis* and *Enterococcus faecalis* lipoteichoic acid. J Endod 38: 351–356.
45. Semple F, Webb S, Li HN, Patel HB, Perretti M, et al (2010) Human beta-defensin 3 has immunosuppressive activity in vitro and in vivo. Eur J Immunol 40: 1073–1078.
46. Suphasiriroj W, Mikami M, Shimomura H, Sato S (2013) Specificity of antimicrobial peptide LL-37 to neutralize periodontopathogenic lipopolysaccharide activity in human oral fibroblasts. J Periodontol 84: 256–264.
47. Bodet C, Chandad F, Grenier D (2006) Anti-inflammatory activity of a high-molecular-weight cranberry fraction on macrophages stimulated by lipopolysaccharides from periodontopathogens. J Dent Res 85: 235–239.
48. Boukamp P, Breitkreutz D, Stark HJ, Fusenig NE (1990) Mesenchyme-mediated and endogenous regulation of growth and differentiation of human skin keratinocytes derived from different body sites. Differentiation 44: 150–161.
49. Smola H, Thiekotter G, Fusenig NE (1993) Mutual induction of growth factor gene expression by epidermal-dermal cell interaction. J Cell Biol 122: 417–429.
50. Grøn B, Stoltze K, Andersson A, Dabelsteen E (2002) Oral fibroblasts produce more HGF and KGF than skin fibroblasts in response to co-culture with keratinocytes. APMIS 110: 892–898.
51. Gorr SU, Abdolhosseini M (2011) Antimicrobial peptides and periodontal disease. J Clin Periodontol 38: 126–141.
52. Larrick JW, Hirata M, Balint RF, Lee J, Zhong J, et al. (1995) Human CAP18: a novel antimicrobial lipopolysaccharide-binding protein. Infect Immun 63: 1291–1297.

53. Rosenfeld Y, Papo N, Shai Y (2006) Endotoxin (lipopolysaccharide) neutralization by innate immunity host-defense peptides: peptide properties and plausible modes of action. J Biol Chem 281: 1636–1643.

54. Doss M, White MR, Tecle T, Hartshorn KL (2010) Human defensins and LL-37 in mucosal immunity. J Leukoc Biol 87: 79–92.

55. Nijnik A, Hancock REW (2009) The roles of cathelicidin LL-37 in immune defences and novel clinical applications. Curr Opin Hematol 16: 41–47.

56. Dunsche A, Acil Y, Dommisch H, Siebert R, Schroder JM, et al. (2002) The novel human beta-defensin-3 is widely expressed in oral tissues. Eur J Oral Sci 110: 121–124.

57. Lu Q, Samaranayake LP, Darveau RP, Jin L (2005) Expression of human beta-defensin-3 in gingival epithelia. J Periodont Res 40: 474–481.

58. Saitoh M, Abiko Y, Shimabukuro S, Kusano K, Nishimura M, et al. (2004) Correlated expression of human beta defensin-1, -2 and -3 mRNAs in gingival tissues of young children. Arch Oral Biol 49: 799–803.

59. Pingel LC, Kohlgraf KG, Hansen CJ, Eastman CG, Dietrich DE, et al. (2008) Human beta-defensin 3 binds to hemagglutinin B (rHagB), a non-fimbrial adhesin from *Porphyromonas gingivalis*, and attenuates a pro-inflammatory cytokine response. Immunol Cell Biol 86: 643–649.

60. Inomata M, Into T, Murakami Y (2010) Suppressive effect of the antimicrobial peptide LL-37 on expression of IL-6, IL-8 and CXCL10 induced by *Porphyromonas gingivalis* cells and extracts in human gingival fibroblasts. Eur J Oral Sci 118: 574–581.

61. Sager R, Anisowicz A, Pike MC, Beckmann P, Smith T (1992) Structural, regulatory, and functional studies of the GRO gene and protein. Cytokines 4: 96–116.

62. Dongari-Bagtzoglou A, Ebersole J (1996) Production of inflammatory mediators and cytokines by human gingival fibroblast following bacterial challenge. J Periodont Res 31: 90–98.

63. Mundy G (1991) Inflammatory mediators and the destruction of bone. J Periodont Res 26: 213–217.

64. Wendell KJ, Stein SH (2001) Regulation of cytokine production in human gingival fibroblasts following treatment with nicotine and lipopolysaccharide. J Periodontol 72: 1038–1044.

65. Almasri A, Wisithphrom K, Windsor IJ, Olson B (2007) Nicotine and lipopolysaccharide affect cytokine expression from gingival fibroblasts. J Periodontol 78: 533–541.

66. Mookherjee N, Brown KL, Bowdish DM, Doria S, Falsafi R, et al. (2006) Modulation of the TLR-mediated inflammatory response by the endogenous human host defense peptide LL-37. J. Immunol 176: 2455–2464.

67. Scott MG, Davidson DJ, Gold MR, Bowdish D, Hancock RE (2002) The human antimicrobial peptide LL-37 is a multifunctional modulator of innate immune responses. J Immunol 169: 3883–3891.

25

General Immune Status and Oral Microbiology in Patients with Different Forms of Periodontitis and Healthy Control Subjects

Jana Schmidt[2]*, Holger Jentsch[2], Catalina-Suzana Stingu[3], Ulrich Sack[1]

1 Institute for Clinical Immunology, University of Leipzig, Leipzig, Germany; Translational Centre for Regenerative Medicine (TRM), University of Leipzig, Leipzig, Germany, 2 Department of Cariology, Endodontology and Periodontology, University of Leipzig, Leipzig, Germany, 3 Institute for Medical Microbiology and Epidemiology of Infectious Diseases, University of Leipzig, Leipzig, Germany

Abstract

Objective: Immunological processes in the etiopathogenesis of periodontitis, especially the aggressive form, are not well understood. This study examined clinical as well as systemic immunological and local microbiological features in healthy controls and patients with different forms of periodontitis.

Materials and Methods: 14 healthy subjects, 15 patients diagnosed with aggressive periodontitis, and 11 patients with chronic periodontitis were recruited. Periodontal examination was performed and peripheral blood was collected from each patient. Lymphocyte populations as well as the release of cytokines by T-helper cells were determined by flow cytometry and enzyme linked immunosorbent spot assay. Subgingival plaque samples were taken from each individual and immediately cultivated for microbiological examination.

Results: When stimulating peripheral blood mononuclear cells (PBMCs) with lipopolysaccharide, a higher IL-1β release was found in patients with moderate chronic periodontitis compared to the other groups ($p < 0.01$). Numbers of B-cells, naïve and transitional B-cells, memory B-cells, and switched memory B-cells were within the reference range for all groups, but patients with chronic periodontitis showed the highest percentage of memory B-cells without class switch ($p = 0.01$). The subgingival plaque differed quantitatively as well as qualitatively with a higher number of Gram-negative anaerobic species in periodontitis patients. *Prevotella denticola* was found more often in patients with aggressive periodontitis ($p < 0.001$) but did not show an association to any of the systemic immunological findings. *Porphyromonas gingivalis*, which was only found in patients with moderate chronic periodontitis, seems to be associated with an activation of the systemic immune response.

Conclusion: Differences between aggressive periodontitis and moderate chronic periodontitis are evident, which raises the question of an inadequate balance between systemic immune response and bacterial infection in aggressive periodontitis.

Editor: Özlem Yilmaz, University of Florida, United States of America

Funding: The work presented in this paper was made possible by funding from the German Federal Ministry of Education and Research (BMBF 1315883). The study was supported by the Translational Centre for Regenerative Medicine (TRM), University of Leipzig, Leipzig, Germany (http://www.trm.uni-leipzig.de/). The funders had no role in study design, data collection and analysis, decision to publish, or preparation of the manuscript.

Competing Interests: The authors have declared that no competing interests exist.

* Email: jana.schmidt@medizin.uni-leipzig.de

Introduction

Periodontitis is an inflammatory disease affected by a variety of factors. Smoking and age as well as diabetes mellitus, which seems to be in a bidirectional relationship with periodontitis [1], and stress are known risk factors. Furthermore, gender [2], education level [3], and immunological diseases such as HIV-infection [4] influence the presentation of periodontal diseases. On the other hand, periodontal inflammation seems to promote cardiovascular diseases, stroke, and pneumonia [5–7]. Therefore, especially severe forms of periodontitis are of common and interdisciplinary interest. Chronic periodontitis is a quite common disease in adult patients characterized by pocket formation and/or recession [8]. While progressive loss of periodontal attachment occurs slowly to moderately [9], local risk factors, e.g. bacterial plaque and calculus, accelerate loss of attachment particularly rapidly [10].

Aggressive periodontitis is characterized by its severe and fast progressing destructive course in young individuals, which often leads to tooth loss early in life followed by the need for prosthetic treatment. Family aggregation is described [11]. Discrepancies between local factors and disease severity are often presented [10]. Diagnosis should be based upon all available information referring to general and special anamnesis and after careful clinical examination of a patient [12].

The microbiological differences between the chronic and aggressive forms of periodontitis are a topic of extensive debate. It is generally accepted that potential pathogenic bacteria belong to the commensal oral microflora [13]. Rescala et al. could not find any differences in the microbial profile between patients with chronic and aggressive periodontitis [14]. Most species, like *Porphyromonas gingivalis*, seem to be associated with probing depth rather than with aggressive or chronic periodontitis [15]. Other authors showed associations between different pathogens (*P. gingivalis, T. forsythia, T. denticola*) and chronic periodontitis [16].

Innate and adaptive immunity are both arms of the immune system defending the organism against pathogens. The first wall of defense against invading pathogens is the innate immunity, which is activated within a few hours. If the innate immunity is not able to limit an infection, adaptive immunity develops accompanied by the development of immunological memory [17]. Lipopolysaccharide (LPS) is a potent stimulator of the immune system due to its endotoxic, highly conserved lipid region (lipid A) [18]. Different Gram-negative bacteria express different forms of LPS on their surface enabling them to activate pattern recognition receptors (PRR) as toll-like-receptors (TLR) [19]. Enterobacteria such as *Escherichia coli* stimulate TLR-4 as does the LPS found on the periodontal pathogen *Porphyromonas gingivalis* [20]. A cluster of cytokines released by peripheral blood mononuclear cells (PBMCs) when stimulated by LPS could give additional information about patients' susceptibility to periodontitis. Cytokines, such as Interleukin (IL)-1β, as well as chemokines, such as IL-8, play an important role in immune regulation, managing the maturation of dendritic cells and leading to the initiation of the transition from innate to adaptive immune response [21]. This transition is mainly initiated in regional lymph nodes by dendritic cells presenting bacterial antigens to naïve T-cells with their corresponding receptor [22]. A suitable T-cell is activated by interaction with an antigen-presenting cell which presents antigen fragments on its major histocompatibility complex (MHC). The MHC-antigen-complex activates the T-cell-receptor, thereby stimulating cytokine release by CD4 T-helper cells or activating cytotoxic T-cells which express CD8 [17]. T-helper cells express receptors, which only interact with MHC-II bound antigens. They play a major role in modulating the immune response without being phagocytic and express only partially cytotoxic activity. Different types of T-helper cells play a role in the pathogenesis of periodontal disease: Th2-cells induce the humoral B-cell response by releasing IL-4, IL-5, and IL-10 on the one hand and suppress the T-cell mediated immune response on the other hand [23]. Therefore, this Th-cell subset is associated with non-protective antibody response resulting in aggressive periodontitis and progression of periodontal lesions. Contrary to the Th2-cells, Th1-cells are associated with stable periodontal lesions [24,25]. This can be explained by the cellular immune response stimulated by IL-12 and IFN-γ, which are characteristic Th-1 cytokines [26], and the inhibition of the differentiation of osteoclasts by self-fusion of macrophages [27]. Furthermore, the immune response mediated by Th1-cells is associated with the generation of specific antibodies [16]. Besides Th1- and Th2-cells, Th17-cells and regulatory Th-cells are described: Th17-cells produce IL-17, which induces the release of IL-6, IL-8, and prostaglandin E$_2$. Furthermore, the activation of osteoclasts by Th17-cells has been shown [16], which leads to the progression of (alveolar) bone loss. Regulatory Th-cells (CD4+ CD25+) were found to have anti-inflammatory and protective effects by which they possibly control gingival inflammation as well as alveolar bone resorption [28]. They were found in periodontal lesions in cases of increasing percentages of B-cells [29].

Memory B-cells express CD27, a member of the TNF-receptor-family, on their surface, which is also expressed by naïve T-cells. CD27 binds CD70, a surface protein of dendritic cells and thereby mediates the interaction between dendritic cells und B-cells [30].

As shown above, different immunological aspects are suspected to play roles in the development of periodontal diseases. Furthermore, microbiological features are reported to determine pathogenesis. In our study, we intended to examine clinical as well as immunological and microbiological features in patients with different forms of periodontitis and healthy controls. We hypothesized that there would be differences in the percentage of CD4+ T-cells producing IL-4 between patients suffering from aggressive periodontitis compared to patients with chronic periodontitis and healthy controls. The Th1/Th2 ratio was expected to be lower in patients with aggressive periodontitis compared to the other groups, because Th1-responses are linked with a potent immune response as explained above. Furthermore, we hypothesized that PBMCs' expression of IL-1β and IL-8 upon stimulation with standardized extracts of bacterial antigens would differentiate the groups. Differences were expected in the microbiological profile between healthy controls and patients, but not between the different groups of patients suffering from moderate chronic periodontitis (CP) or aggressive periodontitis (AP).

Materials and Methods

Ethics statement

We recruited patients for our study from the Department of Cariology, Endodontology, and Periodontology, University of Leipzig, Germany, according to the ethics committee approval of the Ethics Committee of the Faculty of Medicine, University of Leipzig, Germany (registry number 151-2009-06072009, in German). Every patient was informed about the aim and the course of the study and signed a consent form as well as a data protection policy.

Subject selection

Every subject filled out a questionnaire about their medical history and some main aspects of oral hygiene. The subjects included were in good general health (no history of diabetes, hepatitis or HIV infection; no immunosuppressive chemotherapy; no diseases which compromise the immune system) and had at least 20 teeth. All subjects had to be of European descent and non-smokers for at least five years or occasional smokers with a cigarette consumption of up to ten cigarettes per week [31]. Patients were excluded if there was any immunosuppressive therapy in their medical history or if they took antibiotics during the previous six months. Female patients were excluded if pregnant or lactating.

The diagnosis was based on clinical and radiographic parameters and in accordance with the Classification of Periodontal Diseases [32]. We conducted a six-point-measurement of each tooth, recording probing depth (PD), clinical attachment loss (CAL), tooth mobility (TM), and bleeding on probing (BOP). To assess oral hygiene, the Interproximal Plaque Index (IPI) adapted from Lange [33] was assessed after coloring the plaque with "Mira 2 Ton", Hager and Werken (Leimen, Germany). Periodontal measurements were performed by two dentists using the rigid Parodontometer UNC#UNC15, Hu Friedy (Leimen, Germany). The intra- and inter-examiner reproducibility of measurement was tested before commencing the study.

According to the measurement results the subjects were assigned into one of three clinical categories:

(1) Healthy control group (HC): Subjects aged between 21 to 35 years with no history of periodontal disease and no PD >3 mm (excluding third molars) or CAL >1 mm.

(2) Moderate chronic periodontitis (CP): Patients between 30 and 60 years old with tooth sites exhibiting 3 to 4 mm of CAL and ≥4 mm PD, in at least three teeth in two or more different quadrants. Fast progression of periodontal disease led to exclusion.

(3) Aggressive periodontitis (AP): The diagnosis was made before age 35 or retrospectively based on x-ray images made before the 35th birthday of the patient [34]. Rapidly progressive loss of attachment was confirmed and family aggregation likely (not absolutely necessary) in the patients. Patient tooth sites exhibited ≥5 mm PD and CAL in at least two remaining teeth. Radiographic bone loss was at least 50%, in at least two different teeth [34].

Reagents

LPS from *Escherichia coli* (L2654) was obtained from Sigma Aldrich (Saint Louis, Missouri USA) and ultrapure LPS from *Porphyromonas gingivalis* from Invivo Gen (San Diego, USA); CWPS (Pneumococcal-cell-wall-polysaccharide mixture) was obtained from Statens Serum Institute (Copenhagen, Denmark), and CEF peptide pool from R&D Systems (Minneapolis, USA). RPMI 1640 with L-Glutamine, HEPES (N-2-hydroxyethylpiperazine-N′-2-ethanesulfonic acid) and low-endotoxin fetal calf serum (FCS) were purchased from PAA (Pasching, Austria). Pairs of antibodies against IL-1β and IL-8 suitable for enzyme-linked immunosorbent spot (ELISpot) assay were obtained from BioLegend/BIOZOL (Eching, Germany). Streptavidin alkaline phosphatase (Streptavidin-ALP) was from Mabtech (Hamburg, Germany) and BCIP/NBT (5-bromo-4-chloro-3-indolyl-phosphate/nitro blue tetrazolium) substrate was from Sigma Aldrich (Steinheim, Germany).

Cell isolation, freezing procedure, and thawing of cells

Blood was deposited into BD Vacutainer-EDTA-Tubes (REF 368861) and CPT™ Cell Preparation Tubes (two tubes á 9 ml per patient). Deposited heparinized blood from the examined subjects was used as the source of peripheral blood mononuclear cells (PBMCs). After centrifugation at 430×g for 20 minutes at 21°C, the PBMC fraction was collected and washed twice in 50 ml of sterile PBS (phosphate buffered sodium chloride). The cells were suspended in 1500 μl of sterile fetal calf serum (FCS). In three sterile cryo tubes, 400 μl of sterile FCS were prepared and 500 μl of cell solution were added to each of them followed by gradually adding 100 μl of DMSO from Applichem (Darmstadt, Germany) and swinging the closed tube slowly back and forth before freezing it immediately in a Nalgene freezing box in a −80°C refrigerator. Cells were transferred into liquid nitrogen for long-term storage during the following month.

The thawing of the cells was performed according to an established protocol. The cells were counted and their viability was checked using trypan blue (Sigma Aldrich, Steinheim, Germany) exclusion. Cells were thawed and suspended to the desired concentration in cell culture medium, consisting of RPMI enriched with 10% FCS.

Measurement of IL-8 and IL-1β release from PBMCs

The ELISpot protocol to examine the release of IL-8 and IL-1β by PBMCs was based on the work of Smedmann et al., 2009 [35]. As the stimulation by LPS varies depending on the charge, we performed preliminary tests with healthy cells and found 200 ng/ml to be the concentration that lies completely in the linear range under the used culture conditions. According to the manufacturer's specification the LPS contained less than 1% protein and less than 1% RNA. Prior to coating, each of the PVDF (polyvinylidene

difluoride) membrane plates (MSIPS4510 from Millipore) were pre-wetted with 50 μl 35% ethanol/well for 2 minutes and washed five times with 200 μl sterile H₂O/well. Capture antibodies were diluted in sterile PBS to 7.5 μg/ml of which 100 μl was added to each well of the membrane plate. After incubation overnight at + 4°C, the coated wells were washed five times with 200 μl sterile PBS per well followed by blocking the membrane for 30 minutes with 200 μl/well of cell culture medium (RPMI +10% FCS). The medium was then removed and 100 μl/well of the same culture medium with and without stimulant (concentrations: *E. coli* and *Porphyromonas gingivalis* LPS: 200 ng/ml; CWPS: 200 ng/ml; prefabricated solution) were added followed by the addition of 100 μl/well of cell solution (3500 cells per well). We performed double determination. Plates were transferred to a 5% CO₂-incubator and incubated for 5 hours (for IL-8) and 21 hours (for IL-1β). After incubation the cells were removed by washing five times with 200 μl/well of sterile PBS using a multichannel pipette (Eppendorf). The biotinylated antibodies were diluted in PBS with 0.5% FCS to the concentration of 1 μg/ml and 100 μl were added per well. After incubation for 2 hours at room temperature in the case of IL-1β or overnight at +4°C in the case of IL-8, plates were washed as described above and developed as described in Smedmann et al.

Reading and counting of spots were performed with the AID Spot Reader. We divided the number of spots formed in wells without antigen-stimulation by the number of spots in wells with antigen-stimulation to calculate the stimulation-index (SI) for each stimulant.

$$SI = \frac{\text{cytokine release when stimulated with antigen (LPS)}}{\text{cytokine release without stimulation with antigen (blank value)}}$$

Flow cytometry diagnostics

CVID panel. Peripheral B-cell phenotyping was conducted using flow cytometry. 20 μl of normal serum mix consisting of mouse and goat serum (Dako) were pipetted in each FACS vial with the cell suspension, mixed well, and incubated for 10 minutes at room temperature in the dark. Subsequently, 39.5 μl of an antibody mix made of IgD FITC, CD21 PE, CD5 Per-Cy5.5, CD38 PE-Cy7, IgM APC, CD27 APC-H7, CD19 AmCyan (BD Biosciences, San Jose, California, USA), and CD24 Pacific Blue (EXBIO Praha, Vestec u Prahy, Czech Republic) were pipetted into the vials and mixed well. After another 15 minutes of incubation as described above, lysis buffer (BD Biosciences, San Jose, California USA) was added and the vials were incubated for another 10 minutes. After centrifugation at 250×g for 5 minutes, the supernatant was poured off and cells were suspended in 3 ml of PBS and mixed. After another round of washing the supernatant was discarded and the cell pellet was loosened and fixed by adding 250 μl of PBS with 1% formaldehyde. After fixation, measurement was carried out using a FACS Canto II and analyses were performed with BD Facs Diva.

Release of intracellular cytokines in T-helper (Th) cells. After thawing the PBMCs as described above, lymphocytes were stimulated by adding calcium ions, 10 ng/ml phorbol-12-myristate-13-acetate (PMA) (Sigma Aldrich, Steinhein, Germany) and ionomycin (1 μM) (Calbiochem, Merck, Darmstadt, Germany) to activate protein kinase C. To interrupt intracellular protein transport, monensin (2.5 μM) (Sigma Aldrich, Steinheim, Germany) was added. After 5 hours of incubation at 37°C in

CO_2-atmosphere, cells were washed with PBS +10% FCS and fixated for 10 minutes at 4°C. Subsequently, cells were permeabilized and visualization of cell type and cytokine production was conducted simultaneously using CD3 (BD Biosciences, San Jose, California USA), CD4-APC, and CD8-PC5 (IMMUNOTECH SAS, Marseille, France) for visualizing different T-cell-subsets. ALEXA Fluor 647 Mouse anti-Human IL-17A (BD Biosciences, San Diego, California USA), IOTest Anti-IFNγ-PE, and IOTest Anti-IL4-PE (Immunotech, Marseille, France) were used as antibodies to detect the released cytokines. As the percentage of IFN-γ producing T-cells represents the Th1 fraction and IL-4 is a typical Th2 cytokine, we divided the one percentage by the other to illustrate the ratio of Th1 and Th2 cells.

Microbiological diagnostics

Probes were taken from the four teeth with the highest values of PD and CAL, if possible each from another quadrant. One sterile paper point (ISO 50) was used per site and kept in situ for 10 seconds. All four paper points were immersed in an Eppendorf tube with 1 ml Brain Heart Infusion (BHI) Bouillon (Oxoid, Basingstoke, Hants, UK). The pooled probes were vortexed for 30 seconds and 10-fold serially diluted up to 10^{-5} in thioglycolate broth. For cultivation 100 µl of broth dilution (10^{-1} to 10^{-5}) were plated on Columbia blood agar (Oxoid, Basingstoke, Hants, UK) supplemented with or without gentamycin (100 mg) (Oxoid, Basingstoke, Hants, UK). Also, 100 µl aliquots (10^{-1} to 10^{-3}) were cultivated on trypticase soy serum bacitracin vancomycin (TSBV) agar (Oxoid, Basingstoke, Hants, UK) for the selective isolation and counting of A. actinomycetemcomitans. Columbia plates were incubated anaerobically at 37°C for 7 days and TSBV plates at 37°C in 10% CO_2 atmosphere for 3 days. Facultative anaerobic strains were not further included in the analysis while anaerobic strains were identified based on Gram stain, colony morphology, production of catalase, An-Ident disc pattern (Oxoid, Basingstoke, Hants, UK), and biochemical tests using the Rapid ID 32A system (BioMerieux, Lyon, France). A. actinomycetemcomitans was identified by its typical colony morphology (star-like inner structure) and the production of catalase.

Strains which could not be identified were frozen at −80°C for further analysis.

Frozen samples were thawed at room temperature. Subsequently, the templates were generated and analyzed using the DNeasy Blood and Tissue Kit (Qiagen, Hilden, Germany). 2.0 µl template was mixed with 48.0 µl mastermix (consisting of 36.75 µl distilled water, 5.0 µl buffer, 3.0 µl $MgCl_2$, 1.0 µl dNTPs, 1.0 µl BAK, 1.0 µl PC3mod, and 0.25 Taq polymerase). DNA amplification was done with the T-gradient (PCR-blog). 10.0 µl of the thus generated PCR product were plated on an agarose gel to evaluate PCR success. If the characteristic pattern was identified, the product was cleaned using an Invisorb Spin PCRapid Kit (Invitek, Berlin, Germany) according to manufacturer's instructions. The next step of sequencing required production of a mastermix of 8.0 µl distilled water, 4.0 µl marked dNTPs (Interdisciplinary Center for Clinical Research of the Medical Faculty, Leipzig) and 1.0 µl BAK (Biometra, Göttingen, Germany) as a primer. Sequencing was done in the thermocycler using program 3. 2.0 µl of natrium-acetate and 60.0 µl of 96% ethanol were added to the product and incubated for 15 minutes at room temperature followed by another 15 minutes of centrifugation at 1371×g. Subsequently, ethanol was removed carefully and 100.0 µl of 70% ethanol was added and centrifuged as described above. After removing the ethanol the product was dried at room temperature and given to the Interdisciplinary Center for Clinical Research of the Medical Faculty, Leipzig, for further analysis.

Identification was based on the 16S ribosome DNA genes [7] and with the aid of the BLAST database (http://blast.ncbi.nlm.nih.gov.Blast.cgi).

Four individuals were not microbiologically characterized because of internal hospital processes/sample handling.

Statistical analysis

Microsoft Excel 2010 was used for organizing the data. Statistical analyses and graphical display were conducted with SPSS Statistics 14.0 (SPSS Inc.). This program always performs an analysis whether the data follow a Gaussian distribution. Nearly all results did not follow a Gaussian distribution. Therefore, we decided to perform non-parametric analyses for all measurement groups, even in the few ones that did show a Gaussian distribution, because non-parametric tests always deliver accurate results.

We used the Kruskal-Wallis test for analyzing differences between different groups in stimulation indices for IL-8 and IL-1β as determined by ELISpot Assay. Bonferroni adaption was performed and differences were considered to be significant for $p < 0.008$.

Microbiological findings were analyzed using the Chi-Square-test and the Mann-Whitney-U-test. After the Bonferroni correction was applied, $p < 0.001$ was considered significant.

Associations between microbiological and immunological data were investigated with the Mann-Whitney-U-test and the Kruskal-Wallis-Test. Associations with $p < 0.05$ were considered significant and are shown in this article.

Results

As previously defined in the inclusion criteria, patients with aggressive periodontitis showed increased clinical attachment levels (median 3.4 mm) in accordance with advanced radiographic bone loss and pocket probing depths (median 3.2 mm) as displayed in Table 1. All included subjects were non-smokers and none of them reported any of the medical conditions leading to exclusion from the study. Patients suffering from moderate chronic periodontitis revealed worse oral hygiene represented by higher API values (median 36%) compared to patients with aggressive periodontitis (median 25%) and healthy subjects (median 12.5%). On the other hand, clinical signs of inflammation were much more pronounced in patients with aggressive periodontitis as shown by higher bleeding on probing (BOP) (Table 1).

Stimulation index for IL-1β significantly elevated in CP group

In the production of IL-1β by PBMCs, we found no difference between the healthy control (HC) and aggressive periodontitis (AP) groups, as is shown in Figure 1 (grouped boxplots for stimulation index). By contrast, we found significantly elevated stimulation indices in the chronic periodontitis (CP) group when PBMCs were stimulated by both P. gingivalis LPS and E. coli LPS (p = 0.002). Regarding the release of IL-8 we could not find any differences between the groups (no figure shown).

Highest percentage of memory B-cells without class switch in CP group

The results of the CVID-panel revealed that no immunodeficiency was present in any of the examined subjects. Numbers of B-cells, naïve and transitional B-cells, memory B-cells, and switched memory B-cells were within the reference range defined by Warnatz et al. [36].

Table 1. Mean Clinical Parameters of Study Patients.

		Aggressive Periodontitis (n = 15)	Chronic Periodontitis (n = 11)	Healthy Controls (n = 14)
		8 ♀, 7 ♂	5 ♀, 6 ♂	11 ♀, 3 ♂
Age [years]	x̄±σ	32.1±7.1	45.2±8.0	24.9±1.6
	x̃	31.0	46.0	25.0
IPI [%]	x̄±σ	30.7±15.2	35.6±16.4	12.1±5.5
	x̃	25.0	36.0	12.5
BOP [%]	x̄±σ	30.1±20.1	24.8±14.4	13.6±8.9
	x̃	24.6	17.5	17.0
CAL [mm]	x̄±σ	3.4±1.0	2.2±0.8	0.4±0.4
	x̃	3.4	2.2	0.3
PD [mm]	x̄±σ	3.3±1.0	2.7±0.7	2.0±0.3
	x̃	3.1	2.5	2.1
PD (max) [mm]	x̄±σ	7.7±2.7	5.3±1.4	3.6±0.6
	x̃	7.0	5.0	4.0
Bone loss [%]	x̄±σ	66.7±9.8	13.2±4.6	0.0±0.0
	x̃	70.0	15.0	0.0

IPI: interproximal plaque index; PD: probing depth; CAL: clinical attachment level; BOP: bleeding on probing; bone loss: maximum of radiographic bone loss.

Differences between the three groups were found in the percentage of memory B-cells without class switch as shown in Figure 2 with the highest median value in the CP group (33.03%) compared to the AP (15.06%) and HC (19.39) groups. This difference between moderate chronic periodontitis and the other two groups is significant (p = 0.01).

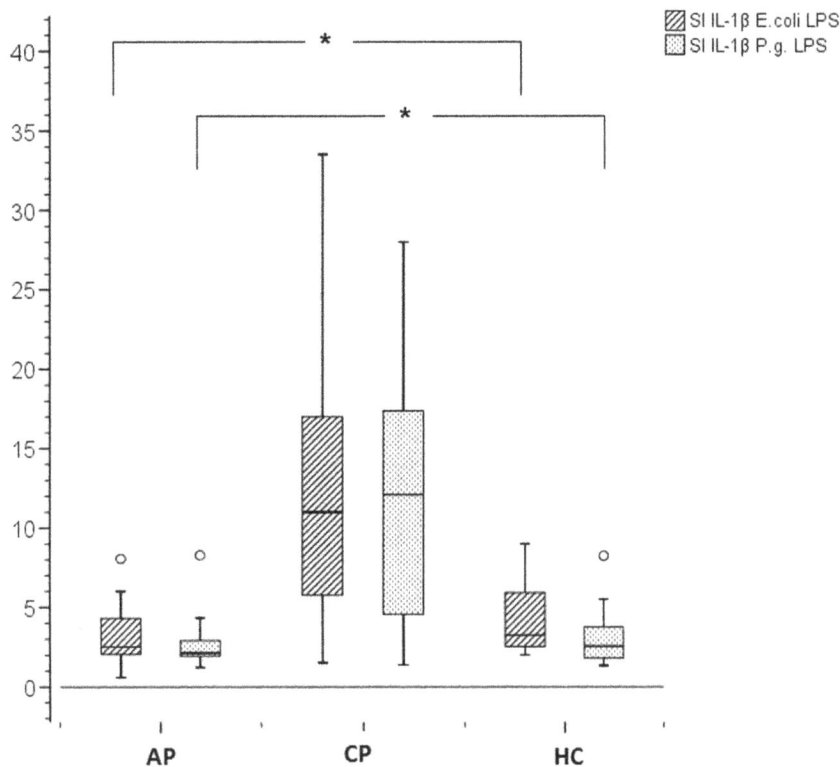

Figure 1. Stimulation Index for IL-1β. PBMCs (3500 cells/well) were stimulated for 20 hours with different forms of LPS (200 ng/ml). Stimulations were run in duplicate. Boxplots represent minimum, first quartile, median, third quartile, and maximum. Differences between the groups were considered to be significant for p<0.008 (Bonferroni adjustment).

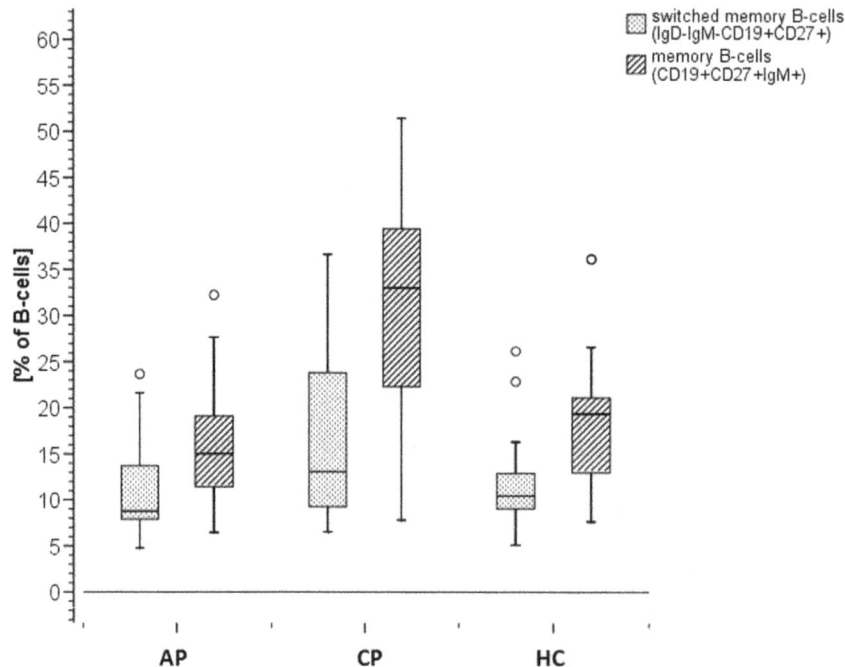

Figure 2. Percentage of Memory B-cells. Memory B-cells as percentage of CD19[+] B-cells measured by flow cytometry. Explorative analysis revealed a higher level of memory B-cells in patients with moderate chronic periodontitis (median of 33.03%) compared with healthy subjects and patients with aggressive periodontitis (median of 19.39%/15.06%). With a median of 19.39% for all subject groups, an increase in memory B-cells in patients with moderate chronic periodontitis is statistically significant (p = 0.01).

Intracellular cytokines showed a slightly reduced Th1 response in AP

As shown in Figure 3, regarding IL-4 and IFN-γ, a slightly higher intracellular cytokine secretion was found in PBMCs of subjects with CP with a median of 1.00% of the cells secreting IL-4 and 10.29% of the cells secreting IFN-γ compared to HC (0.67% and 7.55%) and AP (0.58% and 7.74%). Therefore, Th1/Th2-ratios showed a slightly reduced Th1 response in AP patients defined by a lower Th1/Th2 ratio (8.59) compared to healthy controls (10.93) and CP patients (11.83). No differences in PBMC-release of IL-17 when stimulated by PMA between the three groups were found. In each group the percentage of cells secreting IFN-γ was found to be higher compared to cells secreting IL-4 and IL-17.

Microbiological findings in relation to clinical diagnosis

All patients with chronic periodontitis, 12 of the 15 patients with aggressive periodontitis and 13 of the 14 healthy subjects were microbiologically examined. We identified 236 anaerobic isolates (186 strains from patients, 50 from healthy subjects). 51 different anaerobic species could be identified, with a mean of approximately 8 species per periodontitis patient and almost 4 species per healthy control subject. The detection frequencies of anaerobic bacteria are listed in Table 2. Subjects in whom a given species was detected were considered to be colonized by that species.

Only *Prevotella denticola* was significantly associated with AP and CAL (p = 0.001). All other associations were not statistically significant. *P. intermedia* and *F. nucleatum* were also found in healthy subjects but in lower quantities. We did not detect *A. actinomycetemcomitans* in any of our samples.

Microbiology in relation to immunological findings

We examined associations between immunological and micro-biological findings in an exploratory way to find possible links and generate topics for further research. Findings with p<0.05 are shown in Table 3, irrespective of periodontal diagnosis. For *Prevotella denticola*, which was shown to be associated with aggressive periodontitis, we could not find any association with any of the examined immunological parameters. *P. gingivalis*, which was found only in the CP group, showed an association to higher stimulability of PBMC-release of IL-1β and IL-8. Furthermore, this strain could be associated with the percentage of IFN-γ-releasing T-helper cells, which leads to a higher IFN-γ/IL-4 ratio in relation to intracellular cytokine release in T-helper cells. Additionally, we found that patients who harbor *P. g.* in their subgingival microflora have a shift in CD4/CD8 ratio towards CD8.

For patients harboring *Prevotella disiens* in their subgingival flora, a higher stimulation index (SI) was found for the release of IL-1β when cells were stimulated with *P. g.* LPS, and a higher IFN-γ/IL-4 ratio was also found. Furthermore, *Prevotella intermedia* harboring patients showed a lower percentage of switched memory B-cells.

In summary, as shown in Table 3, we found nine associations for T- and B-cells, which are representative for adaptive immunity, with microbiological strains. Five associations were found for SI of IL-1β release and two associations for SI of IL-8 release, both representing innate immunity.

Discussion

In this study we included patients suffering from aggressive periodontitis as well as patients with chronic periodontitis and healthy subjects. We collected clinical data and isolated the

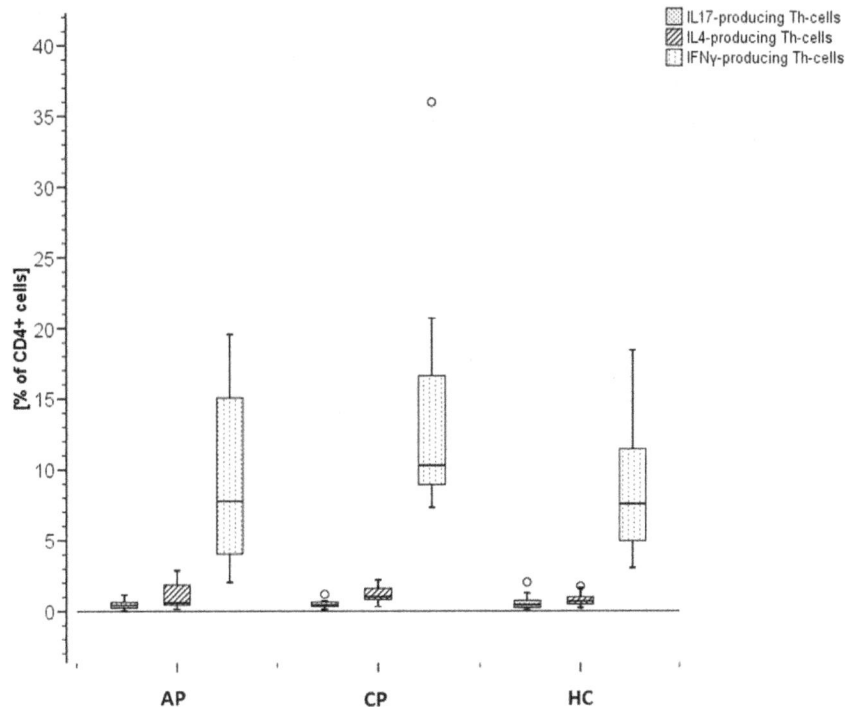

Figure 3. Intracellular Cytokine Release. Production of intracellular cytokines (IL-17, IL-4, IFN-γ) in T-helper cells (Th-cells). Measured by flow cytometry after stimulating CD4+ T-cells with PMA (10 ng/ml).

PBMCs from peripheral blood of each subject in order to examine the reaction to stimulation with standardized extracts of bacterial toxins (LPS from *E. coli* and *P. gingivalis*). Furthermore, we investigated T-cells and B-cells as well as the microbiological composition of patients' subgingival microbiota. Although there are differences in age existing between the three groups according to the inclusion criteria used in this study, they are not large enough to expect them to be the reason for the immunological differences we have found. We have no reason to suspect the unequal proportion of men and women between the groups influenced the study results. A systematic review by Shiau and Reynolds found a greater risk for destructive periodontal disease in men than in women, but without a higher risk for more rapid periodontal destruction [37]. As we performed analyses with the PBMCs in vitro an influence of gender mediated by hormones, biofilm or other factors is not to be expected. No other differences concerning potential risk factors for periodontal diseases exist between the groups.

Generally, immunological investigations of regulatory mechanisms in the pathogenesis of periodontitis can be performed with different types of cells from different origins in the organism. It is important to note that the local immune response is not determined only by PBMCs, but these cells represent the systemic immune status.

Recent studies focused on innate immunity in periodontitis pathogenesis. Production of IL-1 upon bacterial stimulation has been of special interest [38]. As many authors found that most patients suffering from each form of periodontitis have a mixed colonization of subgingival microbiota, we did not use a specific bacterial extract for stimulating PBMCs but two different standardized LPSs (from *E. coli* and *P. gingivalis*). *E. coli* LPS was used as it has a similar structure to LPS of the periodontal pathogen *A. actinomycetemcomitans*, and is a TLR-4 agonist [39]. Ultrapure LPS from *Porphyromonas gingivalis* is an agonist of

TLR-4 as well. The TLR-2 activity of *P. gingivalis* LPS is ascribed to a contaminant lipoprotein [40] which is not present in ultrapure LPS because of the enzymatic treatment. Therefore, an activation of the TLR-2 cannot be assumed. As shown in Figure 1, for both LPSs, a significantly higher stimulation of IL-1β production was found in patients with moderate chronic periodontitis compared to the other groups (p = 0.002), indicating a higher activation of innate immunity in moderate chronic periodontitis. Many studies have investigated IL-1β in gingival tissues and sulcus fluid. They showed a positive association between the local expression of IL-1β and severity of periodontal disease [41,42]. On the other hand, plasma levels of all the interleukins studied (IL-1β, IL-6, IL-11) were not significantly different between study groups (chronic periodontitis, generalized aggressive periodontitis, gingivitis, healthy subjects) [42]. Our results show that IL-1β release by PBMCs after stimulation with LPS in patients with AP is approximately identical to healthy controls, but increased in patients with CP. This finding does not correlate with the fact that patients with CP show a milder disease progression, as IL-1β is a proinflammatory cytokine. In contrast, other authors hypothesized that a reduction in levels of IL-1β could attenuate the host's ability to fight an infection [43]. A possible explanation could be the turnover of neutrophils in gingival tissue, which seems to be reduced in patients with aggressive periodontitis because of less TNF-α [44]. In patients with moderate chronic periodontitis, the immunological homeostasis in relation to neutrophil turnover seems to be sustained, maybe because of IL-1β, which compensates for TNF-α, resulting in limited inflammation.

We did not find differences in the release of IL-8 by PBMCs when stimulated with LPS between the different groups. IL-8 is an important pro-inflammatory chemokine which is regulated by an activator-protein and/or by NF-κB-mediated transcriptional activity and some other stimuli [45]. Goncalves et al. found a

Table 2. Carriers of Individual Cultivated Species among Different Subject Groups.

Bacterial Species	colonized AP (n_total=12)		colonized CP (n_total=11)		colonized HC (n_total=13)		p-value
	n	%	n	%	n	%	
Prevotella intermedia *	9	75.00	9	81.82	5	38.46	0.046
Fusobacterium nucleatum	7	58.33	8	72.73	5	38.46	0.355
Prevotella oralis *	7	58.33	6	54.55	1	7.69	0.013
Prevotella denticola **	7	58.33	1	9.09	0	0	0.001
Veillonella species	7	58.33	2	18.18	5	38.46	0.116
Actinomyces meyeri	5	47.92	2	18.18	4	30.78	0.682
Prevotella loeschii	5	47.92	4	36.36	3	23.08	0.618
Micromonas micros *	5	47.92	2	18.18	0	0	0.042
Anaerococcus prevotii *	4	33.33	0	0.00	0	0	0.011
Fusobacterium necrogenes	3	25.00	1	9.09	1	7.69	0.377
Bacteroides ureolyticus	3	25.00	3	27.27	1	7.69	0.449
Prevotella buccae	3	25.00	6	54.55	3	23.08	0.295
Selenomonas spp.	3	25.00	2	18.18	0	0	0.037
Eggerthella lenta	2	16.67	1	9.09	3	23.08	0.614
Capnocytophaga spp.	2	16.67	3	27.27	6	46.15	0.258
Prevotella melaninogenica	2	16.67	0	0.00	2	15.38	0.349
Gemella morbillorum	2	16.67	5	45.45	2	15.38	0.243
Peptostreptococcus anaerobicus	2	16.67	1	9.09	0	0	0.322
Eubacterium limosum	2	16.67	0	0.00	0	0	0.117
Clostridium histolyticum	2	16.67	0	0.00	0	0	0.117
Campylobacter rectus	2	16.67	0	0.00	0	0	0.117
Clostridium beijerium	2	16.67	1	9.09	0	0	0.307
Actinomyces israelii	1	8.33	1	9.09	2	15.38	0.809
Actinomyces odontolyticus	1	8.33	1	9.09	1	7.46	0.998
Actinomyces naeslundii	1	8.33	0	0.00	0	0	0.353
Fusobacterium varium	1	8.33	1	9.09	0	0	0.573
Fusobacterium necrophorum	1	8.33	0	0.00	1	7.69	0.609
Clostridium bifermentans	1	8.33	0	0.00	0	0	0.353
Prevotella buccalis	1	8.33	1	9.09	0	0	0.573
Propionibacterium acnes	1	8.33	1	9.09	1	7.69	0.998
Propionibacterium propionicus	1	8.33	0	0.00	0	0	0.353
Bacteroides merdae	1	8.33	1	9.09	0	0	0.573
Eubacterium yurii	1	8.33	0	0.00	0	0	0.353
Actinomyces viscosus	0	0.00	1	9.09	0	0	0.353

Table 2. Cont.

Bacterial Species	colonized AP (n_total = 12)		colonized CP (n_total = 11)		colonized HC (n_total = 13)		p-value
	n	%	n	%	n	%	
Actinomyces prevotii	0	0.00	1	9.09	0	0	0.011
Prevotella bivia	0	0.00	0	0.00	1	7.69	0.397
Prevotella disiens *	0	0.00	2	18.18	0	0	0.037
Prevotella tannerae	0	0.00	1	9.09	0	0	0.353
Prevotella nigrescens	0	0.00	0	0.00	1	7.69	0.397
Eubacterium brachy	0	0.00	1	9.09	0	0	0.353
Finegoldia magna	0	0.00	2	18.18	0	0	0.117
Porphyromonas gingivalis *	0	0.00	3	27.27	0	0	0.011
Porphyromonas asaccharolytica	0	0.00	2	18.18	0	0	0.117
Porphyromonas endodontalis	0	0.00	1	9.09	0	0	0.353
Clostridium clostridioforme	0	0.00	1	9.09	0	0	0.117
Clostridium fallax	0	0.00	1	9.09	0	0	0.117
Clostridium tyrobutyricum	0	0.00	1	9.09	0	0	0.117
Clostridium spp.	0	0.00	0	0.00	1	7.69	0.397
Clostridium sordellii	0	0.00	1	9.09	0	0	0.353
Clostridium innocuum	0	0.00	1	9.09	1	7.69	0.609
Clostridium sporogenes	0	0.00	1	9.09	1	7.69	0.609

* < 0.05; ** < 0.001.

Table 3. Associations between Immunological and Microbiological Findings.

Bacterial Species	Immunological Finding	Association	p	Interpretation
P. gingivalis (n = 3)	SI IL-1β E.coli LPS	positive	0.019	1
	SI IL-8 E.coli LPS	positive	0.029	1
	SI IL-8 P.g. LPS	positive	0.015	1
	CD4/CD8 ratio	negative	0.023	1
	IFN-γ producing T-helper cells	positive	0.023	1
	IFN-γ/IL-4 ratio	positive	0.015	1
F. nucleatum (n = 20)	B-cells	negative	0.030	2
	naïve and transitional B-cells	negative	0.050	2
	switched memory B-cells	positive	0.014	2
	memory B-cells	positive	0.018	2
A. prevotii (n = 4)	SI IL-1β E.coli LPS	negative	0.007	3
A. meyeri (n = 12)	B-cells	negative	0.049	4
P. disiens (n = 2)	SI IL-1β P.g. LPS	positive	0.029	5
	IFN-γ/IL-4 ratio	positive	0.029	5
C. rectus (n = 2)	SI IL-1β E.coli LPS	negative	0.038	3
	IFN-γ producing T-helper cells	negative	0.019	3
E. limosum (n = 2)	naïve and transitional B-cells	positive	0.013	2
	B-cells	positive	0.013	2
Finegoldia magna (n = 2)	B-cells	positive	0.013	6
	IFN-γ/IL-4 ratio	negative	0.019	6
	SI IL-8 E.coli LPS	negative	0.038	6
	IL-4 producing T-helper cells	positive	0.038	6
P. oralis (n = 14)	switched memory B-cells	negative	0.035	2
	IFN-γ/IL-4 ratio	negative	0.035	2
P. buccalis (n = 2)	CD4/CD8 ratio	positive	0.003	

n: positive identifications from the 46 microbiologically characterized individuals; SI: stimulation index;
[1] activation of Th1-response;
[2] activation of B-cell-maturation;
[3] negative regulation of innate immunity;
[4] no B-cell stimulation;
[5] positive regulation of innate immunity;
[6] activation of humoral immunity (Th2).

higher LPS-induced release of IL-8 in healthy subjects' PBMCs compared to patients suffering from chronic periodontitis [46]. In contrast to Goncalves, Dias et al. found higher plasma concentrations of IL-8 in patients with severe chronic periodontitis compared to healthy controls [47]. This indicates that local processes do not reflect systemic immune regulation one-to-one.

The final immune response takes place on the local level and is crucial for the regulation of the microbiota by stimulating microenvironmental changes limiting the increase of periodontal pathogens and helping protective bacteria to predominate or by permitting the establishment of a more pathogenic microbial ecology [48]. Most of the local immunological factors belong to the innate immune system with monocytes (CD14+) representing one of the principal peripheral mononuclear cells. When monocytes migrate into the periodontal tissue they convert to macrophages. However, previous studies suggested that a bacteremia that is caused by periodontitis [49] might induce cytokines to change the immune cell function (e.g. developing CD14+ and CD16+ monocytes [50]). On the other hand, these changes might also be triggered by cytokines released from periodontal lesions. Therefore, it was of special interest for us not only to determine

associations between microbiological and clinical but also immunological findings. We showed predominance of known periodontal pathogens in the periodontitis groups (Table 2) and found differences in microbial colonization between healthy and diseased sites in quantity as well as in quality as other authors have described before [51]. In this study, a higher quantity of Gram-negative anaerobic bacteria was detected in periodontitis patients compared to healthy subjects: P. gingivalis, P. intermedia, P. oralis, Parvimonas micra, and Prevotella denticola were associated with periodontitis. These findings support previous results of other research groups who correlated P. gingivalis and P. intermedia with periodontal lesions [51,52]. As shown by other authors and summarized by Mombelli et al. [53], we also found no differences in the microbiological colonization between patients in the AP and CP groups. Furthermore, we found known periodontopathogenic species: Veillonella, Capnocytophaga, F. nucleatum, and P. intermedia in the sulcus of healthy individuals as has been shown before [15,54].

Our microbiological and immunological findings allowed us to identify links between several periodontal pathogens and adaptive as well as innate immune response (Table 3). These associations should be interpreted cautiously because of multiple testing and limited sample sizes, which is why we regard these results as exploratory. We found an association between *P. gingivalis* and Th1-response which is contradictory to a recent study of Moutsopoulos et al. who were able to show that *P. gingivalis* W83 stimulates myeloid antigen presenting cell (APC) differentiation to Th17-cells in vitro by activating NFκB and thereby inducing IL-1β, IL-6, and IL-12p40 [55]. On the other hand, an older study from 2002, which investigated the influence of *P. gingivalis* LPS on the accumulation of IL-12 and IFN-γ in T-cells, suggested an increase in the production of inflammatory cytokines caused by an activation loop with IL-12 and IFN-γ established by *P. gingivalis* [56]. Thus, this study supports our results. As we indicated above, there remains widespread disagreement in the literature regarding the systemic immunopathology of periodontitis.

Considering B-cell maturation, we found the highest percentage of memory B-cells in the CP group as shown in Figure 2, suggesting a stronger antibody-mediated systemic immune response towards infection than in the other groups. This assumption is based on the fact that IL-1β can induce production of IL-6, which leads to the activation of lymphocytes and their release of immunoglobulin [30]. This results in a higher release of IgG in patients with moderate chronic periodontitis than in the other groups. As a reduced production of IgG could be associated with severity of periodontitis [57], this could be an explanation for the milder progress of illness in patients with moderate chronic periodontitis and an illustration for the interaction between innate and adaptive immunity.

One of the main strengths of this study is that we determined well-defined cohorts with numbers of individuals that were adapted to the incidence of aggressive periodontitis. Furthermore, we collected periodontological, microbiological and functional as well as phenotypic immunological data, which enabled us to characterize the individuals in a comprehensive way. Nevertheless, the number of individuals is relatively low. Therefore, some of the results can only be considered as exploratory and a direct connection between local and systemic immunological factors cannot be assumed. Therefore, these points represent limitations of our study. Further studies should follow-up the immunological and microbiological results described in our study, preferably on the basis of an appropriate number of individuals, to characterize the connection between systemic factors and local factors in the periodontium more precisely.

Overall Conclusions

The results of this study provide evidence for possible associations between clinical diagnosis, immunological findings, and periodontal pathogens. Considering systemic immune status we found a significantly higher activation of innate and adaptive immunity in patients with moderate chronic periodontitis compared to the other groups, represented by the significantly higher stimulability of PBMCs in IL-1β release and the elevated percentage of memory B-cells compared to the other groups. Furthermore, we were able to show an association between the presence of bacteria typical for periodontal disease and the systemic immune response. The results indicate that in periodontal disease there is some kind of self-limitation of inflammation in patients diagnosed with moderate chronic periodontitis. In such instances, a clearly milder disease progression is observed as compared to patients with aggressive periodontitis.

Acknowledgments

The work presented in this paper was made possible by funding from the German Federal Ministry of Education and Research (BMBF 1315883).

The authors thank P. Petz for his support with the examination and the collection of test material in participants of this study; H. Knaack, K. Bauer, F. Kahlenberg for their support in laboratory work; A. Braun for proofreading the manuscript.

Author Contributions

Conceived and designed the experiments: JS US C-SS. Performed the experiments: JS C-SS. Analyzed the data: JS US. Contributed reagents/materials/analysis tools: JS US C-SS. Wrote the paper: JS HJ C-SS US.

References

1. Chi AC, Neville BW, Krayer JW, Gonsalves WC (2010) Oral manifestations of systemic disease. Am Fam Physician 82 (11): 1381–1388.
2. Timmerman MF, van der Weijden GA (2006) Risk factors for periodontitis. Int J Dent Hyg 4 (1): 2–7.
3. van der Weijden F, Slot DE (2011) Oral hygiene in the prevention of periodontal diseases: the evidence. Periodontol 2000 55 (1): 104–123.
4. Imai K, Ochiai K (2011) Role of histone modification on transcriptional regulation and HIV-1 gene expression: possible mechanisms of periodontal diseases in AIDS progression. J Oral Sci 53 (1): 1–13.
5. Brown LJ, Johns BA, Wall TP (2002) The economics of periodontal diseases. Periodontol 2000 29: 223–234.
6. Salvi GE, Carollo-Bittel B, Lang NP (2008) Effects of diabetes mellitus on periodontal and peri-implant conditions: update on associations and risks. J Clin Periodontol 35 (8 Suppl): 398–409.
7. Dewhirst FE, Chen T, Izard J, Paster BJ, Tanner ACR, et al. (2010) The Human Oral Microbiome. J Bacteriol 192 (19): 5002–5017.
8. Albandar JM (2011) Underestimation of periodontitis in NHANES surveys. J Periodontol 82 (3): 337–341.
9. Lindhe J, Ranney R, Lamster I, Charles A, Chung C, et al. (1999) Consensus Report: Chronic Periodontitis. Ann Periodontol 4 (1): 38.
10. Smith M, Seymour GJ, Cullinan MP (2010) Histopathological features of chronic and aggressive periodontitis. Periodontol 2000 53: 45–54.
11. Marazita ML, Burmeister JA, Gunsolley JC, Koertge TE, Lake K, et al. (1994) Evidence for autosomal dominant inheritance and race-specific heterogeneity in early-onset periodontitis. J Periodontol 65 (6): 623–630.
12. Armitage GC, Cullinan MP (2010) Comparison of the clinical features of chronic and aggressive periodontitis. Periodontol 2000 53: 12–27.
13. Papaioannou W, Gizani S, Haffajee AD, Quirynen M, Mamai-Homata E, et al. (2009) The microbiota on different oral surfaces in healthy children. Oral Microbiol Immunol 24 (3): 183–189.
14. Rescala B, Rosalem W, Teles RP, Fischer RG, Haffajee AD, et al. (2010) Immunologic and microbiologic profiles of chronic and aggressive periodontitis subjects. J Periodontol 81 (9): 1308–1316.
15. Riep B, Edesi-Neuss L, Claessen F, Skarabis H, Ehmke B, et al. (2009) Are putative periodontal pathogens reliable diagnostic markers? J Clin Microbiol 47 (6): 1705–1711.
16. Ohlrich EJ, Cullinan MP, Seymour GJ (2009) The immunopathogenesis of periodontal disease. Aust Dent J 54 Suppl 1: S2–10.
17. Warrington R, Watson W, Kim HL, Antonetti FR (2011) An introduction to immunology and immunopathology. Allergy Asthma Clin Immunol 7 Suppl 1: S1.
18. Berezow AB, Ernst RK, Coats SR, Braham PH, Karimi-Naser LM, et al. (2009) The structurally similar, penta-acylated lipopolysaccharides of Porphyromonas gingivalis and Bacteroides elicit strikingly different innate immune responses. Microb Pathog 47 (2): 68–77.
19. Kumar H, Kawai T, Akira S (2009) Toll-like receptors and innate immunity. Biochem Biophys Res Commun 388 (4): 621–625.
20. Darveau RP, Pham TT, Lemley K, Reife RA, Bainbridge BW, et al. (2004) Porphyromonas gingivalis lipopolysaccharide contains multiple lipid A species that functionally interact with both toll-like receptors 2 and 4. Infect Immun 72 (9): 5041–5051.
21. Turvey SE, Broide DH (2010) Innate immunity. J Allergy Clin Immunol 125 (2 Suppl 2): S24–32.
22. Steinman RM, Hemmi H (2006) Dendritic cells: translating innate to adaptive immunity. Curr Top Microbiol Immunol 311: 17–58.
23. Modlin RL, Nutman TB (1993) Type 2 cytokines and negative immune regulation in human infections. Curr Opin Immunol 5 (4): 511–517.
24. Ford PJ, Gamonal J, Seymour GJ (2010) Immunological differences and similarities between chronic periodontitis and aggressive periodontitis. Periodontol 2000 53: 111–123.

25. Garlet GP (2010) Destructive and protective roles of cytokines in periodontitis: a re-appraisal from host defense and tissue destruction viewpoints. J Dent Res 89 (12): 1349–1363.

26. Taylor JJ (2010) Cytokine regulation of immune responses to Porphyromonas gingivalis. Periodontol 2000 54 (1): 160–194.

27. Gaffen SL, Hajishengallis G (2008) A new inflammatory cytokine on the block: re-thinking periodontal disease and the Th1/Th2 paradigm in the context of Th17 cells and IL-17. J Dent Res 87 (9): 817–828.

28. Kobayashi R, Kono T, Bolerjack BA, Fukuyama Y, Gilbert RS, et al. (2011) Induction of IL-10-producing CD4+ T-cells in chronic periodontitis. J Dent Res 90 (5): 653–658.

29. Nakajima T, Ueki-Maruyama K, Oda T, Ohsawa Y, Ito H, et al. (2005) Regulatory T-cells infiltrate periodontal disease tissues. J Dent Res 84 (7): 639–643.

30. Kenneth Murphy (2012) Janeway's Immunobiology. New York: Garland Science.

31. Gonzales JR, Mann M, Stelzig J, Bödeker RH, Meyle J (2007) Single-nucleotide polymorphisms in the IL-4 and IL-13 promoter region in aggressive periodontitis. J Clin Periodontol 34 (6): 473–479.

32. Armitage GC (1999) Development of a classification system for periodontal diseases and conditions. Ann Periodontol 4 (1): 1–6.

33. Lange DE, Plagmann HC, Eenboom A, Promesberger A (1977) Klinische Bewertungsverahren zur Objektivierung der Mundhygiene. Dtsch Zahnarztl Z 32 (1): 44–47.

34. Guentsch A, Puklo M, Preshaw PM, Glockmann E, Pfister W, et al. (2009) Neutrophils in chronic and aggressive periodontitis in interaction with Porphyromonas gingivalis and Aggregatibacter actinomycetemcomitans. J Periodont Res 44 (3): 368–377.

35. Smedman C, Gårdlund B, Nihlmark K, Gille-Johnson P, Andersson J, et al. (2009) ELISpot analysis of LPS-stimulated leukocytes: human granulocytes selectively secrete IL-8, MIP-1beta and TNF-alpha. J Immunol Methods 346 (1–2): 1–8.

36. Warnatz K, Schlesier M (2008) Flowcytometric phenotyping of common variable immunodeficiency. Cytometry B Clin Cytom 74 (5): 261–271.

37. Shiau HJ, Reynolds MA (2010) Sex differences in destructive periodontal disease: a systematic review. J Periodontol 81 (10): 1379–1389.

38. Preshaw PM, Taylor JJ (2011) How has research into cytokine interactions and their role in driving immune responses impacted our understanding of periodontitis. J Clin Periodontol 38 Suppl 11: 60–84.

39. Li X, Zhou L, Takai H, Sasaki Y, Mezawa M, et al. (2012) Aggregatibacter actinomycetemcomitans lipopolysaccharide regulates bone sialoprotein gene transcription. J Cell Biochem 113 (9): 2822–2834.

40. Ogawa T, Asai Y, Makimura Y, Tamai R (2007) Chemical structure and immunobiological activity of Porphyromonas gingivalis lipid A. Front Biosci 12: 3795–3812.

41. Scheres N, Laine ML, Vries TJ de, Everts V, van Winkelhoff AJ (2010) Gingival and periodontal ligament fibroblasts differ in their inflammatory response to viable Porphyromonas gingivalis. J Periodont Res 45 (2): 262–270.

42. Becerik S, Ozgen Öztürk V, Atmaca H, Atilla G, Emingil G (2012) Gingival Crevicular Fluid and Plasma Acute Phase Cytokine Levels in Different Periodontal Diseases. J Periodontol 83 (10):1304–13.

43. Bostanci N, Allaker R, Johansson U, Rangarajan M, Curtis MA, et al. (2007) Interleukin-1alpha stimulation in monocytes by periodontal bacteria: antagonistic effects of Porphyromonas gingivalis. Oral Microbiol Immunol 22 (1): 52–60.

44. Zaric S, Shelburne C, Darveau R, Quinn DJ, Weldon S, et al. (2010) Impaired immune tolerance to Porphyromonas gingivalis lipopolysaccharide promotes neutrophil migration and decreased apoptosis. Infect Immun 78 (10): 4151–4156.

45. Waugh DJJ, Wilson C (2008) The Interleukin-8 Pathway in Cancer. Clin Cancer Res 14 (21): 6735–6741.

46. Goncalves TO, Costa D, Brodskyn CI, Duarte PM, Cesar NJB, et al. (2010) Release of cytokines by stimulated peripheral blood mononuclear cells in chronic periodontitis. Arch Oral Biol 55 (12): 975–980.

47. Dias IH, Matthews JB, Chapple IL, Wright HJ, Dunston CR, et al. (2011) Activation of the neutrophil respiratory burst by plasma from periodontitis patients is mediated by pro-inflammatory cytokines. J Clin Periodontol 38 (1): 1–7.

48. Ebersole JL, Dawson DR, Morford LA, Peyyala R, Miller CS, et al. (2013) Periodontal disease immunology: 'double indemnity' in protecting the host. Periodontol 2000 62 (1): 163–202.

49. Slots J (2003) Update on general health risk of periodontal disease. Int Dent J 53 Suppl 3: 200–207.

50. Nagasawa T, Kobayashi H, Aramaki M, Kiji M, Oda S, et al. (2004) Expression of CD14, CD16 and CD45RA on monocytes from periodontitis patients. J Periodont Res 39 (1): 72–78.

51. Darveau RP (2009) The oral microbial consortium's interaction with the periodontal innate defense system. DNA Cell Biol 28 (8): 389–395.

52. Lafaurie GI, Contreras A, Barón A, Botero J, Mayorga-Fayad I, et al. (2007) Demographic, clinical, and microbial aspects of chronic and aggressive periodontitis in Colombia: a multicenter study. J Periodontol 78 (4): 629–639.

53. Mombelli A, Casagni F, Madianos PN (2002) Can presence or absence of periodontal pathogens distinguish between subjects with chronic and aggressive periodontitis? A systematic review. J Clin Periodontol 29 Suppl 3: 10–21; discussion 37–8.

54. Stingu CS, Jentsch H, Eick S, Schaumann R, Knofler G, et al. (2012) Microbial profile of patients with periodontitis compared with healthy subjects. Quintessence Int 43 (2): e23–31.

55. Moutsopoulos NM, Kling HM, Angelov N, Jin W, Palmer RJ, et al. (2012) Porphyromonas gingivalis promotes Th17 inducing pathways in chronic periodontitis. J Autoimmun 39 (4): 294–303.

56. Yun PLW, DeCarlo AA, Collyer C, Hunter N (2002) Modulation of an interleukin-12 and gamma interferon synergistic feedback regulatory cycle of T-cell and monocyte cocultures by Porphyromonas gingivalis lipopolysaccharide in the absence or presence of cysteine proteinases. Infect Immun 70 (10): 5695–5705.

57. Sugita N, Iwanaga R, Kobayashi T, Yoshie H (2012) Association of the FcγRIIB-nt645+25A/G polymorphism with the expression level of the FcγRIIb receptor, the antibody response to Porphyromonas gingivalis and the severity of periodontitis. J Periodont Res 47 (1): 105–113.

Permissions

The contributors of this book come from diverse backgrounds, making this book a truly international effort. This book will bring forth new frontiers with its revolutionizing research information and detailed analysis of the nascent developments around the world.

We would like to thank all the contributing authors for lending their expertise to make the book truly unique. They have played a crucial role in the development of this book. Without their invaluable contributions this book wouldn't have been possible. They have made vital efforts to compile up to date information on the varied aspects of this subject to make this book a valuable addition to the collection of many professionals and students.

This book was conceptualized with the vision of imparting up-to-date information and advanced data in this field. To ensure the same, a matchless editorial board was set up. Every individual on the board went through rigorous rounds of assessment to prove their worth. After which they invested a large part of their time researching and compiling the most relevant data for our readers.

The editorial board has been involved in producing this book since its inception. They have spent rigorous hours researching and exploring the diverse topics which have resulted in the successful publishing of this book. They have passed on their knowledge of decades through this book. To expedite this challenging task, the publisher supported the team at every step. A small team of assistant editors was also appointed to further simplify the editing procedure and attain best results for the readers.

Apart from the editorial board, the designing team has also invested a significant amount of their time in understanding the subject and creating the most relevant covers. They scrutinized every image to scout for the most suitable representation of the subject and create an appropriate cover for the book.

The publishing team has been an ardent support to the editorial, designing and production team. Their endless efforts to recruit the best for this project, has resulted in the accomplishment of this book. They are a veteran in the field of academics and their pool of knowledge is as vast as their experience in printing. Their expertise and guidance has proved useful at every step. Their uncompromising quality standards have made this book an exceptional effort. Their encouragement from time to time has been an inspiration for everyone.

The publisher and the editorial board hope that this book will prove to be a valuable piece of knowledge for researchers, students, practitioners and scholars across the globe.

List of Contributors

Qisheng Tu and Liming Yu
Division of Oral Biology, Tufts University School of Dental Medicine, Boston, Massachusetts, United States of America

Lan Zhang, Shu Meng, and Yin Tang
Division of Oral Biology, Tufts University School of Dental Medicine, Boston, Massachusetts, United States of America
Key Laboratory of Oral Diseases, West China Hospital of Stomatology, Sichuan University, Chengdu, Sichuan, China

Jake Chen
Division of Oral Biology, Tufts University School of Dental Medicine, Boston, Massachusetts, United States of America
Department of Anatomy and Cell Biology, Tufts University School of Medicine, Sackler School of Graduate Biomedical Sciences, Boston, Massachusetts, United States of America

Xuedong Zhou
Key Laboratory of Oral Diseases, West China Hospital of Stomatology, Sichuan University, Chengdu, Sichuan, China

Michel M. Dard
Periodontology and Implant Dentistry, New York University College of Dentistry, New York, New York, United States of America,

Sung-Hoon Kim
Cancer Preventive Material Development Research Center (CPMDRC) and Institute, College of Oriental Medicine, Kyung Hee University, Dongdaemun-gu, Seoul, Korea

Paloma Valverde
Department of Sciences, Wentworth Institute of Technology, Boston, Massachusetts, United States of America

Søren Jepsen and James Deschner
Department of Periodontology, Operative and Preventive Dentistry, University of Bonn, Bonn, Germany

Moritz Kebschull
Department of Periodontology, Operative and Preventive Dentistry, University of Bonn, Bonn, Germany

Department of Internal Medicine II, University of Bonn, Bonn, Germany

Manuela Haupt, Georg Nickenig and Nikos Werner
Department of Internal Medicine II, University of Bonn, Bonn, Germany

Adriana L. Santos and Alexandre S. Rosado
Institute of Microbiology Prof. Paulo de Góes, Federal University of Rio de Janeiro, Rio de Janeiro, Brazil,

José F. Siqueira Jr. and Isabela N. R ôças
Department of Endodontics and Molecular Microbiology Laboratory, Esta´cio de Sa´ University, Rio de Janeiro, Brazil,

James M. Tiedje
Center for Microbial Ecology, Michigan State University, East Lansing, Michigan, United States of America,

Ederson C. Jesus
Laboratory of Soil Microbiology, EMBRAPA, Serope´dica, Brazil

Haleh Davanian, Tove Båge and Tülay Yucel-Lindberg
Division of Periodontology, Department of Dental Medicine, Karolinska Institutet, Huddinge, Sweden

Henrik Stranneheim and Joakim Lundeberg
Science for Life Laboratory, Division of Gene Technology, School of Biotechnology, Royal Institute of Technology (KTH), Solna, Sweden

Maria Lagervall and Leif Jansson
Department of Periodontology at Skanstull, Stockholm County Council Sweden, Stockholm, Sweden

Wei Luo and Lijian Jin
Faculty of Dentistry, The University of Hong Kong, Hong Kong SAR, China,

Cun-Yu Wang
University of California Los Angeles, School of Dentistry, Los Angeles, California, United States of America

Neville Gully, Richard Bright, Victor Marino, Ceilidh Marchant and Mark Bartold
Colgate Australian Clinical Dental Research, School of Dentistry, University of Adelaide, Adelaide, South Australia, Australia

Melissa Cantley and David Haynes
Discipline of Anatomy and Pathology, School of Medical Sciences, University of Adelaide, Adelaide, South Australia, Australia

Catherine Butler, Stuart Dashper and Eric Reynolds
Oral Health Collaborative Research Centre, Melbourne Dental School, The University of Melbourne, Melbourne, Victoria, Australia

Jörg Eberhard, Wieland Heuer, Nico Stumpp and Meike Stiesch
Department of Prosthetic Dentistry and Biomaterials Science, Hannover Medical School, Hannover, Germany

Karsten Grote., Maren Luchtefeld, Harald Schuett, Dimitar Divchev and Bernhard Schieffer
Department of Cardiology and Angiology, Hannover Medical School, Hannover, Germany

Ralph Scherer
Department of Medical Statistics, Hannover Medical School, Hannover, Germany

Ingmar Staufenbiel
Department of Operative Dentistry and Periodontology, Hannover Medical School, Hannover, Germany

Ruth Schmitz-Streit and Daniela Langfeldt
Institute for Microbiology, Christian-Albrechts-University Kiel, Kiel, Germany

Peter Durand Skottrup, Grete Sørensen and Erik Riise
Biomolecular Interaction Group, Department of Drug Design and Pharmacology, Faculty of Health and Medical Sciences, University of Copenhagen, Copenhagen, Denmark

Miroslaw Ksiazek
Department of Microbiology, Faculty of Biochemistry, Biophysics and Biotechnology, Jagiellonian University, Krakow, Poland

Jan Potempa
Department of Microbiology, Faculty of Biochemistry, Biophysics and Biotechnology, Jagiellonian University, Krakow, Poland
Oral Health and Systemic Diseases Research Group, University of Louisville, School of Dentistry, Louisville, Kentucky, United States of America

Dandan Li., Qi Cai., Junqing Ma, Weibing Zhang, Yongchu Pan and Lin Wang
Institute of Stomatology, Nanjing Medical University, Nanjing, China

Lan Ma and Meilin Wang
Institute of Stomatology, Nanjing Medical University, Nanjing, China
Department of Epidemiology, Nanjing Medical University, Nanjing, China

Daniel D. Sommer
Center for Bioinformatics and Computational Biology, University of Maryland, College Park, Maryland, United States of America

Bo Liu and Mohammad Ghodsi
Center for Bioinformatics and Computational Biology, University of Maryland, College Park, Maryland, United States of America
Department of Computer Science, University of Maryland, College Park, Maryland, United States of America

Mihai Pop
Center for Bioinformatics and Computational Biology, University of Maryland, College Park, Maryland, United States of America
Department of Computer Science, University of Maryland, College Park, Maryland, United States of America
Biological Sciences Graduate Program, University of Maryland, College Park, Maryland, United States of America

Theodore R. Gibbons
Center for Bioinformatics and Computational Biology, University of Maryland, College Park, Maryland, United States of America
Biological Sciences Graduate Program, University of Maryland, College Park, Maryland, United States of America

Todd J. Treangen
Center for Bioinformatics and Computational Biology, University of Maryland, College Park, Maryland, United States of America,
The McKusick-Nathans Institute for Genetic Medicine, The Johns Hopkins University School of Medicine, Baltimore, Maryland, United States of America

Niels Klitgord, Varun Mazumdar and Yi-Chien Chang
Bioinformatics Program, Boston University, Boston, Massachusetts, United States of America

Daniel Segre
Bioinformatics Program, Boston University, Boston, Massachusetts, United States of America
Department of Biology, Boston University, Boston, Massachusetts, United States of America

Department of Biomedical Engineering, Boston University, Boston, Massachusetts, United States of America

Simon Kasif
Bioinformatics Program, Boston University, Boston, Massachusetts, United States of America
Department of Biomedical Engineering, Boston University, Boston, Massachusetts, United States of America
Children's Informatics Program, Harvard-Massachusetts Institute of Technology Division of Health Sciences and Technology, Boston, Massachusetts, United States of America

Salomon Amar
Bioinformatics Program, Boston University, Boston, Massachusetts, United States of America,
Center for Anti-Inflammatory Therapeutics; Boston University Goldman School of Dental Medicine, Boston, Massachusetts, United States of America

Shan Li and O. Colin Stine
Department of Epidemiology and Public Health, University of Maryland School of Medicine, Baltimore, Maryland, United States of America

Hatice Hasturk
The Forsyth Institute, Department of Periodontology, Cambridge, Massachusetts, United States of America

Heng Yang and Qi Wang
State Key Laboratory of Oral Diseases, Sichuan University, Chengdu, Sichuan, China,

Raydolfo M. Aprecio, Xiaodong Zhou, Wu Zhang and Yiming Li
Center for Dental Research, Loma Linda University School of Dentistry, Loma Linda, California, United States of America

Yi Ding
Department of Periodontology, West China Hospital of Stomatology, Sichuan University, Chengdu, Sichuan, China

Karen Schwarzberg, Rosalin Le and Scott T.Kelley
Department of Biology, San Diego State University, San Diego, California, United States of America

Balambal Bharti and Suzanne Lindsay
Graduate School of Public Health, San Diego State University, San Diego, California, United States of America

Giorgio Casaburi and Francesco Salvatore
CEINGE-Biotecnologie Avanzate, Napoli, Italy

Dipartimento di Medicina Molecolare e Biotecnologie Mediche, Universita` di Napoli Federico II, Napoli, Italy

Mohamed H. Saber and Faisal Alonaizan
Section of Endodontics, Herman Ostrow School of Dentistry of USC, Los Angeles, California, United States of America

Jørgen Slots
Professor of Dentistry and Microbiology, Herman Ostrow School of Dentistry of USC, Los Angeles, California, United States of America

Roberta A. Gottlieb
BioScience Center, San Diego State University, San Diego, California, United States of America

J. Gregory Caporaso
Department of Biological Sciences, Northern Arizona University, Flagstaff, Arizona, United States of America
Institute for Genomics and Systems Biology, Argonne National Laboratory, Argonne, Illinois, United States of America

Mi-Fang Yang
Institute of Stomatology, Nanjing Medical University, Nanjing, China

Ying Sun, Hui Li, Meng-Jun Sun and Yan Xu
Institute of Stomatology, Nanjing Medical University, Nanjing, China
Department of Periodontology, Stomatology Hospital affiliated t o N anjing M edical U niversity, Nanjing, China

Wei Shu
Department of Periodontology, Stomatology Hospital affiliated to Nanjing Medical University, Nanjing, China

Frank C. Nichols and Erica Knee
Department of Oral Health and Diagnostic Sciences, University of Connecticut School of Dental Medicine, Farmington, Connecticut, United States of America

Xudong Yao and Bekim Bajrami
Department of Chemistry, University of Connecticut, Storrs, Connecticut, United States of America

Julia Downes and Sydney M. Finegold
Division of Infectious Diseases, VA Greater Los Angeles Healthcare System, Los Angeles, California, United States of America

James J. Gallagher
Department of Surgery, University of Connecticut School of Medicine, Farmington, Connecticut, United States of America

Connecticut Vascular Institute, Hartford, Connecticut, United States of America

William J. Housley and Robert B.Clark
Departments of Immunology and Medicine, School of Medicine, University of Connecticut, Farmington, Connecticut, United States of America

Kaining Liu, Huanxin Meng and Jianxia Hou
Department of Periodontology, Peking University School and Hospital of Stomatology, Beijing, China

Srinivas Ayilavarapu, Hatice Hasturk and Thomas E. Van Dyke
Department of Periodontology, The Forsyth Institute, Cambridge, Massachusetts, United States of America

Gabrielle Fredman
Department of Periodontology, The Forsyth Institute, Cambridge, Massachusetts, United States of America
Department of Anesthesiology, Perioperative, and Pain Medicine, Center for Experimental Therapeutics and Reperfusion Injury, Brigham and Women's Hospital Harvard Medical School, Boston, Massachusetts, United States of America

Sungwhan F. Oh and Charles N. Serhan
Department of Anesthesiology, Perioperative, and Pain Medicine, Center for Experimental Therapeutics and Reperfusion Injury, Brigham and Women's Hospital Harvard Medical School, Boston, Massachusetts, United States of America

Oleh Andrukhov
Division of Oral Biology, Bernhard Gottlieb School of Dentistry, Medical University of Vienna, Vienna, Austria

Ulamnemekh Hulan
Division of Oral Biology, Bernhard Gottlieb School of Dentistry, Medical University of Vienna, Vienna, Austria
Department of Restorative Science, School of Dentistry, Health Science University of Mongolia, Ulan Bator, Mongolia

Yan Tang
Division of Oral Biology, Bernhard Gottlieb School of Dentistry, Medical University of Vienna, Vienna, Austria
Department of Stomatology, Xuanwu Hospital, Capital Medical University, Beijing, China

Xiaohui Rausch-Fan
Division of Oral Biology, Bernhard Gottlieb School of Dentistry, Medical University of Vienna, Vienna, Austria

Division of Orthodontics, Bernhard Gottlieb School of Dentistry, Medical University of Vienna, Vienna, Austria

Olena Andrukhova
Department of Biomedical Science, University of Veterinary Medicine, Vienna, Austria

Hans-Peter Bantleon
Division of Orthodontics, Bernhard Gottlieb School of Dentistry, Medical University of Vienna, Vienna, Austria

Xingxing Wang, Xu Han Xiaolong Luo and Dalin Wang
Department of Stomatology, Changhai Hospital, The Second Military Medical University, Shanghai, China

Xiaojing Guo
Department of Health Statistics, The Second Military Medical University, Shanghai, China

Na An
Department of General Dentistry II, School and Hospital of Stomatology, Peking University, Beijing, China

Oleh Andrukhov
Division of Oral Biology, Bernhard Gottlieb School of Dentistry, Medical University of Vienna, Vienna, Austria

Yan Tang
Division of Oral Biology, Bernhard Gottlieb School of Dentistry, Medical University of Vienna, Vienna, Austria
Department of Stomatology, Xuanwu Hospital, Capital Medical University, Beijing, China

Xiaohui Rausch-Fan
Division of Oral Biology, Bernhard Gottlieb School of Dentistry, Medical University of Vienna, Vienna, Austria
Division of Orthodontics, Bernhard Gottlieb School of Dentistry, Medical University of Vienna, Vienna, Austria

Frank Falkensammer4 and Hans-Peter Bantleon
Division of Orthodontics, Bernhard Gottlieb School of Dentistry, Medical University of Vienna, Vienna, Austria

Xiangying Ouyang
Department of Periodontology, School and Hospital of Stomatology, Peking University, Beijing, China

Nan Zhang
Department of Dentistry, the First Affiliated Hospital, College of Medicine, Xi'an Jiaotong University, Xi'an, China

Yuehong Xu
Key Laboratory of Environment and Genes Related to Diseases, College of Medicine, Xi'an Jiaotong University, Xi'an, China

Bo Zhang
School of Life Science and Technology, Xi'an Jiaotong University, Xi'an, China

Dexing Zhong
School of Electronic and Information Engineering, Xi'an Jiaotong University, Xi'an, China

Tianxiao Zhang
Department of Psychiatry, Washington University in Saint Louis, Saint Louis, Missouri, United States of America

Bao Zhang and Zufei Feng
Key Laboratory of National Ministry of Health for Forensic Sciences, College of Medicine, Xi'an Jiaotong University, Xi'an, China

Haojie Yang
The Second Department of Orthopedics, the Second Affiliated Hospital, College of Medicine, Xi'an Jiaotong University, Xi'an, China

Burcu Özdemir
Department of Periodontology, Faculty of Dentistry, Gazi University, Ankara, Turkey
Division of Oral Biology, Bernhard Gottlieb School of Dentistry, Medical University, Vienna, Austria

Oleh Andrukhov
Division of Oral Biology, Bernhard Gottlieb School of Dentistry, Medical University, Vienna, Austria

Rausch-Fan
Division of Oral Biology, Bernhard Gottlieb School of Dentistry, Medical University, Vienna, Austria
Division of Orthodontics, Bernhard Gottlieb School of Dentistry, Medical University, Vienna, Austria

Bin Shi
Division of Oral Biology, Bernhard Gottlieb School of Dentistry, Medical University, Vienna, Austria
Department of Oral Surgery, First Affiliated Hospital of Fujian Medical University, Fuzhou, China

Hans Peter Bantleon
Division of Orthodontics, Bernhard Gottlieb School of Dentistry, Medical University, Vienna, Austria

Andreas Moritz
Division of Conservative Dentistry, Periodontology and Prophylaxis, Bernhard Gottlieb School of Dentistry, Medical University, Vienna, Austria

Yifei Zhang, Jianwei Hu, Ning Du and Feng Chen
Central Laboratory, School of Stomatology, Peking University, Beijing, P. R. China,

Yunfei Zheng
Department of Periodontology, School of Stomatology, Peking University, Beijing, P. R. China

Shingo Matsuura, Kinuyo Ohara, Hiroki Komiya and Tetsuro Watase
Department of Endodontics, Nihon University School of Dentistry, Tokyo, Japan

Kohei Shimizu, Bunnai Ogiso and Keisuke Hatori
Department of Endodontics, Nihon University School of Dentistry, Tokyo, Japan
Divisions of Advanced Dental Treatment, Dental Research Center, Nihon University School of Dentistry, Tokyo, Japan

Kunihito Matsumoto
Department of Radiology, Nihon University School of Dentistry, Tokyo, Japan
Divisions of Advanced Dental Treatment, Dental Research Center, Nihon University School of Dentistry, Tokyo, Japan

Yuka Nakaya
Department of Oral Diagnosis, Nihon University School of Dentistry, Tokyo, Japan

Noboru Noma
Department of Oral Diagnosis, Nihon University School of Dentistry, Tokyo, Japan
Divisions of Clinical Research, Dental Research Center, Nihon University School of Dentistry, Tokyo, Japan

Yoshiyuki Tsuboi and Masamichi Shinoda
Department of Physiology, Nihon University School of Dentistry, Tokyo, Japan
Division of Functional Morphology, Dental Research Center, Nihon University School of Dentistry, Tokyo, Japan

Koichi Iwata
Department of Physiology, Nihon University School of Dentistry, Tokyo, Japan
Division of Functional Morphology, Dental Research Center, Nihon University School of Dentistry, Tokyo, Japan
Division of Applied System Neuroscience Advanced Medical Research Center, Nihon University Graduate School of Medical Science, Tokyo, Japan

Telma Blanca Lombardo Bedran
Department of Oral Diagnosis and Surgery, Araraquara Dental School, State University of São Paulo, São Paulo, Brazil

Márcia Pinto Alves Mayer
Department of Microbiology, Institute of Biomedical Sciences, University of São Paulo, São Paulo, Brazil,

Denise Palomari Spolidorio
Department of Physiology and Pathology, Araraquara Dental School, State University of São Paulo, São Paulo, Brazil

Daniel Grenier
Oral Ecology Research Group, Faculty of Dentistry, Universite´ Laval, Quebec City, QC, Canada

Moïse Desvarieux
Department of Epidemiology, Mailman School of Public Health, Columbia University, New York, New York, United States of America
Centre de recherche Epide´miologies et Biostatistique, INSERM U1153, Equipe: Me´thodes en e´valuation the´rapeutique des maladies chroniques, Paris, France

Panos N. Papapanou
Division of Periodontics, Sectiono f Oral and Diagnostic Sciences, College of Dental Medicine, Columbia University, New York, New York, United States of America

Feng-Yen Lin, Chun-Yao Huang, Chun-Ming Shih and Nen-Chung Chang
Division of Cardiology, Taipei Medical University Hospital, Taipei, Taiwan
Cardiovascular Research Center, Taipei Medical University Hospital, Taipei, Taiwan
Department of Internal Medicine, School of Medicine, College of Medicine, Taipei Medical University, Taipei, Taiwan

Yi-Wen Lin
Department of Internal Medicine, School of Medicine, College of Medicine, Taipei Medical University, Taipei, Taiwan
Institute of Oral Biology, National Yang-MingU niversity, Taipei, Taiwan

Fung-Ping Hsiao
Institute of Oral Biology, National Yang-MingU niversity, Taipei, Taiwan

Shan-Ling Hung
Institute of Oral Biology, National Yang-MingU niversity, Taipei, Taiwan
Department of Stomatology, Taipei Veterans General Hospital, Taipei, Taiwan

Nai-Wen Tsao
Division of Cardiovascular Surgery, Taipei Medical University Hospital, Taipei, Taiwan

Chien- Sung Tsai
Division of Cardiovascular Surgery, Tri-Service General Hospital, National Defense Medical Center, Taipei, Taiwan

Shue-Fen Yang
Department of Dentistry, National Yang-Ming University, Taipei, Taiwan
Department of Stomatology, Taipei Veterans General Hospital, Taipei, Taiwan

Qichao Tu, Zhili He, Ye Deng, Christopher L. Hemme, Tong Yuan, Joy D. Van Nostrand and Liyou Wu
Department of Microbiology and Plant Biology, Institute for Environmental Genomics, University of Oklahoma, Norman, Oklahoma, United States of America

Jizhong Zhou
Department of Microbiology and Plant Biology, Institute for Environmental Genomics, University of Oklahoma, Norman, Oklahoma, United States of America
Earth Science Division, Lawrence Berkeley National Laboratory, Berkeley, California, United States of America
State Key Joint Laboratory of Environment Simulation and Pollution Control, School of Environment, Tsinghua University, Beijing, China

Yan Li and Xuedong Zhou
State Key Laboratory of Oral Diseases, West China Hospital of Stomatology, Sichuan University, Chengdu, China

Yanfei Chen and Lanjuan Li
State Key Laboratory for Diagnosis and Treatment of Infectious Disease, The First Affiliated Hospital, Zhejiang University, Hangzhou, China

Lu Lin and Jian Xu
Chinese Academy of Sciences, Qingdao Institute of Bioenergy and Bioprocess Technology, Qingdao, Shandong, China

Wenyuan Shi
UCLA School of Dentistry, University of California Los Angeles, Los Angeles, California, United States of America

Wagner Serra e Silva Filho
Federal University of Piauí, Piauí, Brazil

Renato C. V. Casarin
Paulista University, São Paulo, Brazil

Eduardo L. Nicolela Junior and Humberto M. Passos
Center of Hemodynamics, Emcor, Piracicaba, Brazil

Antônio W. Sallum
Piracicaba Dental School, State University of Campinas, São Paulo, Brazil

Reginaldo B. Gonçalves
Groupe de Recherche en Ecologie Bucale, Universite´ Laval, Quebec, Canada

Yvonne Jockel-Schneider, Imme Haubitz, Stefan Fickl, Martin Eigenthaler, and Ulrich Schlagenhauf
Department of Periodontology, University Hospital Wuerzburg, Wuerzburg, Germany

Inga Harks
Department of Periodontology, University Hospital Muenster, Muenster, Germany

Johannes Baulmann
Clinic of Internal Medicine II, University Hospital Schleswig-Holstein, Luebeck, Germany

Ashley Thai and Ryan T. Demmer
Department of Epidemiology, Mailman School of Public Health, Columbia University, New York, New York, United States of America

David R. Jacobs Jr.
Division of Epidemiology and Community Health, School of Public Health, University of Minnesota, Minneapolis, Minnesota, United States of America
Department of Nutrition, University of Oslo, Oslo, Norway

Ulrich Sack
Institute for Clinical Immunology, University of Leipzig, Leipzig, Germany; Translational Centre for Regenerative Medicine (TRM), University of Leipzig, Leipzig, Germany

Jana Schmidt and Holger Jentsch
Department of Cariology, Endodontology and Periodontology, University of Leipzig, Leipzig, Germany

Catalina-Suzana Stingu
Institute for Medical Microbiology and Epidemiology of Infectious Diseases, University of Leipzig, Leipzig, Germany

Index

www.ingramcontent.com/pod-product-compliance
Lightning Source LLC
Chambersburg PA
CBHW080505200326
41458CB00012B/4098